AF753388

# Obstetrics and Gynecology Advances

**Ectopic Pregnancy: Endless Challenges**
Elisa Picardo (Editor)
Marco Mitidieri (Editor)
Saverio Danese (Editor)
2023. ISBN: 978-1-68507-979-6 (Softcover)
2023. ISBN: 979-8-88697-513-0 (eBook)

**Endometrial Cancer: Current Epidemiology, Detection and Management (Second Edition)**
Samir A. Farghaly, M.D., PhD (Editor)
2022. ISBN: 978-1-68507-964-2 (Hardcover)
2022. ISBN: 979-8-88697-405-8 (eBook)

**Hormonal Treatments in Gynaecology**
Jose Miguel García Cebrian, MD (Editor)
María Teresa Gómez García, PhD (Editor)
2022. ISBN: 978-1-68507-784-6 (Hardcover)
2022. ISBN: 979-8-88697-629-8 (eBook)

**A Closer Look at Pregnancy and Childbirth**
Louise J. Salgado (Editor)
2022. ISBN: 978-1-68507-658-0 (Hardcover)
2022. ISBN: 978-1-68507-667-2 (eBook)

**Cancer and Pregnancy: A Practical Approach for the Gynecologist**
Elisa Picardo, MD, Marco Mitidieri, MD and Saverio Danese, MD (Editors) 2021. ISBN: 978-1-53619-844-7 (Hardcover)
2021. ISBN: 978-1-53619-928-4 (eBook)

More information about this series can be found at https://novapublishers.com/product-category/series/obstetrics-and-gynecology-advances/

**Obstetrics and Gynecology Advances**

nova
Medicine & Health
New York

**Arpita Roy**
**Gowhar Rashid**
**and Nihad Ashraf Khan**
Editors

# Polycystic Ovarian Syndrome (PCOS) and Our Biological Clock

nova
Medicine & Health
New York

**Copyright © 2023 by Nova Science Publishers, Inc.**

**All rights reserved.** No part of this book may be reproduced, stored in a retrieval system or transmitted in any form or by any means: electronic, electrostatic, magnetic, tape, mechanical photocopying, recording or otherwise without the written permission of the Publisher.

We have partnered with Copyright Clearance Center to make it easy for you to obtain permissions to reuse content from this publication. Please visit copyright.com and search by Title, ISBN, or ISSN.

For further questions about using the service on copyright.com, please contact:

Copyright Clearance Center
Phone: +1-(978) 750-8400 Fax: +1-(978) 750-4470 E-mail: info@copyright.com

## NOTICE TO THE READER

The Publisher has taken reasonable care in the preparation of this book but makes no expressed or implied warranty of any kind and assumes no responsibility for any errors or omissions. No liability is assumed for incidental or consequential damages in connection with or arising out of information contained in this book. The Publisher shall not be liable for any special, consequential, or exemplary damages resulting, in whole or in part, from the readers' use of, or reliance upon, this material. Any parts of this book based on government reports are so indicated and copyright is claimed for those parts to the extent applicable to compilations of such works.

Independent verification should be sought for any data, advice or recommendations contained in this book. In addition, no responsibility is assumed by the Publisher for any injury and/or damage to persons or property arising from any methods, products, instructions, ideas or otherwise contained in this publication.

This publication is designed to provide accurate and authoritative information with regards to the subject matter covered herein. It is sold with the clear understanding that the Publisher is not engaged in rendering legal or any other professional services. If legal or any other expert assistance is required, the services of a competent person should be sought. FROM A DECLARATION OF PARTICIPANTS JOINTLY ADOPTED BY A COMMITTEE OF THE AMERICAN BAR ASSOCIATION AND A COMMITTEE OF PUBLISHERS.

**Library of Congress Cataloging-in-Publication Data**

ISBN: 979-8-89113-100-2

Published by Nova Science Publishers, Inc. † New York

# Contents

# Preface

Polycystic Ovarian Syndrome (PCOS), a lifestyle disorder which is related with the imbalance in our Biological Clock. Several endocrine hormones play a critical role in the manifestation of PCOS which can be avoided, prevented or cured by setting our biological clock on track. This book will provide a close insight into our biological system. It will have a collection of all the endocrine hormones involved in the PCOS and their impact on human body. An overview right from the normal functioning of a hormone to its imbalance and effect on signal pathways of other hormones will be discussed in a finely crafted manner.

Many women having PCOS now have lost the hope of setting their life back on track because of the various repercussions of this disorder. Little they know the complexity of their body and connection of one hormone with the other. The obesity, hair loss, diabetes, depression and anxiety along with infertility problems have taken a great toll over a women's mind with PCOS.

Chapter 1 and 2 discuss about the Transition from Historical to Current Advancements in PCOS and impact of FSH and LH on menstrual health.

Chapter 3 and 4 deals with the increased androgen levels and its impact on PCOS and imbalance and Impact of Melatonin Hormone

Chapter 5-11 discuss about association of PCOS with other diseases like Obesity, role OF ACTH, Insulin resistance, Osteoporosis, Anti-Mullerian hormone, Polymorphisms, genetical inheritance

Chapter 12 and 13 discuss about Several Diagnostic tools and tests for analysis of PCOS and Holistic Approach Towards Several Biomarkers for Early Detection of PCOS

Chapter 15 and 16 discuss about the novel approaches towards PCOS and Epigenetic markers in the pathogenesis of PCOS

# Chapter 1

# An Overview: The Transition from Historical to Current Advancements in Polycystic Ovarian Syndrome

**Mansi Gupta**[1]
**and Nihad Ashraf Khan**[2,*]
[1]Department of Biotechnology, Maharishi Dayanand University, Rohtak, India
[2]Department of Biosciences, Faculty of Natural Sciences, Jamia Milia Islamia, Delhi, India

## Abstract

Polycystic ovary syndrome (PCOS) is a complex well acknowledge disorder that affects females during adolescence. Approximately 25% of females in recent years have been diagnosed with the following disorder which manifests several signs and symptoms of menstrual dysfunctioning, acne, obesity, and many more. The disease is commonly diagnosed with hyperandrogenism and chronic ovulation dysfunction, also known as PCOS. According to three organizations criteria have been set that identifies the following disorder which includes chronic oligo/anovulation, the menstrual cycle happens from less than 21 days or more than 35 days, hyperandrogenism, and morphology of polycystic ovary, but these subsets were recognized that can rule out the anovulation or androgen excess conditions before PCOS confirmations. Several chronic metabolic ailments are predisposed to risk factors like insulin resistance (IR), endothelial dysfunction, dyslipidemia, and systemic inflammation. The prevalence of disease in reproductive age is about 5-18% which poses a higher risk for metabolic disorders, obesity, metabolic syndrome, cardiovascular events, etc. The main characteristics of PCOS are a disruption in anovulation and hypothalamic-pituitary-ovarian axis (HPOA) which is indeed marked by follicle development and reduced hormone production that differs from other ovulation issues. The most prominent feature of this is levels of Luteinizing hormone (LH) in serum, which results in Hyperandrogenism and altered Follicle-stimulating hormone (FSH). Hence, in this chapter, several aspects of PCOS have been discussed with the approaches to managing PCOS.

**Keywords:** polycystic ovarian syndrome (PCOS), endocrinological, anovulation, hyperandrogenism, chronic ovulation, insulin resistance (IR), dyslipidemia, hypothalamic-

---

* Corresponding Author's Email: nihadashraf5@gmail.com.

In: Polycystic Ovarian Syndrome (PCOS) and Our Biological Clock
Editors: Arpita Roy, Gowhar Rashid and Nihad Ashraf Khan
ISBN: 979-8-89113-100-2
© 2023 Nova Science Publishers, Inc.

pituitary-ovarian axis (HPOA), luteinizing hormone (LH), follicle-stimulating hormone (FSH)

## 1. Introduction

Infertility in females is the inability to conceive a child due to the production of abnormal levels of hormones and androgen synthesis where, among all the issues disease Polycystic ovary syndrome (PCOS) has a high degree of heterogeneity and is characterized by an increased in androgen biosynthesis, anovulation, etc. As a chronic disorder, it shows symptoms such as infertility, hirsutism, and dysfunctioning in menstruation. Several institutions and organizations such as the National Institute of Health, Rotterdam, and Androgen excess society (AES) set some criteria to identify and diagnose the following disorder whereas before confirmation of PCOS diagnosis other disorders ruled out that cause anovulation and hyperandrogenism (Varanasi LS et al., 2018). According to these subsets of criteria, several debates have been done which didn't come to any conclusion that shows that still some issues need to get identified to reveal the actual conditions and mechanisms behind PCOS but after prognosis and diagnosis, scientists and clinicians have found the increased risk of skin alterations (mutations) that are associated with cancer and other related issues, affected metabolic and physiologic processes and these issues when appearing in the body most of the times reveal the case of PCOS. However, these long-term repercussions go far beyond the reproductive years and affect women's health. The prevalence of PCOS is still under debate where results from studies suggest that approximately 8-13% of females are affected by this disease and the prevalence is about 6-26% but some conclusions were drawn from the experiments of Bozdag G et al. 2016 that the prevalence was 5-10% according to the subset criteria. However, this variability in Prevalence depends on several factors that contributed to the alteration of diagnostic conditions also due to a lack of information and studies women could not receive formal diagnosis if they got, several years will take to receive the treatment (Rao, Manisha et al., 2020). The main disorders that characterize PCOS are anovulation and hypothalamic-pituitary-ovarian axis dysfunction, resulting in menstrual issues, infertility, and reduced hormone secretions. Some studies revealed that endometrial hyperplasia, Insulin resistance, and metabolic syndrome are more likely to present in PCOS patients. PCOS is a neuro-endocrine disorder that in contrast to other ovulatory syndromes shows abnormality or non-functionality in ovaries (Akre S, Sharma K et al., 2022). In PCOS menstrual irregularities happen which affects almost 25% of women with main hormonal issues such as an Imbalance of the Gonadotrophin hormone and excess androgen. Theoretically, PCOS results from enlarged ovaries with inflamed theca cells that secrete higher amounts than normal, which is especially the enzymatic overactivity that produces steroids. In PCOS a disturbance in gonadotrophin-releasing hormone (GnRH) takes place that imbalances LH and FSH release hypothalamic-pituitary axis where the release of estrogen plays a critical role in causing the increased release of LH. In healthy women, the ratio of LH to FSH should be between 1 and 2. Whereas, in Polycystic-ovary disease, the ratio has reached 2 and 3. This abnormal release does not allow ovulation to take place in patients (Saadia Z. et al., 2020). Another clinical feature of PCOS is hyperandrogenism and hirsutism which are increased hair growth in males and excess androgen growth. Impaired folliculogenesis characterized by excess androgens is the result of disruption in normal ovarian and adrenal function. This is the early gonadotropin-independent stage that stimulates the growth of primordial follicles and atrial follicles generally it is hypothesized that imbalanced LH and FSH secretions are hallmarks of hyperandrogenism that have the appearance of cysts like beads on a string. This kind of increase in follicles and the expression of key enzymes promotes the synthesis of androgen which is further validated by the fact of improving insulin resistance and decreasing hyperandrogenism (Ashraf, S et al., 2019). It is worth noting that females with PCOS suffer from a sleep disorder like irregular sleep patterns which can be called a circadian rhythm disorder this shows the delayed offset of melatonin related to the clock and sleep time also high serum-free testosterone levels are depicted. Current studies reveal the serum melatonin concentration in PCOS women with a high direct metabolite of melatonin α-MT6s in the urine along with circadian and circannual variations are found in the follicular fluid that indicates the effect of arrhythmia in PCOS patients at the follicular level. However, only a few reports support the data of melatonin levels in the follicular fluid which limits the understanding of the concept and the therapeutic effects of melatonin on PCOS infertility are evaluated to reveal the changes in melatonin level, sleep disorder, etc. (Li H, Liu M et al., 2022). PCOS is a premenopausal reproductive condition that poses a high risk for metabolic disorders such as obesity as in some reported cases more than 50 % of women have increased abdominal fat. Adipose tissue is an endocrine organ that is metabolically active and the excess adiposity factor is associated with hyperinsulinemia, synthesis of decreased sex-hormone binding 90 globulin protein, and hyper androgenemia this visceral obesity increases impaired glucose tolerance, Diabetes mellitus (Type2), and cardiovascular issues. Worst metabolic profiles with high triglyceride levels at an early age have been illustrated which somewhere may be independent of obesity. Other than this several severe outcomes are associated with obesity (Ollila MM et al., 2016). The presence of varying symptoms and biochemical heterogeneity leads to a variety of phenotypes that have negative impacts on physical and psychological aspects of life. Asthma is a bronchial obstruction associated with hyperresponsiveness of airway inflammation. The prevalence of asthma in PCOS is related to obesity which has shown that menstrual irregularities are associated with the severity of asthma which indeed suggests that there is some hormonal component as possible evidence for the cause of the pathogenesis of asthma the pieces of evidence are still uncertain whether this relationship between asthma and PCOS are independent risk factors or not (Htet TDet al., 2017). A few mediators were described that were considered common in PCOS are Insulin resistance and hyperinsulinism which are mainly responsible for increases in androgen secretion. However, insulin acts on the ovary similar to gonadotropin and triggers androgen secretion from the adrenal gland (Rodriguez Pari et al., 2019). However, another characteristic of PCOS described is a familial aggregation of PCOS which indicates that a few genetic variations and genetic mutations have been accumulated and replicated in populations which also is influenced by some environmental factors that are already predisposed in the family such as lifestyle modifications that sometimes might benefit the PCOS patients, or sometimes considered harmful (Gu Y, Zhou G, etal., 2022). Several lifestyle changes and body composition intensify the clinical manifestations that cause such disease one more manifestation is. Stress plays a critical role in the development of PCOS pathogenesis in patients Stress-induced anovulation leads to infertility where cortisol is considered a sensitive biomarker for body changes that causes stress. These changes reflect the activation of the Sympathetic-adrenal medullary and hypothalamic-pituitary-adrenal axis. However, few things are known about stress-related PCOS also the association of stress mediators with altered body composition (Basu BR et al. 2018). Although a deficiency in Vitamin D is linked to several metabolic disorders in countries of Middle Eastern Asia and

Africa where obesity is considered one major factor for hypovitaminosis D whose relation with PCOS is well established by the scientists who described that deficiency of Vitamin D as 25 (OH) serum levels <20ng/mL is related with several intracellular regulatory mechanisms such as apoptotic pathways (intrinsic) in ovaries (Kumar A et al., 2017). The deficiency or insufficiency of Vitamin D may not participate in pathophysiology but participates indirectly in lower mineral density in the body which results in poor body balance, and fragile fractures as it stimulates differentiation and development of Granulosa cells and has a direct effect on anti-mullerian hormones to influence the follicular maturation (Di Bari F et al., 2021). Some scientific studies reveal that there is evidence of female fetuses exposed to a high risk of congenital hyperplasia which is due to a 21-OHase enzyme deficiency that after growth develops into PCOS. This pathological condition appears even after eliminating hyperandrogenemia with post-natal therapies. It is also said that defects in the p450 aromatase enzyme that helps in the conversion of estrogen may also develop PCOS in adulthood. Recent advancements it has shown that PCOS may develop in adulthood if a female fetus possesses some hormone deficiency (Gur EB et al., 2015). The genetic contribution also results in the developing PCOS in patients which is the case of complicated and ambiguous pathogenesis. Data from studies reveal that genetic polymorphism is associated with genetic instability which in turn leads to disrupted steroid biosynthesis, gonadotropin secretion, and folliculogenesis. Several genes such as Steroidogenic acute regulatory gene (StAR) Gonadotropin-Releasing Hormone Receptor (GnRhR) Follicle-stimulating hormone receptor (FSHR), Interleukin-1β/IL-1 receptor antagonist (IL-1β/il-1rα) shows polymorphism and pathogenesis of PCOS (Chen Y et al. 2018). The maternal inheritance of these genes causes alteration in the genome of a fetus that ultimately results in the development of symptoms in adulthood. Therefore, to diagnose and manage this common disease in countries several approaches are used and with the help of the development of several tools and techniques, the preventive measure taken to control the increasing number of female Infertility. The clinical features of PCOS can easily be identified by conducting pelvic tests, and transvaginal ultrasounds, and hence still there is controversy regarding the specific diagnostic tools for PCOS.

## 2. History of Poly-Cystic Ovary Syndrome

In history, the first description of PCOS was given by Stein and Leventhal scientists but it was a medical scientist, and physician named Vallisneri who in 1721, described a woman with a case of infertility having large-sized ovaries as same as the pigeon eggs. In 1884, the fibrous and sclerotic lesions in ovaries were shown by Chereau and Rokitansk. Later, Bulius and Kretschmar gave Hyperthecosis concept. After several studies in 1879, Lawson Tait suggested the need for treatment of symptomatic cystic degeneration. In 1902, a review paper was published to raise the voice regarding this critical issue of PCOS where a scientist McGlinn 1915, suggested a method to treat the disease by just ‘puncturing the ovary cyst on the surface rather than resection.’ Later this stein and Leventhal, in 1935 presented women with disturbance in the menstrual cycle, hirsutism, and enlarged ovaries with small follicles where by using the ovary resection method they were the first to describe the increased volume of ovaries in women with a lack of menstrual cycle and after this treatment women again got pregnant and regain their menstruation (Manti, M. et al., 2020). However, with the availability of treatments like Follicle stimulating hormones and urinary sources, the use of surgical treatments ends. Initially, PCOS was described as distinct masculinization and luteinization syndrome but Stein and Leventhal in their report described that cyst in ovaries results from hormonal stimulation abnormalities. After this statement given by the scientists, that the adrenal gland not only produces androgens but ovaries too then in 1953, to treat sclerotic ovaries cortisone therapy was done by using testosterone. For the diagnosis of PCOS 3 investigators investigated the increased level of LH and 17-Ketosteroids in the urine of patients with cystic ovaries which were considered the key regulators in mediating normal fertility in women (Azziz R, et al., 2010). Later the irregularity in the release of gonadotropin and androgen was confirmed, but the theory of abnormal concentration of gonadotropins in PCOS was discarded due to the increase in testosterone levels that ultimately leads to increase in the circulating androgens in patients with PCOS. Due to the lack of clinical advancements, in the diagnosis of PCOS several women without the conformation of hormone release disorder met the criteria of PCOS which shows a pulsative nature of hormones i.e., maximum and minimal concentration differs during the daytime and especially in females with low androgen levels that mislead the disease identification (Silva M. S. B. et al., 2022). Several tools came into advancement that benefitted the PCOS prognosis and diagnosis. However, recent advancements in ultrasound examination have benefited the medical field due to its non-invasive approach, repeatability, simplicity, and precision in ovary follicles which was highly appreciated. Later Swanson for the first time described the structure of ovaries with PCOS by using ultrasonography. Another scientist after looking at the Swanson technique aimed the use of transvaginal and transabdominal ultrasound that proved the presence of false negative results in the case of abdominal lining examination. The use of advanced technology has provided a new way to diagnose the disease and ultrasound progress is the one that has made prognosis easy by identifying the localization of PCOS where the ratio of ovarian stroma to the total has been considered the best condition of diagnosis and prognosis. Several women in the population were examined ultrasonically in case cyst appearance took place with no clinical symptoms. After several studies on PCOS, some criteria had been set by the NIH which were widely accepted in the research and clinical community. These criteria explained hyperandrogenic anovulation in PCOS where if the women consist of symptoms of excess androgens, rare chances of ovulation may occur excluding other disorders. Therefore, diagnostic features of PCOS are still under study. But in later studies, Rotterdam set the criteria of size and morphology of the ovary. Therefore, the presence of 2 out of 3 rare ovulation, excess androgen activity, and polycystic ovaries after other pathology exclusion decides the PCOS. Hirsutism is considered the clinical features of hyperandrogenemia that could be assessed according to the Ferriman-Gallwey score, seborrheic disease, etc. Additionally, the concentration analysis of testosterone, 17-OH progesterone, and other hormones are useful in excess androgen assessment. A debate on ultrasound criteria raised a question about the diagnostic criteria of ultrasound. The answer which was provided is if the diagnosis is made by transvaginal ultrasound during the follicular phase where more than 12 follicles of diameter with size <10mm are visible or the volume of the ovary has increased. Other questions were raised on the importance of technique and why lesions don't have to be bilateral. In Rotterdam and NIH definitions the main difference was the use of patients with biochemical hyperandrogenemia was necessary for PCOS diagnosis. However, the Rotterdam criteria faced criticism due to the involvement of mild phenotypes for the combination of cystic ovaries with oligomenorrhea but the results of nor androgenic patients can be extrapolated here (Chang S et al., 2021). The presence of these additional phenotypes led to the generalization of clinical trials which might also increase the prevalence of PCOS. Now, in 2006 Androgen Excess Society (AES) delivered a statement on criteria where the sign of a non-diagnostic condition in combination with other syndromes was established. The main focus of AES is to eliminate some mild phenotypes such as excess androgen and menstruation disorder based on both the syndrome's reproductive and metabolic symptoms. However, there is a need to work more on PCOS to get the appropriate medicine, studies, and treatment because it not only causes menstrual disorders and others but also cardiovascular disease and reproductive cancer. The puzzled etiology of PCOS is now accepted that suggest that PCOS is multifactorial and partly genetic. Indeed, several genes were identified among women with PCOS but were not included in the diagnosis. As compared to healthy patients with PCOS the cardiovascular risk and carbohydrate metabolism disturbance are increased which can be treated based on the modification of lifestyle (Parker J et al., 2022). Several sensitizing agents that not only restore ovulation but facilitate weight loss, counter androgenic symptoms, prevent long-term complications, and decreased the risk of early pregnancy loss and hyperstimulation syndrome were used to improve the outcomes of in-vitro fertilization therapies. The potential consequences and mechanisms of intrauterine androgen exposure and anti-mullerian hormone action are investigated in further research and studies (Abbott DH et al., 2019).

## 3. Epidemiology of PCOS

The prevalence of PCOS in India and other countries is widely studied where in these countries a higher proportion is seen in urban areas than in women of rural areas. A study conducted in a medical school found a common disorder among participants of PCOS where a high incidence rate of mood swings is reported. According to Vidya Bharathi et al. depending on three criteria the prevalence of PCOS is found to be variable in patients which might be a reason for the disparity in widespread presence rates which in India ranges to 8.2% percent in comparison to other countries (Ganie MA et al., 2019). According to three criteria set by the organizations, it states that PCOS is a common endocrinopathy that affects 4-8% of women of reproductive age. A descriptive table of data from several countries is depicted below in Table 1 which illustrates the prevalence rates of PCOS in most countries.

**Table 1.** This table depicts data from some countries where the prevalence of PCOS is commonly seen in recent studies conducted. Among all the countries Australia consists of highest prevalence rate of 55% in the age period of 18-45 whereas, the lowest rate is shown by Beijing which reveals the health status of women in the country

| S. no | Countries | PCOS prevalence rate | Age of females | References |
|---|---|---|---|---|
| 1. | India | 8.2% | 17-24 | Gupta M et al., 2018 |
| 2. | Denmark | 16.6% | 20-40 | Lauritsen MP et al., 2014 |
| 3. | USA | 53% | 18-45 | Clark N M et al., 2014 |
| 4. | Beijing | 5.6%1 | 9-45 | Deswal R et al., 2020 |
| 5. | Iran | 7.1 | 18-45 | Tehrani FR et al.,2011 |

Some countries are reported to have a prevalence rate of 2-4% whereas countries like China, Beijing, and Sri Lanka have 5-10% but after a comparison of all countries, the prevalence rate is higher in Australia, Denmark, and Turkey. Family history is one of the risk factors for this disease which by clustering case study reveal that it is a heritable disorder. The high prevalence and its features are suggestive of genetic influences. However, monozygotic and dizygotic twins have been reported where the mode of inheritance remains elusive. Several issues which need to be discussed are the heterogeneity of phenotypes, handling, and obtaining of large sampling size. Some shreds of evidence from studies suggest that PCOS is an ancient disorder that originates in Africa before the migration of humans. The history of weight gain, followed by a healthy lifestyle illustrated to reduce body weight, and abdominal fat, improve insulin resistance, and decreased hirsutism. According to experimental data, it was suggested that obese women had a prevalence of 28.3 %. However, rates for varying weight categories were 8.2%, 9.8%,9.9%and 11.5% through which it was concluded that obesity is the factor that can increase the risk of PCOS irrespective of its effect which was modest. In epilepsy, the frequency of reproductive disorders has been considered high, also some antiepileptic drugs increase the risk of PCOS. Insulin resistance or diabetes is another PCOS risk factor. These several other factors are there which may increase the prevalence rate of PCOS and this is most prominently found in children where some of the factors are apparent in childhood (Sirmans SM et al., 2013).

## 4. Etiology

Etiology is the study of a variety of factors that cause disease or are responsible to cause the symptom of disease here is Polycystic Ovary Syndrome, which is discussed in detail in further chapters but the overview of some risk factors or causes is mentioned here. Although a variety of factors involves in oligogenic disorder with a common familial link that represents an autosomal dominant pattern which is still unclear, a rather modified lifestyle has caused obesity in females which could be one reason behind increasing insulin resistance and diabetes in PCOS (Ndefo UA et al., 2013). According to the International based and American College of Obstetricians and Gynecologists, Other prevalence factors share anomalies with hormones such as thyroid, prolactin, androgen-secreting tumors (Teede H J et al., 2018, Christopherson, R.et al., 2016)). Lifestyle factors influence overall health by regulating metabolism and maintaining a healthy weight. Being overweight is a major factor in PCOS. Other than this genetics, environmental factors, excess androgen, and reproductive system abnormalities are some major and common factors that cause PCOS. However, the exact causes are not yet understood very well (Shannon M, et al., 2012). Low-grade inflammation refers to when white blood cells make substances in response to any pathogenic infection that scientist has considered the cause of PCOS to produce androgens. Reproductive system abnormalities stand for the abnormal level of androgen production that interferes with the ovaries' functions. In PCOS menstrual cycle abnormality produce multiple follicles of smaller size less than 10 mm in diameter. The smaller size leads to anovulation and imbalance of hormones. The adrenal gland and ovaries generally produce androgens that include testosterone, andro-testosterone, and dihydro-epiandrosterone (DHEA). The high levels of LH increase androgen levels in women. Moreover, when glucose levels are uncontrolled with increased or decreased amounts of insulin condition is called diabetes (Type 1 and Type2). Insulin resistance and hyperinsulinemia occur in both normal and overweight women with PCOS indeed, in obese women it appears to be a three-fold increase and approximately 35% of women develop glucose intolerance. Some causes are described here as there are no certain causes for PCOS.

## 5. Pathophysiology of PCOS

PCOS is a mechanism that impacts fertility in women and has not been completely understood to date. When the diagnosis has been established it represented a self-perpetuating vicious cycle that acted on ovaries and endometrium including dysfunctioning in the neuroendocrinal system with a multi-prolonged pathogenesis and abnormal gonadotropin-releasing hormone (GnRH) regulation that ultimately leads to increased Luteinizing hormone (LH) and decreased Follicle-stimulating hormone (FSH) levels in the body. Including these other mechanisms such as an increase in anti-mullerian hormone (AMH), *f*ollicular arrest, increased testosterone, estradiol, and dehydro-epiandrosterone (DHEA) (Gambineri A et al., 2002). The major predisposing factor that scientists said is another major cause of PCOS is obesity which is the major expression of insulin resistance and metabolic phenotype in the disease. Epigenetics and several environmental factors influence the interactions between multiple proteins and genes. Other biochemical and hormonal aspects studied by scientists are under investigation. However, in the adolescent stage, it starts developing, and during these early puberty years when recent clinical, experimental, and genetics data is collected scientists concluded the emphasis on neuroendocrine development in the pathophysiology of PCOS. Leptin is a major intermediary compound whose high level has been found to associate with a marker of IR. Also, it positively correlates with serum testosterone levels. However, from case studies, it was difficult to ascertain the causes and effective relationships between leptin and hyperandrogenemia. Singh et al. in their case studies demonstrated that adiponectin levels were found to be altered in obese women when compared to normal and healthy women but independent of obese status women may have accumulated intra-abdominal fat and unhealthy metabolic profiles which all are represented in Figure1.

In large-scale studies, proteomics, genomics, and metabolomics found altered levels of proteins, hormones, genes, and compounds. Altered levels of several proteins that play critical roles in extracellular matrix modeling, dysfunctioning of complement proteins, fibrinolysis, and many more reflected the molecular defects in folliculogenesis (Ambekar AS et al., 2015). However, in reproductive disease and conditions oxidative stress and autoimmunity are other factors that play a critical role in the pathogenesis of PCOS where plasma amino acid levels are found to be deranged in women and scientists suggest this unregulated level can be a marker of metabolic and oxidative stress in PCOS women. It also has been suspected to have some components of autoimmune origin. The presence of a large number of antithyroglobulin antibodies in PCOS suggested a possible role of autoimmunity (Arora et al., 2016). Some studies have suggested the role of vitamin D deficiency in metabolic abnormalities which are found common in India and in other countries of East Asia that do not alter the metabolic phenotype of PCOS but play a role in pathogenesis (Kumar A et al., 2017). The various components of PCOS including obesity-related cytokines and oxidative stress markers evaluated the pathogenesis and highlighted the multifaceted nature and the need to further research to understand and delineate the contribution of each. However, the overall pathophysiology of PCOS is illustrated below with the help of Figure 2.

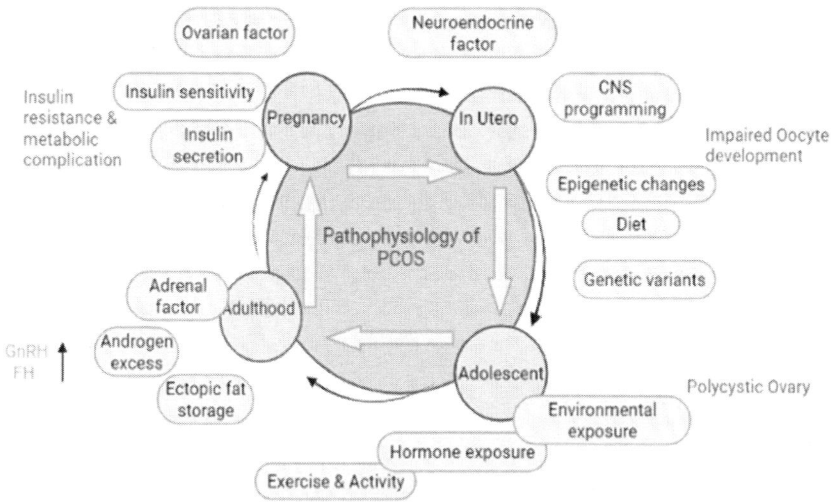


**Figure 1.** In this figure, several factors are depicted that cause PCOS. In the Adolescent stage environmental exposure is the main factor that disrupts hormone regulation which in adulthood leads to an increase in androgen excess by the abnormal release of LH and FSH. This abnormal release of hormones causes insulin resistance & other complications which in later ages can cause issues in the neuroendocrine system.

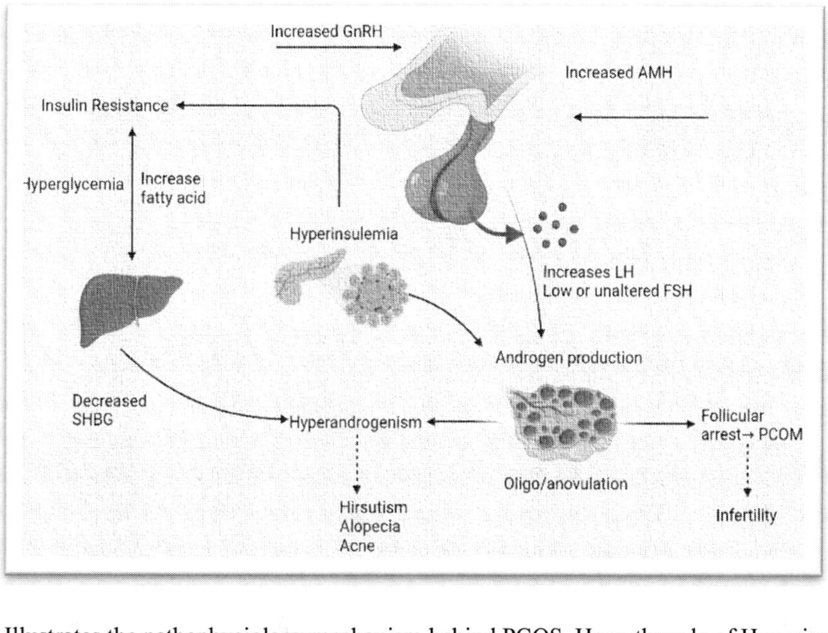


**Figure 2.** Illustrates the pathophysiology mechanism behind PCOS. Here, the role of Hyperinsulinemia is depicted that results in insulin resistance, and Increased levels of GnRH and Anti-mullerian hormone (AMH) from the anterior pituitary lead to abnormal LH levels of LH that interrupt follicular formation and cause infertility in women.

## 6. PCOS at Different Stages of Life

During menstruation, every month ovulation takes place through which the egg is released and the fertility of females decides on that process. But women with PCOS do not ovulate and find difficulty in pregnancy. The progression of this in different stages of life is not well understood due to the dearth of studies. According to experimental studies, the comparison of clinical and biochemical parameters was investigated where investigation criteria were associated with the menstrual cycle, the decrease in androgen level, and insulin resistance. The PCOS manifestations in specific age groups are described as early and late symptoms of life.

### 6.1. Early Symptoms of PCOS

In recent medical conditions, multi-specialist vision is required for effective management and treatment, but initially, signs and symptoms of disorders are necessary to understand therefore, scientists have studied clinical symptoms of PCOS in the early life stage of females. During childhood, some interactions between environmental conditions and genetic predisposition play a role in the pathogenesis of PCOS (Bellver J et al., 2018). In the adolescent stage, the increased risk of PCOS could be due to the intrauterine growth retardation and excess androgen that produces large amounts of glucocorticoids which induces epigenetic modification and increased risk for disease. Menstrual cycle irregularity, hirsutism, acne, a family history of overweight, low birth weight, obesity, IR risk developing the syndrome. Strict criteria have been set which require moderate to severe hirsutism and the constant elevation of testosterone levels in serum, and ovary dysfunctioning to find exact management and mechanism. Recent studies have shown that adolescents having PCOS possess a high risk for MS in addition dietary factors are there to affect the lifestyle of females and affect the reproductive system (Witchel SF et al., 2015, Rocha AL et al., 2019). Unhealthy mothers who are diagnosed with PCOS contribute prenatal hyperandrogenic milieu to their daughters, which is considered to play a reprogramming role in female offspring (Risal S et al., 2019). Additionally, injuries in the fetoplacental unit such as hypertension, and Type-2 diabetes mellitus may have some influence on weight birth reprogramming. This metabolic memory induces a non-genetic inheritance that is linked to overweight and abdominal obesity. Apart from these female fetuses have subtle signs of compromised cardiometabolic health which is linked to pervasive developmental disabilities (Gunning MN et al., 2020). However, polycystic ovary syndrome is difficult to diagnose in infancy and childhood due to missing symptoms and the measurement of anti-mullerian hormone represents a reliable proxy, indeed the values are higher among girls at puberty and multi-follicular ovarian morphology that results from enhanced recruitment or decreased growth or arrest correlates with the LH and plasma testosterone levels. However, the actual diagnosis is difficult to identify the real contribution of PCOS mothers to offspring development where increased glucose-stimulated insulin levels are found in some constant phenotype categories in daughters with PCOS (Bell GA et al., 2018).

### 6.2. Late Symptoms of PCOS

During childhood, the problems and issues faced by females continue to the adult stage such as infrequent menstrual cycle (oligomenorrhea), acne, and amenorrhea (primary, secondary) leads to severe consequences like infertility, overweight, hirsutism (excess hair on chest, the nipple, and abdomen), pelvic pain, acanthosis nigricans (dark leathery lines on the skin behind the neck, under the breast), depression, anxiety, the birth of a baby before 37-month completion, etc. all physical symptoms are due to hormonal imbalance and dysregulation. Apart from this severe increased-risk symptoms include which appears due to hormone dysregulation is Type-2 diabetes which is a lifelong condition that causes high blood sugar level in the body, High blood pressure, and cholesterol leading to obesity, cardiovascular risk, and stroke conditions, sleep apnea overweight women develop this disorder due to the interrupted breathing during sleep. Tumor development is also one of the consequences of PCOS (Aversa A et al., 2020). Several meta-analyses revealed the increased risk for gestational diabetes mellitus (GDM) with miscarriage. Indeed, this factor is in contrast not affected mainly by PCOS rather other factors contribute to it. Significantly women have obesity increases insulin resistance and results in hyperinsulinemia that further leads to altered adipogenesis and lipolysis. Also, obesity increases the LH stimulation from theca cells resulting in hyperandrogenism (Glueck CJ et al., 2019). Although, BMI is thought to be independent of glucose prevalence and continues to increase in the late reproductive stage. Meta-analysis has revealed that there is a two-fold increase in Metabolic syndrome. However, clustering of metabolic risk in a family of PCOS females is reported where fathers, brothers, and sisters are exposed to lipidemia and hypertension. Although postmenopausal phenotypes are less and not well understood (Rubin KH et al., 2017, Yilmaz B et al., 2018). This creates long-term adverse health effects in patients. However, menopause is a stage that occurs at 50-52 years of age that shows limited phenotypes due to age changes as aging in PCOS patients associate with a reduced number or loss of follicles and the disappearance of PCOM (Day FR et al., 2015). In conclusion, the Postmenopausal persistence of this disorder continues to show shreds of evidence of hyperandrogenism and irregular menstrual cycles (Teede HJ et al., 2018).

## 7. Biomarkers Presentation by Cells for Diagnosis in PCOS

Recent studies have found several biological markers that are responsible for the alteration and cause of PCOS. Several agents cause PCOS and represent autosomal dominant inheritance patterns such as genetic, and environmental factors. However, PCOS is known as a heterogenic syndrome and shows a relationship with disorders like hyperinsulinemia and androgenemia. Several genes that regulate insulin functions and androgen synthesis are found to be associated with PCOS (Sharif E et al., 2019). The pathogenesis of PCOS is depicted by insulin production and signaling via receptors where the activation of these polymorphic receptors like INSR, and IGF-1 is mediated by insulin that triggers tyrosine kinase activation and further signaling. Studies found that there are some defects associated with post-signaling cascade and a few markers are D19S884 and IRS polymorphism which is associated with PCOS cases in other countries Italy, Japan, Greek, etc (Nuzhat Shaikh et al., 2014). ENPP1, Calpain-10, and PPARy are some other polymorphic markers that associate with insulin resistance. CYP17 shows a correlation with hyperandrogenism which is due to overexpression of theca cells this marker is located on the 10q24.3 chromosome and transcribes the p450c-17α enzyme. The polymorphism in CYP17 manifests the PCOS although the marker is still in debate. miRNA is another marker that plays a role in the formation of the primordial follicle and regulates follicular development with a significant increase which manifests in follicular fluid and serum of patients (Eisenberg I, et al., 2017). According to scientists there exist a relation between marker (PPARGC1A) located on mitochondrial DNA, the amount of which in PCOS depleted to a certain level. This marker shows an epigenetic modification alteration that causes hypermethylation of promoters and increases the metabolic risk in females. Panda PK et al. demonstrated a few genes that act as a PCOS marker with their locus on chromosomes. Some steroidogenic markers P450scc (CYP11α) and p450arom (CYP19) were considered potential candidates for involvement in PCOS. The association of these genes demonstrates that allelic variation mediates the development of hyperandrogenemia, PCOS, and hirsutism. The lack of ovulatory status indicates that it also plays a role in the development of hirsutism in PCOS. This variation is sufficient to cause altered ovarian morphology. Some non-invasive markers used in the diagnosis of PCOS such as zonulin regulate the permeability of the gut and correspond to PCOS insulin resistance, dyslipidemia, and menstrual disorder (Polak K 2017). Adiponectin is an adipocytokine produced by adipocytes the levels of which go down in obese patients. Investigations suggest that this marker is linked with Type-2 DM in PCOS patients it has been confirmed the relation between adiponectin concentration and insulin resistance that obstruct the functioning of beta cells. Apelin, a biologically active peptide considered a biomarker for the diagnosis of PCOS irrespective of the fact that it is involved in cardiovascular disease and dyslipidemia. This peptide is found in body organs including the heart, brain, and kidney. etc. Different levels of this enzyme are associated with different stages of ovarian follicles also it affects the intake of water and the hypothalami-hypophyseal axis (Sun X et al. 2015). Although PCOS is caused by folliculogenesis that in turn leads to oligo-ovulatory cycles and activated granulosa cells to produce high anti-mullein hormones (AMH) secreted by granulosa cells. The decreased levels of AMH follows the development of follicles and vice versa happens due to the proliferation of pre-antral follicle (Deveer M et al. 2015). In contrast, it is, therefore, concluded that levels of AMH in addition to LH and FSH ratio increase. The ratio of testosterone to dihydrotestosterone is an adequate biomarker in PCOS diagnosis. Copeptin resembles arginine vasopressin known to stabilize vascular tone and fluid balance. As being more sensitive and stable, this shows an association with insulin resistance and cardiometabolic complications. Irisin is responsible for white fat and glucose tolerance. It is a myokine found in serum and plasma and cannot be considered a definitive marker in PCOS. Ghrelin is a glycopeptide that possesses multi-functions influence the pituitary gland by secreting hormones. Same gene codes for another hormone i.e., Obestatin the alteration in levels of these two helps in the diagnosis of PCOS (Kruszewska J et al., 2022). Metastin is involved in multi-metabolic diseases and is also named Kisspeptin encoded by the Kiss-1 gene. The high levels of this hormone increase the LH and elucidated role is mentioned in non-obese PCOS patients. Proteomic studies it is revealed that there is a correlation exist between haptoglobin and PCOS. It is a positive marker for inflammation that prevents oxidative damage and is involved in the development of PCOS. There are several other potential biomarkers for which insufficient knowledge exist and due to instability and easily degradable nature, they could not be described. Moreover, most of the described markers are easily distinguished and useful in prognosis and disease monitoring (Sharif E et al., 2019).

## 8. Diagnosis and Tools for PCOS

Various methods are used to prognose and diagnose the heterogenous nature of PCOS where for the first time Stein and Leventhal used a method to diagnose the presence of enlarged multicystic ovary by using the technique pneumo-roentgenography or laparotomy in women who possess either anovulation or hirsutism, or both (Rui wang et al., 2017). In past years the only option for clinicians to detect multiple cysts in ovaries is to examine the vaginal and rectal area repeatedly. The presence of cysts in PCOS is confirmed by administering the air into the peritoneum cavity via an intersection in the abdomen this confirms the presence of polycystic ovaries only when the image of ovaries appears to be three-quarters the size of the shadow on an X-ray. Several examples of this technique are shown in Stein and Leventhal's publication where a lot of advantages and disadvantages are also mentioned which were faced during the examination of PCOS. Lipiodol drug administration was done concurrently to define the structure of the uterus in women. However, this approach is not widely accepted and laparotomy and wedge biopsy were employed for the diagnosis as standard methods (Rui wang et al., 2017). An increase in urinary LH levels with bilateral PCOM was reported in 1958 by three scientists named McArthur, Ingersoll, and Worcester whereas, early during the 1970s and 80s increased hormone levels in serum were considered the basis of diagnosis (Rosenfield RL et al., 2016). Although the ratio of LH and FSH in the late 80s was considered to be the markers of PCOS diagnosis which later found of no use only if no exact values were obtained if the absolute values were obtained then it would be considered for the diagnostic purpose. After the invention of the ultrasound technique, Swanson et al. 1981 used it for the first time to detect polycystic ovaries afterward the technique was named ultrasonography (USG). However, the ultrasound examination of ovaries is considered simple, and non-invasive with multiple measurements. Follicular structures located below the surface of the ovaries can be visualized and diagnosed easily which illustrates the increased density of cells in stroma (Ali I H et al., 2016). In conclusion, PCOS manifests in a variety of clinical ways whose etiology is still unknown, while the pathophysiology of PCOS is complex and difficult to diagnose. There has been a significant amount of scientific debate found in the literature regarding the standardization of diagnostic criteria. After so many debates and discussions in 1990, the National Institute of Health (NIH) laid down the diagnostic criteria for PCOS. Subsequently, in a workshop held in 2003, Rotterdam developed a novel criterion for diagnosis that came to be known as the Rotterdam criteria. As per these criteria set, if any of the two characteristics mentioned below is present during diagnosis and prognosis confirmation of PCOS is done (Richard S et al., 2013).

1) Irregular menstrual cycles
2) Clinical/biochemical hyperandrogenism, and
3) Multiple cysts in ovaries having more than 12 follicles in each ovary measuring between 2 and 9 millimeters).

Later after the Rotterdam criteria, the Androgen Excess Society (AES) revised the diagnostic criteria in 2006 which necessitates the presence of a certain character i.e clinical/biochemical hyperandrogenism that combines with either oligo-ovulation or irregular menstruation (Bani Mohammad et al., 2017). Figure 3 below illustrates the various diagnostic criteria for PCOS.

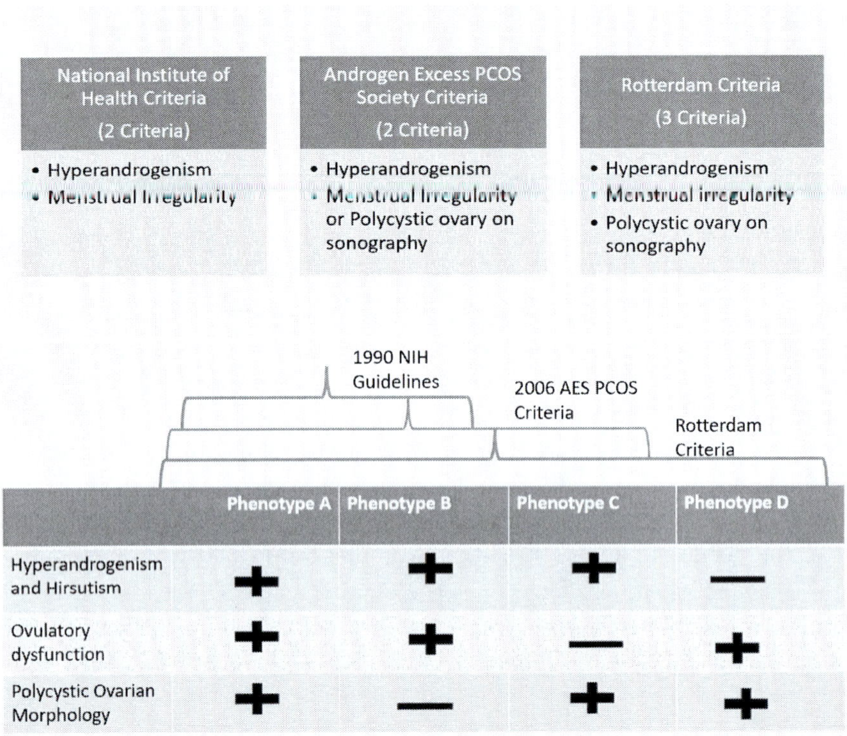


**Figure 3.** During the diagnosis of PCOS several criteria were set by the organizations to detect the factors responsible to cause the disease and depending on the three criteria mentioned above abnormal phenotypes related to Hyperandrogenism, Hirsutism, ovulatory dysfunctioning, and Polycystic ovarian morphology can be diagnosed. The + sign dictates the presence of Character.

However, there are a few roadblocks that interfere with deciding the process of standardizing PCOS diagnosis. Firstly, ovulation is frequently unpredictable in the years leading up to the onset of menarche. Because of this, anovulation cannot be regarded as an unquestionable proof of the presence of the syndrome.

- Second, transvaginal ultrasounds are difficult in the adolescent stage, due to which the capacity of visualization of ovaries eliminates and restricts the possibility of an invasive diagnosis of polycystic ovarian morphology.
- Third, there is no or very less agreement on the biochemical levels of hyperandrogenism available in a similar manner less information is registered in the literature on normal androgen levels in adolescents. Therefore, both issues contribute to the lack of information, and determining whether an individual has an abnormal level of androgens is, therefore, a difficult task.
- Fourth, it is difficult to differentiate multimolecular ovaries from polycystic ovaries, even though the former may be a normal occurrence in adolescent girls.

Other than these several recent advancements have already been done with the use of a Deep sequence learning system that distinguishes the PCOS symptoms in adult and childhood stages with the identification of several biomarkers.

## 9. Complications Associated with PCOS

According to studies from the literature, it is suggested that women with PCOS in the adult (18-45) stage are more prone to many short & long-term health complications such as infertility, obstetric complications, and other chronic issues such as cardiovascular risks, metabolic issues, and oncological ailments. However, it is still unclear to determine the exact cause of these complications due to the heterogeneity of the syndrome and its ambiguous pathology. Obesity also serves as a confounding factor in understanding the pretext of these complications. Because of the syndrome's heterogeneity, unclear pathogenetic mechanisms, and the presence of confounding factors such as obesity, determining the precise extent of these complications is extremely difficult. The presentation of PCOS phenotypes varies during the life of the female which leads to alterations in ovarian & metabolic functions thereby, altering the disease expression and & lead to other co-morbidities later in life. This section discusses some of the most common PCOS complications.

### 9.1. Early-Term Complications

#### *9.1.1. Infertility*

During epidemiological studies, PCOS is reported as a common cause of ovulatory dysfunction that can further lead to infertility (inability to conceive a child). However, the case of primary infertility was reported in almost 50% of the diseased women with PCOS, while secondary infertility was reported in 25% of the women. This case study is an eye-catching point for identifying primary infertility as a major reason to develop PCOS. Few comorbidities such as IR and obesity associated with PCOS may also contribute to the effect of fertility. Both comorbidities in turn found to be linked to an enhanced abortion risk, lowered chances of pregnancy, and birth rates. Another co-morbidity associated with PCOS; is endometrial abnormalities that affect implantation. Follicular vascularity and the fluid environment are other abnormalities that influence fertility (Palomba S et al., 2015).

However, literature has suggested the improvement of PCOM females over time with the regulation of the menstrual cycle with increasing age. Although the reproductive outcomes in PCOS women were found to be similar in non-PCOS women rather, a condition of a longer reproductive window can be seen in PCOS women only due to the preserved nature of ovarian reserves. Studies on miscarriage in women with PCOS are scarce and according to scientists, this complication can be excluded which makes PCOS not a potential cause of miscarriages in women. Additionally, according to the most recent guidelines of the Endocrine Society (AES)-appointed Task Force of Experts, PCOS can lead to infertility only if oligo ovulation is present and it was suggested to screen ovulatory status and menstrual history in women with PCOS that can get help with infertility issues (Legro R S et al., 2013).

#### *9.1.2. Obstetric Complications*

Ovulatory infertility links PCOS and today, in the past few years, the focus has shifted towards reproductive issues including obstetrics complications. Furthermore, the relationship between obesity, IR, diabetes, and cardiovascular health issues leads to the generation of obstetric risk in PCOS. However, further complications related to multiple pregnancies create higher chances of infertility in mid-aged women and the change in guidelines declared by AES for the prognosis, diagnosis, and treatment has already proved that PCOS women are at high risk of pregnancy complications, and pre-conceptual assessment of BMI, blood pressure, and glucose tolerance are recommended to detect and diagnose the further links between them (Palomba S et al., 2014). According to the Endocrine Society women those who are at an increased risk of pregnancy complications are initially screened to test blood pressure, weight, and blood sugar level in the body.

The medications given for ovulation are thought to decrease the risk of miscarriage still there is an ambiguity regarding the risk of miscarriage when compares to healthy women. According to studies, two comparable points suggest the rates of miscarriage. During meta-analytic studies, the comparison of PCOS women with healthy women who undergoes in-vitro fertilization was found to be reported no significant differences. Other studies have found a relationship between hypertension and PCOS where scientists concluded that there is a three-fold increase in pregnancy-induced hypertension or preeclampsia and also an absolute risk of 6-15% with gestational diabetes described PCOS complication in pregnancy (Qin J Z et al., 2013).

## 9.2. Long-Term Complications of PCOS

### *9.2.1. Cardiovascular Risk*

Cardiovascular disease has gained interest in the diagnosis of PCOS due to increased prevalence and other factors such as hypertension, dyslipidemia, diabetes, and obesity. Some other non-classic factors are C-reactive protein (CRP), homocysteine, and tumor necrosis factor (TNF-α). CVD markers at any age are associated with an increased risk of PCOS that can be presented due to non-obesity in women (Conway G et al., 2014). According to inter-heart studies, published in 2004, some potentially identifiable risk factors have accounted for 94% of risks of first myocardial infarction in women; factors included smoking, hypertension, diabetes, visceral obesity, psychological factors, and less fruit and vegetable consumption. Alcohol consumption etc. The majority of these can be seen in PCOS women. According to experimental studies, when compared to controls, the prevalence of each risk factor is estimated to be double that of normal in women with PCOS while during comparison it is 1.5 times higher in BMI-matched studies during adolescence (Fauser B C et al., 2012). There is also an increased risk of hypertension that can be explained by IR and hyperinsulinemia, through which alterations in smooth muscle cells can be studied which results in hypertrophy of the vascular muscle wall with reduced compliance as well as interference with endothelium-dependent vasodilation mechanism. High testosterone levels, except sex hormone-binding globulin (SHBG) levels, also associates with an increased risk of hypertension (Scicchitano P et al., 2012). In studies, the absence of a hypertensive state continues to show some significant cardiovascular issues as an increase in daytime systolic blood pressure, mean arterial blood pressure, and pulse rate. Dyslipidemia is manifested by hypertriglyceridemia, low high-density lipoprotein (HDL), cholesterol levels, and small low-density lipoprotein (LDL) particles which are similar to type-2 diabetes mellitus (T2DM) and typical IR states. However, the increased LDL cholesterol levels are less dependent on body weight and may relate to hyperandrogenism. Higher non-HDL cholesterol levels common in PCOS women reflect altered Apolipoprotein

B/A1 ratios that are considered to be the important risk factors for CVD (Palomba S et al., 2015).

### 9.2.2. Metabolic Risk

Based on the seriousness and rapid spreading of obesity in the global population scientists called it an epidemic disorder in children and adolescents. PCOS women are usually found overweight than healthy women (BMI 2.5kg/m$^2$ and obese (BMI.30 kg/m2) with a typical central distribution of adipose tissue, up to 61%. Although the prevalence of this condition varies widely across several countries and ethnicities (Lim SS et al., 2012). However, the role is unknown where cultural, lifestyle, and ethnic factors are supposed to play important roles in these conditions. According to literature studies conducted obesity is thought to be associated with severe reproductive phenotypes that are distinguished by chronic anovulation and hyperandrogenism where lean women were found to have mild reproductive phenotypes when compared to those women who were overweight, this implies that obesity can intensify the reproductive phenotypes of PCOS (Stepto NK et al., 2013). Obesity shows a bidirectional relationship with PCOS, as with the increasing weight prevalence increases. Even for upper body fat distribution women with PCOS are more likely to have it in the absence of obesity and regardless of BMI (Teede HJ et al.,2018). One most metabolically important adipose tissue is the distribution of fat around the abdominal area which appears like the shape of an apple. Indeed, the most serious health consequences of PCOS are associated with excess weight and abdominal area, because increased visceral adiposity is associated with increased IR, which is thought to be one of the symptoms and most important metabolic pathogenetic keys. Excess central adiposity is also linked to a worsening dyslipidaemic profile, with higher triglyceride levels and lower HDL cholesterol levels (Peigné M, Dewailly D et al., 2014).

Being a key etiological factor in PCOS, IR has traditionally been linked to obesity. Furthermore, it is demonstrated that the presence of IR in PCOS is evidenced by abnormalities in insulin signaling and excessive phosphorylation of serine residues on receptors, and defects in post-receptor signaling molecules. The cellular and molecular mechanisms of IR in PCOS are distinct from those seen in other metabolic diseases such as T2DM and obesity. However, the synergistic effect of obesity on insulin action is well-known in PCOS, as hepatic IR is only found in obese PCOS women. IR can occur without obesity also, and its prevalence in thin women with PCOS is approximately 75%. Obesity and overweight, however, are said to increase the risk of developing T2DM in PCOS women, even though we can say that PCOS is an independent risk factor for T2DM, as previously reported. The syndrome, in particular, is thought to be a significant risk factor for the development of diabetes both later in life and young overweight, or obese women with PCOS (Garima K, Anju S 2017).

### 9.2.3. Oncology Risk

Due to the chronic multisystemic and multifaceted nature of PCOS, the reproductive and metabolic changes characterize the syndrome that might be linked to an increased risk of developing cancers of endometrial, ovarian, and breast cancer, through which hormonal and metabolic pathogenetic mechanisms can be recognized. Obesity is linked with endometrial cancer and is considered a known risk factor. According to the authors of several kinds of literature, the most recent meta-analysis recognizes that the heightened risk of cancer in PCOS women may be due to obesity. T2DM is another potential confounding factor that is more common in PCOS women and is linked to an increased risk of endometrial cancer, possibly due to hyperinsulinemia, hyperglycemia, and inflammation (Harris et al. 2016). However, it is in debate whether the increased risk of endometrial cancer is due to different metabolic risk factors or PCOS itself or not, which is defined by multiple metabolic and reproductive complications that may lead to an increased endometrial oncology risk.

### *9.2.4. Other Disorders*

In addition to the well-known cardiovascular and metabolic disease patients with PCOS faced impairment of psychological problems and decreased quality of life (QoL) in comparison to healthy women. There is mounting evidence that women with PCOS are more likely to be prone to mood disorders. The underlying causes/mechanisms remain unknown; however, factors such as obesity, insulin resistance, high androgen levels, and clinical features such as hirsutism-related distress, weight gain, acne, and infertility are other influencers (Dokras A et al., 2012). Here Figure 4: briefly illustrates various diagnostic criteria that cause, implications and complications related to PCOS.

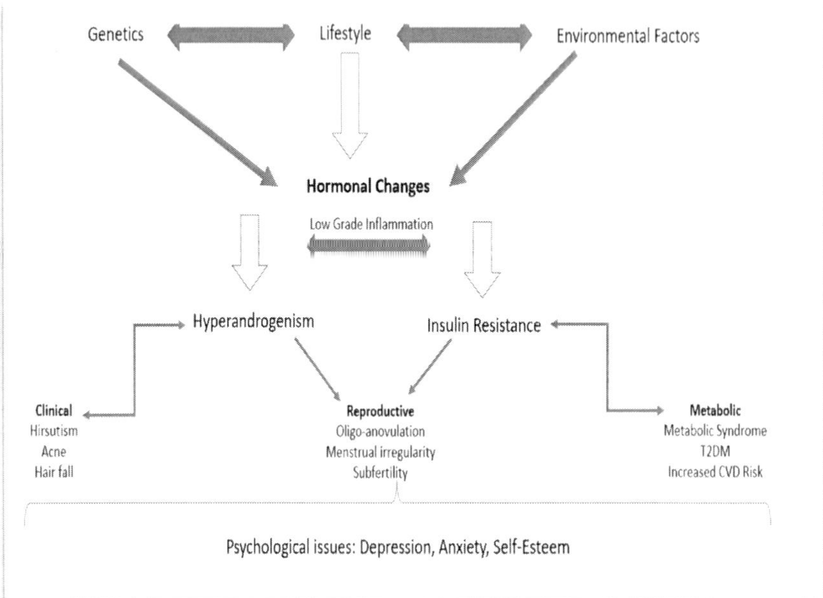


**Figure 4.** Explains the issues associated with Hormonal changes, low-grade inflammation that results from Lifestyle and environmental factors that affect the normal working and mechanism of androgens and Insulin hormone and leads to psychological issues, Depression, Anxiety, and Self-Esteem.

## 10. Trends in the Management of PCOS

The modality in treatment for diseased women is completely based on the symptoms presented where the different strategies are utilized for the management of women where to date no clear guidelines are depicted for PCOS. Based on the recent trends in advancements treatments can be modified for the comfort, compliance, and safety of patients. Several trends in the treatment of disease are discussed below.

### 10.1. Trends in the Treatment of Hyperandrogenic Features

Acne, hirsutism, and alopecia are the most common androgen-related reports of PCOS. The symptoms vary from patient to patient; some present with only one or two symptoms, while others complain of all three. The first-line pharmacologic treatment in terms of oral contraceptive pills (OCPs) is typically used for hirsutism in premenopausal women. Other techniques like laser hair removal and other mechanical hair removal methods are also used as pharmacologic treatments that do not provide the desired results and the associated disadvantage is it is time-consuming. Because of the cycle of hair growth, it usually takes at least 6 months of treatment to see a response; if there is no progress after six months of medication, anti-androgens can be added (Orio F et al., 2014).

In the treatment of acne anti-androgens and OCPs, both are effective. However, in severe acne, Isotretinoin is commonly used in patients which consists of limited data on alopecia treatment, but OCPs and androgen inhibitors are found to be beneficial in the same. For patients who do not want to become pregnant, combined hormonal contraceptives (CHC) OCPs are a good treatment choice, and they are frequently in the treatment of PCOS-related hirsutism and acne. Although, CHCs cause negative feedback on LH production, resulting in decreased androgen synthesis by the ovaries. Reduction in androgens is shown by other mechanisms by which CHCs include:

1) Increasing SHBG production in the liver;
2) Reducing androgen secretion by the adrenal gland and,
3) Obstructing the conversion of testosterone to dihydrotestosterone and binding of it to androgen receptors (Franik S et al., 2014).

### 10.2. Trends in Treatment of Menstrual Disorders

In addition to menstrual irregularities, chronic anovulation associated with PCOS can make patients more susceptible to developing endometrial hyperplasia and carcinoma where this endometrial proliferation can be inhibited by using cyclic progestin or a low-dose CHC containing estrogen and progestin. For PCOS-related menstrual disorders and improved menstrual regularity, low-dose CHCs are the most prescribed primary recommended treatment option.

For numerous metabolic advantages weight loss provides an efficient way and can aid in improving circulating androgen levels, thereby easing many manifestations of PCOS. However, after the loss of 5% initial weight actual weight loss benefits can be seen in patients. Acupuncture is another treatment that is gaining popularity. It is found to be beneficial in regulating androgen levels and ameliorating menstrual irregularity.

#### *10.2.1. Treatment of Infertility*

The standard approach for overweight and obese women is to reduce weight mainly infertile women. In most cases, it was seen that obesity is linked to anovulation and pregnancy loss and a poor response to fertility treatment with clomiphene citrate, gonadotropins, and laparoscopic ovarian diathermy. Data from observational studies show that a 5%-10% weight loss can increase the chances of ovulation and pregnancies. Bariatric surgery, however, has been demonstrated to improve cycle regularity and increase ovulation, and spontaneous conception.

For inducing ovulation in women with PCOS, Clomiphene is considered the first investment where clomiphene citrate is a modulator of the partially selective estrogen receptors. Its activity against estrogen at the hypothalamus causes a change in the GnRH pulse frequency, resulting in the increased pituitary gland release of FSH (Orio F et al., 2016).

### 10.3. On-Pharmacological Interventions for the Management of PCOS

Many non-pharmacological interventions are also advised for the management of PCOS. Some of these are described below with a table of the most preferable medications.

a) Lifestyle Modifications

PCOS women are often obese which is found to be associated with IR. Hence, for the management of PCOS weight loss becomes an important part of it also It has resulted in the restoration of spontaneous ovulation and a higher fertility rate. In the management of obese pregnancies, an aggressive weight-loss strategy, including pharmacological strategies, contraception, and high-dose folic acid has been found helpful. With lifestyle modification programs there are low compliance and high dropout rate are found to be associated which highlights the need for more structured and feasible exercise training programs for obese females with PCOS. Even though the cumulative pregnancy rate was similar between the two approaches, structured exercise training resulted in higher menstrual frequency and ovulation. In terms of the pregnancy rate, lifestyle modifications were more effective than drugs such as clomiphene citrate (CC) and metformin. A comparative study reported that 20% more pregnancies were reported with PCOS women who were given CC, metformin, and lifestyle modification as compared to 12.2% reported after CC alone, 14.4% reported after metformin, and 14.8% after CC with metformin. Data on PCOS management through therapy and medication refers to in Table 2.

**Table 2.** The table describes the drug treatment to find the cure for the disease PCOS. A lot of pharmacological testing found useful results for the cure of diseases. Synthetic and natural drugs are tested against most of the symptoms such as Hyperandrogenism, anovulation, etc,and show effective results

| S. no | Drugs used in the management of PCOS | Effect | Kind of Therapy |
|---|---|---|---|
| 1. | Metformin | Nausea, vomiting, Diarrhoea | Hyperinsulinemia, Androgen excess, Anovulation |
| 2. | Clomiphene Citrate | Mood swing, fluid retention, gestation | Ovulation indication |
| 3. | Vitamin D | Weight loss or poor appetite | Regular menstrual cycles, hyperandrogenism |
| 4. | Calcium | Dry mouth, headache | Menstrual regulation, anovulation |
| 5. | Eflornithine | Acne, swollen patches, dry or tingling skin | Hirsutism |
| 6. | Licorice | Mineralocorticoid excess, high blood pressure | Hyperandrogenism |
| 7. | Holy basil | Diarrhea, hypoglycemia (large doses), nausea | Hyperandrogenism, Hyperinsulinemia |
| 8. | Flax seeds | Loose stools, delayed clotting time | Hyperandrogenism, regulation of menstrual cycles |

b) Yoga and Naturopathy

Various drugs are there for the current line of treatment for polycystic ovarian syndrome and hormonal menstrual disorders as ovulation induction, weight management insulin resistance. However, these drugs may have few side effects when consumed for a longer duration. Thereby, alternative therapies such as herbal medicine, proper diet, lifestyle modification, exercises, and yoga and stress relief techniques become potential options for the management of PCOS. Yoga can serve as a complementary and alternative therapy as it aids in weight loss relaxes the body and mind, relieves stress, regulates blood circulation, and increases the body and metabolism. Some special and important Asanas are mentioned in traditional yogic texts ("Gherand Samhita, Shiva Samhita, and Hatha Yoga Pradipika") that impact reproductive organs, like the ovaries, and uterus, as well as digestion.

## Conclusion

Stein and Leventhal were the first to describe PCOS in 1935. Since then, a lot of research has been done on the causes, manifestations, complications, and treatment of PCOS. It is a widespread, heterogeneous, heritable disorder that affects women throughout their lives. Hyperandrogenism, ovulatory dysfunction, and polycystic ovaries are all symptoms of PCOS. There is, however, a significant interindividual variation seen in the manifestation of these symptoms. Insulin resistance and hyperinsulinemia are common and make women suffering from PCOS more vulnerable to diabetes and cardiovascular disease. However, most of the cases of PCOS are due to steroidogenesis dysregulation that sensitizes hormonal imbalance and androgen biosynthesis where the hyperresponsiveness of FOH and its association with a higher prevalence of glucose intolerance in the presence of increased insulin resistance is still a matter of debate. Accordingly, the insulin resistance factor is independent of obesity but the excess release of it stimulates adipogenesis and lipogenesis somewhat contributing to obesity in PCOS. To some extent, inflammatory cytokines play a role in obesity and PCOS for which improved comprehension is necessary to facilitate prognosis and diagnosis. The elucidation of specific markers enables the identification of specific genetic predisposing factors which gets hampered by non-specific criteria in current use. Recent genome-wide association technique has screened unrecognized protein variant in androgen-producing cells which involves untransformed human cell line transformations that facilitate the knowledge of normal or abnormal steroidogenesis. One major mystery about PCOS is the link that connects ovarian hyperandrogenism, obesity, and insulin resistance to decode this more research is necessary. According to results obtained by many scientists, PCOS women possess a high risk of complications in comparison to non-PCOS women with different intensities for which the mechanism of early-term and long-term complications in pathogenesis is not completely known. Also, the exact mechanisms need to be elucidated for hormonal and metabolic features. Several factors that influence PCOS are race, and ethnicity which differ in both metabolic phenotypes and social behavioral models both of these have impacted the lives of women the most. During menopausal transitions, a plateau has reached some metabolic disorders. However, the studies are somewhat lacking in discussing PCOS from adolescent studies which are still conflicting among scientists. A subsequent decrease in testosterone is observed in post-menopausal and improved menstrual cyclicity phenotypes. Although Fetal exposure to a variety of environmental factors leads to epigenetic changes and confers the susceptibility to develop derangement in offspring of PCOS. Several therapies in the treatment of PCOS have focussed on the use of inositol, stains, and other drugs that shows promising results in less time still more clinical inventions need advancement addition of laser and cosmetic intervention has shown great results in the improvement of physical appearance in patients. Treatment of PCOS in a better way and with technological advancement can pave the way for better regimens that can finally improve the quality of life and prevent the development of comorbidities. Conclusively PCOS has now become a global threat for women that has been raised due to multiple factors the reasons of which are unknown and to answer all the questions related to the onset complications of this disease are under investigation. As a result, PCOS hurts endocrine, metabolic, and cardiovascular health. Various pharmacological and non-pharmacological treatment options are available for managing PCOS and its associated risks.

## References


Abbott, D. H., Kraynak, M, Dumesic, D. A, & Levine, J. E. (2019). In utero androgen excess: a developmental commonality preceding polycystic ovary syndrome? *Hyperandrogenism in Women*, 53, 1-17.

AGill, H., Tiwari, P, & Dabadghao, P. (2012). Prevalence of polycystic ovary syndrome in young women from North India: A Community-based study. *Indian Journal of Endocrinology and Metabolism*, 16(Suppl 2), S389.

Akre, S., Sharma, K., Chakole, S., & Wanjari, M. B. (2022). Recent advances in the management of polycystic ovary syndrome: a review article. *Cureus*, 14(8).

Ali, H. I, Elsadawy, M. E., & Khater, N. H. (2016). Ultrasound assessment of polycystic ovaries: ovarian volume and morphology; which is more accurate in making the diagnosis? *The Egyptian Journal of Radiology and nuclear medicine*, 47(1), 347-350.

Ambekar, A. S., Kelkar, D. S., Pinto, S. M., Sharma, R., Hinduja, I., Zaveri, K & Mukherjee, S. (2015). Proteomics of follicular fluid from women with polycystic ovary syndrome suggests molecular defects in follicular development. *The Journal of Clinical Endocrinology & Metabolism*, 100(2), 744-753.

Arora, S., Sinha, K., Kolte, S., & Mandal, A. (2016). Endocrinal and autoimmune linkage: evidence from a controlled study of subjects with polycystic ovarian syndrome. *Journal of Human Reproductive Sciences*, 9(1), 18.

Ashraf, S., Nabi, M., Rashid, F., & Amin, S. (2019). Hyperandrogenism in polycystic ovarian syndrome and role of CYP gene variants: a review. *Egyptian Journal of Medical Human Genetics*, 20(1), 1-10.

Aversa, A., La Vignera, S., Rago, R., Gambineri, A., Nappi, R. E., Calogero, A. E., & Ferlin, A. (2020). Fundamental concepts and novel aspects of the polycystic ovarian syndrome: expert consensus resolutions. *Frontiers in endocrinology*, 11, 516.

Azziz, R., Dumesic, D. A., & Goodarzi, M. O. (2011). Polycystic ovary syndrome. *Fertility and Sterility,* 95(5), 1544-1548.

Basu, B. R., Chowdhury, O., & Saha, S. K. (2018). Possible link between stress-related factors and altered body composition in women with polycystic ovarian syndrome. *Journal of Human Reproductive Sciences*, 11(1), 10.

Bell, G. A., Sundaram, R., Mumford, S. L., Park, H., Mills, J., Bell, E. M, & Yeung, E. H. (2018). Maternal polycystic ovarian syndrome and early offspring development. *Human Reproduction*, 33(7), 1307-1315.

Bellver, J., Rodríguez-Tabernero, L., Robles, A., Muñoz, E., Martínez, F., Landeras, J, & Group of interest in Reproductive Endocrinology (GIER) of the Spanish Fertility Society (SEF). (2018). Polycystic ovary syndrome throughout a woman's life. *Journal of assisted reproduction and genetics*, 35, 25-39.

Bharathi, R. V., Swetha, S., Neerajaa, J., Madhavica, J. V., Janani, D. M., Rekha, S. N, & Usha, B. (2017). An epidemiological survey: Effect of predisposing factors for PCOS in Indian urban and rural population. *Middle East Fertility Society Journal*, 22(4), 313-316.

Bozdag, G., Mumusoglu, S., Zengin, D., Karabulut, E., & Yildiz, B. O. (2016). The prevalence and phenotypic features of polycystic ovary syndrome: a systematic review and meta-analysis. *Human reproduction*, 31(12), 2841-2855.

Chang, S., & Dunaif, A. (2021). Diagnosis of polycystic ovary syndrome: which criteria to use and when? *Endocrinology, and Metabolism Clinics*, 50(1), 11-23.

Chen, Y., & Fang, S. Y. (2018). Potential genetic polymorphisms predicting polycystic ovary syndrome. *Endocrine connections*, 7(5), R187.

Christopherson, R. (2016). *Polycystic Ovary Syndrome Metabolic Comorbidities: A Critical Appraisal of the Evidence with Practice Recommendations.*

Clark, N. M., Podolski, A. J., Brooks, E. D., Chizen, D. R., Pierson, R. A., Lehotay, D. C., & Lujan, M. E. (2014). Prevalence of polycystic ovary syndrome phenotypes using updated criteria for polycystic ovarian morphology: an assessment of over 100 consecutive women self-reporting features of polycystic ovary syndrome. *Reproductive Sciences*, 21, 1034-1043.

Conway, G., Dewailly, D., Diamanti-Kandarakis, E., Escobar-Morreale, H. F., Franks, S., Gambineri, A. & Yildiz, B. O. (2014). The polycystic ovary syndrome: a position statement from the European Society of Endocrinology. *European Journal of Endocrinology*, 171(4), P1-P29.

Day, F. R., Hinds, D. A., Tung, J. Y., Stolk, L., Styrkarsdottir, U., Saxena, R., & Perry, J. R. (2015). Causal mechanisms and balancing selection inferred from genetic associations with polycystic ovary syndrome. *Nature communications*, 6(1), 8464.

Deswal, R., Narwal, V., Dang, A., & Pundir, C. S. (2020). The prevalence of polycystic ovary syndrome: a brief systematic review. *Journal of human reproductive sciences*, 13(4), 261.

Deveer, M., Deveer, R., Basaran, O., Turkcu, U. O., Akbaba, E., Cullu, N., & Kasap, B. (2015). Serum copeptin, pentraxin 3, anti-mullerian hormone levels with echocardiography and carotid artery intima-media thickness in adolescents with polycystic ovary syndrome. *Journal of clinical medicine research*, 7(12), 989.

Di Bari, F., Catalano, A., Bellone, F., Martino, G., & Benvenga, S. (2021). Vitamin D, bone metabolism, and fracture risk in polycystic ovary syndrome. *Metabolites*, 11(2), 116.

Dokras, A., Clifton, S., Futterweit, W., & Wild, R. (2012). Increased prevalence of anxiety symptoms in women with polycystic ovary syndrome: systematic review and meta-analysis. *Fertility and sterility*, 97(1), 225-230.

Eisenberg, I., Nahmias, N., Persky, M. N., Greenfield, C., Goldman-Wohl, D., Hurwitz, A.& Imbar, T. (2017). Elevated circulating micro-ribonucleic acid (miRNA)-200b and miRNA-429 levels in anovulatory women. *Fertility and Sterility*, 107(1), 269-275.

Fan, Q., He, J. F., Wang, Q. R., Cai, H. B., Sun, X. G., Zhou, X. X., & Jia, W. H. (2013). A functional polymorphism in the 5'-UTR of CR2 is associated with susceptibility to nasopharyngeal carcinoma. *Oncology Reports*, 30(1), 11-16.

Fauser, B. C., Tarlatzis, B. C., Rebar, R. W., Legro, R. S., Balen, A. H., Lobo, R.& Barnhart, K. (2012). Consensus on women's health aspects of polycystic ovary syndrome (PCOS): the Amsterdam ESHRE/ASRM-Sponsored 3rd PCOS Consensus Workshop Group. *Fertility and sterility*, 97(1), 28-38.

Franik, S., Kremer, J. A., Nelen, W. L., & Farquhar, C. (2014). Aromatase inhibitors for subfertile women with polycystic ovary syndrome. *Cochrane Database of Systematic Reviews*, (2).

Gambineri, A., Laudisio, D., Marocco, C., Radellini, S., Colao, A., Savastano, S., & Obesity Programs of nutrition, Education, Research and Assessment (OPERA) group. (2019). Female infertility: which role for obesity? *International journal of obesity supplements*, 9(1), 65-72.

Ganie, M. A., Vasudevan, V., Wani, I. A., Baba, M. S., Arif, T., & Rashid, A. (2019). Epidemiology, pathogenesis, genetics & management of polycystic ovary syndrome in India. *The Indian Journal of medical research*, 150(4), 333.

Garima K, Anju S. Long term complications of Polycystic ovary syndrome. Glob J Reprod Med. 2017; 2(1): 555577.

Gautam, A., Gupta, S., Mehndiratta, M., Sharma, M., Singh, K., Kalra, O. P., & Gambhir, J. K (2017). Association of NFKB1 gene polymorphism (rs28362491) with levels of inflammatory biomarkers and susceptibility to diabetic nephropathy in Asian Indians. *World Journal of Diabetes*, 8(2), 66.

Glueck, C. J., & Goldenberg, N. (2019). Characteristics of obesity in polycystic ovary syndrome: Etiology, treatment, and genetics. Metabolism, 92, 108-120.

Gu, Y., Zhou, G., Zhou, F., Wu, Q., Ma, C., Zhang, Y., & Hua, K. (2022). Life modifications and PCOS: old story but new tales. *Frontiers in Endocrinology*, 488.

Gunning, M. N., Sir Petermann, T., Crisosto, N., Van Rijn, B. B., De Wilde, M. A., Christ, J. P.& Fauser, B. C. (2020). Cardiometabolic health in offspring of women with PCOS compared to healthy controls: a systematic review and individual participant data meta-analysis. *Human reproduction update*, 26(1), 104-118.

Gupta, M., Singh, D., Toppo, M., Priya, A., Sethia, S., & Gupta, P. (2018). A cross-sectional study of the polycystic ovarian syndrome among young women in Bhopal, Central India. *Int J Community Med Public Health*, 5(1), 95-100.

Harris, H. R., & Terry, K. L. (2016). Polycystic ovary syndrome and risk of endometrial, ovarian, and breast cancer: a systematic review. *Fertility Research and Practice*, 2(1), 1-9.

Htet, T. D., Teede, H. J., De Courten, B., Loxton, D., Real, F. G., Moran, L. J., & Joham, A. E. (2017). Asthma in reproductive-aged women with polycystic ovary syndrome and association with obesity. *European Respiratory Journal*, 49(5).

Joseph, N., Reddy, A. G., Joy, D., Patel, V., Santhosh, P., Das, S., & Reddy, S. K. (2016). Study on the proportion and determinants of polycystic ovarian syndrome among health sciences students in South India. *Journal of natural science, biology, and Medicine*, 7(2), 166.

Joshi, B., Mukherjee, S., Patil, A., Purandare, A., Chauhan, S., & Vaidya, R. (2014). A cross-sectional study of the polycystic ovarian syndrome among adolescent and young girls in Mumbai, India. *Indian Journal of Endocrinology and Metabolism*, 18(3), 317.

Kruszewska, J., Laudy-Wiaderny, H., & Kunicki, M. (2022). Review of Novel Potential Insulin Resistance Biomarkers in PCOS Patients-The Debate Is Still Open. *International journal of environmental research and public health*, 19(4), 2099.

Kumar, A., Barki, S., Raghav, V., Chaturvedi, A., & Kumar, K. H. (2017). Correlation of Vitamin D with metabolic parameters in polycystic ovarian syndrome. *Journal of Family Medicine and Primary Care*, 6(1), 115.

Lauritsen, M. P., Bentzen, J. G., Pinborg, A., Loft, A., Forman, J. L., Thuesen, L. L., & Nyboe Andersen, A. (2014). The prevalence of polycystic ovary syndrome in a normal population according to the Rotterdam criteria versus revised criteria including anti-Müllerian hormone. *Human reproduction*, 29(4), 791-801.

Legro, R. S., Arslanian, S. A., Ehrmann, D. A., Hoeger, K. M., Murad, M. H., Pasquali, R., & Welt, C. K. (2013). Diagnosis and treatment of polycystic ovary syndrome: an Endocrine Society clinical practice guideline. *The Journal of Clinical Endocrinology & Metabolism*, 98(12), 4565-4592.

Li, H., Liu, M., & Zhang, C. (2022). Women with polycystic ovary syndrome (PCOS) have reduced melatonin concentrations in their follicles and mild sleep disturbances. *BMC Women's Health*, 22(1), 79.

Lim, S. S., Davies, M. J., Norman, R. J., & Moran, L. J. (2012). Overweight, obesity and central obesity in women with polycystic ovary syndrome: a systematic review and meta-analysis. *Human reproduction update*, 18(6), 618-637.

Manti, M. (2020). *Developmental Origins of Polycystic Ovary Syndrome: Role of Early Adverse Life Events on Adult Health* (Doctoral dissertation, Karolinska Institutet (Sweden)).

Mohammad, M. B., & Seghinsara, A. M. (2017). Polycystic ovary syndrome (PCOS), diagnostic criteria, and AMH. *Asian Pacific Journal of cancer prevention: APJCP*, 18(1), 17.

Ndefo, U. A., Eaton, A., & Green, M. R. (2013). Polycystic ovary syndrome: a review of treatment options with a focus on pharmacological approaches. *Pharmacy and therapeutics*, 38(6), 336.

Nidhi, R., Padmalatha, V., Nagarathna, R., & Amritanshu, R. (2011). Prevalence of polycystic ovarian syndrome in Indian adolescents. *Journal of Pediatric and adolescent gynecology*, 24(4), 223-227.

Ollila, M. M. E., Piltonen, T., Puukka, K., Ruokonen, A., Järvelin, M. R., Tapanainen, J. S., & Morin-Papunen, L. (2016). Weight gain and dyslipidemia in early adulthood associate with polycystic ovary syndrome: prospective cohort study. *The Journal of Clinical Endocrinology & Metabolism*, 101(2), 739-747.

Orio, F., Tafuri, D., Ascione, A., Marciano, F., Savastano, S., Colarieti, G & Muscogiuri, G. (2016). Lifestyle changes in the management of adulthood and childhood obesity. *Minerva endocrinologica*, 41(4), 509-515.

Palomba, S., Falbo, A., Chiossi, G., Orio, F., Tolino, A., Colao, A., & Zullo, F. (2014). Low-grade chronic inflammation in pregnant women with polycystic ovary syndrome: a prospective controlled clinical study. *The Journal of Clinical Endocrinology & Metabolism*, 99(8), 2942-2951.

Palomba, S., Santagni, S., Falbo, A., & La Sala, G. B. (2015). Complications and challenges associated with polycystic ovary syndrome: current perspectives. *International journal of women's health*, 745-763.

Panda, P. K., Rane, R., Ravichandran, R., Singh, S., & Panchal, H. (2016). Genetics of PCOS: A systematic bioinformatics approach to unveil the proteins responsible for PCOS. *Genomics data*, 8, 52-60.

Parker, J., O'Brien, C., Hawrelak, J., & Gersh, F. L. (2022). Polycystic ovary syndrome: an evolutionary adaptation to lifestyle and the environment. *International journal of environmental research and public health*, 19(3), 1336.

Peigné, M., & Dewailly, D. (2014, September). Long-term complications of polycystic ovary syndrome (PCOS). In *Annales d'endocrinologie* (Vol. 75, No. 4, pp. 194-199). Elsevier Masson.

Polak, K., Czyzyk, A., Simoncini, T., & Meczekalski, B. (2017). New markers of insulin resistance in polycystic ovary syndrome. *Journal of endocrinological investigation*, 40, 1-8.

Qin, J. Z., Pang, L. H., Li, M. J., Fan, X. J., Huang, R. D., & Chen, H. Y. (2013). Obstetric complications in women with polycystic ovary syndrome: a systematic review and meta-analysis. *Reproductive Biology and Endocrinology*, 11(1), 1-14.

Rao, M., Broughton, K. S., & LeMieux, M. J. (2020). A cross-sectional study on the knowledge and prevalence of PCOS at a multiethnic university. *Progress in Preventive Medicine*, e0028.

Rashid, R., Mir, S. A., Kareem, O., Ali, T., Ara, R., Malik, A.& Bader, G. N. (2022). Polycystic ovarian syndrome-current pharmacotherapy and clinical implications. *Taiwanese Journal of Obstetrics and Gynecology*, 61(1), 40-50.

Risal, S., Pei, Y., Lu, H., Manti, M., Fornes, R., Pui, H. P.& Stener-Victorin, E. (2019). Prenatal androgen exposure and transgenerational susceptibility to polycystic ovary syndrome. *Nature Medicine*, 25(12), 1894-1904.

Rocha, A. L., Oliveira, F. R., Azevedo, R. C., Silva, V. A., Peres, T. M., Candido, A. L.& Reis, F. M. (2019). Recent advances in the understanding and management of polycystic ovary syndrome. *F1000Research*, 8.

Rodriguez Paris, V., & Bertoldo, M. J. (2019). The mechanism of androgen actions in PCOS etiology. *Medical sciences*, 7(9), 89.

Rubin, K. H., Glintborg, D., Nybo, M., Abrahamsen, B., & Andersen, M. (2017). Development and risk factors of type 2 diabetes in a nationwide population of women with polycystic ovary syndrome. *The Journal of Clinical Endocrinology & Metabolism*, 102(10), 3848-3857.

Saadia, Z. (2020). Follicle-stimulating hormone (LH: FSH) ratio in polycystic ovary syndrome (PCOS)-obese vs. Non-obese women. *Medical Archives*, 74(4), 289.

Scicchitano, P., Dentamaro, I., Carbonara, R., Bulzis, G., Dachille, A., Caputo, P & Ciccone, M. M. (2012). Cardiovascular risk in women with PCOS. *International Journal of Endocrinology and Metabolism*, 10(4), 611.

Shaikh, N., Dadachanji, R., & Mukherjee, S. (2014). Genetic markers of polycystic ovary syndrome: emphasis on insulin resistance. *International Journal of Medical Genetics*, 2014.

Shannon, M., & Wang, Y. (2012). Polycystic ovary syndrome: a common but often unrecognized condition. *Journal of Midwifery & Women's Health*, 57(3), 221-230.

Sharif, E., & Alwakeel, M. (2019). *New markers for the detection of polycystic ovary syndrome.*

Silva, M. S., & Campbell, R. E. (2011). Polycystic ovary syndrome and the neuroendocrine consequences of androgen excess. *Comprehensive Physiology*, 12(2), 3347-3369.

Singh, A., Bora, P., & Krishna, A. (2017). Direct action of adiponectin ameliorates increased androgen synthesis and reduces insulin receptor expression in the polycystic ovary. *Biochemical and Biophysical Research Communications*, 488(3), 509-515.

Sirmans, S. M., & Pate, K. A. (2014). Epidemiology, diagnosis, and management of polycystic ovary syndrome. *Clin Epidemiol*. 2014; 6: 1–13.

Stepto, N. K., Cassar, S., Joham, A. E., Hutchison, S. K., Harrison, C. L., Goldstein, R. F., & Teede, H. J. (2013). Women with polycystic ovary syndrome have intrinsic insulin resistance on euglycaemic–hyperinsulinaemic clamp. *Human reproduction*, 28(3), 777-784.

Sun, X., Wu, X., Zhou, Y., Yu, X., & Zhang, W. (2015). Evaluation of apelin and insulin resistance in patients with PCOS and therapeutic effect of drospirenone-ethinylestradiol plus metformin. *Medical science monitor: international medical journal of Experimental and clinical research*, 21, 2547.

Teede, H. J., Misso, M. L., Boyle, J. A., Garad, R. M., McAllister, V., Downes, L & Woolcock, J. (2018). Translation and implementation of the Australian-led PCOS guideline: clinical summary and translation resources from the International Evidence-based Guideline for the Assessment and Management of polycystic ovary syndrome. *Medical Journal of Australia*, 209, S3-S8.

Tehrani, F. R., Simbar, M., Tohidi, M., Hosseinpanah, F., & Azizi, F. (2011). The prevalence of polycystic ovary syndrome in a community sample of Iranian population: Iranian PCOS prevalence study. *Reproductive Biology and Endocrinology*, 9(1), 1-7.

Varanasi, L. C., Subasinghe, A., Jayasinghe, Y. L., Callegari, E. T., Garland, S. M., Gorelik, A., & Wark, J. D. (2018). Polycystic ovarian syndrome: Prevalence and impact on the wellbeing of Australian women aged 16–29 years. *Australian and New Zealand Journal of Obstetrics and Gynaecology*, 58(2), 222-233.

Wang, R., & Mol, B. W. J. (2017). The Rotterdam criteria for polycystic ovary syndrome: evidence-based criteria? *Human Reproduction*, 32(2), 261-264.

Witchel, S. F., Oberfield, S. E., & Peña, A. S. (2019). Polycystic ovary syndrome: pathophysiology, presentation, and treatment with emphasis on adolescent girls. *Journal of the Endocrine Society*, 3(8), 1545-1573.

Yilmaz, B., Vellanki, P., Ata, B., & Yildiz, B. O. (2018). Metabolic syndrome, hypertension, and hyperlipidemia in mothers, fathers, sisters, and brothers of women with polycystic ovary syndrome: a systematic review and meta-analysis. *Fertility and sterility*, 109(2), 356-364.

## Chapter 2

# PCOS and the Rhythmicity of GnRH: The Impact of FSH and LH on Menstrual Health

**Nikhil Maheshwari[1], Toyeeba Hassan[2] and Gowhar Rashid[3,*]**

[1]Department of Biochemistry, Faculty of Life Sciences, Aligarh Muslim University, Aligarh, India
[2]Centre of Research for Development, University of Kashmir, Srinagar, Kashmir, India
[3]Amity Medical School, Amity University Haryana, India

## Abstract

Polycystic ovarian syndrome (PCOS) is a hereditary, endocrine, and metabolic disorder associated with chronic anovulatory, polycystic ovaries, and hyperandrogenism. Ovarian stromal-thecal hyperactivity is the primary endocrine abnormality that affects the energy metabolism of the gonadotropin-releasing hormone (GnRH) pulse generator, which lambast knockdown by ovarian steroids, causing an increase in luteinizing hormone (LH) secretion and a decrease in follicle-stimulating hormone (FSH). This hormonal dysregulation could result in serious biochemical, reproductive, and metabolic dysfunction. Numerous etiological studies reported 5-10% of cases of PCOS in women of reproductive age. The development of the PCOS phenotype and its long-term effects may be significantly influenced by in-utero fetal coding or chronic stress of the hypothalamic-pituitary-gonadotropic axis, which would be mediated by the communication of biologically predetermined hyperandrogenism and external conditions (obesity). Obesity, metabolic changes, and ethnicity all have a significant impact on PCOS symptoms, which can fluctuate over time. The pathophysiology of PCOS has been linked to a number of probable genetic variations in steroid hormone synthesis and metabolism, gonadotropin and gonadal hormone action, obesity and energy balance, insulin secretion and action, and many more. PCOS can be treated with a variety of pharmaceutical drugs, but lifestyle modifications, such as healthy eating and exercise, have been proven to be much more useful and should be considered the very first line of treatment, particularly even though obesity is a major factor in the pathogenesis of the condition. Fighting PCOS and its associated issues should prioritize proactive measures to spot and cure the disease in children before it becomes apparent in adolescence and has an impact on adulthood.

---

* Corresponding Author's Email: gowhar9@gmail.com.

In: Polycystic Ovarian Syndrome (PCOS) and Our Biological Clock
Editors: Arpita Roy, Gowhar Rashid and Nihad Ashraf Khan
ISBN: 979-8-89113-100-2
© 2023 Nova Science Publishers, Inc.

**Keywords:** polycystic ovarian syndrome (PCOS), gonadotropin-releasing hormone (GnRH), luteinizing hormone (LH), follicle-stimulating hormone (FSH), metabolism, reproduction

## 1. Introduction

The genetic, endocrine, and metabolic condition known as polycystic ovarian syndrome (PCOS) is a multifactorial, diverse, complicated disorder. It is characterized by persistent anovulation, menstrual irregularities polycystic ovaries, and biochemical and clinical signs of hyperandrogenism (Franks et al., 2006). Ovarian stromal-thecal hyperactivity in PCOS leads to hyperandrogenism, and gonadotropin-releasing hormone (GnRH) imbalance causing increased luteinizing hormone (LH) metabolism and reduced follicle-stimulating hormone (FSH). This hormonal imbalance may result in serious biochemical, reproductive, and metabolic dysfunction of the ovaries.

The menstrual cycle is normally operated by a series of hormonal signals, and the cycle starts with the release of GnRH from the master gland hypothalamus located in the brain. GnRH then stimulates the pituitary gland to secrete LH and FSH. These two hormones activate the ovary to produce the sex hormones estrogen and progesterone which are directly involved in menstruation (Figure 1). LH causes the maturation of eggs and initiates the process of ovulation by releasing the eggs from the ovary. GnRH is associated with sexual maturity, fertility, and sex drive.

In females who are normally ovulating, a rise in GnRH pulse frequency even during the follicular phase favors the production of LH, whereas a fall in GnRH pulse frequency during the luteal phase due to the progesterone impact favors the production of FSH. It is challenging to pinpoint a single factor for PCOS owing to the disorder's complex underlying causes, evidence of several genes affecting the hormonal and metabolic pathways becoming involved, and the disease's diverse nature.

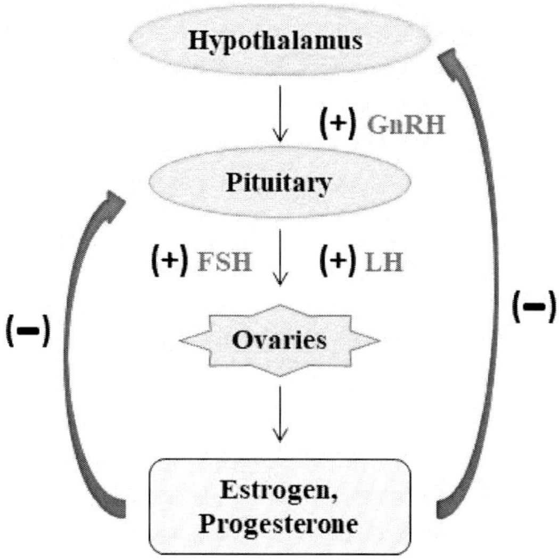


GnRH, gonadotropin-releasing hormone; LH, luteinizing hormone; FSH, follicle-stimulating hormone.

**Figure 1.** Hormonal pathways in ovulation under normal conditions.

## 2. Role of GnRH in PCOS Patients

Recent research suggests that PCOS is characterized by anomalies in the nutrient and reverse communication among ovarian androgens, GnRH, LH, and FSH (Barontini et al., 2001). In PCOS, a steroid-permissive environment and reduced attentiveness of the GnRH exciter to responses suppression by hormonal steroids lead to high GnRH pulse regularity, irregular gonadotropin extravasation, such as LH over secretion, which is characteristic of hyperandrogenism (McCartney et al., 2002) (Figure 2).

Additionally, this might shed light on how PCOS developed during puberty. Patients with PCOS had higher levels of basic LH isoforms, higher frequency and/or duration of LH pulses, greater disorganized LH discharge, and enhanced in vitro LH bioactivity. Adolescents with PCOS were shown to have peak serum levels of immuno-reactive and bioactive LH that were three times (P 0.001) and two times (P = 0.002) higher than those in controls, respectively (Ropelato et al., 1999) (Figure 2).

The insensitivity of the gonadotropin pulse generator following sex hormones reduction throughout fetal growth may be the origin of the perimenarchal anomalies seen in hirsutism teenage girls who look to have initial PCOS symptoms (Marshall et al., 2000). Elevated blood LH levels in women with hyperandrogenemia brought on by 21-hydroxylase deficiency, a prevalent cause of adrenal hyperandrogenism, give more indications for that kind of in utero conditioning of the hypothalamic-pituitary (HP) axial direction in individuals (Legro et al., 1998).

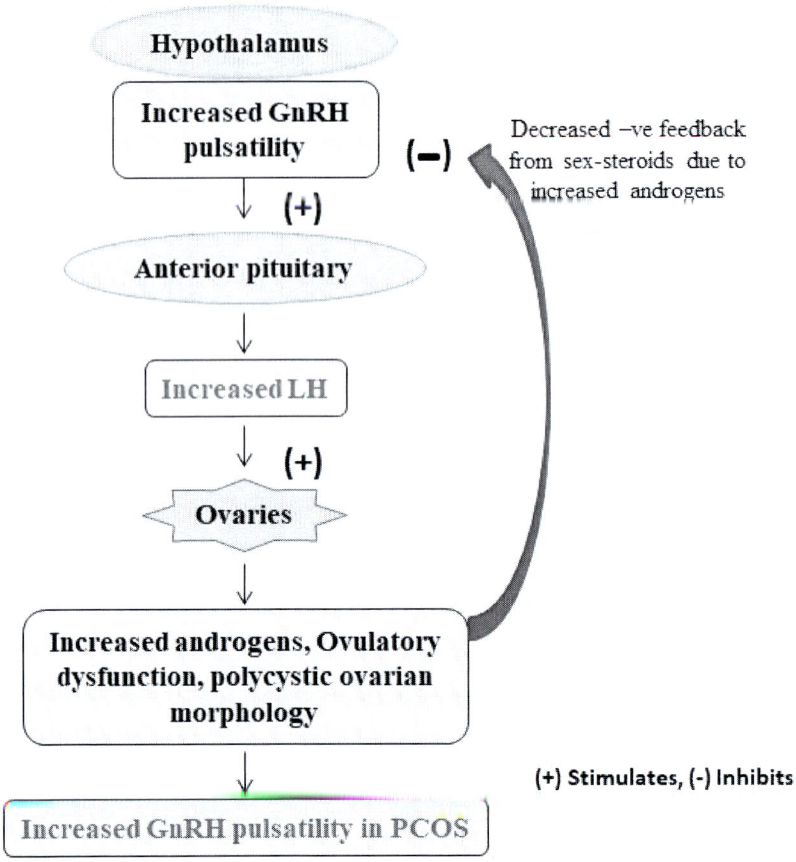


GnRH, gonadotropin-releasing hormone; LH, luteinizing hormone; PCOS, polycystic ovarian syndrome.

**Figure 2** Altered hormonal pathways in ovulation in PCOS.

## 2.1. Hyperandrogenism

Hyperandrogenism is one of the most often shown characteristics of PCOS due to LH overproduction, which is the main clinical expression of steroid production dysregulation in PCOS (Barnes et al., 1998). Elevated serum levels of 17-hydroxyprogesterone, androstenedione, and testosterone are seen in PCOS-affected adolescents and have been positively linked with LH hypersecretion. In cultures of theca cells, steroidogenic enzymes P450c17 and 3b-hydroxysteroid dehydrogenase activity increased by several hundred-fold, and C17,20-lyase activity increased disproportionately. A sensitive way to evaluate hyperandrogenemia is to measure liberated testosterone or the natural hormone ratio (Nelson et al., 2011).

### *2.1.1. Causes of Hyperandrogenism*

1. LH hypersecretion via GnRH.

2. Downregulation of theca cell androgen biosynthesis intrinsic to the ovary because of irregularity in P450c17a or an anomaly in the endocrine variables that regulate P450c17a, the enzyme that regulates the rate of androgen biosynthesis, results in increased production of testosterone precursors.
3. The enhancement of androstenedione synthesis by inhibition as seen in cultured human theca cells.
4. Hyperandrogenism is thought to be primarily caused by hyperinsulinemia. In addition to working as a co-gonadotropin and raising ovarian LH function, it may also do so indirectly by increasing serum LH pulse amplitude, directly by enhancing cytochrome P450c17a action in PCOS-afflicted women's ovaries or adrenals, and indirectly by altering steroidogenesis.
5. An increase in the insulin receptor's serine phosphorylation, which activates the P450c17a enzymes in the adrenal gland and the ovaries and encourages the production of androgen.
6. Genomic differences in genes linked to androgen biosynthesis regulation, function, and androgen accessibility to target tissues, insulin sensitivity, and metabolic disorders may have an impact on the genetic susceptibility to operational hyperandrogenism and PCOS. The occurrence including both hyperandrogenism and hypoestrogenism in PCOS indicates that abnormalities in regional regulators of steroidogenesis have an impact on both theca and granulosa cells. It is impossible to ignore how increased androgen synthesis is aided by LH synthesis and secretion and impaired insulin, and how certain many processes can combine to influence the development of hyperandrogenism (Barnes et al., 1998).

#### *2.1.2. Hyperandrogenism's Outward Physical Symptoms*

The overall effects of hyperandrogenism emerge in genetically susceptible individuals as hirsutism and acne. 70% of women with a PCOS diagnosis have a hormonal imbalance, which is defined by an overgrowth of ending hair in a masculine dispersion on the face and/or other parts of the body (such as the neck and lower belly). Substantial weight gain may result in adaptive hyperinsulinemia and insulin sensitivity, both of which can lower sex hormone binding globulin (SHBG), increase free physiologically active testosterone, and ultimately cause hirsutism. Production must be taken into consideration, and all of these mechanisms may interact to affect the resulting hyperandrogenism. The growth hormones insulin and insulin-like promote 5a reductase activity (Archer et al., 2004). The overproduction of androgen receptors in the pilosebaceous unit (PSU), is the first step in the pathophysiology of acne vulgaris. This leads to an excess of sebum production, follicular keratinization, and cornification, which are all accompanied by poor drainage and, ultimately, comedone formation (Oztan et al., 2021).

## 3. GnRH Abnormalities and Their Impact on PCOS Patients

### 3.1. Reproductive Dysfunction

Reproductive problems in women with PCOS are common. Ovarian function can be altered, leading to aberrant steroidogenesis and folliculogenesis. Although the precise pathophysiology of anovulation is difficult to pinpoint, many potential causes have been hypothesized. Obesity, hypersecretion of LH, hyperandrogenaemia, hyperinsulinemia, hyperinsulinemia, abnormal ovarian and endometrial function have all been linked to the pathophysiology of PCOS women (Oztan et al., 2021).

### 3.2. Menstrual Abnormalities

The most common gynecological symptom of PCOS is irregular menstruation, including oligomenorrhea occurring in up to 85-90% of afflicted women and up to 30–40% of amenorrheic individuals. Low placental and fetal growth, which may be associated with the daughter's more severe PCOS symptoms and frequently results in an early clinical diagnosis of the condition, or increased maternal obesity in late gestation, which may be related to childhood obesity and issues with weight-related reproduction. (Charnvises et al., 2005).

### 3.3. Abnormal Follicular Dynamics

In polycystic ovaries, preantral and antral follicle counts are higher than in healthy ovaries (Nakamura et al., 2018). Hypoestrogenism may be caused by insulin resistance, which leads to increased adipose tissue deposition and enhanced peripheral or granulosa cell aromatization of androgens to estrogens or as a result of numerous follicles. Estradiol hypersecretion may be a sign of the medium-sized antral follicles' accelerated maturation (Adams et al., 1986). Furthermore, it's seen that LH and insulin production and secretion possibly contribute to PCOS differently by worsening the current ovarian dysregulation. LH hypersecretion can halt follicular development by encouraging letting early development of granulosa cells and luteinization or secondarily by generating hyperandrogenism. Insulin production and secretion increase the influence of LH on gonadotropins of separated granulosa cells and that may hinder the formation of moderate antral follicles by causing the granulosa cell to prematurely differentiate by releasing 'preovulatory' levels of cAMP (Franks 2008). Hyperinsulinemia, LH, anomalies in the genes governing androgen biosynthesis, and androgen dysregulation all contribute to hyperandrogenism, which is frequently accompanied by a rise in the number of follicles that evade atresia (Nakamura et al., 2018). A greater proportion of primary follicles in the developing ovary and a slower rate of oocyte loss in late gestation, infancy, and adolescence are signs that the polycystic ovary has a problem with early follicular development (Franks et al., 2006; Forsdike et al., 2007). But it's unproved to date whether this phenomenon results from the ovary's greater exposure to androgens or if it's a result of it. Women having polycystic ovaries or PCOS had a greater rate of spontaneous abortions in the first trimester (25-73%), according to reports (Forsdike et al., 2007).

### 3.4. Infertility

The World Health Organization (WHO) has identified infertility as a problem for the general public's health. Equitable access to superior reproductive health care for all people is one of the primary goals of the 2015 UN Conference Agenda for Action on Human Development and

Population (Piazza 2009). The agency's definition of infertility was the loss of pregnancy following two years of regular sexual activity regardless of the use of any form of contraception. There is consensus, nonetheless, that an evaluation of probable factors implicated should start after a year (Izzo 2008). The ESHRE/ASRM recommends that a counseling session before conception emphasize the significance of lifestyle changes, such as losing weight and exercising regularly in overweight individuals, quitting smoking, and limiting alcohol usage (Barbosa et al., 2016; Dokras et al., 2017). Anatomical changes, ovulatory modifications, immunological issues, and endometriosis are some of the most typical female infertility causes. The woman's age, how often she engages in sexual activity, her weight, and whether or not she smokes are just a few of the variables that can affect her infertility patterns. In this way, many procedures should be used to obtain a precise diagnosis (Barbosa et al., 2016). About 50% of infertile women are obese (Table 1). Abdominal fat is the biggest regional area for the transformation of sex hormones to steroid hormones, which contributes to the production of estrogen and shows the link between overweight and amenorrhoea (Izzo 2008). A secondary screening test that could be utilized is the progesterone dosage.

**Table 1.** Analysis of PCOS and non-PCOS patients in a population

| S.No. | Sample size (n) | PCOS/Non-PCOS | Infertility (%) | BMI | Irregular menstruation (%) | References |
|---|---|---|---|---|---|---|
| 1. | 309 | PCOS | 72 | 27.9 ± 0.4 kg/m2 ($p \leq 0.001$) | 79% | Joham et al., 2015 |
| 2. | 4547 | Non-PCOS | 16 | 25.1 ± 0.1 kg/m2 ($p \leq 0.001$) | 34% | Joham et al., 2015 |

BMI, body mass index; PCOS, Polycystic ovary syndrome.

**Table 2.** Outcome of induction of ovulation in women treated with low-dose gonadotrophin

| S.No. | Sample size (n) | PCOS/ Non-PCOS | Pregnancies (%) | Multiple pregnancies (%) | Miscarriages (%) | References |
|---|---|---|---|---|---|---|
| 1. | 199 | PCOS | 46 | 3 | 21 | Gorry et al., 2006 |

PCOS, Polycystic ovary syndrome.

It's crucial to rule out factors other than anovulation in families whenever the female partner has PCOS. The presence of PCOS suggests metabolic issues, a significant risk of stroke, and, most important, directly affects these people's ability to conceive (Legro et al., 2013). 81% of women who experienced recurrent fetal loss exhibited abnormalities in LH secretion, and increased androgen levels were seen in these women whether or not they had PCOS. Insulin resistance (IR) and obesity are usually discovered to be associated with ovulatory infertility, which is caused by halted folliculogenesis in PCOS (Wickenheisser et al., 2004). The disorder of folliculogenesis, oocyte maturation, steroidogenesis, and endometrial receptivity by a multitude of ovulatory signaling pathways, including insulin-like growth factors (IGF), adenosine monophosphate (AMH), growth differentiation factor 9 (GDF-9), and inhibin, as well as extra ovarian growth factors (GH, IGF-1, and insulin), appears to contribute to anovulation or early pregnancy loss. Being overweight is more closely connected with diseases that can affect pregnant women with multiple miscarriages, birth, and increased birth mass, which is linked to slower fetal growth and more pregnancies ending in miscarriage (Metwally et al., 2007).

However, low-dose gonadotropin therapy proves to be beneficial in PCOS women (Table 2). Kamrava et al., successfully induced ovulation in PCOS patients by giving a daily dose (75 IU) of only a single ampule (Kamrava et al., 1982). According to Gorry et al., in 73% of treatment cycles a 37.5-75 IU dose of gonadotropin and a 150 IU dose of hMG (16 days/cycle) was required in only 4% of cases to produce a dominant follicle (Gorry et al., 2006).

### 3.5. Metabolic Dysfunction

Metabolic syndrome (MBS), also known as syndrome X or IR syndrome, is characterized by insulin resistance, insulin sensitivity, gestational weight gain, hypertension, and atherogenic dyslipidemia (Essah et al., 2007). The major risk factors for acquiring the clinical manifestations of cardiovascular disease are lack of physical activity, atherogenic diet, and belly fat, and mainly characterized by adiposity (Glueck et al., 2006). By a factor of nearly 2, MBS has been observed to occur more commonly in women with PCOS (43%) than in the normal populace. Women with PCOS from the 20-29 age group exhibited a nearly 8-fold higher prevalence of MBS (44.8%) whereas women with PCOS aged 30-39 years would have an approximately 4-fold higher risk when compared to age-matched women in the general population. Also to add, women with MBS had BMI levels that were much higher and were greater likely to show hirsutism (Essah et al., 2007).

In addition to a decrease in high-density lipoprotein (HDL) cholesterol content, these alterations can be detected as an increase in blood total cholesterol, low-density lipoprotein (LDL) cholesterol, and triglycerides (TG). 85% of women with PCOS have dyslipidemia which is a symptom of the MBS as compared to those without the condition.

### 3.6. Insulin Resistance and Hyperinsulinemia

The onset of insulin resistance (IR) is one of the most detrimental impacts of obesity, which is rapidly becoming more prevalent worldwide (Bentley-Lewis et al., 2011). Hyperinsulinemia can be brought on by genetic abnormalities in insulin production, insulin sensitivity, or obesity (Table 3) (Livadas et al., 2022).

In females with early adrenarche during pubertal gonadotropin activation, hyperinsulinemia increases combined adrenal and ovarian cytochrome P450c17a performance and might even underlie the transition to PCOS, whether brought on by weight gain or by innate insulin action irregularities (Chandrashekaran et al., 2007). The amplitude of the LH pulse can be increased, or the actions of LH on ovarian steroidogenesis can be amplified, causing hyperandrogenism. Humans with PCOS experience long-term hyperinsulinemia, which encourages the release of leptin from adipose tissue and has been associated with poor reproductive health (Zargar et al., 2005). More than half of PCOS women are overweight or obese having (BMI >25 kg/m$^2$) (Balen et al., 2002). 7.5% of obese PCOS women will have frank diabetes before turning 40. Obese women experience more extreme hyperandrogenism (Agarwal et al., 1999).

**Table 3.** Cases of dysglycemia in PCOS patients

| S.No. | sample size (n) | Age (yr) | Country | PCOS/T2D Criteria | T2D (%) | IGT (%) | References |
|---|---|---|---|---|---|---|---|
| 1. | 90 | 15-39 | UK | NIH/WHO | 2 | 9 | Rajkhowa et al., 1996 |
| 2. | 254 | 14-44 | USA | NIH/WHO | 7.5 | 31 | Legro et al., 1999 |
| 3. | 122 | 13-40 | USA | NIH/ADA | 10 | 35 | Ehrmann et al., 1999 |
| 4. | 121 | 14-37 | Italy | Rotterdam/WHO | 2.5 | 15.7 | Gambineri et al., 2004 |
| 5. | 71 | 30 ± 6 | USA | NIH/ADA | 10 | 25 | Legro et al., 2005 |
| 6. | 102 | 24.2 ± 6 | China | Rotterdam/WHO | 1.9 | 20.5 | Chen et al., 2006 |
| 7. | 264 | 28 ± 0.4 | Germany | NIH/WHO | 1.5 | 14.3 | Mohlig et al., 2006 |

ADA, American Diabetes Association; IGT, impaired glucose tolerance; NIH, National Institutes of Health; PCOS, Polycystic ovary syndrome; T2DM, Type 2 diabetes mellitus; WHO, World Health Organization.

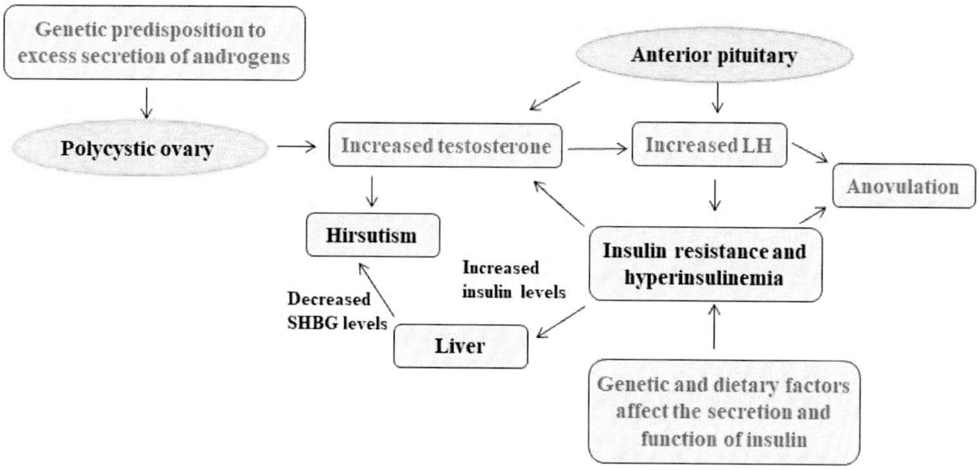


LH, luteinizing hormone; SHBG, sex hormone-binding globulin.

**Figure 3.** The role of hyperandrogenism in insulin sensitivity and secretion.

Hyperandrogenism, independent genetic and dietary factors also alters the function, sensitivity, and release of insulin (Figure 3). Insulin resistance is the prime cause of the enhanced risk of T2DM in PCOS patients (Jayasena and Frank 2014).

Dyslipidaemia is a lipoprotein metabolism malfunctioning that can result in excess or deficiency of lipoproteins. Lipid and lipoprotein irregularities in PCOS women have been connected to hyperinsulinemia brought on by IR. About 25% of PCOS women have lipid changes related to insulin (Legro et al., 1999).

### 3.7. Effect of Androgens on Leptin in PCOS

The blood levels of leptin, a hormone mostly produced by adipose tissue, are influenced by (androgens and estrogens), and insulin peaks. Leptin is a crucial bond between adipose tissue and the hypothalamus-pituitary-gonadal (HPG) axis since it not only regulates the body's energy metabolism but also has important reproductive consequences. Human long-term hyperinsulinemia, as found in PCOS patients, encourages the production of leptin from adipose tissue (Zargar et al., 2005). Based on the serum concentration, leptin could have a highly skewed impact just on the HPG axis; at smaller concentrations, it could have a tolerant threshold effect on the CNS, that also regulates gonadotropin discharge, even though increased plasma leptin levels (leptin resistance), as seen in the in obese people, may have an inhibitory effect on the gonads. Leptin resistance, may be a symptom of human obesity and be brought on by leptin receptor deficiencies (Waterworth et al., 1997).

## Conclusion

PCOS is a complex, heterogeneous metabolic syndrome caused or perpetuated by the interaction of inheritable genetic susceptibilities and vulnerability factors. PCOS causes menstrual cycle anomalies as well as the appearance of clinical symptoms, particularly changes in the LH/FSH ratio. The complex origins and negative results of PCOS on the body's biochemical, reproductive, and metabolic functioning, as well as its potentially fatal implications, necessitate early detection and therapy of this illness. Although it may not be possible to change the genetic algorithms underlying the syndrome, elements can generally be controlled. One such environmental factor is fatness which may also, whether or not interact with genetic factors that play an important role in upsetting the programming underlying multiple organ systems as well as the syndrome's final manifestation. Despite the wide range of available therapies, medicinal therapy should only be used if lifestyle changes are ineffective because obesity plays an important role in the pathophysiology, etiology, and developmental origin of PCOS, and signs can often be improved with straightforward lifestyle changes like counting calories. The optimal treatment option should be regulated by evidence-based therapeutic practice with a patient-tailored strategy. Additionally, research findings on dietary changes have demonstrated that hormonal, metabolic, and reproductive irregularities in women with PCOS can continue improving via lifestyle interventions, suggesting that external conditions like food toxicants, smoking, pollution, and so forth play a significant role in masking biological propensity. Future studies should concentrate on therapeutic methods to improve PCOS women's reproductive outcomes as well as initiatives to lessen inter-generational sensitivity to adulthood PCOS and associated metabolic abnormalities.

## References

Adams J., Polson D. W., Franks S. 1986. Prevalence of polycystic ovaries in women with anovulation and idiopathic hirsutism. *Br Med J* (Clin Res Ed). 293(6543):355-359.

Agarwal S. K., Vogel K., Weitsman S. R., Magoffin D. A. 1999. Leptin antagonizes the insulin-like growth factor-I augmentation of steroidogenesis in granulosa and theca cells of the human ovary. *J Clin Endocrinol Metabol.* 84(3):1072-1076. https://doi.org/10.1210/jcem.84.3.5543.

Archer J. S., Chang R. J. 2004. Hirsutism and acne in polycystic ovary syndrome. *Best Pract Res Clin Obstet Gynaecol.* 18(5):737–754. https://doi.org/10.1016/j.bpobgyn.2004.05.007

Balen A., Michelmore K. 2002. What is polycystic ovary syndrome? Are national views important? *Hum Reprod.* 17(9):2219-2227.

Barbosa G., de Sa L. B. P. C., Rocha D. R. T. W., Arbex A. K. 2016. Polycystic ovary syndrome (PCOS) and fertility. *Open J Endocr Metab Dis.* 6(1):58-65.

Barnes R. B. 1998. The pathogenesis of polycystic ovary syndrome: lessons from ovarian stimulation studies. *J Endocrinol Invest.* 21:567-579.

Barontini M., Garcıia-Rudaz M. C., Veldhuis J. D. 2001. Mechanisms of hypothalamic-pituitary-gonadal disruption in polycystic ovarian syndrome. *Arch Med Res.* 32(6):544-552

Bentley-Lewis R., Seely E., Dunaif A. 2011. Ovarian hypertension: polycystic ovary syndrome. *Endocrinol Metab Clin North Am.* 40(2):433-449.

Chandrashekaran I. R., Yao S., Wang C. C., Bansal P. S., Alewood P. F., Forbes B. E. Wallace J. C., Bach L. A., Norton R. S. 2007. The N-terminal subdomain of insulin-like growth factor (IGF) binding protein 6. Structure and interaction with IGFs. *Biochem.* 46(11):3065-3074.

Charnvises K., Weerakiet S., Tingthanatikul Y., Wansumrith S., Chanprasertyothin S., Rojanasakul A. 2005. Acanthosis nigricans: clinical predictor of abnormal glucose tolerance in Asian women with polycystic ovary syndrome. *Gynecol Endocrinol.* 21(3):161-164.

Chen X., Yang D., Li L., Feng S., Wang L. 2006. Abnormal glucose tolerance in Chinese women with polycystic ovary syndrome. *Hum Reprod.* 21:2027-2032.

Dokras A., Saini S., Gibson-Helm M., Schulkin J., Cooney L., Teede H. 2017. Gaps in knowledge among physicians regarding diagnostic criteria and management of polycystic ovary syndrome. *Fertil Steril.* 107(6):1380-1386.

Dunaif A. 1997. Insulin resistance and the polycystic ovary syndrome: mechanism and implications for pathogenesis. *Endocr Rev.* 18(6):774-800.

Ehrmann D. A., Barnes R. B., Rosenfield R. L., Cavaghan M. K., Imperial J. 1999. Prevalence of impaired glucose tolerance and diabetes in women with polycystic ovary syndrome. *Diabetes Care.* 22:141-146.

Essah P. A., Wickham E. P., Nestler J. E. 2007. The metabolic syndrome in polycystic ovary syndrome. *Clin Obstet Gynecol.* 50(1):205-225.

Forsdike R. A., Hardy K., Bull L., Stark J., Webber L. J., Stubbs S., Robinson J. E., Franks S. 2007. Disordered follicle development in ovaries of prenatally androgenized ewes. *J Endocrinol.* 192(2):421-428.

Franks S., McCarthy M. I., Hardy K. 2006. Development of polycystic ovary syndrome: involvement of genetic and environmental factors. *Int J Androl.* 29(1):278-285.

Franks S. 2008. Polycystic ovary syndrome in adolescents. *Int J Obes.* 32(7):1035-1041.

Gambineri A., Pelusi C., Manicardi E., Vicennati V., Cacciari M., Morselli-Labate A. M., Pagotto U., Pasquali R. 2004. Glucose intolerance in a large cohort of mediterranean women with polycystic ovary syndrome: phenotype and associated factors. *Diabetes.* 53:2353-2358.

Glueck C. J., Aregawi D., Winiarska M. 2006. Metformin-diet ameliorates coronary heart disease risk factors and facilitates resumption of regular menses in adolescents with polycystic ovary syndrome. *J Pedia Endocrinol Metab.* 19(6):831-842.

Gorry A., White D. M., Franks S. 2006. Infertility in polycystic ovary syndrome. Focus on low-dose gonadotropin treatment. *Endocrine.* 30(1):27-33,

Izzo C. R. 2008. Infertilidade de causa hormonal para o ginecologista. *Boletim da SBRH: Artigos Cientificos* 6(2):1-3.

Jayasena C., Franks S. 2014. The management of patients with polycystic ovary syndrome. *Nat Rev Endocrinol.* 10, 624–636.

Joham A. E., Teede H. J., Ranasinha S., Zoungas S., Boyle J. 2015. Prevalence of infertility and use of fertility treatment in women with polycystic ovary syndrome: Data from a large community-based cohort study. *J Women's Health.* doi: https://doi.org/10.1089/jwh.2014.5000.

Kamrava M. M., Seibel M. M., Berger M. J., Thompson I., Taymor M. L. 1982. Reversal of persistent anovulation in polycystic ovarian disease by administration of chronic low-dose follicle-stimulating hormone. *Fertil Steril.* 37(4):520-523.

Legro R. S., Arslanian S. A., Ehrmann D. A., Hoeger K. M., Murad M. H., Pasquali R., Welt C. K. 2013. Diagnosis and treatment of polycystic ovary syndrome: an Endocrine Society clinical practice guideline. *J Clin Endocrinol Metab.* 98(12):4565-4592.

Legro R. S., Driscoll D., Strauss I. J. F., Fox J., Dunaif A. 1998. Evidence for a genetic basis for hyperandrogenemia in polycystic ovary syndrome. *Proc Natl Acad Sci.* 95(25):14956-14960.

Legro R. S., Gnatuk C. L., Kunselman A. R., Dunaif A. 2005. Changes in glucose tolerance over time in women with polycystic ovary syndrome: a controlled study. *J Clin Endocrinol Metab*. 90:3236-3242.

Legro R. S., Kunselman A. R., Dodson W. C., Dunaif A. 1999. Prevalence and predictors of risk for type 2 diabetes mellitus and impaired glucose tolerance in polycystic ovary syndrome: a prospective, controlled study in 254 affected women. *J Clin Endocrinol Metab*. 84(1):165-169. https://doi.org/10.1210/jcem.84.1.5393.

Livadas S., Anagnostis P., Bosdou J. K., Bantouna D., Paparodis R. 2022. Polycystic ovary syndrome and type 2 diabetes mellitus: A state-of-the-art review. *World J Diabetes*. 13(1):5-26.

Marshall J. C., Eagleson C. A. 1999. Neuroendocrine aspects of polycystic ovary syndrome. *Endocrinol Metab Clin North Am. 28*(2):295-324.

McCartney C. R., Eagleson C. A., Marshall J. C. 2002. Regulation of gonadotropin secretion: implications for polycystic ovary syndrome. *Semin Reprod Med.* 20(4):317-326.

Metwally M., Cutting R., Tipton A., Skull J., Ledger W. L., Li T. C. 2007. Effect of increased body mass index on oocyte and embryo quality in IVF patients. *Reprod Biomed Online*. 15(5):532-538.

Mohlig M., Flöter A., Spranger J., Weickert M. O., Schill T., Schlosser H. W., Brabant G., Pfeiffer A. F., Selbig J., Schofl C. 2006. Predicting impaired glucose metabolism in women with polycystic ovary syndrome by decision tree modelling. *Diabetologia.* 49:2572-2579.

Nakamura T., Murase T., Osuka S., Goto M., Iwase A. 2018. The regulation of ovarian follicular growth by anti-Müllerian hormone. *J Mamm Ova Res*. 35(1):13-19.

Nelson V. L., Qin K. N., Rosenfield R. L., Wood J. R., Penning T. M., Legro R. S., Strauss J. F. 3rd, McAllister J. M. 2001. The biochemical basis for increased testosterone production in theca cells propagated from patients with polycystic ovary syndrome. *J Clin Endocrinol Metab.* 86(12):5925-5933.

Oztan O., Erdogan G., Şimşir C., Turksoy V. A., Abuşoglu G., Tutkun L., Deniz S, Alagüney M. E. 2021. Levels of methylated arginines and L-arginine in patients with polycystic ovary syndrome: a promising approach in clinical evaluation. *Anatol Curr Med J.* 3(4):291-299.

Piazza V. 2009. Sindrome dll'ovaio policistico. *Disponívelem*: http://www.vincenzopiazza.it/sindrome_ovaio_policistico.htm.

Rajkhowa M., Talbot J. A., Jones P. W., Clayton R. N. 1996. Polymorphism of glycogen synthetase gene in polycystic ovary syndrome. *Clin Endocrinol* (Oxf), 44:85-90.

Ridker P. M. 2003. Clinical application of C-reactive protein for cardiovascular disease detection and prevention. *Circulation.* 107(3):363-369.

Ropelato M. G., Garcia-Rudaz M. C., Castro-Fernandez C., Ulloa-Aguirre A., Escobar M. E., Barontini M., Veldhuis J. D. 1999. A preponderance of basic luteinizing hormone (LH) isoforms accompanies inappropriate hypersecretion of both basal and pulsatile LH in adolescents with polycystic ovarian syndrome. *J Clin Endo Metab.* 84(12):4629-4636.

Waterworth D. M., Bennett S. T., Gharani N., McCarthy M. I., Hague S., Batty S., Conway G. S., White D., Todd J. A., Franks S., Williamson R. 1997. Linkage and association of insulin gene VNTR regulatory polymorphism with polycystic ovary syndrome. *Lancet.* 349(9057):986-990.

Wickenheisser J. K., Nelson-DeGrave V. L., McAllister J. M. 2004. Dysregulation of cytochrome P450 17α-hydroxylase messenger RNA stability in theca cells isolated from women with polycystic ovary syndrome (PCOS). *J Clin Endocrinol Metab*. 90(3):1720-1727.

Zargar A. H., Gupta V. K., Wani A. I., Masoodi S. R., Bashir M. I., Laway B. A., Ganie M. A., Salahuddin M. 2005. Prevalence of ultrasonography proved polycystic ovaries in North Indian women with type 2 diabetes mellitus. *Reprod Biol Endocrinol.* 3(1):1-7.

# Chapter 3

# PCOS and Increased Androgen Levels: Hirsutism and Its Pathophysiology

**Syed Douhath Yousuf[1]**
**Kulsum Akhtar[1]**
**and Mohammad Ashraf Ganie[2,*]**
[1]Department of Clinical Biochemistry, Sher-i-Kashmir Institute of Medical Sciences, SKIMS, Soura, Srinagar, Jammu and Kashmir, India
[2]Department of Endocrinology, Sher-i-Kashmir Institute of Medical Sciences, SKIMS, Soura, Srinagar, Jammu and Kashmir, India

## Abstract

In the hyperandrogenic condition known as polycystic ovarian syndrome (PCOS), the ovaries overproduce androgens. The most usual symptoms of hyperandrogenism in women are irregular menstruation, infertility, and hirsutism. Hirsutism is the term used to describe excessive facial or body hair development in females. A hirsutism sign is coarse, black hair that can develop on the upper arms, upper legs, chest, abdomen, or back. Hirsutism is a sign of medical conditions linked to androgens. The diagnosis is difficult due to the heterogeneity of the condition and the wide range of its associated characteristics. Classic PCOS affects 10% of reproductive-age women which includes hyperandrogenism plus ovulatory dysfunction. Hyperandrogenism, whether it be clinical, biochemical, or both, is a feature of PCOS. About 60–76% of PCOS women are hirsute, and 75–90% of them have hyperandrogenemia. Hirsutism frequently gets better with medical treatment. It's critical to get medical care right away because putting off treatment might make it more difficult and have long-term effects on your health. This chapter will endeavor to sum up the biochemical and clinical presentations of hyperandrogenism, its pathophysiology and management.

**Keywords:** polycystic ovary syndrome (PCOS), androgens, hyperandrogenism, hirsutism, infertility

---

* Corresponding Author's E-mail: ashraf.endo@gmail.com.

In: Polycystic Ovarian Syndrome (PCOS) and Our Biological Clock
Editors: Arpita Roy, Gowhar Rashid and Nihad Ashraf Khan
ISBN: 979-8-89113-100-2
© 2023 Nova Science Publishers, Inc.

# 1. Introduction

PCOS is the most prevalent endocrine disease which is reported to affect about 5-20% of women of reproductive age. It is characterized by hirsutism, deranged menstruation cycles, and infertility (Asunción et al., 2000; Diamanti-Kandarakis et al., 1999; Dunaif, 1997). Antonio Vallisnerie, an Italian physician first noted it in 1721 when he noticed cystic ovaries in obese infertile women. The phrase "femmes à barbe diabetique" (=diabetic women with beard) was initially used by French doctors Achard and Thiers in 1921 after discovering a correlation between diabetes and hyperandrogenism (Heutling et al., 2007). American gynecologists Irving Stein and Michael Leventhal published the first comprehensive description citing polycystic ovaries, hirsutism, amenorrhea, and obesity in 1935. A disorder known as Stein-Leventhal syndrome has a substantial impact on a woman's reproductive potential, metabolic health, and cardiovascular health (Ehrmann, 2005).

Hirsutism is characterized by the male pattern of terminal hair on the body of the female. Male sexual type is observed in sites that are androgen-sensitive like the chest, breast areola, face, linear alba, lower back, inner legs, buttocks, and external genitalia (Amiri et al., 2022; Randall, 2008). Compared to the general population, where women (4-10%) are affected by hirsutism, it is anticipated that 6-75% of women with PCOS will experience it (Azziz et al., 2016). The degree of androgen excess and individual differences in the pilosebaceous unit's sensitivity to androgens determine how severe the problem is (Escobar-Morreale et al., 2012; Spritzer et al., 2016).

## 1.1. Causes of Hirsutism

Many endocrine disorders are responsible for hirsutism in females (Table 1) Hirsutism results from either excessive androgen production or the hair follicles becoming excessively sensitive to androgens. Men have greater access to androgens, although women also contain these hormones, albeit in lesser amounts. Various male hormones like testosterone promote hair growth, expand the size of the body, and heighten hair growth and pigmentation. Hirsutism may also be facilitated by high insulin levels, a hormone that helps cells to utilize energy from carbohydrates. The ovarian cells may be stimulated by insulin to generate androgens. Insulin resistance (IR) in women, like those who suffer from type 2 diabetes (T2D), may experience this.

Increasing insulin levels can also trigger the insulin-like growth factor-I (IGF-1) receptor in the same cells, escalating the secretion of testosterone. Because it can result in T2D, obesity may be a risk factor for the disease. Elevated cholesterol could also be a factor. A side effect of some drugs is hirsutism. The use of testosterone, DHEA, or the medication Danazol as part of an androgen therapy regimen may result in hirsutism. DHEA is a substance that the body naturally makes and that some individuals supplement their diets with to help prevent age-related diseases like osteoporosis. A synthetic steroid called danazol is occasionally used to treat endometriosis. Both may have the adverse effect of increasing testosterone. In women with regular periods, normal testosterone levels, and no underlying disorders, idiopathic hirsutism is the term defined to characterize excess hair growth. This indicates that there is no known etiology for the condition. Hirsutism is not usually an indicator of a serious medical condition. However, before puberty, if it starts, and is followed by other male-related characteristics like a voice which is deep, or is brought on by a tumor, the person should seek medical attention. Hirsutism can occasionally be triggered by ovary tumors, pituitary glands, or adrenal glands. Nonetheless, hirsutism brought on by this source usually starts sooner and is more severe than hirsutism brought on by hormonal factors.

**Table 1.** Causes of Hirsutism

| Frequent | Random |
|---|---|
| • Polycystic ovary syndrome (PCOS) (>70%)<br>• Idiopathic hirsutism (20%) | • Congenital adrenal hyperplasia (CAH) (due to 21-hydroxylase-deficiency)<br>• Different types of ovarian tumors<br>– Sertoli - leydig cell<br>– Granulosa-theca cell<br>– Hilus cell |

## 1.2. Diagnosing Hirsutism

It is essential to examine if the coarse hairs are found in the male pattern or if there is a generalized rise in the development of hair over the entire body when a female patient reports that her hair is growing faster. (Gilchrist & Hecht, 1995; Hunter & Carek, 2003). The below-mentioned measures should be conducted to know the cause of hirsutism once it has been determined. A thorough medical history should comprise information on the onset age (adolescence, menopause, middle age), onset rate (sudden or gradual), and various symptoms of virilization (voice deepening, deranged menstruation, acne, breast tissue loss, or normal female body contour, enhanced libido, clitoromegal, increasing muscle mass as in the shoulder girdle, malodorous perspiration, etc.). A comprehensive general physical and systemic examination is essential, and part of that process should involve palpating the abdomen to check for any ovarian masses. If a medicine is to blame, drug withdrawal happens to be beneficial. In various other circumstances, a laboratory study of the serum markers should be performed to ascertain the precise cause. The many serum indicators consist of:

A. Testosterone – In cases of benign diseases like PCOS and CAH, serum testosterone may be normal or high, but it would unquestionably be elevated (>200 ng/ml) in cases of malignant tumors of the ovary or adrenal (Lin-Su et al., 2008).
B. Dehydroepiandrosterone sulfate (DHEAS)-Elevated DHEAS (>700 g/dl) is always indicative of a malignant or benign adrenal origin.
C. 17 Hydroxy Progesterone (17-OHP) – CAH has a specific serum marker. The measurement should be done between the hours of 0700 and 0900 during the early follicular phase of the menstrual cycle. Under-200 ng/dl readings rule out the condition. An ACTH stimulation is required for levels that are somewhat increased between 300 and 1,000 ng/dl. Cosyntropin (synthetic ACTH) is administered intravenously in a dose of 250 g, and 17-OHP levels are measured both before and one hour after the injection. Positive test findings are readings >1,000 ng/dl following stimulation (Lin-Su et al., 2008).
D. Women with Cushing's syndrome symptoms and signs should have their 24-hour urine-free cortisol levels checked.

E. A sign of PCOS is a Luteinizing hormone(LH)/Follicle stimulating hormone (FSH) ratio greater than 3 (Chang & Katz, 1999)
F. Prolactin would rise due to a pituitary tumor or a hypothalamic problem, in hyperprolactinemia
G. Elevated serum TSH levels: The cofactor in hirsutism elevating TSH is hypophyseal hypothyroidism (Schmidt et al., 1991).
H. Polycystic ovaries or ovarian neoplasms can be observed by Pelvic ultrasonography.
I. Diagnostic use of CT scan or MRI of the adrenal area.

## 1.3. Scoring Hirsutism

Although traditional techniques of testing androgen levels have been shown to have a limited relationship with hirsutism severity, the majority of women with levels of androgen greater than twice the upper limit of the reference range possess a certain amount of hirsutism (Legro et al., 2010). Females may also develop too much body hair while still having appropriate plasma androgen levels. According to these observations, the most common PCOS diagnostic criteria classify the criteria of hyperandrogenism as either clinical or biochemical (Teede et al., 2018). Particularly in women with normal androgen levels, clinical hyperandrogenism is crucial when defining hyperandrogenism for the diagnosis of PCOS.

The Ferriman-Gallwey (FG) scoring method is mostly employed in clinical practice to evaluate visually excess terminal hair, standardizing hirsutism assessment and facilitating comparison of data(Ferriman & Gallwey, 1961). The modified FG (mFG) score is employed to examine the growth of hair in nine different parts of the body. Scores in each area vary from 0 (no terminal hair) to 4 (male pattern hair), with a maximum value of 36 representing intermediate levels of body hair growth (Figure 1). Based on the authentic data given by Ferriman and Gallwey and accounting for the 95th percentile, the original method's cutoff for hirsutism in the mFG score was increased to 8 (Ferriman & Purdie, 1983; Hatch et al., 1981). Given that self-rating in shaved areas only modestly correlates with assessment by an experienced observer, it can be helpful clinically, mostly for follow-up (Wild et al., 2005).

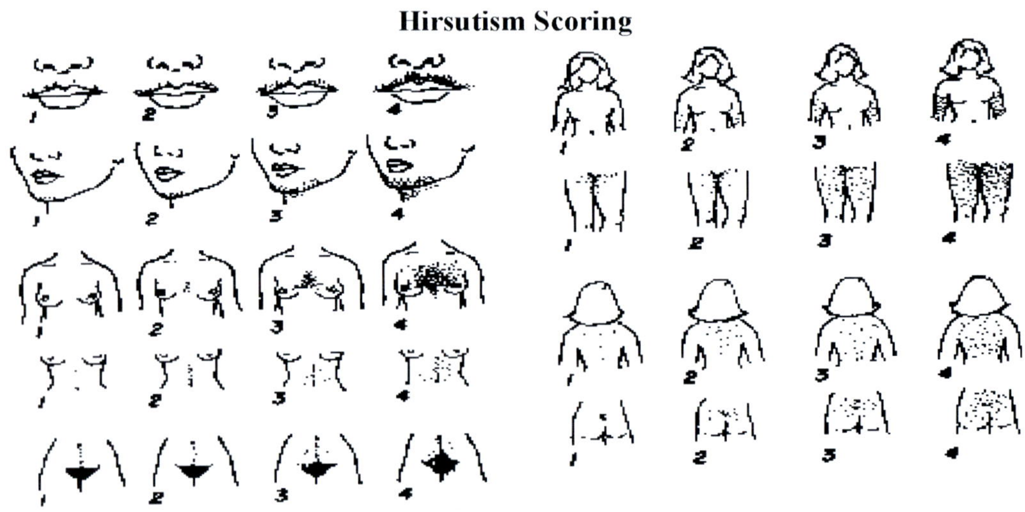


**Figure 1.** Modified Ferrimen Gallway Method.
Each Area = 1-4. Total Score = 36: Significant >8

## 2. Normal Physiology of Androgens in Women

Androgens are essential for female health because they maintain female sexual function, muscle mass, and bone density. DHEA-S and DHEA, as well as testosterone, dihydrotesto-sterone, and androstenedione, among others (DHEA), are examples of androgens. Testosterone and dihydrotestosterone (DHT) are the hormones with the highest physiological activity (Burger, 2002). The adrenal glands (25%), peripheral organs such as the skin, liver, and adipose tissue (50%), and the ovaries (25%). produce androgens (Longcope, 1986). Several research point to the fact that androgen deficiency reduces women's libido and sexual energy even if there is conflicting evidence (Bolour & Braunstein, 2005; Jayasena et al., 2019). The differential diagnosis of hyperandrogenism typically includes ovarian versus adrenal (Cushing syndrome and congenital adrenal hyperplasia) diseases (PCOS, carcinoma, and hyperthecosis). Mild hyperandrogenism symptoms include acne, male-type baldness, and hirsutism; however, severe excess androgen symptoms include virilization (deepening of voice and clitoromegaly), which increases the chance of ovarian hyperthecosis or an androgen-secreting tumour. If the DHEA-S concentration is greater than 700 g/dL (>19.0 mol/L) or the blood total testosterone concentration is more than 150 ng/dL (>5.2 nmol/L), the majority of recommendations advise additional testing(Martin et al., 2018).

A severe case of PCOS has occasionally been compared to ovarian hyperthecosis. This non-neoplastic condition of androgen excess is distinguished by a remarkable and increasing hirsutism or virilization produced by the differentiation of ovarian interstitial cells into active luteinized theca cells capable of producing androstenedione and testosterone. Obesity and hyperinsulinemia are almost universal in women, and their typical testosterone levels are higher than 150 ng/dL. Postmenopausal women are more frequently impacted by it. Histological examination validates the diagnosis (Markopoulos et al., 2015).

## 3. Hair Follicle Cycling

Interaction of the epidermis and dermis leads to the hair follicle development, which are essential skin appendages and microscopic organs. They exhibit a great capacity for regeneration and a regular growth cycle that continues for the whole of the human lifespan. The existence of hair follicles with several stem cell populations causes these characteristics, and a number of signaling pathways are crucial in controlling both the stem cell activity and the development of hair follicles (Ji et al., 2021). Age, environment, and health all play a part in hair follicle tumor development, alopecia areata, and several other conditions which are related, like hirsutism (Lin et al., 2022).

Humans have three different forms of hair: terminal, lanugo, and vellus. The fetal body is covered in the extremely fine hair known as lanugo, which comes off during the initial periods of life. Terminal hair is longer, pigmented, and denser, whereas vellus hair is extremely short, thin, and usually unpigmented. Female body regions where terminal hair is more prevalent are the brows, scalp, axilla, and pubis. Less frequently, terminal hair can grow in females in places associated with supposedly male sexual patterns. Women's hair distribution patterns may be changed by hormones, which could result in uncontrollable hair growth (Lin et al., 2022; Spritzer et al., 2016).

Anagen, catagen, and telogen are the three main stages of the hair follicle cycle that represent the continuous cycles of growth, involution, and rest respectively. The most active stage of hair follicle development is the anagen, during which the hair grows quickly and completely matures into a hair shaft. Epithelial cell differentiation and hair coloring occur during this period. Hair length is maintained by the anagen stage, which is associated with the ongoing differentiation and proliferation of stromal cells at the base of hair follicles (Lin et al., 2022; Spritzer et al., 2016; Yang et al., 2021). At the catagen phase, the hair follicles mostly stop the growth and have atrophied by the time this stage is complete. The catagen stage begins when the availability of matrix cells decreases as the differentiation of the hair shaft and inner root sheath diminishes (apoptosis-driven regression) (Lin et al., 2022; Yang et al., 2021). Following regression, the hair follicle is said to have entered the telogen stage, also referred to as the resting period. This stage is characterized by a reduction in the hair shaft and low biological potency of the follicle. The follicle stays in the telogen stage unless stimulated. The activity and expression of the main regulatory factors that control the cyclical growth of the hair follicle will significantly increase at this stage in order to prepare for the start of the ensuing anagen phase (Lin et al., 2022; Spritzer et al., 2016; Yang et al., 2021).

### 3.1. Metabolism and Actions of Androgens in the Hair Follicle

Hamilton and colleagues discovered the function of androgens in human hair growth in the 1950s when they discovered that castration before puberty hampered beard and axillary hair development while castration after puberty caused axillary hair atrophy and beard (Hamilton, 1951). Pubic or axillary hairlessness is another sign of androgen insensitivity. Since then, research has shown that androgens increase the number of hair follicles in various body parts, the width of hair, and the amount of time that hair is in the anagen stage (Deplewski & Rosenfield, 2000).

It is critical to record that the intensity and frequency of hirsutism are both related to hair follicle androgen sensitivity. Together with the fact that they widely express androgen receptors in response to androgens, hair follicles really have androgen-metabolizing enzymes that are crucial for the regulation of the amount of androgens present in the hair follicle(Grymowicz et al., 2020). Type 2 17-hydroxysteroid dehydrogenase (17-HSD), which converts testosterone into androstenedione, and 5-reductase, which changes testosterone into dihydrotestosterone, are the two main enzymes. Androstenedione and testosterone are converted to estrogens (17-estradiol and estrone, respectively) by the enzyme cytochrome P450 aromatase (DHT). As a result, a changing expression of these enzymes may be associated to a raised or decreased activity of androgens in the hair follicle.

According to recent research, the type 2 17-HSD gene is expressed differentially in the sub-umbilical region and arm skin of hirsute women than in those who do not (Oliveira et al., 2003; Taheri et al., 2015). These reports imply that type 2 17-HSD, an enzyme that causes the oxidation of stronger sex hormones (such as testosterone), may have a crucial part to play in the development of hirsutism. (Oliveira et al., 2003). Further gene expression studies using 5-reductase were used to confirm that females have isotype 1 on the vertex of their scalps, but there was little change in the expression types between females without and with hirsutism (Oliveira et al., 2003). The expression of the 5'-reductase type 1 and 2 genes in dermal papillae from the lower abdomen did not correspond with the degree of hirsutism (Oliveira et al., 2003).

While, changes in the gene encoding 5'-reductase type 1 were related to hirsutism in PCOS females (Goodarzi et al., 2006).

Although androgen activity in the hair follicle is reflected in hirsutism, local factors such as androgen sensitivity, exposure duration, and testosterone conversion to a much more effective androgen, DHT, via 5-reductase may be more significant than androgen levels in plasma(Mihailidis et al., 2017; Paus & Cotsarelis, 1999). L-ornithine decarboxylase activity, an enzyme involved in the synthesis of polyamines involved in cell migration, proliferation, differentiation of hair follicles, the concentration of androgen receptor, as well as 17-HSD and 5-reductase activities, is one of the factors that have a role in growth and hair follicle development (Yildiz et al., 2010).

## 4. Biochemical and Clinical Hyperandrogenism

Hyperandrogenemia is a biological trait of PCOS. Levels of Androgen are high in 75–90% of PCOS individuals with oligomenorrhea, and they usually increase as the phenotypic severity increases (Azziz et al., 2009; Huang et al., 2010; Pasquali et al., 2016). A free/total testosterone, androstenedione, and/or DHEA-S amount greater than the top 95th percentile in 98 healthy, non-hirsute eumenorrheic women is defined as hyperandrogenemia (Knochenhauer et al., 1998). At the lower levels observed in PCOS women, tests for free or total testosterone have poor specificity and sensitivity. The optimal moment to test total testosterone levels is early in the morning, near the start of the follicular phase of the menstrual cycle. Mass spectrometric measurements of total testosterone may be more accurate than those made by other clinical assays (Rosner et al., 2007). The calculated free testosterone or free androgen index (FAI) [(total testosterone 100)/sex hormone-binding globulin (SHBG)] improves diagnostic precision even further. Under 6 FAI is regarded as abnormal. Androstenedione levels happen to be a more accurate indicator of androgen excess than levels of testosterone (O'Reilly et al., 2014). A study comprising of 86 PCOS women, who satisfied the Rotterdam criteria found that 88% had above the reference range of serum androstenedione concentrations and that 65% had elevated blood testosterone levels. Although PCOS hyperandrogenemia is mostly caused by the ovaries, 25–35% of these women also exhibit escalated levels of adrenal DHEA-S (Azziz et al., 2009; Huang et al., 2010; Rosenfield, 1999).

Hirsutism, androgenic alopecia, and acne are all clinical manifestations of hyperandrogenemia. Hirsutism is a much more severe symptom of hyperandrogenism than alopecia and acne. Hirsutism is described as an excess of terminal hair in females that grows in a masculine pattern (Figure 2). The FG scale is used to examine the growth of hair at various sites which are androgen sensitive. A lady is considered hirsute if she gets an 8 FG score or higher (Rosenfield, 2005). Understanding the FG score is made more challenging by racial and ethnic variances. Scores above 15 indicate moderate or severe hirsutism, whereas those between 8 and 15 indicate mild hirsutism. 60–76% of patients with PCOS are often hirsute, with an average score of 8–5 (Azziz et al., 2004; Shapiro, 2007). Hirsutism is caused by the interplay of the sensitivity of hair follicles to androgen and its levels (Rosenfield, 2005)

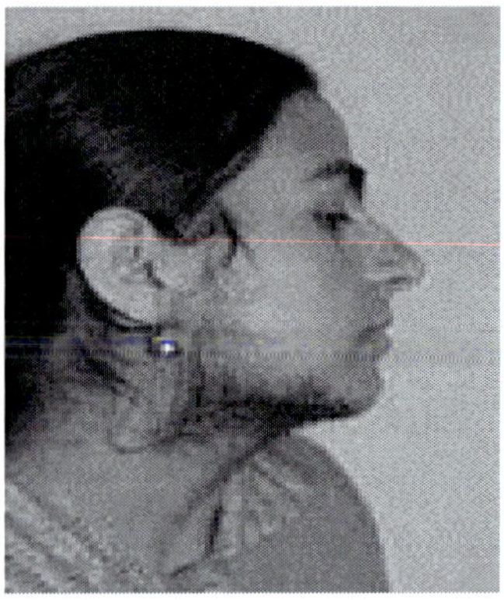

**Figure 2.** Facial Hirsutism (Clinical Hyperandrogenism).

## 5. Hyperandrogenemia and Hyperinsulinism

The fundamental PCOS pathophysiology is still a mystery. Physicians and scientists have disagreed over if the main event is caused by pituitary, ovarian, or hypothalamic origins rather than obesity and the associated hyperinsulinism. PCOS is distinguished by rising LH production and pulsatility of increased gonadotropin-releasing hormone (GnRH) (Haisenleder et al., 1991). The stimulation of several steroidogenic enzymes by LH leads to theca cell hyperplasia and the rising production of testosterone (Hughesdon, 1982). Due to a relative deficiency of FSH, the granulosa cells do not fully aromatize and degrade testosterone. A negative feedback loop in the hypothalamus that occurs as testosterone levels rise limits estradiol and progesterone's ability to diminish GnRH pulse frequency (Diamanti-Kandarakis & Dunaif, 2012). In PCOS, the ovaries do not seem to be the main abnormality, despite the fact that they may respond fast to gonadotropin secretion changes and ovulation happens as a result of the spike in FSH secretion induced by clomiphene citrate. Moreover, shedding pounds reduces insulin and estrone levels in obese individuals, normalizes gonadotropin output, and menstrual cycles are regulated in PCOS-affected females (Benito et al., 2020; McKenna, 1988).

The selective inhibitory effect of estrogen on FSH release, as well as a comparative lack of sensitivity of the release of FSH, explain the pathophysiology of PCOS, which may have its origins primarily at the pituitary level. According to the study, women who were postmenopausal and had PCOS had decreased levels of FSH, SHBG, and free androgen index (FAI) than controls who were similar to them in terms of weight, body mass index (BMI), and waist-to-hip ratio (WHR). LH, DHEA-S, androstenedione, total testosterone, estradiol, and estrone levels were comparable between the two groups (Pinola et al., 2015; Schmidt et al., 2011).

Also, the largest and most extensive association research of PCOS genotype discovered a favorable correlation between mutations in the FSH-beta gene region and a rise in the amount of circulating LH (Hayes et al., 2015). The primary issue in PCOS does not appear to be LH release, as there is proof of a positive feedback mechanism of estrogen on LH release and surge. (Rebar et al., 1976).

Another significant factor in PCOS patients is hyperinsulinemia, which is made worse by the buildup of visceral fat caused by hyperandrogenism (Diamanti-Kandarakis & Dunaif,

2012). Hyperinsulinemia stimulates the hypothalamic-pituitary-adrenal axis both peripherally and centrally, increasing the production of adrenal androgen. DHEA-S levels in PCOS women are related to IR (Barbieri et al., 1984; Brennan et al., 2009; Chan et al., 2005).In addition to increasing free testosterone levels, insulin, and testosterone block the synthesis of SHBG in the liver. As a result, testosterone reduces the sensitivity of the feedback effects of estradiol and progesterone on the hypothalamus and pituitary (Shapiro, 2007).

When the body is insulin resistant, it produces more of the hormone because it is less able to balance its effects on glucose metabolism. Fasting glucose, the homeostasis model assessment (HOMA), the oral glucose tolerance test (OGTT), the frequently sampled intravenous glucose tolerance test (FSIVGTT), and the euglycemic hyperinsulinemic clamp are all used to evaluate insulin sensitivity (Diamanti-Kandarakis & Dunaif, 2012). IR, deranged glucose tolerance, and T2D were found in 53%, 23-35%, and 4%-10% of PCOS women, respectively, according to the modified FSIVGTT. When compared to reproductively healthy control women of comparable age and weight, the rise in insulin responses during the OGTT was twice as large (Legro et al., 1998) (Diamanti-Kandarakis & Dunaif, 2012).

## 6. Psychological Aspects of Hirsutism

The effects of hirsutism, especially unwelcome facial hair, can be extensive. Some women only find it to be a minor annoyance, but other women may find it to be a serious source of distress. The whole emotional burden of undesired facial hair was revealed in a 2010 online study of 1000 UK women with the condition, who ranged in age from 18 to 72. According to the findings, unwanted facial hair had a substantial impact on self-esteem and women's emotional health: 98% of respondents expressed 8 negative feelings about their facial hair; 80% of women felt embarrassed; 90% said they would feel more confident without facial hair; 43% said their facial hair hampered their capability to make relationships; and 25% said their facial hair prevented them from applying for a job and its promotion.

## 7. Management of Hyperandrogenism

Direct hair removal techniques and medication treatments that block androgen synthesis and action can be used to treat hirsutism. A mechanical way of removing hair (plucking, shaving, and waxing) is suggested for mild hirsutism; if this does not work, pharmaceutical treatment (a combination of oral contraceptive tablets and antiandrogens) is added (Martin et al., 2018).

The standard treatment for PCOS to lower hyperandrogenism through several mechanisms is a combination of oral contraceptives. They boost the SBGH production of the liver, which raises androgen binding and lowers serum-free androgen concentrations, and decrease LH, so reducing ovarian androgen release (Fitzgerald et al., 1999). Furthermore, progesterone boosts testosterone clearance. The FG scores were reduced by 5-7 points for all combined oral contraceptives, and the hirsutism scores were practically as low as those of the non-hirsute control group (Porcile & Gallardo, 1991). After receiving therapy for at least six months, changes in hair thickness become apparent. If there is a poor response after six months, antiandrogen medication can be added (McCartney & Marshall, 2016). Also, there is proof that oral contraceptives help in alleviating the severity of acne in PCOS women (Mathur et al., 2008).

Spironolactone (5-reductase inhibitor), flutamide, and finasteride are all examples of antiandrogen therapies (androgen receptor antagonists). Daily doses of spironolactone 100 mg, finasteride 2.5–5 mg, and flutamide 500 mg reduce FG scores by 2–5 points and by 4 points on average and by 15–40% within 6 months of starting therapy, improving hirsutism ratings in comparison to placebo (Swiglo et al., 2008). The three antiandrogens were equally effective; nevertheless, spironolactone is frequently recommended because to its generally favorable safety profile.

Due to the risk of hepatotoxicity, flutamide is no longer a recommended alternative. After starting treatment, spironolactone's maximum effectiveness starts around 3 months later and lasts for another 12 months (Cumming et al., 1982). Spironolactone might somewhat lower levels of testosterone in the blood, which might help hirsutism gradually go away. Women taking antiandrogens have the risk of feminizing a male fetus; as a result, a trustworthy form of contraception must be employed (Cumming et al., 1982).

As was previously mentioned, in women with PCOS, less severe hirsutism is linked with lower insulin levels and lower androgen levels (Chang et al., 2005). Insulin-lowering medications and insulin sensitizers such as metformin and thiazolidinediones reduce blood testosterone levels by 20-25% in women with PCOS, they are no more successful than a placebo in treating hirsutism. Subgroup studies, however, showed that insulin sensitizers may be more advantageous and effective than a placebo in obese and overweight women treated for more than six months (Cosma et al., 2008; McCartney & Marshall, 2016).

Insulin levels fall as weight reduction occurs. In obese PCOS patients, losing at least 5% of body weight decreases androgen levels (total and free testosterone, FAI, and DHEA-S), raises SHBG, helps improve insulin sensitivity (OGTT, HOMA, fasting glucose, and insulin levels), and reduces hirsutism (Moran et al., 2009). These results are most evident following rapid weight loss, such as that which results from bariatric surgery. In one study, with a mean follow-up of 4 years, 29% of obese women with hirsutism had resolved after losing 35% of their body weight with gastric bypass (Christ & Falcone, 2018; Escobar-Morreale et al., 2005; Jamal et al., 2012).

## Conclusion

In a sizeable portion of hirsute women, PCOS is a highly prevalent and frequently underappreciated illness. It may be difficult to accurately assess hyperandrogenism biochemically due to a number of variables. The issues of which androgens should be tested, which assay techniques should be used, and how reference ranges should be established are prominent among them. The great overlap between results obtained from PCOS-affected women and controls, as well as the accessibility to and availability of high-quality assays, are also of current interest. Regarding clinical evaluation, the majority of PCOS patients exhibit clinical signs of hyperandrogenism, which are easy to detect and just call for trained, attentive doctors. Assessment is impacted by hirsutism medicinal and cosmetic treatments. A concurrent interdisciplinary and personalized therapy is necessary to treat complicated metabolic and hormonal abnormalities.

## Future Scope

Exploring new therapeutic targets to address hyperandrogenism in PCOS is another avenue for future research. This could involve investigating the efficacy of existing drugs targeting androgen production or action, as well as developing novel pharmacological agents that specifically address the excess androgens in PCOS.

Future research could also focus on identifying and validating new biomarkers that can aid in the diagnosis and assessment of hyperandrogenism in PCOS women. This could involve exploring genetic markers, epigenetic modifications, or specific hormone profiles that can provide more accurate and reliable diagnostic information.

## References

Amiri, M., Fallahzadeh, A., Sheidaei, A., Mahboobifard, F., & Ramezani Tehrani, F. (2022). Prevalence of idiopathic hirsutism: A systematic review and meta-analysis. *J Cosmet Dermatol*, *21*(4), 1419-1427. https://doi.org/10.1111/jocd.14313

Asunción, M., Calvo, R. M., San Millán, J. L., Sancho, J., Avila, S., & Escobar-Morreale, H. F. (2000). A prospective study of the prevalence of the polycystic ovary syndrome in unselected Caucasian women from Spain. *J Clin Endocrinol Metab*, *85*(7), 2434-2438. https://doi.org/10.1210/jcem.85.7.6682

Azziz, R., Carmina, E., Chen, Z., Dunaif, A., Laven, J. S., Legro, R. S., Lizneva, D., Natterson-Horowtiz, B., Teede, H. J., & Yildiz, B. O. (2016). Polycystic ovary syndrome. *Nat Rev Dis Primers*, *2*, 16057. https://doi.org/10.1038/nrdp.2016.57

Azziz, R., Carmina, E., Dewailly, D., Diamanti-Kandarakis, E., Escobar-Morreale, H. F., Futterweit, W., Janssen, O. E., Legro, R. S., Norman, R. J., & Taylor, A. E. (2009). Task Force on the Phenotype of the Polycystic Ovary Syndrome of The Androgen Excess and PCOS Society. The Androgen Excess and PCOS Society criteria for the polycystic ovary syndrome: the complete task force report. *Fertil Steril*, *91*(2), 456-488.

Azziz, R., Sanchez, L. A., Knochenhauer, E. S., Moran, C., Lazenby, J., Stephens, K. C., Taylor, K., & Boots, L. R. (2004). Androgen excess in women: experience with over 1000 consecutive patients. *J Clin Endocrinol Metab*, *89*(2), 453-462. https://doi.org/10.1210/jc.2003-031122

Barbieri, R. L., Makris, A., & Ryan, K. J. (1984). Insulin stimulates androgen accumulation in incubations of human ovarian stroma and theca. *Obstetrics and Gynecology*, *64*(3 Suppl), 73S-80S.

Benito, E., Gómez-Martin, J. M., Vega-Piñero, B., Priego, P., Galindo, J., Escobar-Morreale, H. F., & Botella-Carretero, J. I. (2020). Fertility and Pregnancy Outcomes in Women with Polycystic Ovary Syndrome Following Bariatric Surgery. *J Clin Endocrinol Metab*, *105*(9). https://doi.org/10.1210/clinem/dgaa439

Bolour, S., & Braunstein, G. (2005). Testosterone therapy in women: a review. *International journal of impotence research*, *17*(5), 399-408.

Brennan, K., Huang, A., & Azziz, R. (2009). Dehydroepiandrosterone sulfate and insulin resistance in patients with polycystic ovary syndrome. *Fertil Steril*, *91*(5), 1848-1852. https://doi.org/10.1016/j.fertnstert.2008.02.101

Burger, H. G. (2002). Androgen production in women. *Fertility and sterility*, *77*, 3-5.

Chan, O., Inouye, K., Akirav, E., Park, E., Riddell, M. C., Vranic, M., & Matthews, S. G. (2005). Insulin alone increases hypothalamo-pituitary-adrenal activity, and diabetes lowers peak stress responses. *Endocrinology*, *146*(3), 1382-1390. https://doi.org/10.1210/en.2004-0607

Chang, R. J., & Katz, S. E. (1999). Diagnosis of polycystic ovary syndrome. *Endocrinol Metab Clin North Am*, *28*(2), 397-408, vii. https://doi.org/10.1016/s0889-8529(05)70076-1

Chang, W. Y., Knochenhauer, E. S., Bartolucci, A. A., & Azziz, R. (2005). Phenotypic spectrum of polycystic ovary syndrome: clinical and biochemical characterization of the three major clinical subgroups. *Fertility and sterility*, *83*(6), 1717-1723.

Christ, J. P., & Falcone, T. (2018). Bariatric Surgery Improves Hyperandrogenism, Menstrual Irregularities, and Metabolic Dysfunction Among Women with Polycystic Ovary Syndrome (PCOS). *Obes Surg*, *28*(8), 2171-2177. https://doi.org/10.1007/s11695-018-3155-6

Cosma, M., Swiglo, B. A., Flynn, D. N., Kurtz, D. M., Labella, M. L., Mullan, R. J., Elamin, M. B., Erwin, P. J., & Montori, V. M. (2008). Clinical review: Insulin sensitizers for the treatment of hirsutism: a systematic review and metaanalyses of randomized controlled trials. *J Clin Endocrinol Metab*, *93*(4), 1135-1142. https://doi.org/10.1210/jc.2007-2429

Cumming, D. C., Yang, J. C., Rebar, R. W., & Yen, S. S. (1982). Treatment of hirsutism with spironolactone. *Jama*, *247*(9), 1295-1298.

Deplewski, D., & Rosenfield, R. L. (2000). Role of hormones in pilosebaceous unit development. *Endocr Rev*, *21*(4), 363-392. https://doi.org/10.1210/edrv.21.4.0404

Diamanti-Kandarakis, E., & Dunaif, A. (2012). Insulin resistance and the polycystic ovary syndrome revisited: an update on mechanisms and implications. *Endocr Rev*, *33*(6), 981-1030. https://doi.org/10.1210/er.2011-1034

Diamanti-Kandarakis, E., Kouli, C. R., Bergiele, A. T., Filandra, F. A., Tsianateli, T. C., Spina, G. G., Zapanti, E. D., & Bartzis, M. I. (1999). A survey of the polycystic ovary syndrome in the Greek island of Lesbos: hormonal and metabolic profile. *J Clin Endocrinol Metab*, *84*(11), 4006-4011. https://doi.org/10.1210/jcem.84.11.6148

Dunaif, A. (1997). Insulin resistance and the polycystic ovary syndrome: mechanism and implications for pathogenesis. *Endocr Rev*, *18*(6), 774-800. https://doi.org/10.1210/edrv.18.6.0318

Ehrmann, D. A. (2005). Polycystic ovary syndrome. *N Engl J Med*, *352*(12), 1223-1236. https://doi.org/10.1056/NEJMra041536

Escobar-Morreale, H. F., Botella-Carretero, J. I., Alvarez-Blasco, F., Sancho, J., & San Millán, J. L. (2005). The polycystic ovary syndrome associated with morbid obesity may resolve after weight loss induced by bariatric surgery. *J Clin Endocrinol Metab*, *90*(12), 6364-6369. https://doi.org/10.1210/jc.2005-1490

Escobar-Morreale, H. F., Carmina, E., Dewailly, D., Gambineri, A., Kelestimur, F., Moghetti, P., Pugeat, M., Qiao, J., Wijeyaratne, C. N., Witchel, S. F., & Norman, R. J. (2012). Epidemiology, diagnosis and management of hirsutism: a consensus statement by the Androgen Excess and Polycystic Ovary Syndrome Society. *Hum Reprod Update*, *18*(2), 146-170. https://doi.org/10.1093/humupd/dmr042

Ferriman, D., & Gallwey, J. D. (1961). Clinical assessment of body hair growth in women. *J Clin Endocrinol Metab*, *21*, 1440-1447. https://doi.org/10.1210/jcem-21-11-1440

Ferriman, D., & Purdie, A. W. (1983). The aetiology of oligomenorrhoea and/or hirsuties: a study of 467 patients. *Postgrad Med J*, *59*(687), 17-20. https://doi.org/10.1136/pgmj.59.687.17

Fitzgerald, C., Elstein, M., & Spona, J. (1999). Effect of age on the response of the hypothalamo-pituitary-ovarian axis to a combined oral contraceptive. *Fertility and sterility*, *71*(6), 1079-1084.

Gilchrist, V., & Hecht, B. (1995). A practical approach to hirsutism. *American family physician*, *52*(6), 1837-1846.

Goodarzi, M. O., Shah, N. A., Antoine, H. J., Pall, M., Guo, X., & Azziz, R. (2006). Variants in the 5alpha-reductase type 1 and type 2 genes are associated with polycystic ovary syndrome and the severity of hirsutism in affected women. *J Clin Endocrinol Metab*, *91*(10), 4085-4091. https://doi.org/10.1210/jc.2006-0227

Grymowicz, M., Rudnicka, E., Podfigurna, A., Napierala, P., Smolarczyk, R., Smolarczyk, K., & Meczekalski, B. (2020). Hormonal Effects on Hair Follicles. *Int J Mol Sci*, *21*(15). https://doi.org/10.3390/ijms21155342

Haisenleder, D. J., Dalkin, A. C., Ortolano, G. A., Marshall, J. C., & Shupnik, M. A. (1991). A pulsatile gonadotropin-releasing hormone stimulus is required to increase transcription of the gonadotropin subunit genes: evidence for differential regulation of transcription by pulse frequency in vivo. *Endocrinology*, *128*(1), 509-517. https://doi.org/10.1210/endo-128-1-509

Hamilton, J. B. (1951). Quantitative measurement of a secondary sex character, axillary hair. *Ann N Y Acad Sci*, *53*(3), 585-599. https://doi.org/10.1111/j.1749-6632.1951.tb31960.x

Hatch, R., Rosenfield, R. L., Kim, M. H., & Tredway, D. (1981). Hirsutism: implications, etiology, and management. *Am J Obstet Gynecol*, *140*(7), 815-830. https://doi.org/10.1016/0002-9378(81)90746-8

Hayes, M., Urbanek, M., Ehrmann, D., Armstrong, L., Lee, J., Sisk, R., Karaderi, T., Barber, T., McCarthy, M., & Franks, S. (2015). Reproductive Medicine Network. Genome-wide association of polycystic ovary syndrome implicates alterations in gonadotropin secretion in European ancestry populations. *Nat Commun*, *6*(1), 7502.

Heutling, D., Schulz, H., Randeva, H., Dodt, C., & Lehnert, H. (2007). Polycystic ovary syndrome. Prototype of a cardio-metabolic syndrome. *Internist (Berl)*, *48*(2), 144-153. https://doi.org/10.1007/s00108-006-1776-7 (Das polyzystische Ovarsyndrom. Prototyp eines kardiometabolischen Syndroms.)

Huang, A., Brennan, K., & Azziz, R. (2010). Prevalence of hyperandrogenemia in the polycystic ovary syndrome diagnosed by the National Institutes of Health 1990 criteria. *Fertility and sterility*, *93*(6), 1938-1941.

Hughesdon, P. E. (1982). Morphology and morphogenesis of the Stein-Leventhal ovary and of so-called "hyperthecosis". *Obstet Gynecol Surv*, *37*(2), 59-77. https://doi.org/10.1097/00006254-198202000-00001

Hunter, M. H., & Carek, P. J. (2003). Evaluation and treatment of women with hirsutism. *American family physician*, *67*(12), 2565-2572.

Jamal, M., Gunay, Y., Capper, A., Eid, A., Heitshusen, D., & Samuel, I. (2012). Roux-en-Y gastric bypass ameliorates polycystic ovary syndrome and dramatically improves conception rates: a 9-year analysis. *Surgery for Obesity and Related Diseases*, *8*(4), 440-444.

Jayasena, C. N., Alkaabi, F. M., Liebers, C. S., Handley, T., Franks, S., & Dhillo, W. S. (2019). A systematic review of randomized controlled trials investigating the efficacy and safety of testosterone therapy for female sexual dysfunction in postmenopausal women. *Clinical endocrinology*, *90*(3), 391-414.

Ji, S., Zhu, Z., Sun, X., & Fu, X. (2021). Functional hair follicle regeneration: an updated review. *Signal Transduct Target Ther*, *6*(1), 66. https://doi.org/10.1038/s41392-020-00441-y

Knochenhauer, E., Key, T., Kahsar-Miller, M., Waggoner, W., Boots, L., & Azziz, R. (1998). Prevalence of the polycystic ovary syndrome in unselected black and white women of the southeastern United States: a prospective study. *The Journal of Clinical Endocrinology & Metabolism*, *83*(9), 3078-3082.

Legro, R. S., Finegood, D., & Dunaif, A. (1998). A fasting glucose to insulin ratio is a useful measure of insulin sensitivity in women with polycystic ovary syndrome. *J Clin Endocrinol Metab*, *83*(8), 2694-2698. https://doi.org/10.1210/jcem.83.8.5054

Legro, R. S., Schlaff, W. D., Diamond, M. P., Coutifaris, C., Casson, P. R., Brzyski, R. G., Christman, G. M., Trussell, J. C., Krawetz, S. A., Snyder, P. J., Ohl, D., Carson, S. A., Steinkampf, M. P., Carr, B. R., McGovern, P. G., Cataldo, N. A., Gosman, G. G., Nestler, J. E., Myers, E. R., Santoro, N., Eisenberg, E., Zhang, M., & Zhang, H. (2010). Total testosterone assays in women with polycystic ovary syndrome: precision and correlation with hirsutism. *J Clin Endocrinol Metab*, *95*(12), 5305-5313. https://doi.org/10.1210/jc.2010-1123

Lin-Su, K., Nimkarn, S., & New, M. I. (2008). Congenital adrenal hyperplasia in adolescents: diagnosis and management. *Ann N Y Acad Sci*, *1135*, 95-98. https://doi.org/10.1196/annals.1429.021

Lin, X., Zhu, L., & He, J. (2022). Morphogenesis, Growth Cycle and Molecular Regulation of Hair Follicles. *Front Cell Dev Biol*, *10*, 899095. https://doi.org/10.3389/fcell.2022.899095

Longcope, C. (1986). 1 Adrenal and gonadal androgen secretion in normal females. *Clinics in endocrinology and metabolism*, *15*(2), 213-228.

Markopoulos, M. C., Kassi, E., Alexandraki, K. I., Mastorakos, G., & Kaltsas, G. (2015). Management of endocrine disease: hyperandrogenism after menopause. *European journal of endocrinology*, *172*(2), R79-R91.

Martin, K. A., Anderson, R. R., Chang, R. J., Ehrmann, D. A., Lobo, R. A., Murad, M. H., Pugeat, M. M., & Rosenfield, R. L. (2018). Evaluation and treatment of hirsutism in premenopausal women: an Endocrine Society clinical practice guideline. *The Journal of Clinical Endocrinology & Metabolism*, *103*(4), 1233-1257.

Mathur, R., Levin, O., & Azziz, R. (2008). Use of ethinylestradiol/drospirenone combination in patients with the polycystic ovary syndrome. *Therapeutics and clinical risk management*, *4*(2), 487-492.

McCartney, C. R., & Marshall, J. C. (2016). CLINICAL PRACTICE. Polycystic Ovary Syndrome. *N Engl J Med*, *375*(1), 54-64. https://doi.org/10.1056/NEJMcp1514916

McKenna, T. J. (1988). Pathogenesis and treatment of polycystic ovary syndrome. *N Engl J Med*, *318*(9), 558-562. https://doi.org/10.1056/nejm198803033180906

Mihailidis, J., Dermesropian, R., Taxel, P., Luthra, P., & Grant-Kels, J. M. (2017). Endocrine evaluation of hirsutism. *Int J Womens Dermatol*, *3*(1 Suppl), S6-s10. https://doi.org/10.1016/j.ijwd.2017.02.007

Moran, L. J., Pasquali, R., Teede, H. J., Hoeger, K. M., & Norman, R. J. (2009). Treatment of obesity in polycystic ovary syndrome: a position statement of the Androgen Excess and Polycystic Ovary Syndrome Society. *Fertil Steril*, *92*(6), 1966-1982. https://doi.org/10.1016/j.fertnstert.2008.09.018

O'Reilly, M. W., Taylor, A. E., Crabtree, N. J., Hughes, B. A., Capper, F., Crowley, R. K., Stewart, P. M., Tomlinson, J. W., & Arlt, W. (2014). Hyperandrogenemia predicts metabolic phenotype in polycystic ovary syndrome: the utility of serum androstenedione. *The journal of clinical endocrinology & metabolism*, *99*(3), 1027-1036.

Oliveira, I. O., Lhullier, C., Brum, I. S., & Spritzer, P. M. (2003). Gene expression of type 2 17 beta hydroxysteroid dehydrogenase in scalp hairs of hirsute women. *Steroids*, *68*(7-8), 641-649. https://doi.org/10.1016/s0039-128x(03)00093-x

Pasquali, R., Zanotti, L., Fanelli, F., Mezzullo, M., Fazzini, A., Morselli Labate, A. M., Repaci, A., Ribichini, D., & Gambineri, A. (2016). Defining hyperandrogenism in women with polycystic ovary syndrome: a challenging perspective. *The Journal of Clinical Endocrinology & Metabolism*, *101*(5), 2013-2022.

Paus, R., & Cotsarelis, G. (1999). The biology of hair follicles. *N Engl J Med*, *341*(7), 491-497. https://doi.org/10.1056/nejm199908123410706

Pinola, P., Piltonen, T. T., Puurunen, J., Vanky, E., Sundström-Poromaa, I., Stener-Victorin, E., Ruokonen, A., Puukka, K., Tapanainen, J. S., & Morin-Papunen, L. C. (2015). Androgen Profile Through Life in Women With Polycystic Ovary Syndrome: A Nordic Multicenter Collaboration Study. *J Clin Endocrinol Metab*, *100*(9), 3400-3407. https://doi.org/10.1210/jc.2015-2123

Porcile, A., & Gallardo, E. (1991). Long-term treatment of hirsutism: desogestrel compared with cyproterone acetate in oral contraceptives. *Fertility and sterility*, *55*(5), 877-881.

Randall, V. A. (2008). Androgens and hair growth. *Dermatol Ther*, *21*(5), 314-328. https://doi.org/10.1111/j.1529-8019.2008.00214.x

Rebar, R., Judd, H. L., Yen, S. S., Rakoff, J., Vandenberg, G., & Naftolin, F. (1976). Characterization of the inappropriate gonadotropin secretion in polycystic ovary syndrome. *J Clin Invest*, *57*(5), 1320-1329. https://doi.org/10.1172/jci108400

Rosenfield, R. L. (1999). Ovarian and adrenal function in polycystic ovary syndrome. *Endocrinology and metabolism clinics of North America*, *28*(2), 265-293.

Rosenfield, R. L. (2005). Clinical practice. Hirsutism. *N Engl J Med*, *353*(24), 2578-2588. https://doi.org/10.1056/NEJMcp033496

Rosner, W., Auchus, R. J., Azziz, R., Sluss, P. M., & Raff, H. (2007). Utility, limitations, and pitfalls in measuring testosterone: an Endocrine Society position statement. *The Journal of Clinical Endocrinology & Metabolism*, *92*(2), 405-413.

Schmidt, J., Brännström, M., Landin-Wilhelmsen, K., & Dahlgren, E. (2011). Reproductive hormone levels and anthropometry in postmenopausal women with polycystic ovary syndrome (PCOS): a 21-year follow-up study of women diagnosed with PCOS around 50 years ago and their age-matched controls. *J Clin Endocrinol Metab*, *96*(7), 2178-2185. https://doi.org/10.1210/jc.2010-2959

Schmidt, J. B., Lindmaier, A., & Spona, J. (1991). Hyperprolactinemia and hypophyseal hypothyroidism as cofactors in hirsutism and androgen-induced alopecia in women. *Hautarzt*, *42*(3), 168-172. (Hyperprolaktinämie und hypophysäre Hypothyreose als Kofaktoren bei Hirsutismus und androgenem Haarausfall der Frau.)

Shapiro, J. (2007). Clinical practice. Hair loss in women. *N Engl J Med*, *357*(16), 1620-1630. https://doi.org/10.1056/NEJMcp072110

Spritzer, P. M., Barone, C. R., & Oliveira, F. B. (2016). Hirsutism in Polycystic Ovary Syndrome: Pathophysiology and Management. *Curr Pharm Des*, *22*(36), 5603-5613. https://doi.org/10.2174/1381612822666160720151243

Swiglo, B. A., Cosma, M., Flynn, D. N., Kurtz, D. M., Labella, M. L., Mullan, R. J., Erwin, P. J., & Montori, V. M. (2008). Clinical review: Antiandrogens for the treatment of hirsutism: a systematic review and metaanalyses of randomized controlled trials. *J Clin Endocrinol Metab*, *93*(4), 1153-1160. https://doi.org/10.1210/jc.2007-2430

Taheri, S., Zararsiz, G., Karaburgu, S., Borlu, M., Ozgun, M. T., Karaca, Z., Tanriverdi, F., Dundar, M., Kelestimur, F., & Unluhizarci, K. (2015). Is idiopathic hirsutism (IH) really idiopathic? mRNA expressions of skin steroidogenic enzymes in women with IH. *Eur J Endocrinol*, *173*(4), 447-454. https://doi.org/10.1530/eje-15-0460

Teede, H. J., Misso, M. L., Costello, M. F., Dokras, A., Laven, J., Moran, L., Piltonen, T., & Norman, R. J. (2018). Recommendations from the international evidence-based guideline for the assessment and management of polycystic ovary syndrome. *Clin Endocrinol (Oxf)*, *89*(3), 251-268. https://doi.org/10.1111/cen.13795

Wild, R. A., Vesely, S., Beebe, L., Whitsett, T., & Owen, W. (2005). Ferriman Gallwey self-scoring I: performance assessment in women with polycystic ovary syndrome. *J Clin Endocrinol Metab*, *90*(7), 4112-4114. https://doi.org/10.1210/jc.2004-2243

Yang, M., Weng, T., Zhang, W., Zhang, M., He, X., Han, C., & Wang, X. (2021). The Roles of Non-coding RNA in the Development and Regeneration of Hair Follicles: Current Status and Further Perspectives. *Front Cell Dev Biol*, *9*, 720879. https://doi.org/10.3389/fcell.2021.720879

Yildiz, B. O., Bolour, S., Woods, K., Moore, A., & Azziz, R. (2010). Visually scoring hirsutism. *Hum Reprod Update*, *16*(1), 51-64. https://doi.org/10.1093/humupd/dmp024

# Chapter 4

# PCOS and Circadian Rhythm: The Imbalance and Impact of the Melatonin Hormone

**Nihad Ashraf Khan[1,*]**
**Sagnik Das[2]**
**Vitasta Jad[3]**
**and Namrata Seth[4]**
[1]Department of Biosciences, Faculty of Natural Science, Jamia Millia Islamia, Delhi, India
[2]Department of Environmental Studies, University of Delhi, New Delhi, India
[3]Department of Marine Biotechnology, University of Goa, Goa, India
[4]Department of Biotechnology, Indian Institute of Science and Technology, Bhopal, India

## Abstract

Melatonin is an indoleamine that serves as the primary hormone produced by the pineal gland for the regulation of circadian rhythm. It also plays a role in regulating various endocrine hormones associated with polycystic ovarian syndrome (PCOS). PCOS is characterized by several symptoms such as hyperandrogenism, insulin resistance (IR), obesity, menstrual irregularities, and anovulation. Maintaining the normal functioning of the female reproductive cycle involves various endocrine hormones such as luteinizing hormone, follicle-stimulating hormone, androgens, and progesterone. Imbalances in these hormones have been linked to the onset of PCOS in reproductively mature women. Melatonin is considered a key regulator of these hormones in PCOS conditions. Melatonin receptors present in the ovary and intra-follicular fluid bind with melatonin hormone, which leads to ovarian follicular maturation and protects ovarian follicles from oxidative stress via anti-oxidative activities. Women with PCOS often exhibit an increased imbalance of melatonin hormone, resulting in sleep disturbances and abnormal sleep architecture. Melatonin's ability to act as an antioxidant and free-radical agent makes it a valuable addition to assisted reproductive techniques (ART). The exogenous administration of synthetic melatonin in women with PCOS could potentially mitigate the adverse effects of PCOS and regulate the endocrine hormones. However, the detailed relationship between circulating levels of melatonin, biomarkers of oxidative stress, and sleep quality in women with PCOS remains unclear.

---

* Corresponding Author's Email: nihadashraf5@gmail.com.

In: Polycystic Ovarian Syndrome (PCOS) and Our Biological Clock
Editors: Arpita Roy, Gowhar Rashid and Nihad Ashraf Khan
ISBN: 979-8-89113-100-2
© 2023 Nova Science Publishers, Inc.

**Keywords:** melatonin hormone, circadian rhythm, polycystic ovarian syndrome, hyperandrogenism, insulin resistance, obesity, menstrual irregularities

## 1. Introduction

Melatonin hormone, tryptophan-derived indoleamine, proficient in free radical scavenging is synthesized by a neuroendocrine organ known as the pineal gland. A master pacemaker, the hypothalamic suprachiasmatic nucleus (SCN) governs the synthesis of melatonin hormone. The production and synthesis of melatonin hormone are tightly linked with the light/dark cycle therefore, its duration and production are dependent on the length of the night. Significantly, the production of melatonin is blocked due to light at night, mediated by the retinal melanopsinergic system coupled with a complex neural system that is responsible for the inhibition of the sympathetic projection to the pineal gland (Cipolla-Neto and do Amaral 2018). The imperative role of melatonin involves synchronization by the light/dark cycle thus, nocturnal photoinhibition helps to synchronize an organism's internal temporal order to the external light/dark environment and helps to regulate the sleep cycle.

Sleep which is an essential component is mainly regulated by the melatonin hormone. Disruption in the sleep cycle or circadian rhythm leads to several health ailments such as diabetes, PCOS, cardiovascular disease, neurodegenerative disorders, etc. The regulation and governing of circadian rhythm, a sleep-wake cycle is mediated by the melatonin hormone that plays a prominent role in the manifestation of PCOS in reproductively mature women when dysregulated (Vasey, McBride, and Penta 2021). Polycystic ovarian syndrome (PCOS) is a heterogeneous endocrine disorder affecting mainly females of reproductive age. PCOS is characterized by anovulation, infertility, hyperandrogenism, insulin resistance, obesity, and cardiovascular problems (Patel 2018). Dysregulation in reproductive hormones such as increased LH: FSH ratio and increased androgen levels are responsible for causing PCOS whereas melatonin hormone, a sleep-regulating hormone also exhibits an essential role in synchronizing reproductive hormones in women. Hence, the disruption of the melatonin hormone has a direct link with the manifestation of PCOS in reproductively mature women (Cipolla-Neto and do Amaral 2018). Disruption in melatonin rhythm has been reported in women with PCOS and its concentration along with other metabolites can be found in the serum and urine of PCOS women (F. Wang et al., 2021).

Mammalian ovaries are the main site for follicular development which displays robust circadian rhythms significantly coordinated by light and endocrine signals. CLOCK and BMAL1 and STAR (steroidogenic acute regulatory protein) along with peroxisome proliferator-activated receptor gamma coactivator 1-alpha regarded as clock genes are involved in ovary-specific rhythms and hence, are regulated in the ovary (F. Wang et al. 2021). Interestingly, a shift from the study of melatonin secretion in cancer development and neurodegenerative disease toward reproductive disorders shows a positive correlation between melatonin secretion and clock gene expression in the development of PCOS. The decrease in the per1 and per2 levels is associated with the development of PCOS whereas decreased expression of clock genes mediates the increase in androgen levels leading to hyperandrogenism and insulin resistance (Brzezinski et al., 2021). Thus, irregular sleeping patterns and changing lifestyles correspond to disruption in circadian rhythm therefore, abnormal secretion of reproductive and gonadotropin hormones regulated due to dysregulation in the expression of clock genes and melatonin secretion is predominantly associated with the pathological features of PCOS in reproductively mature women (Brzezinski et al., 2021)

Significantly, restoration of disrupted circadian rhythm under the effect of melatonin in ovarian cells of PCOS patients has been investigated with successful results. Thus, the melatonin hormone, a rhythm synchronizer regulates the central and peripheral clock genes. Additionally, melatonin has been reported to have a direct and immediate local effect in the ovary due to the presence of melatonin receptors in the human granulosa cell membrane therefore, it can be possibly used in ART (Assisted reproductive technology) to treat PCOS in reproductively aged women.

## 2. PCOS and Circadian Rhythm

### 2.1. Clock Genes

Several endogenous and exogenous factors are responsible for the rhythmic variations in maintaining physiological and behavioral processes. Clock and biological pacemakers contribute to the endogenous factors that are capable of maintaining strong self-sustaining periodic rhythms even in the absence of external stimuli. The biological clock with an endogenous period of 24-h known as a circadian clock has been documented from a prokaryotic cell to a multi-cellular eukaryotic cell to complex organisms such as flies, humans, and rodents (Piggins 2009) The arrhythmic circadian clock is responsible for reproductive dysfunction and several other underlying metabolic disorders whereas their involvement in polycystic ovarian syndrome (PCOS) is less understood (S. Li et al., 2020). The dysfunction of circadian rhythm and poorer sleep has been reported in women with PCOS thereby, portraying circadian rhythm and proper sleep as one of the targets of treatment (Simon et al. 2019). Several prominent biological clock genes identified play a critical role in regulating and modulating the circadian rhythm. BMAL1, a biological clock gene is significantly downregulated in granulosa cells of PCOS patients when compared with the non-PCOS group whereas nuclear receptors REV-ERBα and REV-ERBβ are key circadian rhythm regulators responsible for inhibiting apoptosis in granulosa cells and promotes proliferation (L. Sun et al., 2021). The core clock genes associated with PCOS are CLOCK and PER1/2 genes which show a close interaction with reproduction in women. Dysfunction in the Bmal1 gene impairs hormone synthesis and causes apoptosis in porcine granulosa cells whereas normal functioning of BMAL1 and SIRT1 is essential for the normal development of follicles and biosynthesis of estrogen (Brzezinski et al., 2021). Li et al. noticed a reduction in Bmal1, per1, and per 2 in constant darkness that leads to PCOS. Interestingly, Per1 and Per 2 clock genes are responsible for the optimum surge of LH, associated with ovulation in ovaries and Bmal1 is responsible for maintaining the androgen levels therefore, decreased expression leads to hyperandrogenism in PCOS women (S. Li et al., 2020). Additionally, decreased expression of ARNT-like protein 1 has also been reported which contributes to hyperandrogenism and insulin resistance in PCOS women (Zhai et al., 2020).

Changing lifestyle and irregular sleeping pattern has a direct influence on the circadian rhythm and disruption of the normal functioning of clock genes that explain some of the basic pathologies associated with PCOS. Hence, exogenous administration of melatonin messenger would play a critical role in restoring the circadian rhythm (Tamura et al., 2009).

## 2.2. Melatonin as an Anti-Oxidant

Oxidative stress is a significant factor in various disorders of the female reproductive system, including infertility, PCOS, and endometriosis. Research indicates that women with PCOS have a higher level of oxidative stress compared to healthy women. Furthermore, prolonged exposure to light has been linked to the development of PCOS, which can increase levels of lipid peroxidation, pro-oxidant enzymes, and pro-inflammatory cytokines, leading to higher oxidative stress. However, melatonin, a hormone produced by the pineal gland, can act as an antioxidant and inhibit pro-oxidant enzymes, thus promoting a healthy female reproductive system. (Mojaverrostami, Asghari, Khamisabadi, and Heidari Khoei 2019).

Melatonin hormone an effective anti-oxidant directs the free radical scavenging and activates a series of scavenging mechanisms which include transcription and activation of anti-oxidative enzymes. Melatonin also plays an important role in protecting lipids, proteins, and DNA from oxidative damage. Due to cellular respiration free radicals are formed in abundance in mitochondria. Thus, the higher concentration of melatonin in mitochondria helps in scavenging these free radicals and plays a critical role in various mitochondrial functions (Cipolla-Neto and do Amaral 2018). Therefore, melatonin has been regarded as a delaying ovarian aging hormone that significantly reduces the mRNA levels of LC3a and LC3b in melatonin-treated aged mice (Tamura et al., 2017). The degradation of mitochondrial function with age affects the ovarian reserves and triggers ovarian. Hence, the effect of melatonin on mitochondrial membrane potential via the MT1/AMPK pathway *in vitro* has been proven to reduce ROS levels (L. Zhang et al. 2019). Interestingly, melatonin has also demonstrated a reverse in the meiosis-deficient phenotype in aged mice via SIRT1/SOD2, a major antioxidant enzyme in oocytes (M. Zhang et al., 2020). Furthermore, melatonin can effectively reduce mitochondrial oxidative damage via SIRT3/FOZO3a pathway (Song et al., 2016).

Reports show that women with PCOS have higher levels of lipid peroxides in their serum and follicular fluid (FF), leading to an abundance of MDA. MDA can be responsible for DNA damage and apoptosis in oocytes. Increased oxidative stress is also linked to spindle disorders, organelle degeneration, cytoplasmic heterogeneity, and reduced mitochondrial function in oocytes, ultimately leading to poorer fertilization rates, lower high-quality blastocyst rates, and worse pregnancy outcomes. The concentration of melatonin in FF plays a crucial role in maintaining oxidative stress homeostasis and preventing follicular damage. When melatonin concentration is lower, oocyte quality can be negatively impacted, leading to difficulties in ovulation (Yang et al., 2018).

Additionally, melatonin could potentially induce the synthesis of certain enzymes which helps in the conversion of reactive oxygen species (ROS) into harmless molecules and could also potentially induce the synthesis of other endogenous antioxidants such as SOD, GPX, and glutathione reductase. The production of a large amount of ROS during ovulation thus affects the quality of an oocyte which can be quenched by melatonin and its metabolites thereby, inducing the expression of SOD and GPX (Korkmaz, Rosales-Corral, and Reiter 2012).

# 3. The Trilogy of Androgens, Insulin, and Melatonin in PCOS

Polycystic Ovarian Syndrome (PCOS) is a disorder characterized by hyperandrogenism, insulin resistance and related compensatory hyperinsulinemia, obesity, anovulation, oligoovulation, polycystic ovarian morphology, and ovulatory dysfunction (Bogari 2020; Jain et al., 2022) owes its existence to an array of hormonal interplay, their imbalances, and cascades of biochemical and cytological interactions. Though such characteristics are intricately associated with PCOS yet not all of them are well pronounced in terms of their manifestation among PCOS patients owing to the existence of PCOS phenotypes. Therefore, in 1990 NIH listed oligo/anovulation, hyperandrogenism, and ovulatory dysfunction as the chief diagnostic criteria but later adopted the Rotterdam criteria in 2003 necessitating the presence of any 2/3 criteria for diagnosis (Jain et al., 2022). This hormonal imbalance-induced ailment could further accelerate a lot of co-morbidities such as cardiovascular diseases like atherosclerosis, renal disorders (Ye et al., 2021), metabolic disorders such as Type II Diabetes Mellitus (T2DM) (Bogari 2020), reproductive failure (Yang et al., 2018), etc. all these ailments are consciously interconnected to either of the phenomena namely insulin resistance (IR), Hyperandrogenism (HA) and/or Obesity. And three of these operate among themselves in an extremely complex yet intriguing manner thereby alternatively assuming the domains of cause and effect. Sleep and circadian rhythm-associated hormone melatonin (Shreeve et al., 2013), glucose metabolism hormone insulin (Maqbool et al., 2019), and male sex hormone testosterone (Ye et al., 2021) are primary players in the endocrinological phenomena and their related effects in PCOS because of the crossovers of signaling pathways.

### 3.1. Insulin Resistance (IR) and Hyperinsulinemia

Insulin resistance is the phenomenon by which there is a disruption in the sensitivity of the insulin receptors of the peripheral tissues as a result of which the blood insulin levels surge given that there is lower glucose uptake further leading to compensatory hyperinsulinemia. The lay explanation of this condition is that there exists an incompatibility between the key i.e., insulin, and the lock i.e., the receptor thereby increasing the overall blood insulin and glucose levels which subsequently entrains the receptor to be resistant to insulin thereby aggravating IR and hyperinsulinemia and could further lead to metabolic disorders such as T2DM (Maqbool et al., 2019). Insulin resistance can usher disorders like PCOS, acanthosis nigricans, T2DM (Maqbool et al., 2019), atherosclerosis, obesity, HA (Baptiste et al., 2010), etc., and lead to an array of secondary disorders as well. IR with or without the presence of compensatory hyperinsulinemia (Spinedi and Cardinali 2018) marks its presence in the case of PCOS though it is not characteristic of all the phenotypes (Jain et al., 2022).

IR especially in the case of PCOS can be caused by

- Defects in Insulin-receptor signaling (Baptiste et al., 2010)
- Hyperandrogenism (J. Wang et al., 2019)
- Obesity (Glueck and Goldenberg 2019)
- Oxidative stress (Farid and Diamanti-Kandarakis 2009)
- Alterations in the expression of Clock gene Bmal-1 (Brzezinski et al., 2021)

The cell receptor for insulin comprises two sub-units namely, α and β connected by a disulfide bond, and tyrosine phosphorylation is initiated when a ligand binds to the subunit β generating intrinsic tyrosine activity (since the subunit β is intracellular) (Xu and Qiao 2022). Any alterations in the biochemical morphology can disable insulin receptor binding. Most of the studies on ovarian, muscle, and adipocyte tissues suggested discrepancies in the post-binding signaling pathway as the underlying factor in causing IR which mostly include the early steps in insulin signaling (maximal rate of glucose uptake, the abundance of GLUT4, inhibition of lipolysis stimulated by insulin). Further studies on the skeletal muscle of obese PCOS women demonstrated impaired insulin signaling involving Akt and AS160 leading to decreased insulin action on peripheral glucose metabolism. Akt acts as a mediator in glucose transport and insulin-stimulated GLUT4 translocation (Baptiste et al., 2010). Further serine phosphorylation of the receptors owing to intrinsic or extrinsic factors could degrade the efficiency of the receptors (J. Wang et al., 2019). Free fatty acids such as diacylglycerols and ceramides may activate intracellular serine/threonine kinases and protein phosphatases in the cell thereby causing IR in peripheral muscles. It could be one of the factors for serine phosphorylation (Zeng et al., 2020) operating by inducing P450c17 activity (Baptiste et al., 2010). Excess free fatty acids can further deactivate enzymes such as pyruvate dehydrogenase thereby decreasing glucose transport activity and uptake by reducing insulin sensitivity in cells (J. Wang et al., 2019). In the case of PCOS, there is an overall decrease of about 30-40% in insulin sensitivity (Baptiste et al., 2010). Apart from defective insulin-receptor signaling pathways affecting insulin uptake in adipocytes and skeletal muscles, some studies have also pointed to glucose-stimulated insulin release by β-cells thereby suggesting defects in β-cell functioning contributing to hyperinsulinemia.

Testosterone can inhibit the proliferation and differentiation of cells into mature adipocytes and also inhibit glucose uptake in cells thereby contributing to IR (Spinedi and Cardinali 2018). HA can interfere with the expression of GLUT-4 which inhibits insulin degradation by the liver (J. Wang et al., 2019). IR is a multigenetic phenomenon (Bogari 2020) involving crossovers with pathways of melatonin and circadian rhythm signaling (Owino et al., 2019). IR can also be aggravated by factors such as increased cortisol levels that could induce adipocyte differentiation thereby increasing visceral adipocyte concentrations (J. Wang et al., 2019).

This phenomenon is more pronounced in the case of obese women since intra-abdominal fat tissue undergoes greater lipolysis thereby releasing a greater quantity of free fatty acid in the circulation that aggravates IR (Baptiste et al., 2010). IR on the other hand can cause Leptin resistance and decrease adiponectin levels (Guan et al. 2022) thereby lowering fatty acid oxidation and inducing lipotoxicity (Baptiste et al., 2010). Studies on PCOS patients pointed to higher gene expression levels of CD11c (ITGAX) and tumor necrosis factor-alpha (TNFα) which may aggravate the development of IR in women with PCOS (J. Wang et al., 2019). Higher blood levels of Insulin can induce increased androgen production by lowering Sex hormone Binding Globulin (SHBG) in the liver and further IR (Xu and Qiao 2022). Apart from this in the case of obese people, SHBG is substantially low (Baptiste et al., 2010) thereby increasing levels of free androgen in circulation. In the case of women, testosterone promotes lipogenesis and inhibits lipolysis (Glueck and Goldenberg 2019), especially in visceral adipocytes which may thereby promote increased IR by the excess release of free fatty acid and related mechanisms. Obesity and body muscle mass also affect Insulin sensitivity (Maqbool et al., 2019).

### 3.2. Hyperandrogenism

Hyperandrogenism is the increased levels of androgen in circulation manifested by acne, hirsutism, or frontal alopecia. About 60% of the androgen production in PCOS patients is accounted for by the ovaries and 40% by the adrenal glands. Suppression of one source of production aggravates the production by the other (Baptiste et al., 2010). Apart from clinical hyperandrogenism, two androgen markers namely- serum total testosterone and Free Androgen Index (FAI) are often used in PCOS diagnosis. Though HA is one of the necessary features for PCOS diagnosis as per Rotterdam Criteria 2003, there is a benchmark quantitative value for the diagnosis of the same owing to demographic heterogeneity. It is also poorly related in the case of Asians (Jain et al., 2022).

HA may be caused due to

- Genetic mutations/polymorphisms (J. Wang et al., 2019)
- Defects in androgen synthesis pathways (Baptiste et al., 2010)
- Hyperinsulinemia and IR (Maqbool et al., 2019)
- Obesity (Zeng et al., 2020)

According to Wang et. al. (J. Wang et al., 2019) CAG repeat polymorphisms in the AR gene, PDE8A, the SNP rs3797297 from 121 follistatin (FST) gene could contribute to HA. HA is also associated with decreased expression of the Bmal1 gene (clock gene). (Brzezinski et al. 2021). Androgen synthesis in the theca cells of the ovary can occur through various pathways, including the GPCR/cAMP/PKA pathway, the PI3K/AKT pathway, the MAPK signal pathway, and the Wnt signal pathway (Baptiste et al., 2010), Overactivated PI3K/AKT signals mediated by LH could lead to androgen excess and ovarian dysfunction that could induce/aggravate IR and PCOS. CYP17A1 an important enzyme in androgen synthesis (and highly produced in cases of PCOS) and 17α-hydroxylase are also involved in insulin-induced testosterone biosynthesis in theca cells through PI3K pathway and the coactivation of the cAMP signaling. ERK1/2 a sub-type of MAPK signal pathway is highly involved in androgen and estrogen metabolism and defects in the same could lead to the production of excess androgen (Ye et al., 2021).

Insulin can directly stimulate the hypothalamus and pituitary gland to synthesize defective levels of gonadotropin (Zeng et al., 2020; Maqbool et al., 2019) or act as a cofactor in ACTH-mediated androgen production by altering the sensitivity of the adrenal glands to ACTH. Insulin has also been demonstrated to synergistically collaborate with LH in exacerbating steroidogenesis by increased P450c17 activity (Baptiste et al., 2010) in the theca and granulosa cells of the ovary (Maqbool et al., 2019). Also, IR may directly increase CYP17A1 activity (by PI3K pathway (Ye et al., 2021)) in the theca cells thereby enhancing androstenedione and testosterone production and contributing to HA (Zeng et al., 2020). SHBG and IR are negatively related (Baptiste et al., 2010) since increased levels of insulin inhibit SHBG synthesis which in turn results in increased free androgen in circulation thereby causing hyperandrogenemia (Xu and Qiao 2022) which manifests in the form of acne, alopecia, and hirsutism (Bulsara et al., 2021).

Obesity especially visceral adiposity is known to contribute significantly to HA with a positive correlation between Visceral Adipose Tissue and total androgen levels. In this regard, the relative abundance of free fatty acids in the case of PCOS patients can induce IR (Zeng et al., 2020) which in turn induces HA. Furthermore, leptin and adiponectin produced by adipose tissue regulate androgen levels. Leptin often known as the satiety hormone (Jain et al. 2022) is encoded by the obesity gene. In Granulosa cells of PCOS patients, High leptin concentrations inhibit aromatase mRNA expression thereby disabling the conversion of androgen to estrogen and promoting HA (Zeng et al., 2020). Leptin resistance (common in obesity) (Jain et al., 2022) and reduced adiponectin levels induced by IR may reduce fatty acid oxidation and promote lipo-toxicity thereby exacerbating HA. Apart from this, obese women with PCOS have any way reported lower SHBG levels (Baptiste et al., 2010).

### 3.3. Obesity and Type II Diabetes Meletus (T2DM)

Obesity is a central factor in PCOS although phenotypes with lean women suffering from PCOS are existent (Jain et al., 2022). Obesity is associated with the abnormal functioning of the Hypothalamus-pituitary-ovarian axis in terms of PCOS. Though a myriad of factors is responsible for obesity yet dysfunctional insulin-receptor signaling pathways and hyperandrogenism are the primary causal factors in the case of PCOS. Impaired insulin-stimulated glucose transport in the subcutaneous adipocytes of PCOS patients owing to decreased expression of GLUT-4 and impaired insulin-stimulated phosphorylation of IRS-1 are factors contributing to obesity (Farid and Diamanti-Kandarakis 2009).

Androgens induce abdominal adipose accumulation thereby causing adipose tissue dysfunction as Testosterone based impaired phosphorylation of protein kinase C inhibits insulin-stimulated glucose uptake in adipocytes, which is a primary factor in the case of obesity (Zeng et al., 2020). Despite the enigmatic interaction between androgen and female adipocytes, some studies indicate that androgens in collaboration with overactivated CMKLR1 signaling could simultaneously activate APOBEC3b (apolipoprotein B mRNA editing enzyme catalytic subunit 3B), CCNA2 (cyclin A2) and PRC1 (protein regulator of cytokinesis 1) ushering proliferation of visceral preadipocytes and lipid accumulation. Further local activation of androgen in adipocytes could induce fat mass expansion (Ye et al., 2021). Testosterone inhibits adipocyte maturation, and cell differentiation and reduces glucose uptake in adipocytes. But despite restricting adipogenesis, it causes hypertrophic expansion of White Adipose Tissue by enlargement of individual cell size that in turn produces adipocytokines like TNF-α that can cause IR which could induce further lipid accumulation as discussed earlier (Spinedi and Cardinali 2018).

Type 2 Diabetes Mellitus (T2DM), a metabolic disorder associated with PCOS owes its existence to IR, HA, and Obesity. HA (Rodriguez Paris and Bertoldo 2019) and Obesity can induce impaired glucose tolerance which can directly or indirectly contribute to T2DM (Bogari 2020); (Bulsara et al., 2021); (Glueck and Goldenberg 2019). About 30-40% of PCOS women have impaired glucose tolerance with 10% of them susceptible to T2DM (Jain et al. 2022). A positive correlation between glycosylated hemoglobin (HbA1c), serum insulin levels, and free androgen and a negative correlation of free androgen with insulin sensitivity and β-cell function is suggestive of an intimate relationship between T2DM and PCOS (Ye et al.,2021).

### 3.4. The Crossover of Pathways: Melatonin in IR, HA, and Obesity

Melatonin marks its presence throughout the body with its receptors MT1 and MT2 which are associated with several metabolic disorders such as Type 2 Diabetes Mellitus (T2DM), gestational diabetes mellitus (GDM), and obesity. Melatonin concentration is elevated in ovarian cells vis-à-vis plasma in the case of non-PCOS patients (Jain et al. 2022) thereby paving its therapeutic role in and association with PCOS (Mojaverrostami, Asghari, Khamisabadi, and Khoei 2019). Studies have laid special emphasis on the gene MTNR1B that encodes MT2 (Owino et al., 2019).

Several pinealectomy studies have demonstrated Glucose intolerance (GI) and IR owing to the absence of melatonin thereby revealing the involvement of melatonin in IR, T2DM, and Hyperinsulinemia since the administration of exogenous melatonin reversed the effects. Two prominent variants of MTNR1B - SNPs rs1387153 and rs10830963 have exhibited their role in the modulation of pancreatic β-cells for insulin secretion (Owino et al., 2019). Also, polymorphism in MT1 encoding gene MTNR1A - rs2119882 is said to have a role in PCOS pathogenesis (Spinedi and Cardinali 2018). Knocking out of MT1 in mice displayed impaired glucose uptake in adipose tissue and skeletal muscle along with reduced liver insulin sensitivity which is postulated to be mediated by aberrations in phosphatidylinositol-3-kinase (PI3K)-protein kinase B (AKT) pathways which are also involved in androgen synthesis (Owino et al. 2019). The necessity of melatonin in PI3K-AKT activity is now established (Guan et al. 2022). Melatonin through IRS1/PI-3-kinase pathway can also stimulate glucose transport in skeletal muscles and can sensitize β-cells through cAMP signaling owing to the presence of MT1 and MT2 on β-cells. There is evidence of inhibition of cAMP-stimulated insulin-secretion and cGMP-stimulated insulin-secretion by melatonin mediated through MT1 and MT2 respectively (Espino 2011) along with the downstream Ras-associated factor-1 (Raf-1)-extracellular signal-regulated kinase (ERK) signaling pathway (Guan et al. 2022). It can also trigger insulin release by inducing $Ca^{2+}$ from intracellular storage (Espino 2011) and interacts with pancreatic α-cells for glucagon (Guan et al. 2022) secretion highlighting its role in IR and obesity. Studies have also reported increased insulin receptor substrate 1 (IRS1) phosphorylation by melatonin-enhanced insulin receptor kinase activity, revealing the potential existence of melatonin and insulin crosstalk. Insulin and Melatonin interact antagonistically during the day and night since insulin levels elevate and melatonin levels lower during the day while it works the other way at night (Espino 2011). Disruption of the same can induce IR and T2DM (McMullan et al. 2013) through MT1 (Guan et al., 2022).

Studies have demonstrated Testosterone and estrogen regulates melatonin levels in the body (Mojaverrostami et al., 2019) by modulating steroidogenesis. Melatonin may modulate Steroidogenesis by inhibiting the expression of steroidogenic acute regulatory protein and the second messenger cAMP in granulosa cells or acting as a free radical scavenger. Activation of MT1 and MT2 decreases cAMP levels (Tagliaferri et al., 2018) thereby modulating leptin production (which is related to obesity and HA) in adipocytes (Tamura et al., 2009). In the case of PCOS, there exists a positive correlation in levels of melatonin, testosterone, and LH-FSH ratio further substantiated by the co-relation between SNP rs10830963 (MT2 variant) and the testosterone concentration. Melatonin is also known to regulate androgen synthesis in thecal cells by modulation of GnRH levels (Mojaverrostami et al., 2019) (since GnRH can stimulate LH to induce androgen production). HA and IR are associated with decreased expression of Bmal1 clock genes (Brzezinski et al., 2021).

Melatonin has also demonstrated its role in reducing body weight by inducing lipolysis involving elements of androgen synthesizing pathways - extracellular signal-regulated kinase (ERK) 1/2 and protein kinase A (PKA) (Owino et al., 2019). Lipolysis of adipocytes and up-regulation of lipolytic genes and proteins expression via MT2 and reduction of oxidative stress can be induced by melatonin. Pinealectomy-based studies have demonstrated induction of Leptin resistance (Guan et al., 2022) that impaired body weight regulation (Owino et al., 2019) and contributed to HA (Zeng et al., 2020) and lipotoxicity (Baptiste et al., 2010). Melatonin can reduce muscle mass loss and aid in controlling obesity (Guan et al., 2022). All these suggest that there exists an interplay between androgens, insulin, and melatonin in the case of PCOS, (***Figure 1)***

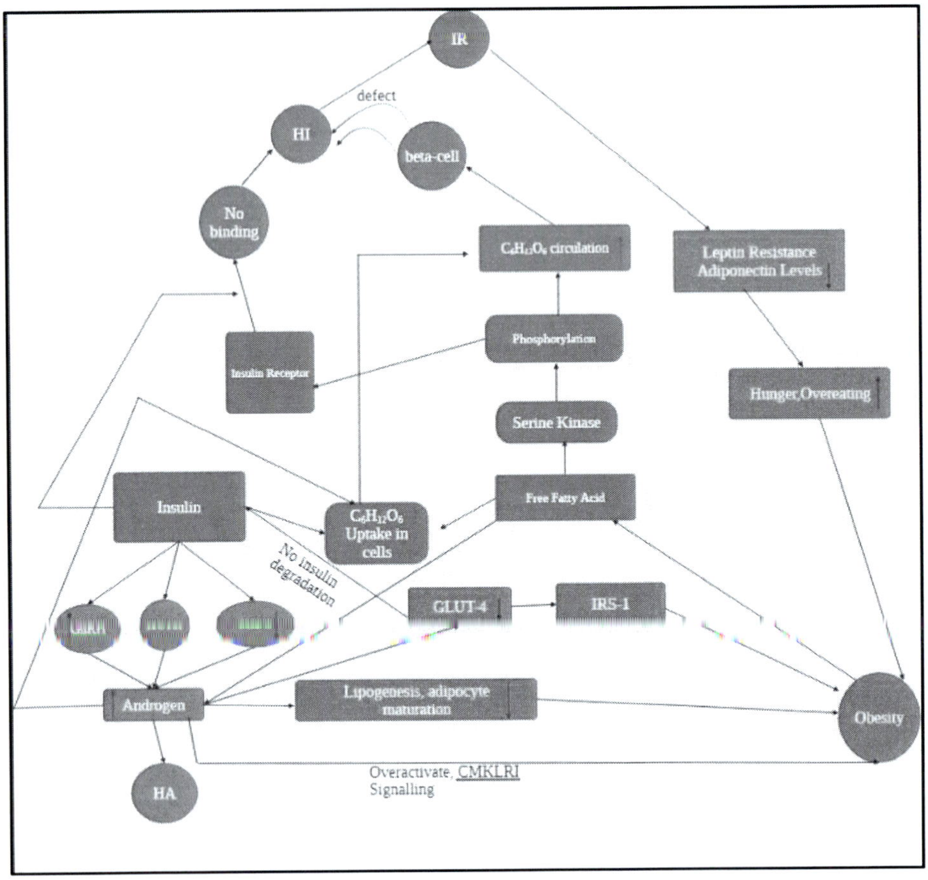


**Figure 1.** The interplay of Insulin Resistance (IR), Hyperandrogenism (HA), and Obesity.

## 4. Melatonin and the Ovary

### 4.1. Role of Melatonin in the Histology of Ovary

Melatonin is one of the most documented biomolecules, well-known for its diverse pharmacological properties (Tamura et al., 2009). Melatonin and its metabolites remove pro-oxidants and help regulate the expression of many antioxidant enzymes protecting other biomolecules from oxidative stress and subsequent damage caused by reactive oxygen and nitrogen species (Ahmadi et al., 2017). Melatonin positively impacts the HPG (Hypothalamic-pituitary-gonadal) axis. Owing to its pleiotropic nature, it helps maintain normal ovarian function and histology (Maganhin et al., 2013). Ovarian follicles actively take up melatonin from the circulating serum and the neighboring reproductive cells such as the oocyte and the granulosa cells which can secrete it. As a result, melatonin found in a normal woman's preovulatory FF (follicular fluid) is almost triple that in blood, and its concentration increases with the size of the follicle (H. Li, Liu, and Zhang 2022). This increase of melatonin within the immature follicle aids in scavenging toxic oxygen species and reducing the formation of free radicals (Cruz et al., 2014; Ahmadi et al., 2017).

Recent studies have demonstrated that melatonin treatment results in an increased number of primordial follicles, primary follicles, and corpus luteum while reducing the number of cystic follicles (Ahmadi et al., 2017). The cytoprotective ability of melatonin also helps delay ovarian aging. Ovarian aging can be marked by a gradual loss of ovarian follicles, especially after the age of 38. Melatonin helps forestall it by preventing the deleterious effects of ROS and RNS which are considered one of the major influencing factors for ovarian aging ***(Figure 2)*** (Tamura et al., 2017).

Melatonin suppresses autophagy and follicular atresia via inducing SIRT1 and SIRT3 (known members of the sirtuin gene family) signaling pathways (Tamura et al. 2017). SIRT1 also known as SOD2 (superoxide dismutase 2) is a key antioxidant enzyme found in human oocytes whereas SIRT3 is a mitochondrial enzyme- histone deacetylase which is found in the Mt matrix and takes part in regulating cellular metabolism and apoptosis. Microarray analysis of patients undergoing melatonin treatment has shown an up-regulation in ribosome-related genes suggesting its role in delaying cell senescence (Tamura et al., 2017).

### 4.2. Ovarian Receptors of Melatonin

Melatonin affects reproductive function by directly binding ovarian granulosa cells, activating, and exerting other effects on the HPO (hypothalamic-pituitary-ovarian) axis (Tamura et al., 2017) (Guo et al., 2021) MT receptors are present in our brain, liver, cardiovascular system, breasts, as well as the myometrium (T. C. Sun et al., 2020).

MT binding sites have been identified within the membrane of mammalian granulosa cells including humans. The melatonin receptors are divided into – membrane-bound receptors and nuclear receptors which mediate certain specific actions (Tamura et al., 2009) (Guo et al. 2021). Three main types of membrane MT receptors have been identified in mammalian ovarian cells namely MT1, MT2, and MT3. Out of these, MT1 and MT2 receptors are encoded by the MTNR1A gene which is present on chromosome 4, and the MTNR1B gene present on chromosome 11 respectively (Guo et al., 2021). Both are members of the GPCR (G-protein coupled receptors) family and have been found to express in human granulosa cells and luteal cells (Tamura et al., 2009) (M Woo et al., 2001). MT3 is a cytosolic receptor and has been identified as an enzyme known as quinone reductase 2 which in some animals possesses the attributes of an MT receptor. Nuclear binding sites, although very less known, are mainly related to some members of the ROR/RZR superfamily of nuclear receptors (Mor et al., 1999).

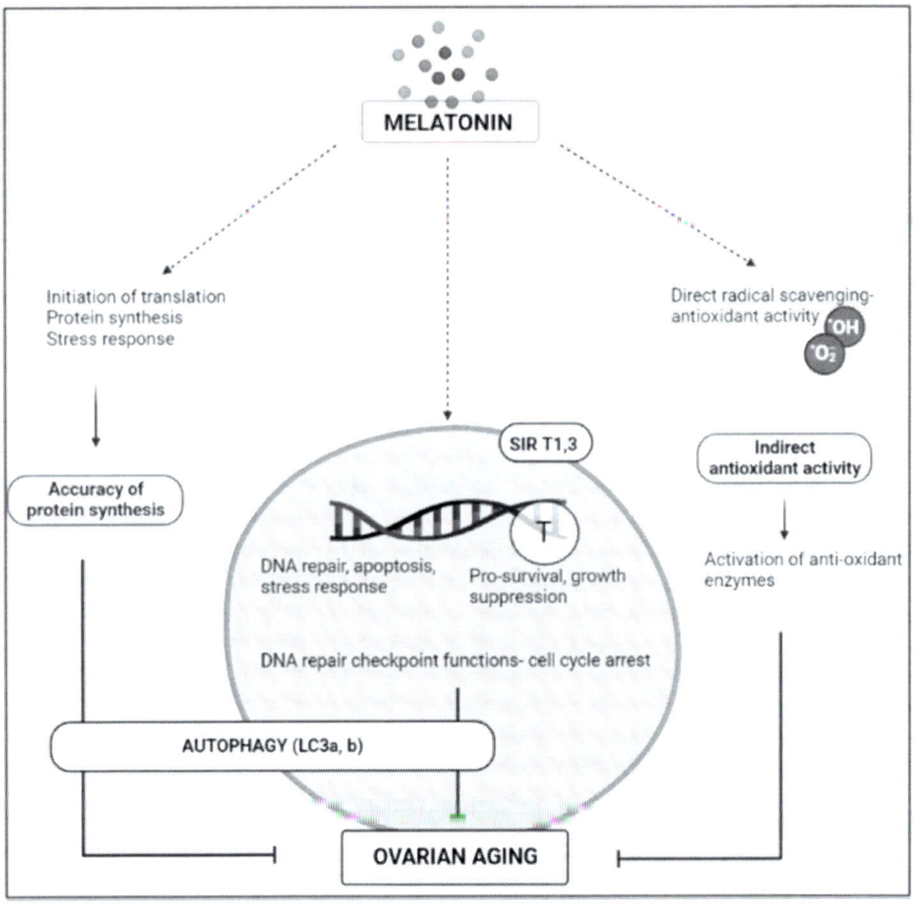


**Figure 2.** Melatonin's mechanism to prevent ovarian aging. Melatonin reduces ovarian oxidative damage via its dual action- as a direct antioxidant, by scavenging free radicals, and as an indirect antioxidant, by enhancing the activity of other antioxidant enzymes. Melatonin boosts eukaryotic initiation factor 2 signaling, which is quite important for the initiation of translation and protein synthesis in ribosomes, and DNA-damage signaling, which is involved in DNA repair and checkpoint functions. MT also helps suppress autophagy-related proteins (light-chain 3a, 3b, LC3a, LC3b). The expression of genes of the sirtuin family (SIRT1,3) and telomere length are also improved (Tamura et al., 2020).

### *4.2.1. Molecular Aspects of Melatonin Receptors*

MT1 receptors are composed of 350 amino acids while MT2 receptors are made up of 363 amino acids. About 60% of their sequences are homologous with similar binding site structures for melatonin The binding of melatonin to both these receptors (MT1 and MT2) mediates different physiological effects via a variety of signaling pathways as shown in ***Figure 3***, including the AC (adenylate cyclase- cAMP), mitogen-activated protein kinase (MAPK)-extracellular signal-regulated kinase (ERK), phosphatidyl inositol-3-kinase (PI-3-K) and other signaling pathways (Tamura et al., 2017).

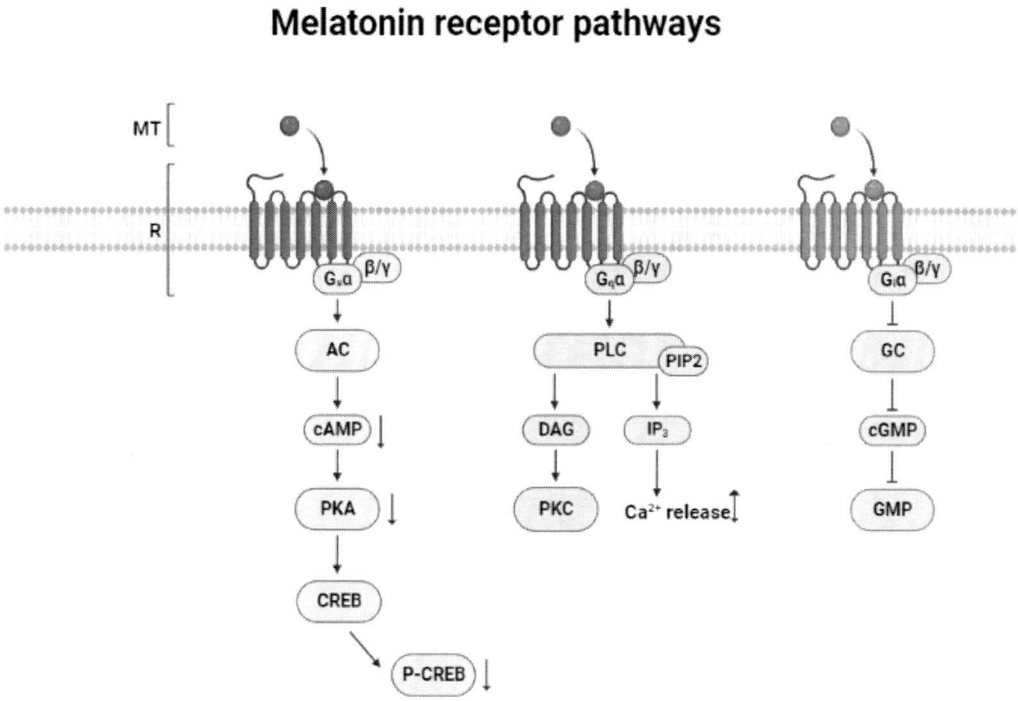


**Figure 3.** showing MT receptors & their signal transduction pathways (Dubocovich et al. 2003). Abbreviations: MT (melatonin), R (MT receptor), cAMP (cyclic adenosine monophosphate), DAG (diacylglycerol), IP3 (inositol triphosphate), CREB (responsive element binding protein), PKA (protein kinase A), ATP (adenosine triphosphate), GTP (guanosine triphosphate), GMP (guanosine monophosphate), cGMP (cyclic guanosine monophosphate), PKC (protein kinase C), PLC (phospholipase C), PIP2 (phosphotidylinositol4,5-bisphosphate), AC (adenylyl cyclase), CG (guanylyl cyclase).

The binding of melatonin to MT1 receptors down-regulates the activity of intracellular PK-A and reduces CREB phosphorylation, thereby inhibiting the cAMP transduction pathway (Zhao et al., 2021). Once activated, the MT1 receptor brings about a transient but notable increase in the cytosolic calcium ions [$Ca^{2+}$] and inositol phosphate concentrations. MT2 receptors transmit signals corresponding to various signaling pathways including its self-activation to improve the production of phosphoinositol along with subsequent inhibition of adenylate as well as guanylate cyclase which helps regulate the downstream pathways ((Mohamed et al. 2021; (Zhao et al., 2021).

Besides its receptor-mediated effects on ovarian clock regulation, a direct effect of melatonin includes as a free radical scavenger and indirectly as an antioxidant to further stimulate the activity of antioxidant enzymes including SOD and GPX that benefit reproductive physiology (Tamura et al., 2017; Guo et al., 2021).

## 4.3. Ovulation and Follicle Maturation

Follicular growth and ovulation are detailed yet complicated events in the process of reproduction. The rupture of the pre-ovulatory follicular wall to release a fertilizable oocyte into the oviduct is modeled as a brief inflammatory process (Yao et al., 2007). At the time of ovulation, a local increase in the concentrations of certain substances in the follicle is seen which can induce oxidative stress; these include free radical generating agents such as prostaglandins, histamine, bradykinin, angiotensin II, eicosanoids, nitric oxide, and superoxides, etc. (Acosta et al., 2000).

The molecular and biochemical pathways amid follicle formation regulated by oxidative species lead to oocyte damage and follicular atresia. ROS produced during the ovulatory process is detrimental to the oocyte and a leading cause of poor oocyte quality and lower fertilization rates (Tamura et al., 2009). Melatonin, which is present in elevated levels within the human follicular fluid can attenuate and eliminate these stressors protecting the oocytes and granulosa cells ***(Figure 4)*** (Ezzati, Velaei, and Kheirjou 2021). It affects the ovarian microenvironment by balancing out the pro and antioxidant structure which helps promote follicular maturation and ovulation (H. Li, Liu, and Zhang 2022).

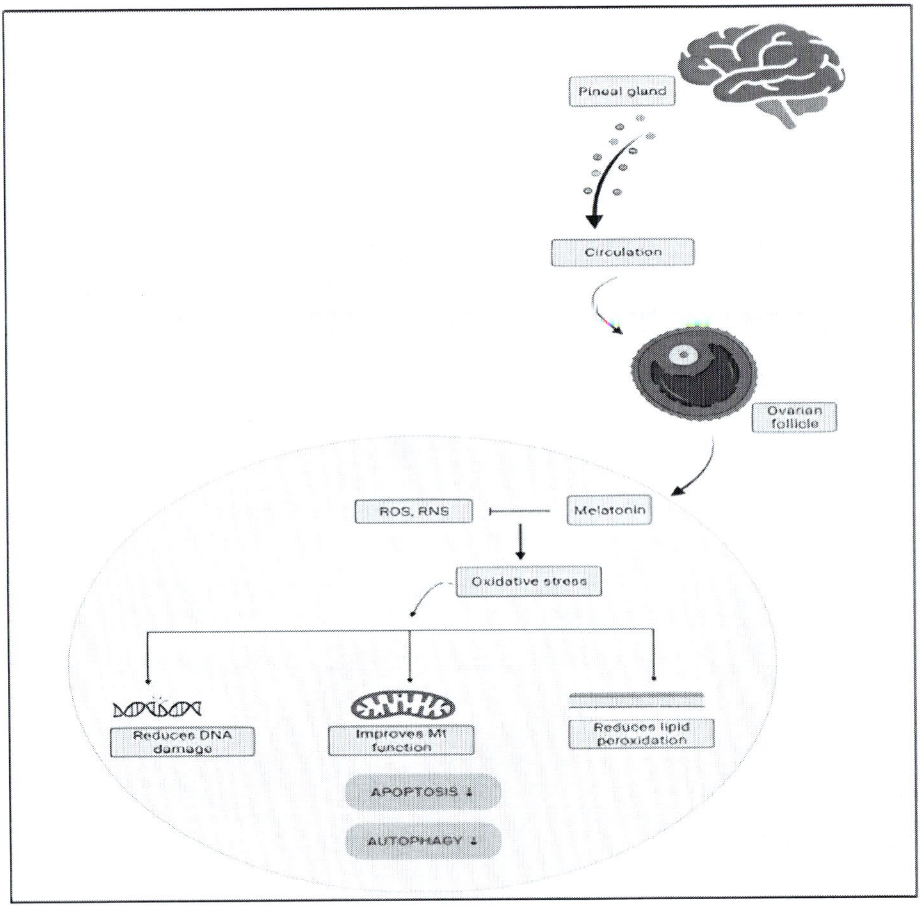


**Figure 4.** Action of MT within the ovarian follicle. Follicles take up the MT circulating in the blood, which is secreted by the pineal gland. The reactive derivatives such as superoxides and peroxides generated during the process of ovulation are actively scavenged by melatonin. It also helps reduce stress-related DNA damage, lipid peroxidation, mitochondrial affliction as well as apoptosis (Tamura et al. 2020).

Melatonin increases glutathione synthesis in human endothelial cells and helps prevent endogenous mitochondrial apoptotic pathways by inducing Bcl-2 expression and reducing caspase-3 activity. Thus, it helps protect the cells from oxidative damage. Melatonin can lower oxidative damage in the follicles when administered exogenously, thereby improving fertilization and pregnancy rates (Ezzati, Velaei, and Kheirjou 2021).

Melatonin, an amphiphilic molecule is considered much more efficient in shielding against oxidative damage than its counterparts which allows it to enter any organ and metabolize harmful partly reduced oxygen derivatives to harmless molecules or induce the synthesis of other beneficial antioxidant molecules (Cruz et al., 2014).

#### *4.3.1. Melatonin and Follicular Development*

Melatonin plays an instrumental role in maintaining a healthy follicle (Maganhin et al. 2013). The expression of melatonin receptors (MT1 and MT2) in granulosa and luteal cells indicates that it plays a pivotal role in the regulation of the reproductive process in mammals. Thus, regulating steroidogenesis and follicular function in humans and rodents. Folliculogenesis can be defined as the process of formation of ovarian follicles. It is highly dependent on the FSH levels. The proper formation of ovarian follicles is supported by low levels of ROS and any increment in its levels can produce oxidative stress which then causes damage to the granulosa cells and oocytes (Haldar and Chowdhury 2020). Therefore, by maintaining the delicate pro-oxidant-antioxidant balance within the oocyte, melatonin protects the female gamete against oxidative stress and regulates healthy folliculogenesis. (Cosme et al., 2022).

The ovarian microenvironment, follicular cells, and oocytes are the main site for the production of ROS. Mammalian oocytes being most vulnerable to lipid peroxidation and DNA fragmentation account for the prominent amount of easily oxidizable lipids. Moreover, Melatonin modulates the follicular response by enhancing the mRNA expression of LH receptors in granulosa cells that influences follicular selection (M Woo et al., 2001).

High concentrations of this neurohormone within the follicular fluid stimulate granulosa cells to proliferate via MAPK activation (mitogen-activated protein kinases) (van Voorhis et al. 1994) and during the pre-ovulatory phase it has been associated with progesterone production, leading to luteinization and hence successful ovulation. Furthermore, the discovery of melatonin receptors in the human granulosa cells also suggests that it stimulates progesterone release (Cosme et al., 2022).

#### *4.3.2. Melatonin and Luteal Phase*

During the luteal phase, melatonin levels are higher than those during the follicular phase, suggesting its modulatory properties. It has been shown that high levels of melatonin in larger follicles correlate with appropriate luteinization, which leads to the production of progesterone (Cosme et al., 2022). Also, melatonin acts as a balance between the luteotrophic and the luteolytic regulators by reducing the luteolytic modulator PgF2α and enhancing the production of luteotrophic prostaglandin PgE2 (Scarinci et al., 2019). It also inhibits the expression of GnRH (Gonadotropin-releasing hormone) and its receptors by up-regulating the expression of LH receptor mRNAs. GnRH modulates the luteinizing hormone and follicle-stimulating hormone secretions, which regulate reproductive function at the gonadal level and help maintain the corpus luteum during a pregnancy (Adriaens et al., 2006).

### *4.3.3. Melatonin and Embryo Development*

In the mammalian reproduction process, oocyte maturation is a prerequisite for successful fertilization and development of the embryo. Owing to its powerful antioxidative capabilities, melatonin is advantageous for oocyte maturation and embryo growth (Y. Li et al., 2019). As per clinical reports orally administered melatonin can not only reduce the concentration of 8-OHdG (a marker for DNA damage due to oxidative stress) in the oocytes obtained from infertile women but increase the fertilization rate through ART (Adriaens et al., 2006). Accumulating studies have demonstrated that melatonin's antioxidant function helps reduce the rigidity of the plasma membrane, promoting human oocyte maturation and early embryonic development by enhancing the CME (reticulin-mediated endocytosis) (Guo et al., 2021). By means of the SIRT3-SOD2 pathway, melatonin enhances the characteristics of oocytes that have been impaired due to maternal obesity, thus inhibiting chromosomal abnormalities in initial-stage embryos (Hu et al., 2020).

Among infertile women, melatonin therapy has become increasingly popular as a way to improve the quality and functioning of their ovarian system, and embryo development, especially if they are about to reach the end of their childbearing age or cannot get pregnant due to poor oocyte quality (Ishizuka et al., 2000).

## 5. Melatonin and the Interplay of Reproductive Hormones

The significant role of melatonin in reproductive physiology is highlighted by its local synthesis, the existence of melatonin receptors in ovarian cells, and the interconnection of pathways with reproductive hormones. Melatonin is involved in oocyte quality regulation, follicular atresia, ovulation, apoptosis, steroidogenesis, follicular function, etc. A greater concentration of melatonin in follicular fluid as compared to serum plasma levels suggests its immense role in follicular functioning (Tamura et al., 2008). The core involvement of clock genes such as PER1 (GnRH AND LH surge), PER2 (LH receptor expression, follicle selection), BMAL1 (GnRH secretion timings) and CLOCK (defects can cause anovulation) indicate the interplay of melatonin with reproductive hormones (Brzezinski et al., 2021).

The process of ovulation results in the release of free radicals hailing as Reactive Nitrogen Species (RNS) and Reactive Oxygen Species (ROS) (Tamura et al., 2008) that participate in the much-needed redox balance (Vitale et al., 2016) which acts by regulating several physiological activities such as oocyte maturation and follicular wall rupture in the body but, access of the same could lead to poor oocyte quality and ovarian cell apoptosis (Tamura et al., 2009). Melatonin acts as a savior of follicular cells by

1. Free radical scavenging through a "scavenging cascade reaction," wherein it generates several stable antioxidant end-products (Vitale et al., 2016) by neutralizing the free radicals through electron donation (Guo Ming Yi et al. 2021). The byproducts of this process, including cyclic 3-hydroxy melatonin, N1-acetyl-N2-formyl-5-methoxykynuramine (AFMK), and N1-acetyl-5-methoxykynuramine (AMK), act as highly effective agents for eliminating free radicals. (Tamura et al., 2009).
2. Synergistically collaborating with other nonenzymatic antioxidants to stimulate antioxidant enzyme synthesis through its receptors (Vitale et al., 2016).

Most of the free radicals are formed inside the mitochondria (Guo Ming Yi et al., 2021) whose DNA (mtDNA) is extremely vulnerable to damage owing to a lack of DNA repair activity. Melatonin can directly act in mitochondria thereby ameliorating oocyte quality (Tamura et al., 2009). This capacity of melatonin in reducing oxidative stress is receptor-independent (Guo Ming Yi et al., 2021).

In reproductive physiology, any shift in the LH: FSH ratio could lead to disorders such as PCOS. While FSH is responsible for follicular growth, LH is responsible for ovulation, steroidogenesis, etc. (Shaaban et al., 2019). In the case of PCOS, there is an increase in the pulse frequency and amplitude of LH secretion which depends on GnRH pulse in the pituitary gland and an inverse correlation exists between in LH: FSH ratio and melatonin levels (Mojaverrostami et al., 2019). The lower concentration of melatonin in the follicular fluid is mainly due to decreased absorption from circulation and decreased ovarian section owing to follicular atresia (H. Li, Liu, and Zhang 2022). Though the elevation of GnRH pulse frequency and amplitude which form the core etiology of PCOS is poorly understood yet certain hypotheses explaining the possible causes are as follows,

1. Hyperinsulinemia elevates GnRH levels by action on GnRH neurons.
2. Low levels of serum progesterone cease the negative feedback by progesterone on GnRH release.
3. HA affects negative feedback of steroid hormones which reduces GnRH antagonist GnIH (Gonadotropin Inhibitory Hormone) (Shaaban et al., 2019).

This results in increased LH secretion thereby increasing the LH: FSH ratio and causing a series of anomalies. In PCOS, chronic LH stimulation reduces FSH receptor mRNA expression leading to loss of response in antral follicles and hampering follicular growth. This in turn reduces the expression of CYP19A1 by inactivating the cAMP-PKA-CREB pathway resulting in arrested follicular development (Zeng et al. 2020) and ovarian cysts (Shaaban et al., 2019). Further, a constant surge of LH diminishes the relative LH peak necessary for menstruation leading to anovulation and HA (J. Wang et al., 2019).

FSH and LH release induced by GnRH can be inhibited by melatonin which interacts with GnRH through the Hypothalamus-Pituitary-Ovarian axis (Cipolla-Neto et al., 2022). Melatonin inhibits GnRH-induced Ca2+ pathways of LH release by inhibiting GnRH-induced phospholipase C activity. Ca2+ release from the endoplasmic reticulum is induced by diacylglycerol and inositol trisphosphate (IP3) which are metabolized by Phospholipase C. Melatonin can also achieve similar results by hyperpolarization of the plasma membrane by inhibiting Na+ influx into gonadotrophs which results in closing of the voltage-sensitive channels thereby inhibiting Ca2+ influx (Vanecek 1999). GnRH function can also be inhibited by melatonin through the up-regulation of LH receptor expression (Guo Ming Yi et al., 2021). PCOS marked by lower FSH levels can thus be ameliorated by melatonin administration, **(Figure 5).**

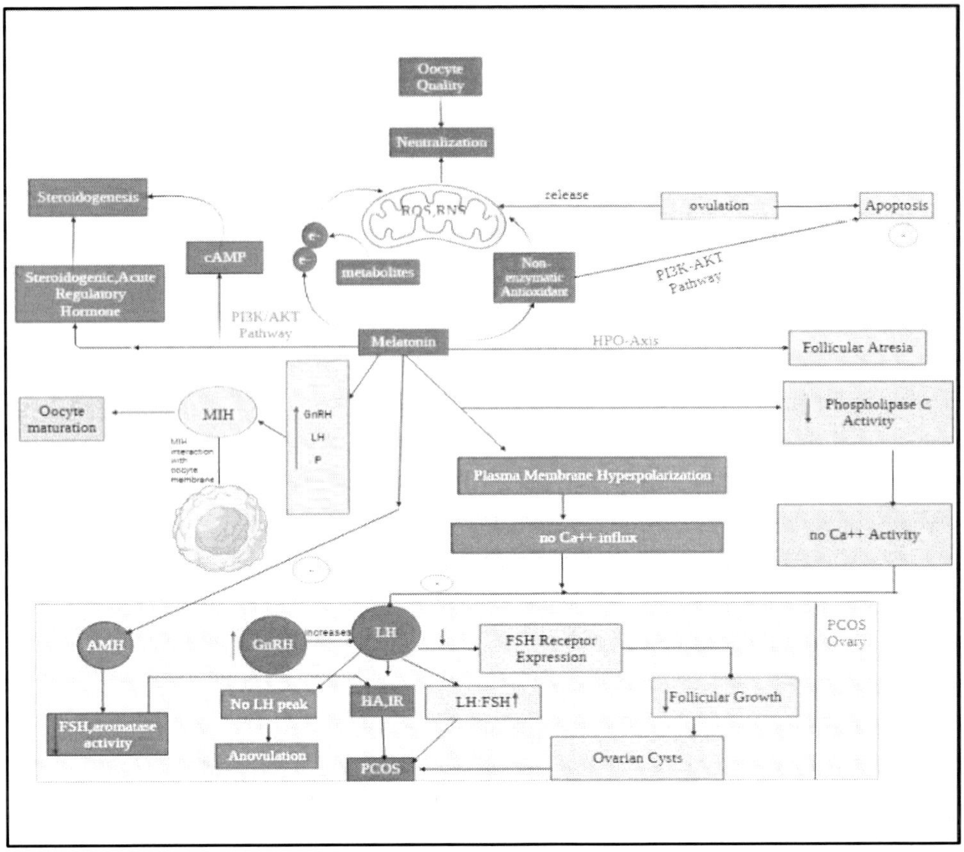


**Figure 5**. Role of Melatonin in Ovarian function modulation.

The presence of reproductive hormone receptors on pineal glands suggests the potential role of reproductive hormones in melatonin secretion, release, and circulation. Estrogen can alter cAMP signaling by acting on melatonin receptors. Melatonin, in turn, affects the reproductive hormones by acting on the hypothalamic GnRH neurons, the pituitary, and the gonads/reproductive organs (Cipolla-Neto et al., 2022). Melatonin can induce progesterone production, GnRH, and LH receptor expression via the mitogen-activated protein kinase (MPK) pathway (Yang et al., 2018). A positive correlation exists between progesterone and melatonin levels in follicular fluid with greater concentrations in larger follicles. Further, higher melatonin levels in preovulatory follicles could aggravate progesterone production and induce ovulation and luteinization. In luteal cells, melatonin induces HCG-stimulated progesterone release by increased LH expression and is known to regulate the expression of several biochemicals that can induce/suppress progesterone production (Tamura et al., 2009). Melatonin is also known to regulate the biosynthesis of estrogen (Cipolla-Neto et al., 2022).

Anti-Mullerian Hormone (AMH) synthesized by the granulosa cells of developing follicles (Jain et al. 2022) is usually high in cases of PCOS because of premature arrest in the development of small antral follicles (Tagliaferri et al., 2018). This can lower FSH and aromatase activity thereby disabling the conversion of androgen to estrogen (Zeng et al., 2020). Melatonin administration has been shown to disrupt the cyclicity of hyperandrogenism, follicular atresia, hyperAMH, and anovulation, especially in the case of PCOS (Tagliaferri et al., 2018).

Maturation Inducing Hormone (17a, 20b-dihydroxy-4- pregnen-3-one) interacts with the oocyte membrane receptor to activate a maturation-promoting factor aiding in oocyte maturation(Tamura et al., 2008) wherein Melatonin is known to stimulate Maturation Inducing Hormone through progesterone(Guo Ming Yi et al., 2021). Lower levels of melatonin can advance follicular atresia (He et al., 2016) which is substantiated by pinealectomy studies (Tamura et al., 2008). Melatonin can affect follicular growth by regulating FSH levels through the Hypothalamus-Pituitary-Ovarian axis (H. Li, Liu, and Zhang 2022). Melatonin regulates steroidogenesis and apoptosis through PI3K/AKT pathway and MT2 receptor (Cipolla-Neto et al., 2022).

## 6. Melatonin as a Therapeutic

### 6.1. Melatonin in ART

Infertility can be defined as the inability to conceive for over a year while subfertility is reduced fertility with a delay in conception for a prolonged time (Gnoth et al. 2005). Both are common conditions affecting 10-20% of women at reproductive ages and can be corrected with the help of ART (Assisted Reproductive Technology). ART includes interventions such as IVF-ET (In-vitro fertilization and embryo transfer) that require in-vitro handling of human gametes intending to achieve a full-term pregnancy. It has helped countless infertile couples to conceive successfully, however, the conception rates or chances of achieving a live birth are close to 30% which is not satisfactory (Seko et al., 2014). The success rate of ART cycles is majorly hampered by oxidative stress caused by ROS in the ovarian follicles, which are a leading cause of poor oocyte quality, reduced fertilization rates, and frequent miscarriages (Hu et al., 2020).

There is a higher risk of oxidative stress in ART procedures because of a variety of extrinsic factors **(Figure 6)** and a lack of physiological defense mechanisms (Cosme et al. 2022). Accumulating studies including randomized trials have supplied evidence of potential therapeutic applications of melatonin in ART by reversing the inhibitory effects of oxidation in improved oocyte quality and greater possibility of a full-term pregnancy. Reducing intrafollicular oxidative damage is, thus, important for the successful outcomes of IVF-ET, and not just that, it can prove beneficial in preventing fetal chromosomal abnormalities (Tamura et al., 2020)

#### *6.1.1. Function of Melatonin in Reproductive Physiology*

Melatonin executes a multitude of physiological functions which includes regulation of central and peripheral activities about circadian rhythm as well as reproduction (Yang et al., 2018).

It has already been discussed in the preceding topics how melatonin acts directly on the ovary, accumulating in high concentrations in the follicular fluid, and carrying out key antioxidant functions thereby protecting ovarian follicles, oocytes, and granulosa cells from oxidative stress caused due to ROS (H. Li, Liu, and Zhang 2022). Melatonin concentration in the ovarian follicle increases as a function of its size, with larger follicles taking up more melatonin from the circulation and exhibiting phasic variations like that in the pineal gland (Tamura et al., 2014).

Numerous studies on short-day breeders have associated elevated melatonin levels with pro-gonadotrophic behavior, while studies on long-day breeders have referred it to as anti-gonadal or antigonadotrophic. However, it is neither anti nor pro-gonadal. In the case of mammals such as humans, the photoperiodic melatonin rhythm is used by the HPO (Hypothalamic-pituitary-ovarian) axis to effectively regulate ovarian physiology, such as steroidogenesis, folliculogenesis, oocyte maturation, and development, among other processes (Reiter et al., 2009).

Melatonin also plays a pivotal role in enhancing HCG secretion, luteinization of granulosa cells, progesterone production, and HVT differentiation (human villous trophoblast) which improves fertilization as well as pregnancy rates (Yang et al., 2018). Being present in such high concentrations in preovulatory FF (follicular fluid), its physiological role during ovulation is that of a broad-spectrum radical scavenger and antioxidant (Tamura et al., 2014).

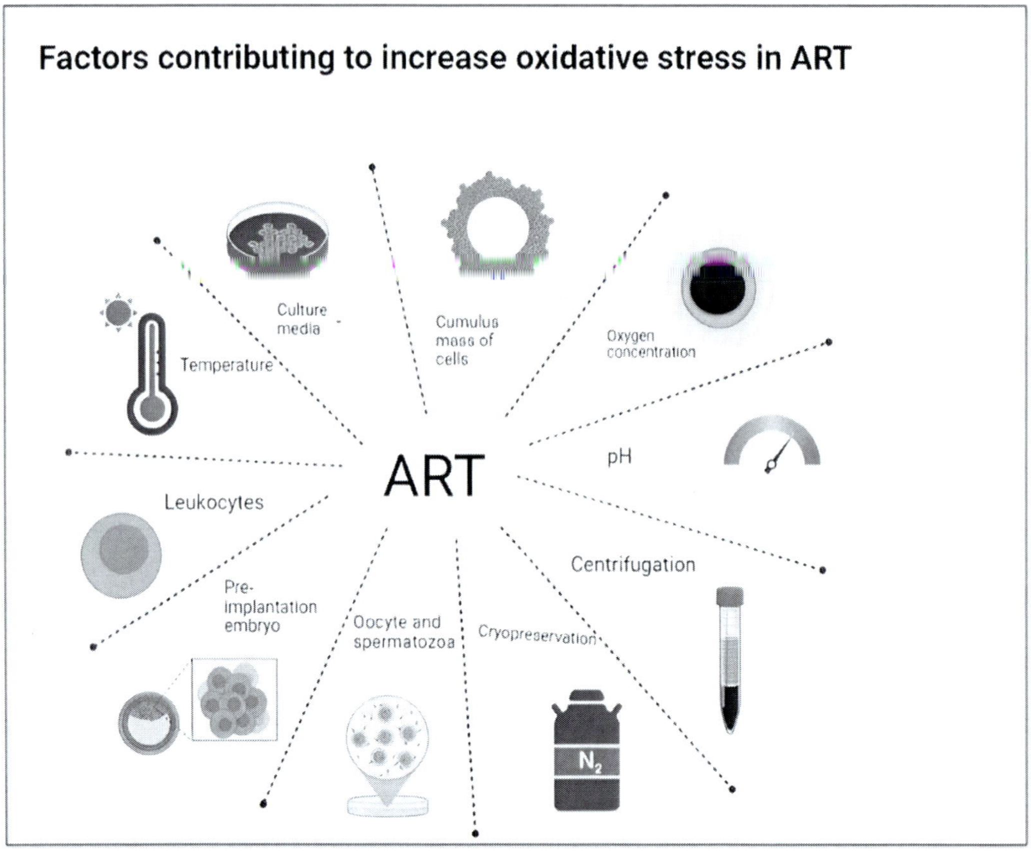


**Figure 6.** Factors contributing to increased oxidative stress in ART (Cosme et al., 2022).

### *6.1.2. Administration of Melatonin Exogenously to Treat PCOS*

Oxidative stress and immune dysregulation can be attributed as notable causes of polycystic ovary syndrome (PCOS) (Yang et al., 2018) which clinically manifests itself as a heterogeneous combination of irregular menstrual cycles, in or sub-fertility, hirsutism, etc. (Tagliaferri et al. 2018). Chronic anovulation is another physio-pathological basis for deviation from a regular menstrual cycle leading to irregularities (Tagliaferri et al., 2018).

Studies have shown the potential of melatonin as a therapeutic agent in treating PCOS. It helps mitigate some of the crucial PCOS hallmarks such as follicular atresia, hyper AMH, and anovulation by actively scavenging ROS, regulating antioxidant activity, and coordinating anti and pro-apoptotic gene expression. It was also found that melatonin helps rescue follicles from atresia by improving the nuclear maturation rate of PCOS oocytes ensuring prospective fertilization (Yang et al., 2018).

Additionally, the administration of exogenous melatonin in infertile women during IVF-ET cycles reduces the intrafollicular concentrations of 8-OHdG and HEL enhancing fertilization as well as pregnancy rates. Reportedly oral melatonin has no negative aftereffects, can significantly increase circulating FSH levels, and is well-continued in thousands of patients with a 3mg/day dose (Tamura et al., 2008) (H. Li, Liu, and Zhang 2022).

In another study conducted by Tagliaferri et al, about 6 months of melatonin treatment for women struggling with PCOS visibly improved their menstrual cyclicity along with a reduction in serum androgen and AMH levels, indicating its beneficiary role in immune-mediated ovarian pathophysiology (Tagliaferri et al., 2018). Melatonin aids PCOS treatment through its regulatory effects on steroidogenesis (Yang et al., 2018). It is emerging as a medicine/drug of choice for women with PCOS/infertility (Tamura et al., 2020).

### *6.1.3. Recent Implementations*

The decline in fertility is intricately linked with ovarian aging, largely characterized by poor oocyte quality and quantity. Melatonin along with other protective adjuvants such as Vitamin E and cysteine has been shown to delay the physiological aging of ovaries, control autophagy within the ovary, support different mitochondrial functions, and significantly improve fertility in many species including humans.

In addition to its existing applications in ART, as shown in ***(Figure 7),*** recent studies have highlighted the remarkable antioxidative properties of melatonin for its application as a potent cryoprotectant during the vitrification (fast-freezing) process to improve the clinical outcomes by enhancing the survivability of gametes and embryos (Choi and Jang 2022). It not only combats oxidative stress, lipid peroxidation, and DNA damage during gamete/embryo freezing but also has an inhibitory effect on apoptosis (Choi and Jang 2022).

Melatonin has demonstrated epigenetic efficacy in several medical conditions such as sleep disorders, hypertension, and even in diseases like cancer.

Endometriosis (EMS) is a frequently recurring gynecological issue, which involves the growth of endometrial tissue outside the uterus and is associated with chronic inflammation. Melatonin has been observed to play a role in the development of EMS. Intraperitoneal melatonin administration has been found to decrease adhesions and induce the degeneration and shrinkage of ectopic lesions by reducing oxidative stress. Studies have demonstrated that melatonin down-regulates the expression of proMMP-9 and elevates TIMP-1 levels, thereby controlling the activity of matrix metalloproteinases (MMPs), which are crucial diagnostic markers and preventing the onset of endometriosis (Özçelik et al., 2003).

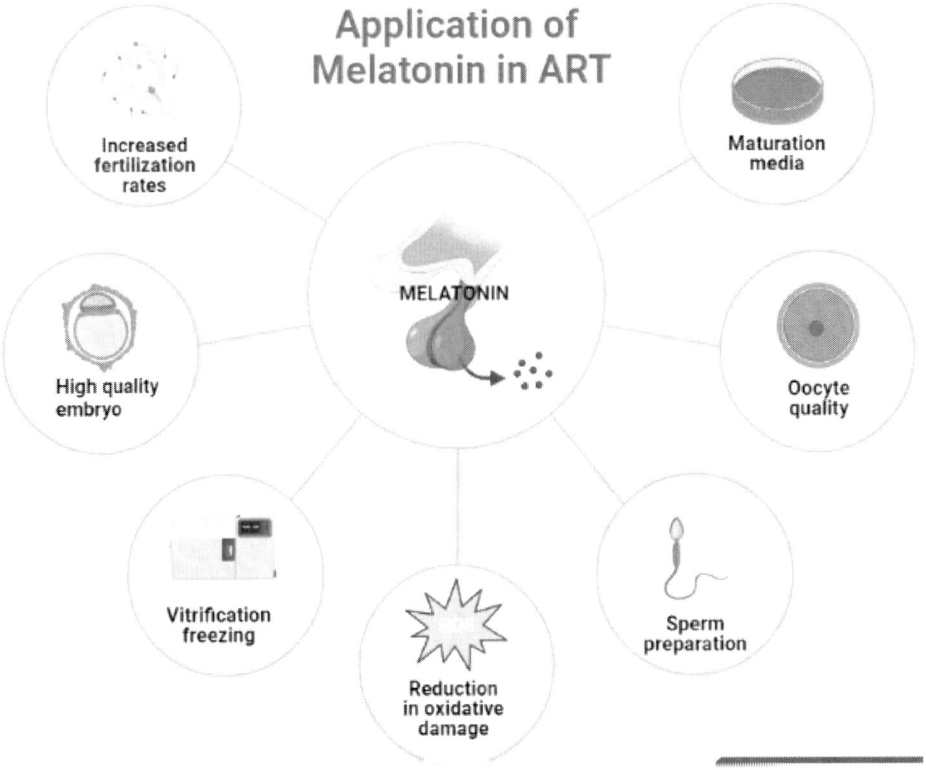


**Figure 7.** Melatonin applications in ART (Cosme et al., 2022).

Some chemotherapeutic agents such as doxorubicin and cisplatin induce ROS generation in the mitochondria affecting the structure and function of GCs (Granulosa cells) and oocytes. Melatonin promotes cancer cell apoptosis and is highly effective in counteracting chemotherapy-induced cytotoxicity via its antioxidant action. It worked synergistically with other chemotherapeutic agents and when administered in patients undergoing cancer treatment, showed a reduction in neuro and cardiotoxicity along with lesser frequent thrombocytopenia (Reiter et al., 2010).

The clinical uses of melatonin in human reproductive medicine have been explored and are numerous. Several findings have paved the way for novel opportunities to effectively manage diseases such as cancer, implying enormous potential in a therapeutic setting (Tamura et al., 2017).

## 7. Conclusion

A polycystic ovarian syndrome characterized by anovulation, hyperandrogenism, insulin resistance, infertility, obesity, and acne is associated with a lifestyle disorder affecting mostly women of reproductive age. Furthermore, the melatonin hormone released by the pineal gland is responsible for synchronizing our 24-h biological clock, known as the circadian rhythm. The imbalance and dysfunction of the melatonin hormone have been correlated with the manifestation of PCOS in women. Additionally, a poorer sleep cycle has also been found in women with PCOS justifying the relationship between melatonin hormone and endocrine hormones. Melatonin hormone, an antioxidant plays a prominent role in scavenging free radicals in the female reproductive system. The abundance of free radicals produced in the mitochondria of an ovarian cell due to various cellular respiration processes is responsible for apoptosis and also limits the development of follicles in an ovary. Thus, the higher concentration of melatonin in mitochondria and melatonin-binding receptors found on the membrane of granulosa cells plays a critical role in preventing the oxidation of ovarian follicles thereby, promoting the growth and differentiation of follicles. Additionally, exogenous administration of melatonin in rat models has improved growth, ovulation, follicular growth, and follicular cycle quality. Hence, promoting the use of melatonin among women with PCOS undergoing ART.

## References

Acosta, T. J., Ozawa, T., Kobayashi, S., Hayashi, K., Ohtani, M., Kraetzl, W. D., Sato, K., Schams, D., and and Miyamoto, A. (2000). "Periovulatory Changes in the Local Release of Vasoactive Peptides, Prostaglandin F 2, and Steroid Hormones from Bovine Mature Follicles *In Vivo* 1." *BIOLOGY OF REPRODUCTION*. Vol. 63.

Adriaens, I., Jacquet, P., Cortvrindt, R., Janssen, K., and Smitz, J. (2006). "Melatonin Has Dose-Dependent Effects on Folliculogenesis, Oocyte Maturation Capacity and Steroidogenesis." *Toxicology*, 228 (2–3): 333–43. https://doi.org/10.1016/j.tox.2006.09.018.

Baptiste, Catherine G., Marie Claude Battista, Andréanne Trottier, and Jean Patrice Baillargeon. (2010). "Insulin and Hyperandrogenism in Women with Polycystic Ovary Syndrome." *Journal of Steroid Biochemistry and Molecular Biology*. https://doi.org/10.1016/j.jsbmb.2009.12.010.

Bogari, Neda M. (2020). "Genetic Construction between Polycystic Ovarian Syndrome and Type 2 Diabetes." *Saudi Journal of Biological Sciences*. Elsevier B.V. https://doi.org/10.1016/j.sjbs.2020.05.004.

Brzezinski, Amnon, Seema Rai, Adyasha Purohit, and Seithikurippu R. Pandi-Perumal. (2021). "Melatonin, Clock Genes, and Mammalian Reproduction: What Is the Link?" *International Journal of Molecular Sciences*, 2021, Vol. 22, Page 13240 22 (24), 13240. https://doi.org/10.3390/IJMS222413240.

Bulsara, Jeshica, Priyanshi Patel, Arun Soni, and Sanjeev Acharya. (2021). "A Review: Brief Insight into Polycystic Ovarian Syndrome." *Endocrine and Metabolic Science*. Elsevier Ltd. https://doi.org/10.1016/j.endmts.2021.100085.

Cipolla-Neto, José, and Fernanda Gaspar do Amaral. (2018). "Melatonin as a Hormone: New Physiological and Clinical Insights." *Endocrine Reviews*, 39 (6), 990–1028. https://doi.org/10.1210/er.2018-00084.

Cosme, Patricia, Ana B. Rodríguez, María Garrido, and Javier Espino. (2022). "Coping with Oxidative Stress in Reproductive Pathophysiology and Assisted Reproduction: Melatonin as an Emerging Therapeutical Tool." *Antioxidants*, 12 (1), 86. https://doi.org/10.3390/antiox12010086.

Cruz, M. H. C., Leal, C. L. V., Cruz, J. F., Tan, D. X., and Reiter, R. J. (2014). "Essential Actions of Melatonin in Protecting the Ovary from Oxidative Damage." *Theriogenology*. Elsevier Inc. https://doi.org/10.1016/j.theriogenology.2014.07.011.

Dubocovich, Margarita L, Moises A Rivera-Bermudez, Matthew J Gerdin, and Monica I Masana. (2003). "Introduction 3. Melatonin Receptors 3.1. MT 1 and MT 2 Melatonin Receptors 3.1.1. Molecular Structure 3.1.2." *Frontiers in Bioscience*., Vol. 8.

Espino, Javier. (2011). "Role of Melatonin on Diabetes-Related Metabolic Disorders." *World Journal of Diabetes*, 2 (6), 82. https://doi.org/10.4239/wjd.v2.i6.82.

Ezzati, Maryam, Kobra Velaei, and Raziyeh Kheirjou. (2021). "Melatonin and Its Mechanism of Action in the Female Reproductive System and Related Malignancies." *Molecular and Cellular Biochemistry*. Springer. https://doi.org/10.1007/s11010-021-04151-z.

Farid, Nadir R., and Evanthia Diamanti-Kandarakis. (2009). *Diagnosis and Management of Polycystic Ovary Syndrome. Diagnosis and Management of Polycystic Ovary Syndrome*. Springer US. https://doi.org/10.1007/978-0-387-09718-3.

Glueck, Charles J., and Naila Goldenberg. (2019). "Characteristics of Obesity in Polycystic Ovary Syndrome: Etiology, Treatment, and Genetics." *Metabolism: Clinical and Experimental*. W.B. Saunders. https://doi.org/10.1016/j.metabol.2018.11.002.

Gnoth, C., Godehardt, E., Frank-Herrmann, P., Friol, Jürgen Tigges, K., and Freundl, G. (2005). "Definition and Prevalence of Subfertility and Infertility." *Human Reproduction*, 20 (5), 1144–47. https://doi.org/10.1093/humrep/deh870.

Guan, Qingyun, Zixu Wang, Jing Cao, Yulan Dong, and Yaoxing Chen. (2022). "Mechanisms of Melatonin in Obesity: A Review." *International Journal of Molecular Sciences*. MDPI. https://doi.org/10.3390/ijms23010218.

Haldar, Chandana, and Jayita Pal Chowdhury. (2020). "Management of Ovarian Functions by Melatonin." *Journal of Reproductive Healthcare and Medicine*, 2, 16. https://doi.org/10.25259/JRHM_39_2020.

Hu, Kai Lun, Xiaohang Ye, Siwen Wang, and Dan Zhang. (2020). "Melatonin Application in Assisted Reproductive Technology: A Systematic Review and Meta-Analysis of Randomized Trials." *Frontiers in Endocrinology*. Frontiers Media S.A. https://doi.org/10.3389/fendo.2020.00160.

Ishizuka, Bunpei, Yasushi Kuribayashi, Kunihiko Murai, Akira Amemiya, and Masanori T Itoh. (2000). "The Effect of Melatonin on *in Vitro* Fertilization and Embryo Development in Mice." *J. Pineal Res*., Vol. 28.

Jain, Manish, Ashutosh Halder, Hemant Kumar, Priyal Sharma, and Mona Sharma. (2022). "Polycystic Ovary Syndrome (PCOS): An Overview and Our Experience." *J Endocrinol Reprod*, 26 (3), 127–52. https://doi.org/10.18311/jer/2022/30241.

Korkmaz, Ahmet, Sergio Rosales-Corral, and Russel J. Reiter. (2012). "Gene Regulation by Melatonin Linked to Epigenetic Phenomena." *Gene*, 503 (1), 1–11. https://doi.org/10.1016/J.GENE.2012.04.040.

Li, Hongwanyu, Mei Liu, and Cong Zhang. (2022). "Women with Polycystic Ovary Syndrome (PCOS) Have Reduced Melatonin Concentrations in Their Follicles and Have Mild Sleep Disturbances." *BMC Women's Health*, 22 (1). https://doi.org/10.1186/s12905-022-01661-w

Li, Shang, Junyu Zhai, Weiwei Chu, Xueying Geng, Zi Jiang Chen, and Yanzhi Du. (2020). "Altered Circadian Clock as a Novel Therapeutic Target for Constant Darkness-Induced Insulin Resistance and Hyperandrogenism of Polycystic Ovary Syndrome." *Translational Research: The Journal of Laboratory and Clinical Medicine*, 219 (May), 13–29. https://doi.org/10.1016/J.TRSL.2020.02.003.

Li, Yue, Hui Liu, Keliang Wu, Hongbin Liu, Tao Huang, Zi Jiang Chen, Shigang Zhao, Jinlong Ma, and Han Zhao. (2019). "Melatonin Promotes Human Oocyte Maturation and Early Embryo Development by Enhancing Clathrin-Mediated Endocytosis." *Journal of Pineal Research*, 67 (3), https://doi.org/10.1111/jpi.12601.

Maganhin, Carla Cristina, Luiz Fernando Portugal Fuchs, Ricardo Santos Simões, Ricardo Martins Oliveira-Filho, Manuel de Jesus Simões, Edmund Chada Baracat, and José Maria Soares. (2013). "Effects of Melatonin on Ovarian Follicles." *European Journal of Obstetrics and Gynecology and Reproductive Biology*, 166 (2), 178–84. https://doi.org/10.1016/j.ejogrb.2012.10.006.

Maqbool, Mudasir, Mohmad Amin Dar, Imran Gani, and Mohammad Ishaq Geer. (2019). "Insulin Resistance and Polycystic Ovary Syndrome: A Review." *Journal of Drug Delivery and Therapeutics*, 9 (1-s), 433–36. https://doi.org/10.22270/jddt.v9i1-s.2275.

McMullan, Ciaran J., Gary C. Curhan, Eva S. Schernhammer, and John P. Forman. (2013). "Association of Nocturnal Melatonin Secretion with Insulin Resistance in Nondiabetic Young Women." *American Journal of Epidemiology*, 178 (2), 231–38. https://doi.org/10.1093/aje/kws470.

Mohamed, Dina Zakaria, Alaa El Din El Sayed El-Sisi, Samia Salim Sokar, Abdelhadi Mohamed Shebl, and Sally El Sayed Abu-Risha. (2021). "Targeting Autophagy to Modulate Hepatic Ischemia/Reperfusion Injury: A Comparative Study between Octreotide and Melatonin as Autophagy Modulators through AMPK/PI3K/AKT/MTOR/ULK1 and Keap1/Nrf2 Signaling Pathways in Rats." *European Journal of Pharmacology*, 897 (April). https://doi.org/10.1016/j.ejphar.2021.173920.

Mojaverrostami, Sina, Narjes Asghari, Mahsa Khamisabadi, and Heidar Heidari Khoei. (2019). "The Role of Melatonin in Polycystic Ovary Syndrome: A Review." *International Journal of Reproductive Biomedicine*, 17 (12), 865–82. https://doi.org/10.18502/ijrm.v17i12.5789.

Mor, M., Plazzi, P. v., Spadoni, G., and Tarzia, G. (1999). "Melatonin." *Current Medicinal Chemistry*, 6 (6), 501—518. http://europepmc.org/abstract/MED/10213796.

M Woo, Michelle M, Chen-jei Tai, Sung Keun Kang, Parimal S Nathwani, Shiu Fun Pang, and Peter C K Leung. (2001). "Direct Action of Melatonin in Human Granulosa-Luteal Cells."

Owino, Sharon, Daniella D.C. Buonfiglio, Cynthia Tchio, and Gianluca Tosini. (2019). "Melatonin Signaling a Key Regulator of Glucose Homeostasis and Energy Metabolism." *Frontiers in Endocrinology*., Frontiers Media S.A. https://doi.org/10.3389/fendo.2019.00488.

Patel, Seema. (2018). "Polycystic Ovary Syndrome (PCOS), an Inflammatory, Systemic, Lifestyle Endocrinopathy." *Journal of Steroid Biochemistry and Molecular Biology*, 182 (September), 27–36. https://doi.org/10.1016/j.jsbmb.2018.04.008.

Piggins, Hugh D. (2009). "Human Clock Genes." Https://Doi.Org/10.1080/078538902320772142, 34 (5), 394–400. https://doi.org/10.1080/078538902320772142.

Rodriguez Paris, Valentina, and Michael J. Bertoldo. (2019). "The Mechanism of Androgen Actions in PCOS Etiology." *Medical Sciences*, 7 (9), 89. https://doi.org/10.3390/medsci7090089.

Scarinci, E., Tropea, A., Notaristefano, G., Arena, V., Alesiani, O., Fabozzi, S. M., Lanzone, A., and Apa, R. (2019). "'Hormone of Darkness' and Human Reproductive Process: Direct Regulatory Role of Melatonin in Human Corpus Luteum." *Journal of Endocrinological Investigation*, 42 (10), 1191–97. https://doi.org/10.1007/s40618-019-01036-3.

Seko, Ludimila M.D., Rafael M. Moroni, Valeria M.S. Leitao, Danielle M. Teixeira, Carolina O. Nastri, and Wellington P. Martins. (2014). "Melatonin Supplementation during Controlled Ovarian Stimulation for Women Undergoing Assisted Reproductive Technology: Systematic Review and Meta-Analysis of Randomized Controlled Trials." *Fertility and Sterility*, 101 (1). https://doi.org/10.1016/j.fertnstert.2013.09.036.

Shaaban, Zahra, Arezoo Khoradmehr, Mohammad Reza Jafarzadeh Shirazi, and Amin Tamadon. (2019). "Pathophysiological Mechanisms of Gonadotropins- and Steroid Hormones-Related Genes in Etiology of Polycystic Ovary Syndrome." *Iranian Journal of Basic Medical Sciences*. Mashhad University of Medical Sciences. https://doi.org/10.22038/ijbms.2018.31776.7646.

Shreeve, N., Cagampang, F., Sadek, K., Tolhurst, M., Houldey, A., Hill, C. M., Brook, N., MacKlon, N., and Cheong, Y. (2013). "Poor Sleep in PCOS; Is Melatonin the Culprit?" *Human Reproduction*, 28 (5), 1348–53. https://doi.org/10.1093/humrep/det013.

Simon, Stacey L., Laura McWhirter, Cecilia Diniz Behn, Kate M. Bubar, Jill L. Kaar, Laura Pyle, Haseeb Rahat, et al. (2019). "Morning Circadian Misalignment Is Associated with Insulin Resistance in Girls with Obesity and Polycystic Ovarian Syndrome." *Journal of Clinical Endocrinology and Metabolism*, 104 (8), 3525–34. https://doi.org/10.1210/jc.2018-02385.

Song, Chao, Wei Peng, Songna Yin, Jiamin Zhao, Beibei Fu, Jingcheng Zhang, Tingchao Mao, Haibo Wu, and Yong Zhang. (2016). "Melatonin Improves Age-Induced Fertility Decline and Attenuates Ovarian Mitochondrial Oxidative Stress in Mice." *Scientific Reports*, 6 (October). https://doi.org/10.1038/SREP35165.

Spinedi, Eduardo, and Daniel P. Cardinali. (2018). "The Polycystic Ovary Syndrome and the Metabolic Syndrome: A Possible Chronobiotic-Cytoprotective Adjuvant Therapy." *International Journal of Endocrinology*., Hindawi Limited. https://doi.org/10.1155/2018/1349868.

Sun, Lihua, Hui Tian, Songguo Xue, Hongjuan Ye, Xue Xue, Rongxiang Wang, Yu Liu, Caixia Zhang, Qiuju Chen, and Shaorong Gao. (2021). "Circadian Clock Genes REV-ERBs Inhibits Granulosa Cells Apoptosis by Regulating Mitochondrial Biogenesis and Autophagy in Polycystic Ovary Syndrome." *Frontiers in Cell and Developmental Biology*, 9 (August): 2079. https://doi.org/10.3389/FCELL.2021.658112/BIBTEX.

Sun, Tie Cheng, Hui Ying Li, Xiao Yu Li, Kun Yu, Shou Long Deng, and Li Tian. (2020). "Protective Effects of Melatonin on Male Fertility Preservation and Reproductive System." *Cryobiology*., Academic Press Inc. https://doi.org/10.1016/j.cryobiol.2020.01.018.

Tamura, Hiroshi, Mai Jozaki, Manabu Tanabe, Yuichiro Shirafuta, Yumiko Mihara, Masahiro Shinagawa, Isao Tamura, et al. (2020). "Importance of Melatonin in Assisted Reproductive Technology and Ovarian Aging." *International Journal of Molecular Sciences*., MDPI AG. https://doi.org/10.3390/ijms21031135.

Tamura, Hiroshi, Mai Kawamoto, Shun Sato, Isao Tamura, Ryo Maekawa, Toshiaki Taketani, Hiromi Aasada, et al. (2017). "Long-Term Melatonin Treatment Delays Ovarian Aging." *Journal of Pineal Research*, 62 (2). https://doi.org/10.1111/JPI.12381.

Tamura, Hiroshi, Yasuhiko Nakamura, Ahmet Korkmaz, Lucien C. Manchester, Dun Xian Tan, Norihiro Sugino, and Russel J. Reiter. (2009). "Melatonin and the Ovary: Physiological and Pathophysiological Implications." *Fertility and Sterility*, 92 (1): 328–43. https://doi.org/10.1016/J.FERTNSTERT.2008.05.016.

Vasey, Clayton, Jennifer McBride, and Kayla Penta. (2021). "Circadian Rhythm Dysregulation and Restoration: The Role of Melatonin." *Nutrients*, 13 (10). https://doi.org/10.3390/nu13103480.

Voorhis, Bradley J van, Melissa S Dunn, Gary D Snyder, and Carl P Weiner. (1994). "Nitric Oxide: An Autocrine Regulator of Human Granulosa-Luteal Cell Steroidogenesis*." *Endocrinology*. Vol. 135.

Wang, Fangfang, Ningning Xie, Yan Wu, Qing Zhang, Yuhang Zhu, Minchen Dai, Jue Zhou, et al. (2021). "Association between Circadian Rhythm Disruption and Polycystic Ovary Syndrome." *Fertility and Sterility*, 115 (3), 771–81. https://doi.org/10.1016/J.FERTNSTERT.2020.08.1425.

Wang, Juan, Daichao Wu, Hui Guo, and Meixiang Li. (2019). "Hyperandrogenemia and Insulin Resistance: The Chief Culprit of Polycystic Ovary Syndrome." *Life Sciences*., Elsevier Inc. https://doi.org/10.1016/j.lfs.2019.116940.

Xu, Yalan, and Jie Qiao. (2022). "Association of Insulin Resistance and Elevated Androgen Levels with Polycystic Ovarian Syndrome (PCOS): A Review of Literature." *Journal of Healthcare Engineering*., Hindawi Limited. https://doi.org/10.1155/2022/9240569.

Yang, Hui Li, Wen Jie Zhou, Chun Jie Gu, Yu Han Meng, Jun Shao, Da Jin Li, and Ming Qing Li. (2018a). "Pleiotropic Roles of Melatonin in Endometriosis, Recurrent Spontaneous Abortion, and Polycystic Ovary Syndrome." *American Journal of Reproductive Immunology* (New York, N.Y.: 1989), 80 (1). https://doi.org/10.1111/AJI.12839.

Ye, Wenting, Tingting Xie, Yali Song, and Lili Zhou. (2021). "The Role of Androgen and Its Related Signals in PCOS." *Journal of Cellular and Molecular Medicine*. Blackwell Publishing Inc. https://doi.org/10.1111/jcmm.16205.

Zeng, Xin, Yuan jie Xie, Ya ting Liu, Shuang lian Long, and Zhong cheng Mo. (2020). "Polycystic Ovarian Syndrome: Correlation between Hyperandrogenism, Insulin Resistance and Obesity." *Clinica Chimica Acta*., Elsevier B.V. https://doi.org/10.1016/j.cca.2019.11.003.

Zhai, Junyu, Shang Li, Min Hu, Fangfang Di, Jiansheng Liu, and Yanzhi Du. (2020). "Decreased Brain and Muscle ARNT-like Protein 1 Expression Mediated the Contribution of Hyperandrogenism to Insulin Resistance in Polycystic Ovary Syndrome." *Reproductive Biology and Endocrinology: RB&E*, 18 (1). https://doi.org/10.1186/S12958-020-00592-1.

Zhang, Lu, Zhenzhen Zhang, Jing Wang, Dongying Lv, Tianqi Zhu, Feng Wang, Xiuzhi Tian, Yujun Yao, Pengyun Ji, and Guoshi Liu. (2019). "Melatonin Regulates the Activities of Ovary and Delays the Fertility Decline in Female Animals via MT1/AMPK Pathway." *Journal of Pineal Research*, 66 (3). https://doi.org/10.1111/JPI.12550.

Zhang, Mianqun, Yajuan Lu, Ying Chen, Yu Zhang, and Bo Xiong. (2020). "Insufficiency of Melatonin in Follicular Fluid Is a Reversible Cause for Advanced Maternal Age-Related Aneuploidy in Oocytes." *Redox Biology*, 28 (January). https://doi.org/10.1016/J.REDOX.2019.101327.

Zhao, S. Q., Gao, Y., Zhang, Y., Yang, X. P., and Yang, Z. (2021). "CAMP/PKA/CREB Signaling Pathway-Mediated Effects of Melatonin Receptor Genes on Clock Gene Expression in Bactrian Camel Ovarian Granulosa Cells." *Domestic Animal Endocrinology*, 76, (July). https://doi.org/10.1016/j.domaniend.2021.106609.

Chapter 5

# PCOS and Obesity: The Role of TSH on Fat Metabolism and Its Dysfunctional Repercussions

**Bushra Zia[1,*,†]**
**Saima Nisar[2,†]**
**and Samrah Zaki Ansari[2,†]**
[1]Department of Biochemistry, Faculty of Life Sciences, Aligarh Muslim University, Aligarh, India
[2]Department of Zoology, Faculty of Life Sciences, Aligarh Muslim University, Aligarh, India

## Abstract

Polycystic ovarian syndrome and obesity have been intimately linked due to numerous incidences of their coexistence in women worldwide. PCOS has been linked to an elevated risk of a variety of clinical outcomes, including metabolic like insulin resistance, and poor glucose tolerance but may also extend to include type 2 diabetes mellitus and cardiovascular disease, whereas abnormalities associated with reproduction include infertility, significantly higher levels of androgens in the blood and hirsutism. Psychological characteristics include constant complaints of anxiety and depression all of which have poor outcomes when associated with quality of life. Obesity exacerbates various aspects of PCOS, including hyperandrogenism, hirsutism, infertility, and complications associated with pregnancy. Obesity and PCOS have both been associated with an increase in not only incidences of insulin resistance but also diabetes mellitus and cardiovascular diseases, which aggravate the reproductive and metabolic aspects of PCOS. This interdependence can be attributed to the coordination of the hypothalamus-pituitary ovary axis and the hypothalamus-pituitary thyroid axis, as well as their interaction, which influences their functionality. Abnormal levels of thyroid stimulating hormone can affect female metabolism and hence create an imbalance in the proper functioning of the reproductive system. The imbalance in the functioning of the hypothalamus-pituitary-ovary axis caused by endocrine hormone disorders in PCOS patients also affects the pituitary thyroid axis by creating an inconsistency in the serum TSH levels. Both thyroid-related disorders and PCOS have been linked to the hyperactive state of the immune system that is known to induce an imbalance in the harmonious functioning of the two systems. A concurrent result of this is the onset of the preliminary stages of obesity, due to a

* Corresponding Author's Email: bushrazia@gmail.com.
† These authors have contributed equally.

In: Polycystic Ovarian Syndrome (PCOS) and Our Biological Clock
Editors: Arpita Roy, Gowhar Rashid and Nihad Ashraf Khan
ISBN: 979-8-89113-100-2
© 2023 Nova Science Publishers, Inc.

phenomenon known as 'insulin resistance,' which is caused by a very low level of serum thyroid hormones.

**Keywords:** TSH (Thyroid-stimulating hormone), hypothyroidism, insulin resistance, obesity, polycystic ovarian syndrome

# 1. Introduction

The endocrine system plays a vital and inimitable role in regulating the important functions of the body including maintaining a steady rate of metabolism and catering to the needs of the reproductive system in a systematic manner. Some such important hormones that are to be discussed in further detail are the hormones produced by the thyroid gland. These hormones are peptide-based and synthesized by a complex mechanism that is under feedback control. The thyroid hormones (TH), therefore play a prominent role in establishing a steady rate of metabolism. Obesity, cardiovascular diseases, and other fatal diseases are sometimes under the indirect control of these hormones. Thyroid hormones are iodinated dipeptides that undergo a complex series of biochemical reactions before being synthesized, stored, released, and transported. These steps are as follows: a) availability and absorption of iodine; b) iodide uptake into the thyroid; c) iodide oxidation; d) iodination of tyrosine residues within thyroglobulin; e) storage of thyroid hormones in a thyroglobulin-bound form; and f) proteolysis of thyroglobulin and hormone release into the blood (Miot et al. 2015); M DeVito et al. 1999).

## 1.1. The Synthesis and Storage of the Thyroid Hormones

Thyroid hormones (TH) are hydrophobic amine hormones; their production depends on the amino acid tyrosine. Their synthesis occurs predominantly in the thyroid gland at the interface of the surface of polarized thyroid follicular cells facing the lumen and the colloid (Peters, van Trotsenburg, and Schoenmakers 2018). The thyroid gland is a butterfly-shaped structure located in front of the trachea in the lower neck region. It is made up of thyroid follicles, which constitute the thyroid gland's structural and functional unit. Thyroid follicles contain simple cuboidal-shaped epithelial cells which are known as thyroid follicular cells. They store thyroid hormone and allow for the regulated release of the hormone (Braverman et al. 2013) as illustrated in Figure 1. The thyroid hormone is composed of two products released by thyroid follicles. They are the prohormone L-thyroxine (tetraiodothyronine, T4) which constitutes the major product, and the active hormone L-triiodothyronine (T3), the minor product (Miot et al. 2015).

### *1.1.1. Availability and Absorption of Iodine*

Iodine is a necessary micronutrient in human nutrition, necessary for the proper growth and development of the body. Iodine is ingested in food and water in its ion form, i.e., as iodide. It is an essential mineral needed for the production of the thyroid hormones thyroxine (T4) and triiodothyronine (T3), accounting for 65% and 59% of their respective weights. Milk, meat, fish, seaweed, shrimp, dairy products, and eggs are some of the major iodine sources (Miot et al. 2015). The daily intake of iodine in an adult human is 150 μg/day. A woman's iodine requirement rises from 150 to 250 µg/day during pregnancy and lactation. The thyroid gland and kidney remove most iodide from circulation. In typical conditions, dietary iodine is absorbed at a rate greater than 90%. The thyroid preferentially concentrates iodide to the levels required for optimum thyroid hormone production, with the majority of the leftover iodine eliminated in the urine. The thyroid's capacity to concentrate iodide was originally observed in 1915 (Braverman et al. 2013).

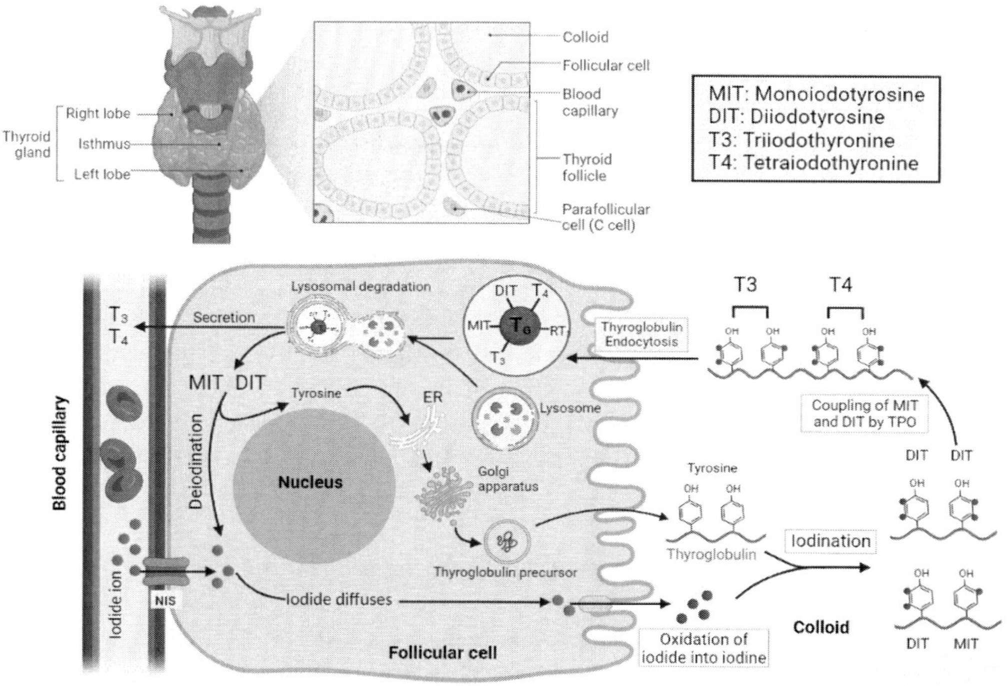


**Figure 1.** Iodide ions are taken up by follicular cells via active transport and are oxidized to iodine which is involved in the iodination of thyroglobulin to synthesize Monoiodotyrosine and Diiodotyrosine which on further coupling will lead to the formation of T3 and T4. The thyroid hormones are endocytosed by the follicular cell and undergo lysosomal degradation to secrete the newly synthesized T3 and T4 hormones, whereas the rest of the substrate is recycled to synthesize thyroglobulin.

### *1.1.2. The Uptake of Iodide into the Thyroid and Its Subsequent Oxidation*

Iodide is the rate-limiting substrate that is actively carried from the blood into the follicular thyroid cells via the thyroidal basal membrane protein sodium/iodide symporter (NIS). It is an integral glycoprotein embedded in the plasma membrane and has a molecular weight of 87 kDa. To ensure that the thyroid gland receives sufficient iodine for hormone production, NIS actively transports iodide into the thyroid gland from the blood circulation at a concentration gradient that is about 20 to 50 times that of the plasma. (Braverman et al. 2013); (Dohán et al. 2003). The Na+/I− symporter couples the transport of sodium and iodide ions. The electrochemical gradient of Na+ created by the Na+/K+ ATPase and the electrical potential across the plasma membrane supply energy for the process, which transports one iodide for every two sodium ions. Because this activity does not employ ATP directly, it is classified as secondary active transport.

Iodide is then passively transferred through the apical plasma membrane by another transporter termed pendrin (PDS) and enters the lumen. Pendrin is a membrane glycoprotein with a molecular weight of 110kDA that is encoded by the PDS gene and has 780 amino acids. (Yoshida et al. 2002); (Miot et al. 2015). Before it is utilized, iodide must be oxidized to a higher oxidation state, i.e., to iodine (I2). In the presence of H2O2, thyroid peroxidase (TPO) catalyzes this reaction. TPO, also known as thyroperoxidase, is a heme-binding glycoprotein found on the apical membrane of the thyrocyte, with its catalytic site towards the lumen (Miot et al. 2015) A membrane-bound NADPH-dependent flavoprotein produces H2O2. It is found in the thyroid follicular lumen and is used as an oxidative agent during thyroid hormone synthesis (Szanto, Pusztaszeri, and Mavromati 2019).

#### *1.1.3. Iodination of Tyrosine Residues within Thyroglobulin*

In addition to catalyzing the oxidation of iodide, TPO is also required for the incorporation of iodide onto tyrosine residues in thyroglobulin, a process known as organification. Thyroglobulin is a large glycoprotein scaffold that is produced and released in the follicular lumen by thyroid epithelial cells. TPO binds iodine to the tyrosine amino acids in thyroglobulin. This is known as iodination, and it results in the formation of the hormone precursors diiodotyrosine (DIT) and monoiodotyrosine (MIT) (Miot et al. 2015)). Thyroperoxidase then catalyzes the intramolecular pairing/coupling of two molecules of diiodotyrosine to create tetraiodothyronine or thyroxine (T4). Triiodothyronine (T3) is produced via a similar pairing of one molecule of monoiodotyrosine and one of diiodotyrosine. T3 and T4 are collectively referred to as thyroid hormones.

#### *1.1.4. Storage of Thyroid Hormones in the Thyroglobulin-Bound Form and Its Ensuing Release into the Bloodstream*

Thyroglobulin, which contains the thyroid hormones, is stored extracellularly in the lumen of the thyroid follicles as a colloid until required. Thyroid hormone stored in follicles is enough to supply thyroid hormones to the body for 2–3 months. When there is a demand for the stored hormone, thyroglobulin enters the thyroid cells as colloid droplets via vesicle-mediated endocytosis. Thyroxine and triiodothyronine are cleaved and released from the thyroglobulin, then delivered in circulation for further activity. Lysosomes in the cell cytoplasm fuse with vesicles containing thyroglobulin (colloid droplets). The lysosome's hydrolytic enzymes digest thyroglobulin molecules, isolating T3 and T4. Thyroxine and triiodothyronine then diffuse out of the follicular epithelial cells into the surrounding capillaries (Nussey S et al. 2001). The MIT and DIT released from the thyroglobulin molecule during the proteolytic breakdown are not secreted in large quantities into circulation. Instead, the deiodinase enzyme cleaves its iodine, making it accessible for the production of thyroid hormones.

### 1.2. Regulation of Thyroid Hormone Production

To ensure that the metabolic levels of the body are optimally maintained, thyroid hormone (TH) should be secreted in the correct amount. So that this optimal level of TH might be attained, the adenohypophysis and the hypothalamus are involved in feedback mechanisms as illustrated in Figure 2.

### *1.2.1. TRH (Thyrotropin Releasing Hormone)*

TRH (Thyrotropin Releasing Hormone) is synthesized in the paraventricular nucleus of the hypothalamus. It moves to the adenohypophysis via the hypophyseal stalk and stimulates the synthesis and release of TSH. (Kim and Mohan 2013). TRH binds to the TRH receptors which are GPCRs and are found on the thyrotropic cells of the pituitary (the cells of the pituitary gland involved in the production and secretion of TSH). This causes the cAMP levels inside the cells to rise and leads to the release of TSH. TRH receptor or TRHR has 398 amino acids and when TRH binds to it, it changes the way it interacts with the G protein. This stimulates the activation of Phospholipase C. The hydrolysis of PI(4,5)P2 to IP3 and DAG is catalyzed by activated PLC. IP3 and DAG initiate a series of reactions, which also include an elevation in the cellular levels of Ca2+ and activation of PKC, which eventually culminate in the production and secretion of TSH (Visser 2018). Dopamine, somatostatin, and leptin modulate the secretion of TSH and act as a central regulator of thyroid hormone release. Kidney failure, starvation, lack of sleep, depression, as well as growth hormone, cortisol, and sex steroids all affect the secretion of TSH as well as its sensitivity to stimulation by TRH (Mullur, Liu, and Brent 2014). The negative feedback mechanism of TH regulates the production followed by the secretion of TRH from the hypothalamus. As TH is involved in the expenditure of energy and heat generation, unsurprisingly, exposure to cold induces secretion of TRH resulting in the stimulation of the HPT axis. Feeding also has an important part to play in the control of the HPT axis, with a significant role played by leptin. Fasting has been reported to be related to the downregulation of the HPT axis. In animals under study, this downregulation is avoided by giving leptin doses to those animals (Visser 2018).

### *1.2.2. TSH (Thyroid Stimulating Hormone)*

A glycoprotein, Thyroid Stimulating Hormone is synthesized in the thyrotropic cells of the adenohypophysis. TSH in humans is composed of 205 amino acids, of which 92 belong to the α subunit and 113 belong to the β subunit. The molecular weight of TSH is 28 kDa. TSH synthesis and release are negatively regulated by somatostatin, dopamine, and cortisol, along with a negative feedback control exerted by TH and also being stimulated by TRH. The receptor for thyroid stimulating hormone called the TSH receptor or TSHR is localized in the thyroid gland, precisely in the follicular cell's plasma membrane. It is a GPCR, composed of 764 amino acids. When Thyroid Stimulating Hormone binds to the receptor, the subunits of the G protein dissociate, as a consequence of which, the adenylate cyclase bound to the membrane is activated, which in turn causes the emergence of cAMP as a secondary messenger. The elevated levels of cAMP culminate in the synthesis followed by the secretion of Thyroid Hormone (Visser 2018). TSH stimulates the production and secretion of T4 (3,5,3′,5′-tetraiodothyronine) and T3 (3,5,3′-L-triiodothyronine). Carrier proteins like TBG (Thyroxine binding globulin), transthyretin, and albumin are involved in binding T3 and T4. Around 0.2% of T3 and 0.02% of T4 occur in the plasma freely. The production and secretion of TRH and TSH are inhibited by TH by means of a nuclear TH receptor found in the hypothalamus and adenohypophysis. This completes a negative feedback loop which helps in maintaining the normal levels of thyroid hormone. The inverse relationship between the levels of circulating T3 and T4 and TSH is also maintained by this negative feedback loop (Kim and Mohan 2013).

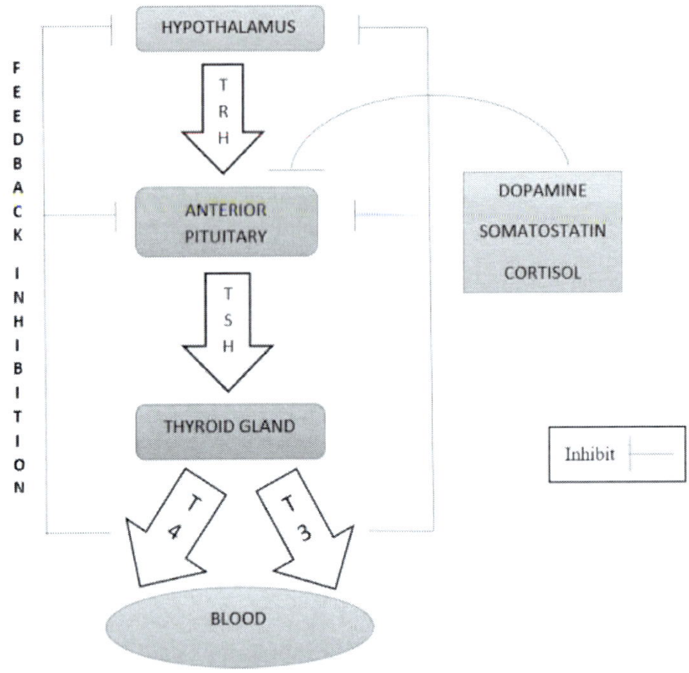


**Figure 2.** Regulation of thyroid hormone production and release.

## 2. Role of TSH on Metabolic and Reproductive Health

The social economy is on the rise in recent decades, and this has led to the advent in the increase of incidences of metabolic disorders that mainly comprise obesity, hypertension, hyperglycemia, diseases that record a higher occurrence of triglycerides and very low levels of high-density lipoproteins cholesterol. Many of which, have a huge impact on the health profile and lifestyle of an individual (Gu et al. 2005). One of the most important organs that significant impact on regulating the metabolism of the body is the thyroid. The thyroid hormones, as discussed above have multiple roles in the regulatory cycles of glucose, lipids, blood circulation, and energy consumption. Thyroid stimulating hormones (TSH) has a regulatory effect on the thyroid hormones. The concentration of TSH in blood plasma will be significantly higher in the case where the individuals have a seemingly lower concentration of thyroid hormones in order to stimulate the synthesis of the thyroid hormones. Hyperthyroidism is a prominent risk factor for hypertension and diabetes whereas hypothyroidism is strongly linked to abdominal obesity and various metabolic disorders. As a result, metabolic syndromes are tightly linked to subclinical hypothyroidism. Kendle, for the first time, reported the case of a young girl with clinically high levels of thyroid hormones who developed precocious puberty (Kendle, 1905). Ever since, strong associations do exist between hypothyroidism and abnormalities associated with reproductive health (Röjdmark, Berg, and Kallner 1988). Studies suggest a decrease in the rate of metabolic clearance of steroid hormones in women with hyperthyroidism (Joshi et al. 1993). Not surprisingly, these metabolic disturbances are resolved once the euthyroid stage is reached. Hypothyroidism has a significant impact on the length and duration of the menstrual cycle of a woman. Additionally, a decrease in the serum levels of clotting factors VII, VIII, IX, and XI has been associated with the abnormalities associated with menstrual cycles mainly menorrhagia and polymenorrhea. Many studies conducted to evaluate the incidences of menstrual irregularities indicate the frequency of these incidences is around three times greater than in the control population (Krassas et al. 1999; Redmond 2004).

On the other hand, the simultaneous appearance of clinical symptoms of metabolic syndrome and thyroid dysfunction is frequently observed. Metabolism-related health problems are often associated with obesity and other risk factors that include cardiovascular diseases, type 2 diabetes, and mortality (Alberti, Zimmet, and Shaw 2005; Hu et al. 2004). There are two major criteria recommended by the International Diabetes Federation and National Cholesterol Education Program includes four main features that outline various physiological characteristics including body adiposity which is measured in terms of the circumference of the waist; serum glucose levels that reflect the diagnosis of diabetes; abnormalities associated with serum levels of triglycerides or 'good' cholesterol and a significant increase in the blood pressure levels.

(Alberti, Zimmet, and Shaw 2005; Expert Panel on Detection and Treatment of High Blood Cholesterol in Adults 2001).

Hence, metabolic syndrome is diagnosed if three or more than three of these features co-exist in the clinical profile of an individual. Another feature that is insulin resistance, characterized by the presence of abnormally high levels of insulin is also cited by some authors. The interrelationship between thyroid dysfunction and metabolic abnormalities can relate both ways, that is, metabolic abnormalities may not necessarily be a consequence of thyroid dysfunction but also vice versa. Therefore, their co-existence makes it difficult to establish the cause-consequence effect. Thyroid hormones and some of their metabolites regulate metabolic rates leading to variations in weight gain and adiposity (Fontenelle M. M. et al. 2016; Laurberg et al. 2012)]. Thyroid hormones play an important role in controlling appetite and sympathetic activity, conversely, the functionality of thyroid hormone is also affected by deposition of adipose tissues (Iwen, Schröder, and Brabant 2013).

## 3. PCOS and Hypothalamic-Pituitary-Thyroid Axis

The hypothalamic-pituitary-ovarian (HPO) axis controls reproductive activity by being involved in the secretion of reproductive hormones. The HPO axis contains three main components – the hypothalamus, the pituitary gland, and the ovaries. The gonadotropin-releasing hormone (GnRH) produced by the hypothalamus acts on the adenohypophysis, better known as the anterior pituitary gland, in response to which the pituitary secretes an assortment of hormones, including LH and FSH. The hormones of the pituitary act on the ovaries, stimulating the release of estrogen and progesterone. The HPO axis and HPT axis are related to each other physiologically. The ovaries bear receptors for the thyroid hormone and estrogen also affects the HPT axis. The increased prevalence of hypothyroidism among patients of PCOS, disturbed levels of leptin, as well as occurrence of insulin resistance in both diseases, denote a prominent link between thyroid disorders and PCOS (Anwaar and Jabeen 2022). The ovarian volume was found to be increased as well as cystic changes were also observed in patients with hypothyroidism (Singla et al. 2015).

The HPT axis controls the level of hormones of the thyroid in the blood. These levels are disturbed in Autoimmune Thyroid Diseases, mainly- Grave's disease and Hashimoto's thyroiditis. Hashimoto's thyroiditis leads to hypothyroidism while Grave's disease leads to hyperthyroidism. An increasing prevalence of PCOS has been reported in females suffering from both hyper- as well as hypothyroidism (Anwaar and Jabeen 2022). Studies were carried out in PCOS patients to note the levels of thyroglobulin antibodies and the levels of the enzyme thyroid peroxidase. Hashimoto's thyroiditis is characteristically diagnosed by the above two mentioned markers. It was found that their levels were elevated in PCOS patients. The thyroid ultrasound of these patients also revealed a pattern resembling that of Hashimoto's thyroiditis (Anwaar and Jabeen 2022).

Hyperthyroidism in Grave's disease leads to thyrotoxicosis-a condition involving high levels of circulating thyroid hormones, which causes elevated levels of testosterone, androstenedione, SHBG, and not to forget, estradiol. Thyrotoxicosis leads to amenorrhea, anovulation, and oligomenorrhea (Nisar et al. 2012). The effects of thyrotoxicosis on the hypothalamic-pituitary axis in adult females lead to fluctuations in the release of gonadotropins and also the amount of SHBG in circulation, that result in altered metabolism of steroids (Anwaar and Jabeen 2022). Hypothyroidism or hyperthyroidism is found to co-exist along with conditions such as a menstrual cycle lacking ovulation, reduction in reproductive capacity, and risky pregnancy. Pituitary hormones, viz., GH, PL, or TSH, can function together along with FSH and LH to assist in the advancement of follicles that lack growth into the growing phase. TRH is another common link between the HPT axis and the HPO axis. TRH is involved in facilitating the secretion of prolactin too, along with TSH. TSH exerts negative feedback control over TRH via a short negative feedback loop. Any increment in levels of TSH leads to a decrease in the release of TRH, consequently inhibiting the secretion of prolactin and TSH. Disturbance in this feedback control may lead to hyperprolactinemia that affects fertility potential negatively by hampering GnRH secretion and thus, leading to disturbed ovulation (P, Ravi, and Sadaria 2021).

## 4. Correlation between hypothyroidism and PCOS

Several research has found a substantial link correlating hypothyroidism and polycystic ovarian syndrome (PCOS). PCOS and hypothyroidism are both prevalent endocrine diseases in the general population. The symptoms of both these hormonal disorders often coincide. Some of these overlapping symptoms include menstrual irregularities, anovulation, weight gain, and increased insulin resistance. Primary hypothyroidism has been related to an increased ovarian volume as well as cystic ovarian abnormalities. Several studies show that there is a significantly higher prevalence of hypothyroidism, especially Hashimoto's thyroiditis (HT) in PCOS-diagnosed women than in women without PCOS (Singla et al. 2015); (Benetti-Pinto et al. 2013) A case study by Hansen et al. reported massive ovarian enlargement and multiple cyst formation in primary hypothyroidism. This ovulatory dysfunction with the formation of cysts in primary hypothyroidism may be due to different factors including abnormal estrogen metabolism, altered metabolism of prolactin, a direct effect on the ovary, etc. (Hansen et al. 1997) as has been depicted in Figure 3.

Hypothyroidism is described as a condition in which the thyroid gland does not produce enough thyroid hormone to fulfill the metabolic demands of the body. Hypothyroidism affects more women than males and worsens with age. PCOS is a prevalent hormonal reproductive disorder that affects 8-20% of reproductive-age women worldwide. At her reproductive age, one out of every ten women has its symptoms (Anwaar and Jabeen 2022). It is characterized by anovulation, hyperandrogenism (an excessive amount of androgens), and polycystic ovarian morphology seen on ultrasound. According to some researchers, a percentage of women with polycystic ovary syndrome may also have an underactive thyroid gland (Elslimani, Elhasi, and Elmhdwi 2016). Different factors are involved in linking these two disorders.

- Autoimmunity: The link between autoimmunity and PCOS in women has received a lot of attention in recent years. Some scientists believe that a chronically overactive immune response may be at the root of both hypothyroidism and PCOS (Romitti et al. 2018).
- Genetic factors: Some research suggests that the FBN3 gene (fibrillin 3) is involved in both these disorders. Gonadotropin-releasing hormone receptor (GnRHR), and CYP1B1 may also be involved. The regulatory T cells (Tregs) are specialized T cells that suppress an overactive immune response. Variations in the FBN3 gene cause it to fail to stimulate Tregs, resulting in unrestrained autoimmune processes and a greater prevalence of hypothyroidism and PCOS (Singh et al. 2020).
- Increased level of testosterone: According to some research, hypothyroidism raises testosterone levels in the body, which causes PCOS symptoms such as irregular periods, excessive face and body hair development, and an irregular polycystic look of the ovaries.

## 4.1. Effect on the Thyroid in PCOS

The result of some previous studies investigating thyroid changes in PCOS showed that PCOS women had higher TSH levels and more autoimmune thyroiditis than non-PCOS women. (Elslimani, Elhasi, and Elmhdwi 2016). Thyroid autoimmunity is more common in PCOS individuals. When compared to controls, PCOS-diagnosed females had higher levels of thyroid antibodies, bigger thyroid volumes, and hypoechogenic thyroid with more hypoechoic nodules (Singla et al. 2015). Multiple studies in PCOS patients have revealed an increase in the levels of antibodies related to the thyroid such as anti-TPO, anti-TSH, and anti-Tg. As a consequence, a rise in estrogen and the estrogen/progesterone ratios was ascribed to an increase in the thyroid autoantibodies observed in PCOS patients (Singh, J et al. 2020). A high estrogen-to-progesterone ratio in PCOS can lead to hypothyroidism. In women with PCOS, estrogen levels are often greater than normal while progesterone levels are lower, increasing the overall estrogen-to-progesterone ratio. Women with PCOS have a greater frequency of hypothyroidism or thyroid autoimmunity, although the pathophysiological mechanism and other reasons behind this association remain unknown.

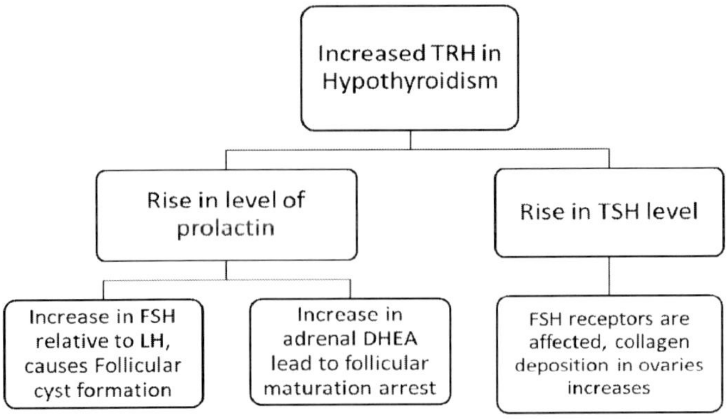


**Figure 3.** Pathophysiology of PCOS in patients with hypothyroidism.

## 5. Impact of TSH Dysregulation on Ovaries

The functioning of the female reproductive system is tightly regulated by the thyroid hormones. Hypothyroidism can cause ovulatory dysfunction, ovarian morphology becomes polycystic and can lead to impaired female fertility (Singla et al. 2015). Animal studies suggest that receptors for the thyroid hormones, thyrotropin-releasing hormone, and thyroid-stimulating hormone are also found in the uterus (Hulchiy et al. 2012). In primary hypothyroidism, a rise in thyrotropin-releasing hormone (TRH) is associated with a rise in the level of prolactin and thyroid-stimulating hormone (TSH). Prolactin inhibits ovulation due to a significant decrease in the ratio of follicle-stimulating hormone (FSH) to luteinizing hormone (LH) and leads to polycystic ovarian morphology. When seen with an ultrasound, a rise in ovarian volume and the development of bilateral multicystic ovaries are frequently observed. Thyroid hormone replacement treatment, in addition to regulating thyroid hormone levels, causes ovarian cysts to retreat and ovarian volume to decrease (Singla et al. 2015); (Elslimani, Elhasi, and Elmhdwi 2016). All of this colludes to one important point which is the significant role of thyroid disorders in affecting the functional reserves of the ovaries. These disorders have been known to cause a diverse range of endocrine problems in the reproductive age and are usually the key factor behind infertility in many cases due to the irregularities in the menstrual and ovulatory cycles caused by them. Though the exact mechanism of action of these thyroid hormones on the ovaries remains unclear, many studies indicate that the relationship may be due to the presence of many receptors of thyroid hormones on the surface of different cells in the ovaries including the granulosa cells, oocytes, and epithelial cells. Additionally, FSH and TSH have a synergistic effect in promoting the proliferation of granulosa cells.

As some studies suggest, follicles are prevented from undergoing apoptosis because of the stimulation of the FSH by TSH. During the formation of follicles, there is a marked increase in the serum TSH level because of the decrease in the free thyroxin level caused due to the binding of thyroid hormones to the thyroid-binding globulin. It is due to this interlinked mechanism, that a dysregulation in the TSH levels may cause direct impairment in the process of the formation of follicles. Apart from this, this hormone also plays an important role in the early phases of development by assisting in the process of implantation because of its effect on the inner lining of the uterus and placenta. Many studies also support the notion that there is a direct relationship between the serum level of TSH hormone and ovarian reserves (Michalakis et al. 2011; Kuroda et al. 2015). But many others contradict this fact and suggest an inverse relationship between the two set parameters (Kabodmehri et al. 2021). Prospective studies with a larger sample set must be carried out in the future to establish the appropriate relationship between the thyroid hormones and their effect on the ovaries and their reserves.

## 6. Role of TSH Dysregulation in Developing Insulin Resistance

Insulin resistance is a glucose homeostasis condition in which a combination of hereditary factors, diet, inactivity, and obesity results in a decreased sensitivity of muscles, liver, adipose tissue, and other body tissues to insulin despite normal blood concentrations (Gierach, Gierach, and Junik 2014). Insulin is a crucial endocrine peptide hormone involved in maintaining glucose homeostasis. Insulin is produced by the pancreas and released into the bloodstream when glucose levels rise following a regular meal. Insulin binds plasma membrane-bound receptors in target cells and enables the uptake of glucose. Insulin also instructs the liver to store blood sugar in the form of glycogen for later usage (Petersen and Shulman 2018). When blood glucose reaches cells, its quantity in circulation lowers, signaling insulin to decrease as well. Insulin resistance occurs when these cells do not react properly to insulin and are unable to utilize blood glucose for energy. To compensate for the cells' increased resistance, the pancreas produces more insulin. Insulin resistance can lead to complications such as diabetes, hypertension, different malignancies, dyslipidemia, atherosclerosis, NASH (nonalcoholic steatohepatitis), and PCOS (polycystic ovarian syndrome).

### 6.1. Thyroid Hormone and TSH in Insulin Resistance

Thyroid hormones, namely T4 and T3 are crucial in glucose metabolism and the development of insulin resistance. The thyroid hormone (TH) acts as both an agonist and antagonist to insulin in various organs. The thyroid hormone inhibits insulin action by promoting hepatic gluconeogenesis and glycogenolysis. TH also increases the expression of GLUT-4 genes and phosphoglycerate kinase, both of which are involved in glucose transport and glycolysis, and hence work in tandem with insulin. This happens in a delicate equilibrium for optimal glucose metabolism. Excess or deficiency of TH can disrupt this balance, causing changes in glucose metabolism (Kapadia, Bhatt, and Shah 2012); (Brenta 2011). TSH regulates thyroid hormone levels, which has a negative feedback effect as has been depicted in Figure 4. TSH receptors have been discovered in a wide range of cell types, including adipocytes. When TSH binds to the receptor present in the adipocytes, it induces the release of interleukin-6, which subsequently mediates preadipocyte and adipocyte proliferation and differentiation, and the secretion of leptin (Zhu, Liu, and Mao 2018). As TSH levels rise, it binds to the TSH receptors on adipocytes, resulting in altered thyroid hormone signaling in adipocytes. This reduces the release of the insulin-sensitizing mediator adiponectin, resulting in insulin resistance (Kumar Ahirwar et al. 2017).

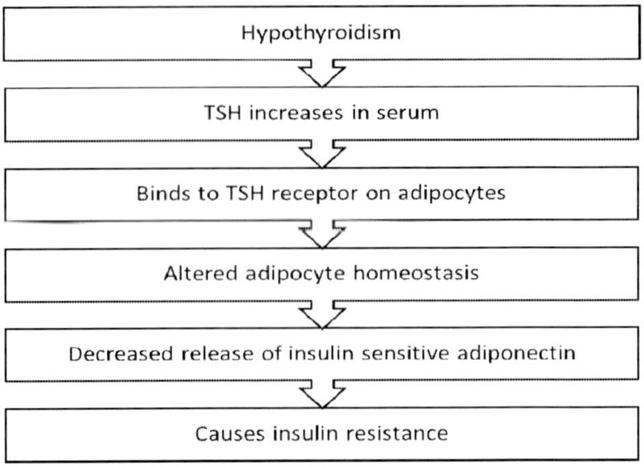


**Figure 4.** Link between thyroid dysfunction and insulin resistance.

## 6.2. Insulin Resistance due to Hypothyroidism

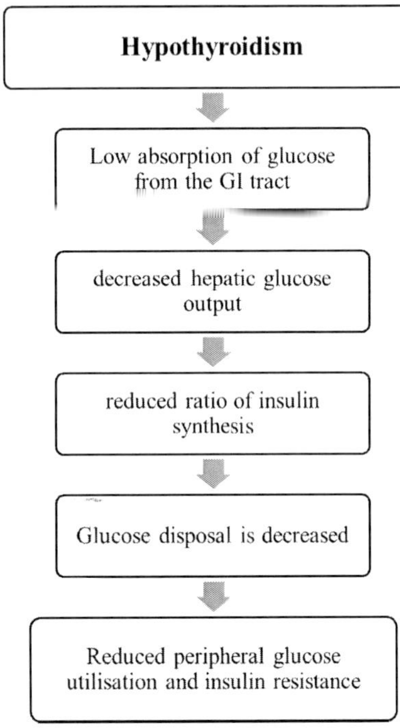


**Figure 5.** Insulin resistance as a consequence of hypothyroidism.

The consequences of hypothyroidism are less obvious. Yet, the evidence suggests that insulin resistance is mostly seen in the peripheral tissues. Thyroid hormones, as previously noted, maintain a delicate balance of glucose metabolism by acting as both insulin agonists and antagonists. Hypothyroidism can disrupt this equilibrium and disrupt glucose homeostasis, leading to insulin resistance as illustrated in Figure 5. Some investigations have found that hypothyroidism has considerably higher insulin levels than controls (Bhongir, 2014) This might be explained by the fact that the lower the level of thyroid hormones in plasma, the poorer the tissue insulin sensitivity. T3 and insulin are known to work together to maintain glucose homeostasis. It may thus be expected that a lower intracellular T3 level would result in poorer insulin-stimulated glucose elimination (Maratou et al. 2009).

### 6.3. Insulin Resistance due to Hyperthyroidism

Excess THs cause hyperglycemia in hyperthyroidism by increasing glucose absorption through the gastrointestinal tract, increasing glucose-stimulated insulin secretion, and increasing peripheral glucose transport and metabolism. It also increases hepatic glucose production, which is a significant factor in the emergence of peripheral insulin resistance (Duntas, Orgiazzi, and Brabant 2011). In hyperthyroid patients, glucose depletion rises to compensate for energy loss, increasing the insulin demand in the peripheral tissues, which is caused by an increase in the rate of insulin-stimulated glucose oxidation as is depicted in Figure 6. This increase in consumption leads to a reduction in insulin sensitivity in the liver (Martinez and Ortiz 2017).

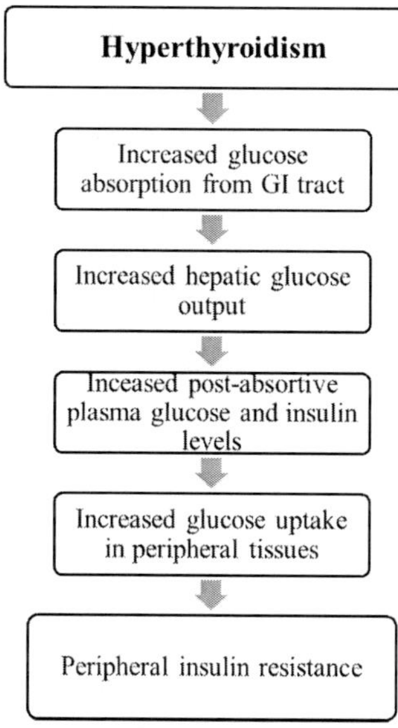


**Figure 6.** Insulin resistance as a consequence of hyperthyroidism.

## 7. The Pathogenetic Mechanism by Which Obesity May Exacerbate or Sustain PCOS

Epidemiological studies express the clear association between PCOS and obesity by revealing that a major portion of women having PCOS, around more than 37% to less than 90%, tend to be obese. This data is supported by the observations that a slight loss of weight, even as low as 5% in such women, can result in better fertility, improved menstrual cycle, and lessened hyperandrogenic clinicobiochemical features (Barber et al. 2015). Obesity might play a pathogenetic role in causing PCOS in those who are vulnerable. Many factors are at play that back the effects that obesity has on PCOS. Obesity might be somewhat accountable for causing resistance to insulin and the resulting hyperinsulinemia in patients. Insulin possesses gonadotrophic action and elevated levels of insulin in the ovarian tissue can lead to hyperandrogenism. Other mechanisms by which obesity promotes the occurrence of hyperandrogenism associated with PCOS include a high rate of estrogen synthesis, elevated activity of the opioid system, hyperactivity of the hypothalamic-pituitary-adrenal axis, reduced synthesis of SHBG, and possibly a greater intake of lipids in the diet (Gambineri et al. 2002).

A major portion of PCOS patients (50-90%) are reported to be insulin resistant. Insulin resistance in PCOS results in compensatory hyperinsulinemia which has further serious repercussions. Insulin leads to increased formation of androgens in ovarian theca cells. The synthesis of SHBG in the liver can be repressed by insulin, as a consequence of which, there will be a rise in the amount of testosterone that occurs in the free and available form. Obesity and further gain of weight can aggravate insulin resistance in PCOS patients (Barber et al. 2019) as illustrated in Figure 7. According to a meta-analysis, levels of serum adiponectin are observed to be lower in patients of PCOS in comparison with BMI-adjusted control women, probably backing insulin resistance. Serum adiponectin is involved in the inhibition of the production of androgens from ovarian theca cells. This makes it quite likely that the hyperandrogenism leading to PCOS might have low levels of serum adiponectin as a contributing factor.

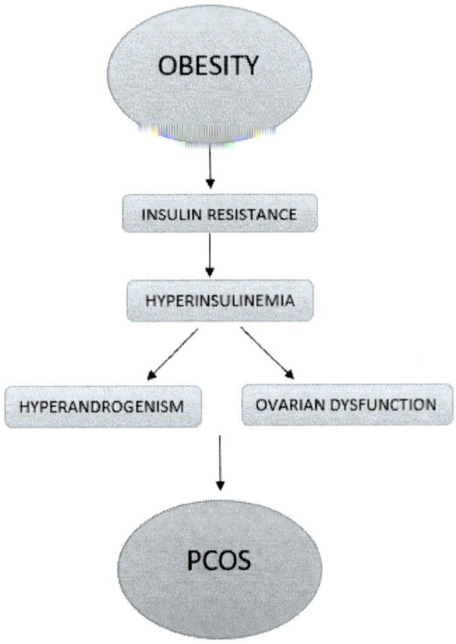


**Figure 7.** A prominent link between obesity and PCOS – Insulin Resistance.

## Conclusion

PCOS is characterized by a culmination of many dysfunctional states including a period of chronic anovulation, irregularities in the menstrual cycle, and increased serum levels of androgens in the bloodstream. Additionally, this syndrome is also associated with metabolic abnormalities. This is indicated by more than normal levels of insulin circulating in the blood of the individuals and progressing towards a condition that is popularly termed as – 'insulin resistance.' An important indicator is however, obesity which is found in more than 50% of women with PCOS, though the inverse is not always true and even women with a normal BMI (Body Mass Index) may be afflicted with PCOS (Diamanti-Kandarakis 2006). Several authors suggest the co-existence of hypothyroidism and the state of insulin resistance in individuals. This is because thyroid hormones may act as not only agonists but also as antagonists of insulin in different cells of the body at the same time. This helps in maintaining a fine balance and establishes a state of normal glucose homeostasis. Any alteration in this fine balance may result in the disruption of the equilibrium. Owing to this, in a state of hypothyroidism, there is a decrease in the production and uptake of glucose, which results in hypoglycemia and insulin resistance at the same time. This may further result in an increase in body fat, lipid levels in blood, and synthesis of steroid hormones, delay in the onset of puberty, and anovulatory cycles. The relationship between PCOS and thyroid dysfunction can also be attributed to autoimmunity. For instance, Autoimmune Thyroiditis is one of the most prominent causes of subclinical hypothyroidism . This results in an imbalance in the levels of estrogen and progesterone in the blood. The immune system is further hyperactivated by estrogen, which is an immune system stimulator. This cycle continues owing to the anovulatory phases which further lead to a marked decrease in the blood levels of progesterone.

Apart from this, the HPO (Hypothalamus-Pituitary-Ovary) and HPT (Hypothalamus-Pituitary-Thyroid) axes are complementary in their action. The link has been established due to the presence of thyroid hormone receptors present on the ovarian follicles. A dip in the level of thyroid hormones may result in an imbalance of estrogen-progesterone ratio as discussed earlier. However, despite the strong consensus regarding the link between hypothyroidism and PCOS, many studies suggest otherwise or conclude that there is no general basis for the stated relationship.

## References


Alberti, K George M M, Paul Zimmet, and Jonathan Shaw. 2005. "The Metabolic Syndrome—a New Worldwide Definition." *The Lancet* 366 (9491): 1059–62. https://doi.org/10.1016/S0140-6736(05)67402-8.

Anwaar, Mariya, and Qaiser Jabeen. 2022. "Thyroid Dysfunction: In Connection with PCOS." In *Polycystic Ovary Syndrome*, edited by Zhengchao Wang, Ch. 2. Rijeka: IntechOpen. https://doi.org/10.5772/intechopen.102492.

Barber, Thomas M, George K Dimitriadis, Avgi Andreou, and Stephen Franks. 2015. "Polycystic Ovary Syndrome: Insight into Pathogenesis and a Common Association with Insulin Resistance." *Clinical Medicine* 15 (Suppl 6): s72. https://doi.org/10.7861/clinmedicine.15-6-s72.

Barber, Thomas M, Petra Hanson, Martin O Weickert, and Stephen Franks. 2019. "Obesity and Polycystic Ovary Syndrome: Implications for Pathogenesis and Novel Management Strategies." *Clinical Medicine Insights: Reproductive Health* 13 (January): 1179558119874042. https://doi.org/10.1177/1179558119874042.

Benetti-Pinto, Cristina Laguna, Vanessa Ribeiro Santana Berini Piccolo, Heraldo Mendes Garmes, and Cássia Raquel Teatin Juliato. 2013. "Subclinical Hypothyroidism in Young Women with Polycystic Ovary Syndrome: An Analysis of Clinical, Hormonal, and Metabolic Parameters." *Fertility and Sterility* 99 (2): 588–92. https://doi.org/10.1016/j.fertnstert.2012.10.006.

Bhongir, Varma. n.d. "*Study of Insulin Resistance in Subclinical Hypothyroidism.*" http://www.medcalc.org.

Braverman, Lewis E, David S Cooper, Sidney C Werner, and Sidney H Ingbar. 2013. *Werner & Ingbar's the Thyroid a Fundamental and Clinical Text. Werner and Ingbar's the Thyroid.* 10th ed. Philadelphia: Wolters Kluwer/Lippincott Williams & Wilkins Health.

Brenta, Gabriela. 2011. "Why Can Insulin Resistance Be a Natural Consequence of Thyroid Dysfunction?" Edited by Masanobu Yamada. *Journal of Thyroid Research* 2011: 152850. https://doi.org/10.4061/2011/152850.

Diamanti-Kandarakis, Evanthia. 2006. "Insulin Resistance in PCOS." *Endocrine* 30 (1): 13–17. https://doi.org/10.1385/ENDO:30:1:13.

Dohán, Orsolya, Antonio de la Vieja, Viktoriya Paroder, Claudia Riedel, Mona Artani, Mia Reed, Christopher S Ginter, and Nancy Carrasco. 2003. "The Sodium/Iodide Symporter (NIS): Characterization, Regulation, and Medical Significance." *Endocrine Reviews* 24 (1): 48–77. https://doi.org/10.1210/er.2001-0029.

Duntas, Leonidas H, Jacques Orgiazzi, and Georg Brabant. 2011. "The Interface between Thyroid and Diabetes Mellitus." *Clinical Endocrinology* 75 (1): 1–9. https://doi.org/https://doi.org/10.1111/j.1365-2265.2011.04029.x.

Elslimani, Fatma Al-zaroug, Mona Elhasi, and Maraia Farag Elmhdwi. 2016. "The Relation between Hypothyroidism and Polycystic Ovary Syndrome." *Journal of Pharmaceutical and Applied Chemistry* 2 (3): 197–200. https://doi.org/10.18576/jpac/020310.

Expert Panel on Detection and Treatment of High Blood Cholesterol in Adults, Evaluation. 2001. "Executive Summary of the Third Report of the National Cholesterol Education Program (NCEP) Expert Panel on Detection, Evaluation, and Treatment of High Blood Cholesterol in Adults (Adult Treatment Panel III)." *JAMA* 285 (19): 2486–97. https://doi.org/10.1001/jama.285.19.2486.

Fontenelle M. M.; Severo J. S.; Freitas T. E. C.; Morais J. B. S.; Torres-Leal F. L.; Henriques G. S.; do Nascimento Marreiro D., L C.; Feitosa. 2016. "Thyroid Function in Human Obesity: Underlying Mechanisms." *Hormone and Metabolic Research* 48 (12): 787–94. https://doi.org/10.1055/s-0042-121421.

Gambineri, A, C Pelusi, V Vicennati, U Pagotto, and R Pasquali. 2002. "Obesity and the Polycystic Ovary Syndrome." *International Journal of Obesity* 26 (7): 883–96. https://doi.org/10.1038/sj.ijo.0801994.

Gierach, Marcin, Joanna Gierach, and Roman Junik. 2014. "Insulin Resistance and Thyroid Disorders." *Endokrynologia Polska* 65 (1): 70–76. https://doi.org/10.5603/EP.2014.0010.

Gu, Dongfeng, Kristi Reynolds, Xigui Wu, Jing Chen, Xiufang Duan, Robert F Reynolds, Paul K Whelton, and Jiang He. 2005. "Prevalence of the Metabolic Syndrome and Overweight among Adults in China." *The Lancet* 365 (9468): 1398–1405. https://doi.org/10.1016/S0140-6736(05)66375-1.

Hansen, Keith A, Sandra P T Tho, Mark Hanly, Richard W Moretuzzo, and Paul G McDonough. 1997. "Massive Ovarian Enlargement in Primary Hypothyroidism." *Fertility and Sterility* 67 (1): 169–71. https://doi.org/https://doi.org/10.1016/S0015-0282(97)81876-6.

Hu, Gang, Qing Qiao, Jaakko Tuomilehto, Beverley Balkau, Knut Borch-Johnsen, Kalevi Pyorala, and for the DECODE Study Group. 2004. "Prevalence of the Metabolic Syndrome and Its Relation to All-Cause and Cardiovascular Mortality in Nondiabetic European Men and Women." *Archives of Internal Medicine* 164 (10): 1066–76. https://doi.org/10.1001/archinte.164.10.1066.

Hulchiy, Mariana, Hua Zhang, J Mark Cline, Angelica Lindén Hirschberg, and Lena Sahlin. 2012. "Receptors for Thyrotropin-Releasing Hormone, Thyroid-Stimulating Hormone, and Thyroid Hormones in the Macaque Uterus: Effects of Long-Term Sex Hormone Treatment." *Menopause* 19 (11). https://journals.lww.com/menopausejournal/Fulltext/2012/11000/Receptors_for_thyrotropin_releasing_hormone,.15.aspx.

Iwen, K Alexander, Erich Schröder, and Georg Brabant. 2013. "Thyroid Hormones and the Metabolic Syndrome." *European Thyroid Journal* 2 (2): 83–92. https://doi.org/10.1159/000351249.

Kabodmehri, Roya, Seyedeh Hajar Sharami, Ziba Zahiri Sorouri, Nasrin Ghanami Gashti, Forozan Milani, Zeinab Chaypaz, and Maryam Ghalandari. 2021. "The Relationship between Thyroid Function and Ovarian Reserve: A Prospective Cross-Sectional Study." *Thyroid Research* 14 (1): 22. https://doi.org/10.1186/s13044-021-00112-2.

Kapadia, Kunal B., Parloop A. Bhatt, and Jigna S. Shah. 2012. "Association between Altered Thyroid State and Insulin Resistance." *Journal of Pharmacology and Pharmacotherapeutics* 3 (2): 156–60. https://doi.org/10.4103/0976-500X.95517.

Kendle, F. W. "Case of Precocious Puberty in a Female Cretin." *BMJ* 1, no. 2301 (1905): 246–46. https://doi.org/10.1136/bmj.1.2301.246.

Kim, Ha-Young, and Subburaman Mohan. 2013. "Role and Mechanisms of Actions of Thyroid Hormone on the Skeletal Development." *Bone Research* 1 (1): 146–61. https://doi.org/10.4248/BR201302004.

Krassas, G E, N Pontikides, Th. Kaltsas, Ph. Papadopoulou, J Paunkovic, N Paunkovic, and L H. Duntas. 1999. "Disturbances of Menstruation in Hypothyroidism." *Clinical Endocrinology* 50 (5): 655–59. https://doi.org/https://doi.org/10.1046/j.1365-2265.1999.00719.x.

Kumar Ahirwar, Ashok, Archana Singh, Anju Jain, Surajeet Kumar, Binita Goswami, M K Bhatnagar, and Jayashree Bhattacharjee. 2017. "Role of Sub Clinical Hypothyroidism in Association with Adiponectin Levels Causing Insulin Resistance in Metabolic Syndrome: A Case Control Study." *Tokai J Exp Clin Med.* Vol. 42.

Kuroda, Keiji, Toyoyoshi Uchida, Saki Nagai, Rie Ozaki, Takashi Yamaguchi, Yuichi Sato, Jan J Brosens, and Satoru Takeda. 2015. "Elevated Serum Thyroid-Stimulating Hormone Is Associated with Decreased Anti-Müllerian Hormone in Infertile Women of Reproductive Age." *Journal of Assisted Reproduction and Genetics* 32 (2): 243–47. https://doi.org/10.1007/s10815-014-0397-7.

Laurberg, Peter, Nils Knudsen, Stig Andersen, Allan Carlé, Inge Bülow Pedersen, and Jesper Karmisholt. 2012. "Thyroid Function and Obesity." *European Thyroid Journal* 1 (3): 159–67. https://doi.org/10.1159/000342994.

Maratou, E., Hadjidakis, D. J., Kollias, A., Tsegka, K., Peppa, M., Alevizaki, M., Mitrou, P., Lambadiari, V., Boutati, E., Nikzas, D., Tountas, N., Economopoulos, T., Raptis, S. A., & Dimitriadis, G. 2009. "Studies of Insulin Resistance in Patients with Clinical and Subclinical Hypothyroidism." *European Journal of Endocrinology* 160 (5): 785–90. https://doi.org/10.1530/EJE-08-0797.

Martinez, Bridget, and Rudy M Ortiz. 2017. "Thyroid Hormone Regulation and Insulin Resistance: Insights from Animals Naturally Adapted to Fasting." *Physiology* 32 (2): 141–51. https://doi.org/10.1152/physiol.00018.2016.

Michalakis, Konstantinos G, Tolga B Mesen, Lynae M Brayboy, Bo Yu, Kevin S Richter, Michael Levy, Eric Widra, and James H Segars. 2011. "Subclinical Elevations of Thyroid-Stimulating Hormone and Assisted Reproductive Technology Outcomes." *Fertility and Sterility* 95 (8): 2634–37. https://doi.org/10.1016/j.fertnstert.2011.02.056.

Miot, Françoise, Corinne Dupuy, Jacques E Dumont, and Bernard Rousset. 2015. "*Chapter 2 Thyroid Hormone Synthesis and Secretion*." In.

Mullur, Rashmi, Yan-Yun Liu, and Gregory A Brent. 2014. "Thyroid Hormone Regulation of Metabolism." *Physiological Reviews* 94 (2): 355–82. https://doi.org/10.1152/physrev.00030.2013.

Nisar, Sobia, ParvezA Shah, MShafi Kuchay, ManzoorA Bhat, Aafia Rashid, Sanjeed Ahmed, and Mohd Ashraf Ganie. 2012. "Association of Polycystic Ovary Syndrome and Graves′ Disease: Is Autoimmunity the Link between the Two Diseases." *Indian Journal of Endocrinology and Metabolism* 16 (6): 982. https://doi.org/10.4103/2230-8210.103006.

Nussey, Stephen, and Saffron A. Whitehead. *Endocrinology: An Integrated Approach*. Oxford England: BIOS Scientific Publishers Ltd., 2002.

Latha, P, B v Ravi, and Roshni Sadaria. 2021. "Study of TSH and Prolactin in PCOS Subjects: A Case Control Study." *International Journal of Clinical Biochemistry and Research* 8 (1): 62–65. https://doi.org/10.18231/j.ijcbr.2021.013.

Peters, C, A S P van Trotsenburg, and N Schoenmakers. 2018. "DIAGNOSIS OF ENDOCRINE DISEASE: Congenital Hypothyroidism: Update and Perspectives." *European Journal of Endocrinology* 179 (6): R297–317. https://doi.org/10.1530/EJE-18-0383.

Petersen, M C, and G I Shulman. 2018. "Mechanisms of Insulin Action and Insulin Resistance." *Physiol Rev* 98: 2133–2223. https://doi.org/10.1152/physrev.

Redmond, Geoffrey P. 2004. "Thyroid Dysfunction and Women's Reproductive Health." *Thyroid* 14 (supplement 1): 5–15. https://doi.org/10.1089/105072504323024543.

Röjdmark, S, A Berg, and G Kallner. 1988. "Hypothalamic-Pituitary-Testicular Axis in Patients with Hyperthyroidism." *Hormone Research in Paediatrics* 29 (5–6): 185–90. https://doi.org/10.1159/000181000.

Romitti, Mírian, Vitor C Fabris, Patricia K Ziegelmann, Ana Luiza Maia, and Poli Mara Spritzer. 2018. "Association between PCOS and Autoimmune Thyroid Disease: A Systematic Review and Meta-Analysis." *Endocrine Connections* 7 (11): 1158–67. https://doi.org/10.1530/EC-18-0309.

Singh, Jaya, Hilda Wong, Nancy Ahluwalia, Ryan M Go, and Michelle A Guerrero-Go. 2020. "Metabolic, Hormonal, Immunologic, and Genetic Factors Associated With the Incidence of Thyroid Disorders in Polycystic Ovarian Syndrome Patients." *Cureus* 12 (11): e11681. https://doi.org/10.7759/cureus.11681.

Singla, Rajiv, Yashdeep Gupta, Manju Khemani, and Sameer Aggarwal. 2015. "Thyroid Disorders and Polycystic Ovary Syndrome: An Emerging Relationship." *Indian Journal of Endocrinology and Metabolism*. Medknow Publications. https://doi.org/10.4103/2230-8210.146860.

Szanto, Ildiko, Marc Pusztaszeri, and Maria Mavromati. 2019. "H2O2 Metabolism in Normal Thyroid Cells and in Thyroid Tumorigenesis: Focus on NADPH Oxidases." *Antioxidants* 8 (5). https://doi.org/10.3390/antiox8050126.

Visser, Theo J. 2018. "Regulation of Thyroid Function, Synthesis and Function of Thyroid Hormones." In *Thyroid Diseases: Pathogenesis, Diagnosis and Treatment*, edited by Paolo Vitti and Laszlo Hegedus, 1–30. Cham: Springer International Publishing. https://doi.org/10.1007/978-3-319-29195-6_1-1.

Yoshida, Akio, Shinichi Taniguchi, Ichiro Hisatome, Ines E Royaux, Eric D Green, Leonard D Kohn, and Koichi Suzuki. 2002. "Pendrin Is an Iodide-Specific Apical Porter Responsible for Iodide Efflux from Thyroid Cells." *The Journal of Clinical Endocrinology & Metabolism* 87 (7): 3356–61. https://doi.org/10.1210/jcem.87.7.8679.

Zhu, Ping, Xinliang Liu, and Xiaoming Mao. 2018. "Thyroid-Stimulating Hormone Levels Are Positively Associated with Insulin Resistance." *Medical Science Monitor* 24: 342–47. https://doi.org/https://dx.doi.org/10.12659/MSM.905774.

## Chapter 6

# PCOS and the Role of ACTH: The Impact of the Cortisol Hormone, a Primary Stress Hormone on Mental Health

**Yasrib Qurishi**[1]
**Mansi Gupta**[2]
**Shruti Awasthi**[3,*]
**and Nihad Ashraf Khan**[4]

[1]School of Allied Healthcare Sciences (SAHS), Jain University, Bangalore, India
[2]Department of Biotechnology, Maharishi Dayanand University, Rohtak, India
[3]Department of Life Sciences, Garden City University, Bangalore, India
[4]Department of Biosciences, Faculty of Natural Science, Jamia Millia Islamia, Delhi, India

## Abstract

Polycystic ovarian Syndrome is the most common cause of infertility affecting women at a very young age. Since it is an endocrine disorder that affects hormones causing amplification in ovary production with small cysts on either side of the border surrounding the ovary. Its approximate prevalence is 6-7% in reproductive-aged women. The causative agent of PCOS is still not clear, but a combination of genetic and environmental factors may be responsible for the same. Although less evidence is in support of the fact that stress (or ACTH) stimulation may be only one of the pathophysiological conditions involved in follicular cyst pathogenesis. Symptoms of PCOS mainly include irregular menstruation, hirsutism, acne, and excessive weight gain. The main line of treatment for PCOS includes the use of birth control pills, and medication like metformin to prevent diabetes as in PCOS there are higher chances of getting lifestyle diseases like diabetes and blood pressure-related issues that can, in turn, lead to higher rates of triglycerides. Although the underlying causes of ACTH and cortisol hormones are just like the two sides of the same coin, much research about its etiology, pathophysiology, and clinical outcome has not yet been postulated.

**Keywords:** infertility, adrenocorticotropic hormone (ACTH), cortisol hormone, diabetes, metformin, pathophysiology, hirsutism, menstruation, triglycerides

* Corresponding Author's Email: shruti.awasthi@gardencity.university.

In: Polycystic Ovarian Syndrome (PCOS) and Our Biological Clock
Editors: Arpita Roy, Gowhar Rashid and Nihad Ashraf Khan
ISBN: 979-8-89113-100-2
© 2023 Nova Science Publishers, Inc.

## 1. Introduction to PCOS

Polycystic ovary syndrome is one of the most predominant endocrine disorders which are caused by interactions between genetic, environmental & intrauterine factors impacting nearly 8–13% of women of fertile age (Teede et al., 2010, Azziz et al., 2016). It is predominantly distinguished by an irregular menstrual cycle and is a global health concern in which ovulation does not occur (Ruta K. et al., 2014). PCOS is nothing but a state where ovaries start synthesizing an excess amount of androgens, generally, they are present in small amounts in females. As we know poly means many so the name PCOS indicates many microscopic cysts that would be formed inside the ovaries as shown in Figure 1. In many cases, women who have PCOS do not have cysts but some women who don't have this disorder develop cysts.

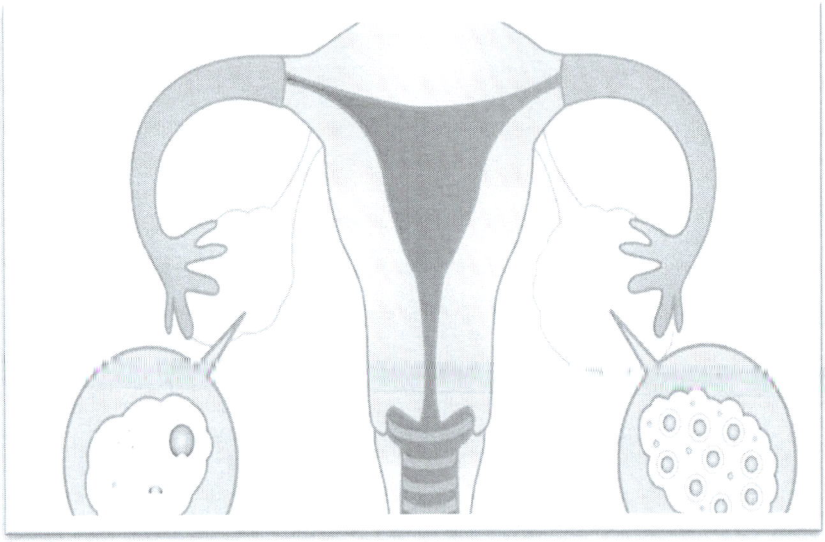

**Figure 1.** Diagram of uterus differentiating normal and cystic ovaries on each side. The right of the uterus depicts multiple cysts in the ovary whereas, the left depicts a normal single follicle in the ovary.

As we know that ovulation is nothing but a portion of our menstrual cycle. The moment eggs start releasing from the ovary possibility is that they may get fertilized and the egg starts moving toward the uterus resulting in pregnancy, and when the eggs are not fertilized it deteriorates and the uterus lining starts peeling off. Now, because of unhealthy lifestyles women are unable to make enough hormones that are needed for ovulation, as a result, the ovaries start developing small cysts these cysts start making excess androgen hormones. PCOS women with this disorder have an elevated range of androgens which is the main reason for the abnormal menstrual cycle in women. Nowadays, everyone is exposed to different types and different conditions of stress depending upon the environment and various physiological conditions that may lead to changes in the serum level of various hormones including glucocorticoids, catecholamines, growth hormone, and prolactin. As a consequence of the changes involved, some reactions are obvious for the fight or flight response to protect oneself. Moreover, due to the stress-induced response, many endocrine disorders can occur (Kumari S. et al.). The release of cortisol from the Adrenocorticotropic hormone results in increased LH activity according to which it is depicted that insulin and LH work synergistically.

Additionally, altered clinical status and stress response can lead to various devastating conditions. Talking from a broader perspective, 'stress' being a generalized term may disturb the equilibrium between the environment and the living systems. In day-to-day life, there are different stressful situations such as the stress of work pressure, student stress from examinations, psychosocial stress, and physical stress due to trauma, surgery, and various medical disorders. As a consequence of stress response, the level of various hormones changes, and the activity is increased which is shown in (Figure 2) the effect of which is to increase the mobilization of energy sources and adapt the individual to the new circumstance. Therefore, this chapter aims to view the role of ACTH and cortisol on the mental health and irregularity or absence in the menstrual cycle of patients who acquires PCOS.

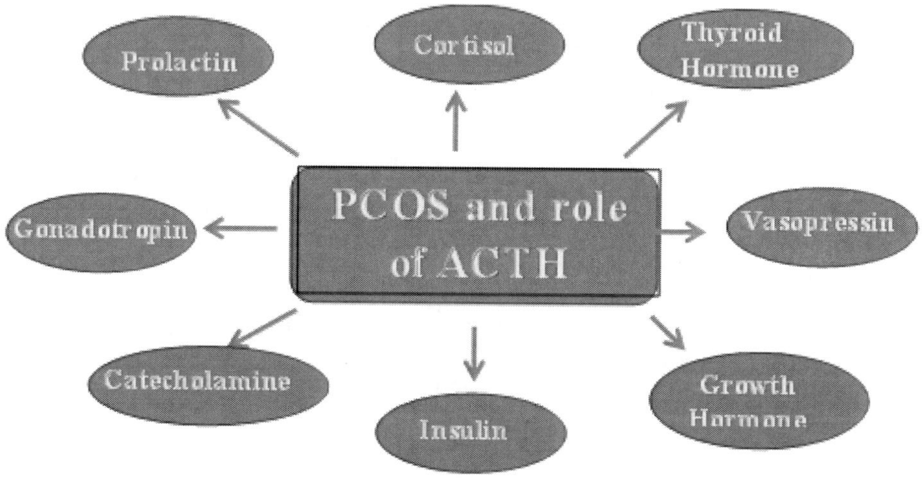


**Figure 2.** Hormonal changes in Polycystic ovarian syndrome are depicted in this figure. The role of Adrenocorticotrophic Hormone illustrates several effects on hormones depicted by the arrow.

## 2. Pathogenesis of PCOS

One of the complex genetic disorders is PCOS which consists of many susceptibility genes having powerful genetic and environmental components (Ehrmann et al., 2005). Research shows that PCOS is more prone in identical twins than fraternal twins. It is also shown that when the mother or the sibling is having PCOS 50% chance is the daughter will also be getting this disease. Much of the research has proved that the female siblings of women with hormonal disorders of PCOS are more accustomed to having insulin resistance than the male sibling of women who do not have this hormonal disorder. However, several gene dysfunctions can be seen in PCOS which are involved to play a critical role in pathogenesis are depicted in Figure 3. Those genes are DENNDIA, THADA, SHBG, FBN3, and many more of these genes after activation starts releasing hormones for biological responses which result in the aggregation of PCOS symptoms (Panda PK et al., 2016, Carmina E et al., 2005). Linkage of genes with PCOS results in insulin resistance and promotes ovulation via an increase in cell surface receptors and a phosphorylation mechanism on receptors that helps in amplifying the signals in cells for various physiological processes (Burgers JA et al., 2010).

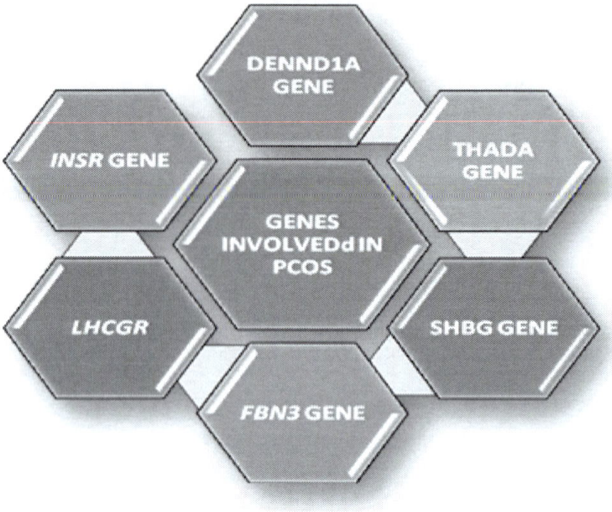


**Figure 3.** Effect of cortisol on PCOD patients. The role of genes involved in PCOS is illustrated in the diagram. INSR, SBHG-like genes show a great impact on the probability of PCOS by showing etiological responses.

## 3. Associated Risk Factors with PCOS

There are many risks factor which help in promoting PCOS like genetic factors, non-genetic factors, and hormonal factors.

### 3.1. Non-Genetic Factors

These factors are not related to genetics, but they arise because of lifestyle and toxins which are present in the environment, as a result, they help in the promotion of PCOS symptoms as shown in Figure 4.

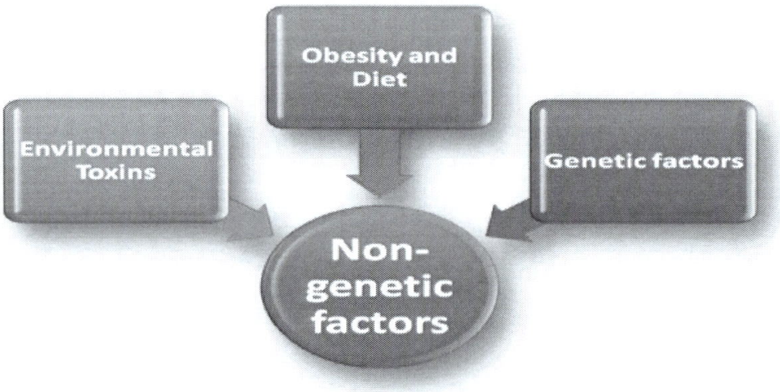


**Figure 4.** The non-genetic factors responsible for the etiology of Polycystic ovary syndrome where genetic, environmental, obesity, and diet factors contribute to it.

### 3.2. Environmental Toxins

The chemical toxins which are present in the environment are called pollutants that cause toxicity to the environment. These pollutants will penetrate the human body either by aspiration or by absorption via mucous membranes and skin (Panidis D et al., 2012). The most common chemical pollutants are tobacco, lead, mercury, and pesticides, and we also get chemical toxins from industrial waste which can hinder the endocrine system, and studies have shown a long-lasting impact on the reproductive system of women (Diamanti et al., 2009).

### 3.3. Obesity and Diet

Adiposity is one of the major threats around the world this risk factors contribute to PCOS among women. The main causes which can inculcate PCOS are diet, stress, and lifestyle which slowly start affecting the reproductive system (Woodruff TJ et al., 2010). The probability of hyperandrogenism, hirsutism, insulin resistance, and infertility is increased in obese PCOS women (Amiri et al., 2020, Balen et al., 2009).

### 3.4. Genetic factors

Researchers have proved that genetic factors contribute to a significant extent to the development of PCOS. Till now no evidence for the genetic makeup of inheritance of PCOS is known. A study advised that first-degree relatives of PCOS patients are at higher risk of development (Van Der Steeg JW et al., 2008). As we know that genes are involved in the biosynthesis and breakdown of ovarian steroidogenesis and if there is any disturbance in the transcription of these genes, that will lead to an increase in the levels of androgen. Many genes that are involved in the ovarian steroidogenesis of PCOS are CYP11A, CYP21, CYP17, CYP19, AR, (figure 5), and sex hormone-binding globulin (SHBG) (Kahsar-Miller MD et al., 2001).

### 3.5. CYP11A

The key enzyme is P450 which is encoded by CYP11A and is responsible for the fusion of fat, steroids, cholesterol, and even for the metabolism of drugs the main role of this enzyme is to convert cholesterol to progesterone which is the reason it is called the slowest step involved in the androgen hormone synthesis (Strachan et al., 1999). Researchers have shown several regions of the world that concluded the alliance of PCOS advancement with CYP11A locus which has a repetitive sequence (Gharani et al., 1997). Furthermore, researchers have shown the important interaction of SNP rs4077582 in CYP11A with the development of PCOS and the androgen level (Reddy et al., 2014).

### 3.6. CYP21

The P45021-hydroxylase is an enzyme that is coded by CYP2. If this enzyme is inactivated it will lead to the futile anabolism of steroidogenesis (Witchel et al.,2000). The engagement of the CYP21 with increased sex hormone ranges has been documented (Peng CY et al., 2014).

### 3.7. CYP17

CYP17 encrypt the enzyme P450 17-hydroxylase/17, 20-desmolase required for the 17-hydroxylase activity which will contribute to abnormal sex hormone level like androgen and triggers the development of PCOS (Carey et al., 1994, Pusalkar et al., 2009).

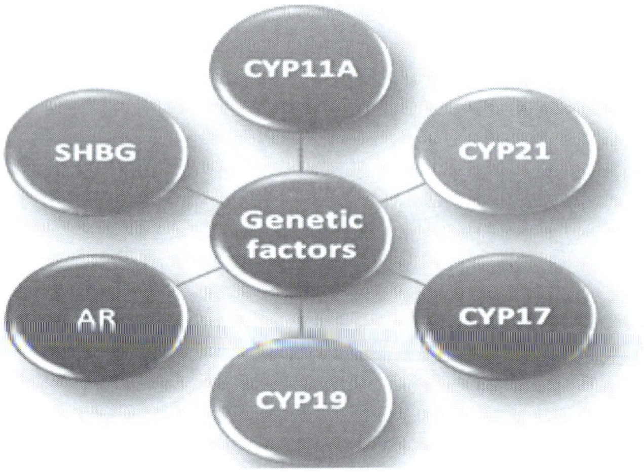


**Figure 5.** Genetic factors that cause disease in females of age 18-45. Several gene mutations in which regulation causes PCOS are responsible to cause PCOS.

### 3.8. CYP19

Aromatase enzyme which is coded by CYP19 help in the production of estrogens (Khan MJ et al.,2019). Researchers have shown that aromatase activity is decreased in women who are lean and obese having PCOS, which is associated with a decrease in androgen level (Dadachanji et al., 2018). Studies showed the association of heterozygous TC by the polymorphism of two genes CYP19 and SNP rs2470152 which were responsible to elevate the testosterone level which is directly involved in the activity of enzyme aromatase (Reddy R et al., 2015).

### 3.9. AR

AR is nothing but an Androgen receptor gene having a site of location on the X chromosome, consisting of an N terminal domain repeat of CAG (Peng CY et al., 2014, Hargreaves et al., 1990, Herman et al., 2003) Studies have shown that if X chromosome is inactivated which will call disturbance in the cellular mechanism increasing androgen level leading to PCOS (Khan MJ et al.,2019).

## 3.10. SHBG

SHBG-encoded protein's main role is to control the sex hormones levels, and they can bind with high-affinity with androgen, estrogens, and testosterone they are also managed by metabolic factors like androgen and insulin (Black PH et al.,1994, Goldstein et al.,1987, Aguilera et al.,2008). Researchers have shown that many proofs show SHBG polymorphism in the association of long TAAAA repeats and contribute to PCOS (Cameron et al.,1997, Salam et al.,2011, Dadachanji et al., 2018). This gene does not result in ovarian steroidogenesis and reproductive dysfunctions as a result many abnormalities in the metabolism are present in women who have PCOS (Dadachanji et al., 2018).

### *3.10.1. Hormonal Factors*

There are several hormonal factors responsible to cause PCOS in females of age 18-45. The modification in a series of genes can cause abnormal secretion of hormones from the hypothalamic-pituitary gland.

### *3.10.2. Hyperandrogenism*

Hyperandrogenism is a condition where changes will happen in the normal functions of the ovarian cell resulting in the overproduction of sex hormones like androgen this condition can be diagnosed by scheming the amount of serum testosterone, sex hormone binding globulin SHBG, 17-hydroxy progesterone, and free androgen index. Research shows that women who have been detected with this condition will have an elevated range of LH and decreased range of FSH during the menstrual cycle. The change in the normal methods will result in an elevated range of LH that stimulate the synthesis of sex hormones like androgen which lower the development in the follicular and if there is a decreased level of FSH that will enhance the growth of the small follicles.

### *3.10.3. Insulin Resistance*

This is a condition in which cells are not able to react to insulin either at the normal or elevated range of insulin. This change in condition leads to abnormalities of metabolism in PCOS. The presence of hyperinsulinemia condition was first reported in PCOS women. Studies have shown that women diagnosed with PCOS are susceptible to intolerance in glucose and abnormalities in the metabolism followed by medical changes like dysfunction in ovulation and hyperandrogenism. Excess of insulin will react as gonadotropin either alone or in combination with LH on the thecal cells and will increase the synthesis of sex hormones when it acts indirectly it will decrease the synthesis of SHBG and IGF-1 whereas when the levels are increased it will stimulate the levels of androgen as well as VAT to synthesize FFA which result to insulin resistance.

## 4. Role of ACTH in the Pathogenesis of PCOS

Adrenocorticotropic hormone (ACTH) is a hormone that is synthesized in the brain its exact position is the anterior pituitary gland. The action of this pituitary ACTH helps in the release of adrenal androgen precursors. This adrenal gland-secreted hormone regulates the steroid hormone as well as cortisol hormone levels. Adrenocorticotropic hormone is a very important hormone that is the prerequisite for the proper functioning of adrenal glands, which stimulate the cortex and start releasing stress hormones known as cortisol (Cussen L. et al. 2022). The ACTH hormone range will vary from individual to individual and with age also. According to the studies, the normal range of ACTH hormones is 6.0 to 7.6 Pg/ml. If the ACTH range is lower than the normal range, then in that condition, that person is diagnosed with hypercortisolism, Adrenal gland receptors can detect variations in the levels of ACTH. The lower range of the adrenocorticotropic hormone is because of hypopituitarism, pituitary gland surgery, and hypercortisolism. The ACTH range is elevated than the normal range, only if the person is having primary adrenal insufficiency. The elevated range of ACTH stimulates the receptors of the adrenal gland for the synthesis of cortisol which will increase the levels of cortisol amount in the blood cells, whereas at the same time, they will decrease the flow of corticotrophin-releasing hormone from the hypothalamus, ACTH and the pituitary gland, in contrast, the ACTH range immediately start falling which is known as a negative feedback cycle. Other factors which then stimulate the ACTH synthesis include both physical and psychological stress. The role of this altered level of ACTH and ultimately cortisol leads to several pathogenic effects in females of 16-45 age. However, the excess of androgen is considered a culprit for PCOS. The higher levels of DHEA, androstenedione, testosterone, and estrone reveal higher levels of blood LH concentration and lower or normal FSH levels which are further included in the etiology of insulin resistance, hirsutism, obesity, and glucose intolerance. The women with a higher ratio of LH: FSH is anovulatory in nature (Yesiladali M et al. 2022).

In early childhood and infancy, the release of excess androgen such as DHEA in optimum levels does not show any significant changes in the ovary related to PCOS but during late stages, the increase in levels of DHEA and testosterone leads to prepubertal changes during adrenarche where the cause of excess androgen secretion is unclear which in contrast coincides with the formation of zona reticularis layer. There are several issues seen in PCOS due to the excess of androgen from the adrenal gland which includes sleep apnea due to the release of stress hormones in the body due to depression or stresses it results in sleep apnea which is the common condition in PCOS patients during stress. Other issues associated are insulin resistance, obesity, glucose intolerance, dyslipidemia, unbalanced LH to FSH ratio, etc. These series of changes are mainly caused by hyperandrogenism which not only promotes PCOS but also negatively interacts with factors that can induce PCOS in females (Zeng, X. et al. 2020). Hyperinsulinism on the other side contributes to increased adrenal androgen by increasing the sensitivity to ACTH action on insulin receptors. Chronic anovulation is another cause of infertility in women where the high levels of LH seem to increase abortion in females despite the fact of lack of studies (Alsadi, B. et al. 2018). In normal women, androgen responses are found to be similar whereas, in PCOS women the responses to ACTH stimulation shows exaggeration in contrast the response of DHEA and androstenedione to ACTH do not show differences in exaggerated and normal women with PCOS. However, hyperresponsiveness to

ACTH is reported to have variable androgen production by the adrenal gland (Maas, K. H. et al. 2016).

### 4.1. Impact of Cortisol Hormone on PCOD Patients

PCOS, one of the most common problems, has fertility issues and causes metabolic dysfunction. The stress mediators which mainly include amylase and cortisol affect young women and have a direct relationship with PCOS. The noteworthy characteristic features of PCOS are oligomenorrhea, hyperandrogenism, central obesity, and Type-2 diabetes.

Moreover, in PCOS, due to the enhanced adrenal gland hormone (ACTH), secretion might contribute to increased adrenal insulin production as shown in Figure 6. On the other hand, previous research methods have been contradictory, and the relationship between heightened HPA axis functioning and phenotypic abnormalities in PCOS is not clear yet. Also, PCOS-diagnosed women have more chances of mood swings, bipolar disorder, attention deficit disorder, or personality disorder.

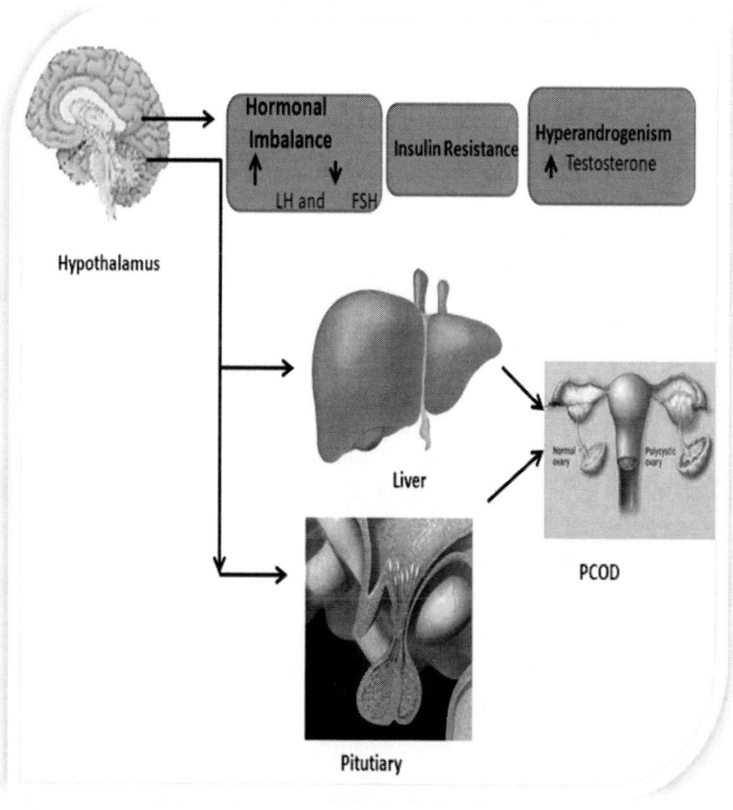


**Figure 6.** The combined effect of cortisol on PCOD patients is depicted in the above figure. Hypothalamus signals the anterior pituitary and liver for the abnormal release of LH/FSH. The imbalance in the ratio leads to cystic ovaries due to the high secretion of androgens.

In addition, the mechanism lying behind the activation of stress response cortisol expression is the sudden threat received by the tiny area of the base of the brain as shown in Figure 5. In women, adrenal glands release adrenaline and cortisol in bulk by a mix of nerve and hormonal impulses. However, not only this but also the activation of these stress response systems regularly and over some time, affects all other systems, leading to women at risk for several pathological conditions that mainly include:

- melancholy
- gastralgia bellyache symptom
- an extremely severe paroxysmal headache
- Muscle rigidity
- Cardiovascular diseases,
- Insomnia
- Gaining weight
- Impairment of memory and focus

### 4.2. Correlation between Increased Cortisol Levels and Dysregulation of FSH and LH Hormone

The adrenal gland consists of the medulla and cortex which is again divided into three different zones and the release of cortisol from the adrenal gland regulates in zona fasciculata by the Hypothalamic- pituitary- axis (HPA). Now this release of cortisol from the pituitary can be imbalanced due to too much stress and depression which leads to the dysfunctional release of LH and FSH again. However, abnormality in a neuroendocrine system where the increased frequency of gonadotropin-releasing hormone signals the pituitary to release Luteinizing hormone (LH) in large amounts while remaining the level of Follicle-stimulating hormone less or normal (Ashraf, S. et al. 2019). This excess LH stimulates ovarian androgen production whereas, the lack or less FSH will impair follicular development. This Hormonal imbalance causes the proliferation of ovarian theca cells which will further lead to an increase in steroidogenesis. The hormonal pathway and their crosstalk are depicted in Figure 7.

The large release of LH is the result of the disrupted feedback mechanism to the pituitary gland and the ovarian hormone estrogen is responsible for this cause of abnormal release and inhibited negative feedback mechanism (Saadia Z. et al. 2020). Thus, high levels of LH are thought to be required for androgen synthesis and when these high levels of LH combine with the FSH and oestradiol synthesis results in anovulation which is prominently due to the absence of dominant follicles in ovaries (Toosy, S. et al. 2018). This absence of mature follicles results in the release of AMH Anti-mullerian hormone that signals the release of GnRH while inhibiting the release of FSH (Franks & Hardy et al. 2020). Hyperandrogenism is the main etiology of increased cortisol metabolism in PCOS patients where the elevated levels and activity of 5α-reductase cause inactivation and impaired regeneration which is still a matter of debate (Krishnan, A. et al. 2017).

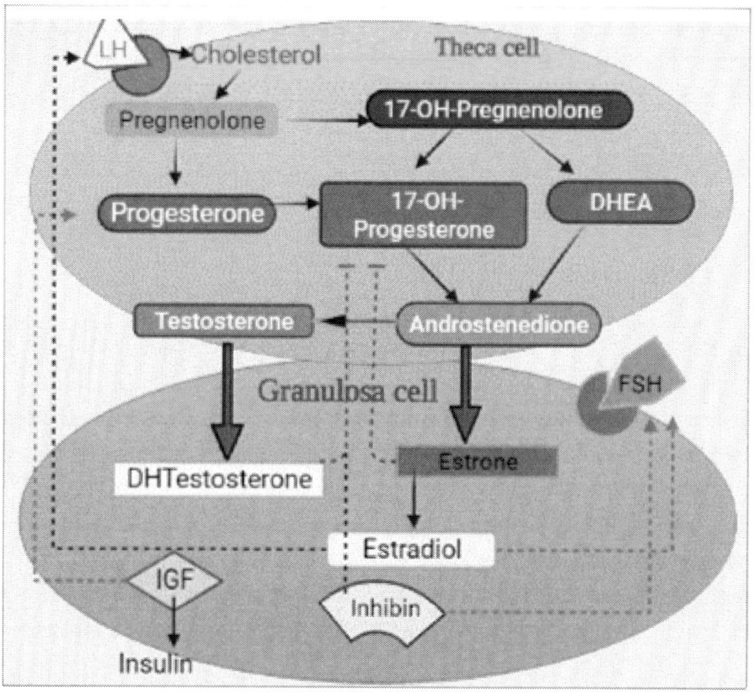


**Figure 7.** This figure depicts the normal hormonal regulation which affects due to the increase in cortisol level by ACTH. The feedback loop of hormones is illustrated in the figure where the negative loop inhibits the secretion of progesterone and LH/FSH secretion in theca cells.

### 4.3. Effect of Cortisol on the Maturation of Ovarian Follicles

Cortisol is a major glucocorticoid released from the adrenal cortex. It is distributed in the body via the bloodstream and plays physiological roles after entering the cells. Some enzymes or hormones regulate the concentration of glucocorticoids in tissues by regulating the Growth Regulators and 11β-hydroxysteroid dehydrogenase. This enzyme regulates follicular development by changing the concentration of cortisol by conversion of non-bioactive cortisone to cortisol (Qin, Y. et al. 2022). High level of cortisol during stress and depression acts directly and indirectly on reproductive functions that result in low reproductive rates and infertility. The increased levels of cortisol hormones reduce the production of estradiol by affecting the granulosa cells present within the follicles, which further deteriorates the quality of oocytes and sometimes leads to the generation of reactive oxygen species in patients which most possibly functions by inducing apoptosis in cells resulting in reduced estradiol 17β biosynthesis in ovaries that however, reduces the growth and development of oocytes follicles and induces oocyte apoptosis (Prasad S. et al. 2016). The complete mechanism of oocyte deterioration by cortisol is depicted in Figure During extreme stress conditions the activity of the hypothalamic-pituitary-gonadal axis is inhibited which can cause late, delayed, or absent periods in patients with PCOS. The rise of cortisol suppresses the GnRH secretion in the hypothalamic-pituitary axis thus reducing the FSH release and LH surge frequency. However, in physiological situations, cortisol is associated with oocyte maturation due to the reason that matured oocyte fluid from follicular cells consists of higher levels of cortisol than immature oocytes (Pontes, J. T. et al. 2019). Therefore, the maturation of follicular cells is inhibited because the presence of large LH receptors on granulosa cells receives more LH and the conversion of androgens into cortisol will be more which disrupts the mechanism of pre-antral to antral follicle maturation in granulosa cells further studies reveal the overexpression of cytochrome P45017 on theca cells which results in excess androgen production.

### 4.4. Effect of Cortisol on Menstrual Health

The most frequent cause of reproductive abnormalities in adolescence and later stages is PCOS. However, menstrual irregularities in females are considered cardinal for PCOS that can manifest as anovulation with irregular menstruation. There are some factors attributed to irregularity, stoppage, or delayed menstruation, and, among all of those cortisol increases is the one that contributes the most (Basu, B. R., et al. 2018). The regulation of the menstrual cycle is done by the hypothalamic-pituitary-gonadal axis. Gonadotropin-releasing hormone from the hypothalamic-pituitary-axis releases FSH and LH that help in the maturation of the egg and coordinate with ovulation which in turn controls the Estrogen and progesterone that further regulates the growth and maturation of eggs and prepares the uterus for pregnancy. Although the release of cortisol from the same axis affects the hormones that are under the control of GnRH. Cortisol can delay ovulation by inhibiting the release of LH which interferes with progesterone regulation and make menstrual flow heavier and longer cycles however, in Contrast, the shortage of cycle depends on the large secretion of progesterone which may stop ovulation and can lead to hypothalamic amenorrhoea with the deposit of fat in the middle of the body. These longer or shorter periods make a stem-loop of feedback and stoppage of it can make the Postmenstrual cycle worsen and also cause a lack of sexual intercourse. The delay in periods is also seen by scientists due to the action of high cortisol on granulosa cells which changes the duration of the cycle by months. However, usually, the levels of cortisol are not high enough during normal menstrual cycles. Several pieces of evidence depict cortisol's effect on menstrual cycle regulation. Some diseases such as Cushing syndrome and hirsutism show some of these symptoms of irregular or delayed menstruation. In the scenario of a feedback loop estrogen elevation leads to the binding of thyroid hormone which dysregulate the B and T cells.

## 5. Correlation between Increased Cortisol Levels and Insulin Resistance

Cortisol release from ACTH also promotes insulin secretion and regulation through granulosa cells in ovaries. According to studies, it was said that cortisol increase can induce insulin resistance by enhancing glucose production from the liver and impeding insulin secretion. Insulin Resistance (IR)is the impairment of insulin action on the target organ. The increase in cortisol through the anterior pituitary leads to abnormal secretion of GnRH decreases the suppressive effects of insulin on glucose production and reduces its uptake in cells. In PCOS patients IR occurs when there is a large quantity of insulin necessary to yield a normal response in cells. However, this does not completely reveal the pathogenicity of molecules associated with insulin. Cortisol leads to increased secretion of LH and binding of it on receptors on theca cells that further stimulates the granulosa cells to secrete insulin for regulating the glucose tolerance in body cells. This insulin in contrast involved with FSH and encourages ovarian thecal-intestinal cell proliferation and differentiation also egg maturation and folliculogenesis are seen as the regulatory mechanism of insulin. The lower concentration of estrogen produced by the action of insulin inhibits LH secretion by creating a negative loop and the increased concentration is responsible for the promotion of LH secretion which creates an LH surge the abnormal level of this surge in hormone creates anovulation also another consequence of insulin production induces hyperresponsiveness which ultimately leads to the inhibition of SHBG resulting in increased androgen production in ovaries (Khan M. S. et al. 2023). The mechanism for insulin resistance, hyperinsulinemia, and Androgen excess is depicted in Figure 8.

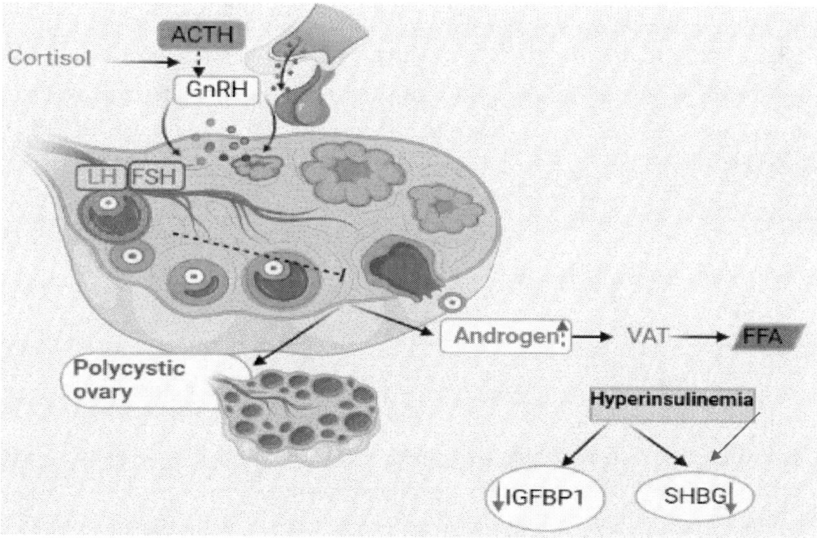


**Figure 8.** The impact of cortisol on insulin resistance and androgen excess in ovaries is illustrated in the diagram where the abnormal release of LH/FSH leads to Polycystic ovary and androgen production that further contributes to Hyperinsulinemia and Insulin resistance by lowering the potential action of Sex Hormone Binding Gene and Insulin-Like Growth Factor Binding Protein-1.

Evidence from studies reveals that IR and Hyperinsulinemia promote the pathogenesis of PCOS. Although, according to studies done on Korean females with PCOS 20% of normoglycemic women had developed type 2 diabetes(T2D) after a period of 3 years which confirms the underlying IR response in PCOS patients.

## 5.1. Effect of Cortisol on Ovarian Follicles Causing Hyperandrogenism

Steroidogenesis in ovaries is a two-celled process which means it requires two cells to complete the synthesis of androgens. Granulosa cells do not contain steroidogenic enzymes, therefore, cannot proceed with the formation but they receive androgens from theca cells to form the substrate for estrogen production. In contrast, Theca cells produce androgens in response to LH stimulation from the pituitary which is further regulated by estrogen. Hyperandrogenism is the condition of producing an excess of androgen in response to LH stimuli which results in the inhibition of Sex Hormone Binding Gene production and increased free androgen level. This free androgen provokes Insulin resistance and further, it is stated that adrenal androgen excess accounts for more than 40% of cases in females with PCOS. Hypothalamus-hypophysis-ovary axis dysregulation is associated with PCOS which depicts that more androgen synthesis in theca cells leads to increased levels of the hormone. Hyperandrogenemia has also been seen to lower the sensitivity to estradiol and progesterone thus, reinforcing the GnRH and LH hypersecretion. HA due to increased cortisol hormone which is a stress hormone leads to the proliferation of theca cells and the absence of their dominance retains hormonal abnormalities which further can be called poly follicular ovarian syndrome in females. For the production of androgen, the increased number of follicular theca cells and enhanced expression of steroidogenic enzymes such as CYP450 in theca cells are observed. Insulin is one of the factors among several that helps to elevate the number of hormones to produce androgen in excess by activating the tyrosine phosphate cascade for glucose utilization (Khan MS et al. 2023). Due to overstimulation of the hypothalamus ratio of LH: FSH disbalances and this imbalanced ratio prevents the development of follicles and enhances androgen release. However, shreds of evidence proved that increased stress leads to an increase in the chances of PCOS etiology and pathophysiology.

## 6. Stress Impacts on Hormones

### 6.1. Cortisol

At the time of stress, the plasma levels of cortisol or corticotrophin-releasing factor (CRF) can increase up to two or fivefold depending upon the severity of the condition (Hargreaves et al.,1990). Moreover, in PCOD patients, stress and in turn, hormonal secretion goes hand in hand that can be brought down to normal levels by exercises such as walking and swimming. Norepinephrine, serotonin, and acetylcholine mediate much of the neurogenic stimulation of CRF production (Herman et al., 2003, Black PH et al., 1994).

### 6.2. Catecholamines

Catecholamine release is instigated by the stimulation of the pituitary-adrenal axis. Due to this, various other complications can arise that can lead to increased glucose flow, bronchiolar dilatation, and behavioral activation can take place (Goldstein et al.,1987).

### 6.3. Vasopressin

- It is also known as Antidiuretic hormone (ADH). Due to vasopressin, the promotion of smooth muscle contraction of the blood vessels can occur. ADH secretion is hyper-activated and detects a change in the concentration of the blood or blood pressure due to PCOS.
- The mechanism lying behind the release of vasopressin lies in the fact that once vasopressin travels to the kidneys thereby preventing water from being lost through

urination. This increases both blood volume and blood pressure. Due to chronic stress-induced activity with corticotrophs, chances of significant expression of hypothalamic vasopressin over CRH can occur (Goldstein et al.,1987).

- *Gonadotropins:*
    - Due to the stress, the release and levels of circulating gonadotropin hormone led to an altered menstrual cycle (Aguilera et al.,2008).

### 6.4. Thyroid Hormones

Due to stress, the levels of thyroid hormones get decreased drastically. Due to the increased levels of stress, TSH secretion gets inhibited through the action of glucocorticoids on the central nervous system.

### 6.5. Growth Hormone

At the time of stress, there is a possibility that growth hormone levels may vary which can lead to either enhanced metabolic activity or it may lead to any kind of defect if there is a prolonged condition of stress.

### 6.6. Prolactin

At the onset of any stressful condition, the levels of prolactin may increase or decrease. At the onset of stress, Vasopressin and peptide histidine isoleucine are involved in the secretion of prolactin (Cameron et al., 1997). However, the teleological significance of the change in the prolactin level is not yet been reported but it may disturb homeostasis and affect the immune system.

### 6.7. Insulin

Insulin may not be directly related to stress (Salam et al., 2011).

## 7. Health Aid in PCOS

Several factors are responsible for the treatment of PCOS. They mainly include the following:

- Change in dietary habits
- Physical activity
- Age
- Severity of symptoms
- Overall health.

The above-mentioned pointers can be considered to get rid of PCOS. If fiber intake is increased in diet and a person is actively involved in workouts and physically more active, PCOD will slowly tend to be treated. Moreover, age has a vital role to play. If a person is diagnosed with PCOS at a very young age, there are chances that it will be taken care of well on time and will be controlled much in advance. Importantly, one has to be very particular about the symptoms of PCOS and consult a gynecologist before the onset of symptoms. Not only PCOS will have a gynecological impact but will lead to weight gain which can lead to other complications. However, the problems encountered during pregnancy by PCOD patients can also lead to twins or multiple births – leading to other complications. And they can cause ovarian hyperstimulation. This condition of hyperstimulation occurs when the ovaries release significantly many hormones that in turn can cause abdominal bloating and pelvic pain (Cowan S et al., 2023).

## Conclusion

PCOS is the most prominent threat to the females in last few years. From 18-45 years of age most females acquire this disease due to unhealthy lifestyles and hormonal imbalance one of the major causes which contributes to the etiology of PCOS is an adrenal hormone which after secretion from the anterior pituitary signals for the release of Growth hormone and due to imbalanced ratio of LH/FSH severe complications takes place such as infertility, acne, hirsutism, etc. It is a very common hormonal imbalance for women, especially those having very high androgen hormonal levels. Women with PCOS do have problems with ovulation and have many small cysts in the ovaries. PCOS can cause missed or irregular menstrual periods, excess hair growth, acne, infertility, and weight gain. Chances of diabetes, hypertension, and weight gain are more prominent in PCOS. The high level of cortisol in the body during stress creates an abnormal androgen section and Hyperinsulinemia that further leads to Insulin resistance and type 2 Diabetes in females. However, It is well known that daughters of PCOS females are mainly affected at an early age after their birth due to genetic issues or gene mutations. Various treatment options were suggested to treat the disorder but the most appropriate way to treat it is to live a healthy lifestyle, keep away from stress and depression situations, eat healthy, and take appropriate and prescribed medications only. The types of treatment for PCOS may depend on the above-mentioned factors.

## References

Aguilera, G., Subburaju, S., Young, S., & Chen, J. (2008). The parvocellular vasopressinergic system and responsiveness of the hypothalamic pituitary adrenal axis during chronic stress. *Progress in brain research,* 170, 29-39.

Alsadi, B. (2018). Polycystic Ovary Syndrome, Pathophysiology, and Reproductive Health Implications. In *Pathophysiology-Altered Physiological States.* IntechOpen.

Amiri, M., & Tehrani, F. R. (2020). Potential adverse effects of female and male obesity on fertility: a narrative review. *International journal of endocrinology and metabolism,* 18(3).

Ashraf, S., Nabi, M., Rashid, F., & Amin, S. (2019). Hyperandrogenism in polycystic ovarian syndrome and role of CYP gene variants: a review. *Egyptian Journal of Medical Human Genetics,* 20(1), 1-10.

Azziz, R., Carmina, E., Chen, Z., Dunaif, A., Laven, J. S., Legro, R. S., ... & Yildiz, B. O. (2016). Polycystic ovary syndrome. *Nature reviews Disease primers,* 2(1), 1-18.

Balen A, Homburg R, Franks S. Defining polycystic ovary syndrome. *BMJ.* 2009;338:a2968.

Basu, B. R., Chowdhury, O., & Saha, S. K. (2018). Possible link between stress-related factors and altered body composition in women with polycystic ovarian syndrome. *Journal of Human Reproductive Sciences,* 11(1), 10.

Black, P. H. (1994). Central nervous system-immune system interactions: psychoneuroendocrinology of stress and its immune consequences. *Antimicrobial agents and chemotherapy,* 38(1), 1-6.

Burgers, J. A., Fong, S. L., Louwers, Y. V., Valkenburg, O., de Jong, F. H., Fauser, B. C., & Laven, J. S. (2010). Oligoovulatory and anovulatory cycles in women with polycystic ovary syndrome (PCOS): what's the difference?. *The Journal of Clinical Endocrinology & Metabolism,* 95(12), E485-E489.

Cameron, J. L. (1997, February). Stress and behaviorally induced reproductive dysfunction in primates. In *Seminars in reproductive endocrinology* (Vol. 15, No. 01, pp. 37-45). Copyright© 1997 by Thieme Medical Publishers, Inc.

Carey, A. H., Waterworth, D., Patel, K., White, D., Little, J., Novelli, P., ... & Williamson, R. (1994). Polycystic ovaries and premature male pattern baldness are associated with one allele of the steroid metabolism gene CYP17. *Human molecular genetics,* 3(10), 1873-1876.

Carmina, E., Chu, M. C., Longo, R. A., Rini, G. B., & Lobo, R. A. (2005). Phenotypic variation in hyperandrogenic women influences the findings of abnormal metabolic and cardiovascular risk parameters. *The Journal of Clinical Endocrinology & Metabolism,* 90(5), 2545-2549.

Cowan, S., Lim, S., Alycia, C., Pirotta, S., Thomson, R., Gibson-Helm, M., ... & Moran, L. (2023). Lifestyle management in polycystic ovary syndrome–beyond diet and physical activity. *BMC Endocrine Disorders,* 23(1), 14.

Cussen, L., McDonnell, T., Bennett, G., Thompson, C. J., Sherlock, M., & O'Reilly, M. W. (2022). Approach to androgen excess in women: Clinical and biochemical insights. *Clinical Endocrinology,* 97(2), 174-186.

Dadachanji, R., Shaikh, N., & Mukherjee, S. (2018). Genetic variants associated with hyperandrogenemia in PCOS pathophysiology. *Genetics research international,* 2018.

Diamanti-Kandarakis, E., Bourguignon, J. P., Giudice, L. C., Hauser, R., Prins, G. S., Soto, A. M., ... & Gore, A. C. (2009). Endocrine-disrupting chemicals: an Endocrine Society scientific statement. *Endocrine reviews,* 30(4), 293-342.

Ehrmann, D. A. (2005). Polycystic ovary syndrome. *New England Journal of Medicine,* 352(12), 1223-1236.

Franks, S., Hardy, K (2020). What causes anovulation in PCOS? *Current opinion in Endocrine & Metabolic Research.* 12, 59-65.

Gharani, N., Waterworth, D. M., Batty, S., White, D., Gilling-Smith, C., Conway, G. S., ... & Williamson, R. (1997). Association of the steroid synthesis gene CYP11a with polycystic ovary syndrome and hyperandrogenism. *Human Molecular Genetics,* 6(3), 397-402.

Goldstein, D. S. (1987). Stress-induced activation of the sympathetic nervous system. *Bailliere's clinical endocrinology and metabolism,* 1(2), 253-278.

Hargreaves, K. M. (1990). Neuroendocrine markers of stress. *Anesthesia progress,* 37(2-3), 99.

Herman, J. P., Figueiredo, H., Mueller, N. K., Ulrich-Lai, Y., Ostrander, M. M., Choi, D. C., & Cullinan, W. E. (2003). Central mechanisms of stress integration: hierarchical circuitry controlling hypothalamo–pituitary–adrenocortical responsiveness. *Frontiers in neuroendocrinology,* 24(3), 151-180.

Kahsar-Miller, M. D., Nixon, C., Boots, L. R., Go, R. C., & Azziz, R. (2001). Prevalence of polycystic ovary syndrome (PCOS) in first-degree relatives of patients with PCOS. *Fertility and sterility,* 75(1), 53-58.

Khan, M. J., Ullah, A., & Basit, S. (2019). Genetic basis of polycystic ovary syndrome (PCOS): current perspectives. *The application of clinical genetics,* 249-260.

Khan, M. S., Kim, H. S., Kim, R., Yoon, S. H., & Kim, S. G. (2023). Dysregulated Liver Metabolism and Polycystic Ovarian Syndrome. *International Journal of Molecular Sciences,* 24(8), 7454.

Krishnan, A., & Muthusami, S. (2017). Hormonal alterations in PCOS and its influence on bone metabolism. *Journal of Endocrinology,* 232(2), R99-R113.

Kumari, S., & Agarwal, R. Comparative study of cortisol level between PCOS women and normal women.

Maas, K. H., Chuan, S., Harrison, E., Cook-Andersen, H., Duleba, A. J., & Chang, R. J. (2016). Androgen responses to adrenocorticotropic hormone infusion among individual women with polycystic ovary syndrome. *Fertility and sterility,* 106(5), 1252-1257.

Panda, P. K., Rane, R., Ravichandran, R., Singh, S., & Panchal, H. (2016). Genetics of PCOS: A systematic bioinformatics approach to unveil the proteins responsible for PCOS. *Genomics data,* 8, 52-60.

Panidis, D., Tziomalos, K., Misichronis, G., Papadakis, E., Betsas, G., Katsikis, I., & Macut, D. (2012). Insulin resistance and endocrine characteristics of the different phenotypes of polycystic ovary syndrome: a prospective study. *Human reproduction,* 27(2), 541-549.

Peng, C. Y., Xie, H. J., Guo, Z. F., Nie, Y. L., Chen, J., Zhou, J. M., & Yin, J. (2014). The association between androgen receptor gene CAG polymorphism and polycystic ovary syndrome: a case-control study and meta-analysis. *Journal of assisted reproduction and genetics,* 31, 1211-1219.

Prasad, S., Tiwari, M., Pandey, A. N., Shrivastav, T. G., & Chaube, S. K. (2016). Impact of stress on oocyte quality and reproductive outcome. *Journal of biomedical science,* 23, 1-5.

Pusalkar M, Meherji P, Gokral J, Chinnaraj S, Maitra A. CYP11A1, and CYP17 promoter polymorphisms associate with hyperandrogenemia in polycystic ovary syndrome. *Fertil Steril.* 2009;92(2):653-9.

Qin, Y., Bai, J., Dai, J., Zhou, J., Zhang, T., Zhang, S., ... & Liu, Y. (2022). Alterations of Cortisol and Melatonin Production by the Theca Interna Cells of Porcine Cystic Ovarian Follicles. *Animals,* 12(3), 357.

Ralph, C. R. Lehman. M N. Goodman. R. L., & Tilbrook, A. J. (2016). Impact of psychological stress on gonadotrophins and sexual behavior in females: a role for cortisol?, *Reproduction,* 152(1), R1-R14.

Reddy, K. R., Deepika, M. L. N., Supriya, K., Latha, K. P., Rao, S. L., Rani, V. U., & Jahan, P. (2014). CYP11A1 microsatellite (tttta) n polymorphism in PCOS women from South India. *Journal of assisted reproduction and genetics,* 31, 857-863.

REDDY[1], K. R., N[1], D. M., LATHA[1], K. P., & R[1], S. S. (2015). Polycystic ovary syndrome: role of aromatase gene variants in South Indian women.

Ruta K. (2014) Contemporary and traditional perspectives of the polycystic ovarian syndrome (PCOS). *Journal of Dental Medical Science,* 13,89-98.

Saadia, Z. (2020). Follicle stimulating hormone (LH: FSH) ratio in polycystic ovary syndrome (PCOS)-obese vs. non-obese women. *Medical Archives,* 74(4), 289.

Salam, R., & Reetu, K. (2011). Stress and hormones. *Indian J Endocrinol Metab,* 15(1), 18-22.

Strachan, T., & Read, A. P. (1999). Instability of the human genome: mutation and DNA repair. *Human Molecular Genetics*, 2, 209-217.

Teede, H., Deeks, A., & Moran, L. (2010). Polycystic ovary syndrome: a complex condition with psychological, reproductive and metabolic manifestations that impacts on health across the lifespan. *BMC medicine,* 8(1), 1-10.

Toosy, S., Sodi, R., & Pappachan, J. M. (2018). Lean polycystic ovary syndrome (PCOS): an evidence-based practical approach. *Journal of Diabetes & Metabolic Disorders,* 17, 277-285.

Van Der Steeg, J. W., Steures, P., Eijkemans, M. J., Habbema, J. D. F., Hompes, P. G., Burggraaff, J. M., ... & Mol, B. W. (2008). Obesity affects spontaneous pregnancy chances in subfertile, ovulatory women. *Human reproduction,* 23(2), 324-328.

Witchel, S. F., & Aston, C. E. (2000). The role of heterozygosity for CYP21 in the polycystic ovary syndrome. *Journal of pediatric endocrinology & metabolism: JPEM,* 13, 1315-1317.

Woodruff, T. J., Janssen, S. J., Guillette Jr, L. J., & Giudice, L. C. (Eds.). (2010). Environmental impacts on reproductive health and fertility. Cambridge University Press.

Yesiladali, M., Yazici, M. G., Attar, E., & Kelestimur, F. (2022). Differentiating polycystic ovary syndrome from adrenal disorders. *Diagnostics,* 12(9), 2045.

Zeng, X., Xie, Y. J., Liu, Y. T., Long, S. L., & Mo, Z. C. (2020). Polycystic ovarian syndrome: correlation between hyperandrogenism, insulin resistance, and obesity. *Clinica chimica acta,* 502, 214-221.

Zhang, T., Liang, W., Fang, M., Yu, J., Ni, Y., & Li, Z. (2013). Association of the CAG repeat polymorphisms in androgen receptor gene with polycystic ovary syndrome: a systemic review and meta-analysis. *Gene,* 524(2), 161-167.

Chapter 7

# PCOS and Insulin Resistance: The Relationship Between Insulin Resistance and Melatonin PI3/AKT Signaling Pathways in Granulosa Cells


**Syed Douhath Yousuf[1]**
**Falak Kayenat[2]**
**Gowhar Rashid[3]**
**and Mohammad Ashraf Ganie[4,*]**

[1]Department of Clinical Biochemistry, Sher-i-Kashmir Institute of Medical Sciences, SKIMS, Soura, Srinagar, Jammu and Kashmir, India
[2]Department of Biotechnology, Jamia Hamdard University, New Delhi, India
[3]Amity Medical School, Amity University Haryana, India
[4]Department of Endocrinology, Sher-i-Kashmir Institute of Medical Sciences, SKIMS, Soura, Srinagar, Jammu and Kashmir, India



## Abstract

Polycystic ovary syndrome (PCOS) is a common endocrine gynecological condition linked with metabolic issues. PCOS is typically characterized by severe insulin resistance (IR) and insulin secretion abnormalities, which plays a significant part in its growth and duration. The PI3K/Akt pathway is an integral component of the complex network that mediates insulin signaling and regulates the impacts of insulin on anabolism in all organisms. It helps promote insulin-mediated glucose uptake in targeted tissues by facilitating the transport of glucose transporter protein type 4 (GLUT4) to the plasmalemma. Melatonin, an essential endogenous hormone, has a positive effect on the female reproductive system. It regulates the expression of GLUT4 and stimulates receptors of insulin, most probably through the PI3K/Akt pathway. Melatonin has been found to significantly increase the expression of GLUT4 and reduce IR in individuals with type-2 diabetes (T2D) and metabolic syndrome. In PCOS individuals, melatonin has been proven to improve mental health metrics, decrease serum insulin levels, and improve PCOS-related pathological changes and insulin-mediated glucose uptake. Therefore, melatonin is an effective agent that can be used to treat several reproductive disorders, including female infertility caused by IR. This chapter intends to review the molecular impact of melatonin



* Corresponding Author's Email: ashraf.endo@gmail.com.



In: Polycystic Ovarian Syndrome (PCOS) and Our Biological Clock
Editors: Arpita Roy, Gowhar Rashid and Nihad Ashraf Khan
ISBN: 979-8-89113-100-2


© 2023 Nova Science Publishers, Inc.

PI3K/Akt signaling pathway on IR in human ovarian granulosa cells (GCs) in women with PCOS.

**Keywords:** polycystic ovary syndrome, PI3K/Akt pathway, GLUT4, insulin resistance, melatonin, granulosa cells

## 1. Introduction

In premenopausal women, polycystic ovary syndrome (PCOS), which has an incidence rate of 5-20%, is the most prevalent endocrine condition and is defined by hirsutism, irregular menstrual cycles, and sterility (Asunción et al., 2000). Insulin resistance (IR) is a crucial contributor in the onset and duration of PCOS, a prevalent endocrine illness associated with metabolic problems (Amato et al., 2015). The hyperinsulinemic-euglycemic glucose clamp or insulin clamp is the benchmark for accurately defining human insulin sensitivity, but it is slow, labor-intensive, costly, and technically challenging (R. A. DeFronzo et al., 1979). The primary technique for measuring IR in scientific research is the homeostatic assessment model analysis of IR (HOMA-IR), as it is straightforward and noninvasive (D. R. Matthews et al., 1985).

Patients having type-2 diabetes (T2D) and people suffering from other conditions distinguished by IR, including obesity and PCOS, are said to have IR if there's a reduction in the uptake of insulin-stimulated glucose into muscle and lipocytes and poor insulin regulation of the production of liver glucose. The term IR was initially used to describe the wide variation in the insulin doses necessary to reduce high sugar concentration in T2D patients, and it was later used to define the extent of variation in blood sugar levels following the introduction of a certain quantity of insulin and glucose. The "described amount of insulin" is crucial because people with IR frequently experience hyperinsulinemia, a state when blood insulin levels are elevated as compared to normal in relation to the proportion of blood sugar concentration including both fasting and fed situation; this hyperinsulinemia corrects for IR in peripheral tissues to bring blood glucose concentrations back to normal (Himsworth, 2013).

A key hormone involved in regulating glucose metabolism, insulin exerts its biological effects via interacting with insulin receptors (Artunc et al., 2016). The PI3K/Akt signaling pathway is essential for controlling the impacts of insulin on anabolism in all organisms and is part of the complex, highly integrated network that mediates the insulin signaling network (C. M. Taniguchi et al., 2006). Once insulin interacts with the receptor, insulin receptor substrate (IRS) recruits as well as stimulates PI3K to produce PIP3, which encourages Akt to recruit and activate. Akt sends signals to downstream pathways that control lipid, glucose, and cell survival (Santoleri & Titchenell, 2019; Titchenell et al., 2017). By encouraging the transport of GLUT4 to the plasma lemma, the PI3K/Akt signaling pathway increases insulin-mediated glucose absorption in target tissues (King et al., 2016). IR is directly associated to the impairment of the PI3K/Akt pathway.

## 2. Pathogenesis of PCOS

Although PCOS is one of the most prevalent endocrinopathies, the full pathophysiological mechanism is yet unknown. Although the description of each relevant pathophysiological mechanism has taken time to develop, the variety of PCOS may suggest the involvement of numerous pathophysiological mechanisms. PCOS is thought to be the outcome of a "vicious cycle" that can start at any of multiple entrance points. An increase in ovarian androgen and anovulation is caused by altered function at any stage in the cycle. A number of hypotheses have been put out to describe the etiology of PCOS, despite the fact that it is a complex condition.

### 2.1. Primary Disordered Gonadotropin Secretion

Disordered secretion of gonadotropin, with a preponderance of luteinizing hormone (LH) to follicle-stimulating hormone (FSH) is the main biochemical anomaly that is known in women with PCOS. This idea clarified hirsutism, anovulation, and ovarian morphology. The pilosebaceous unit is stimulated by the excess androgen in these women, which enhances sebum production, causes terminal hair differentiation, and, seldom, results in pilosbaceous unit atresia and androgenic alopecia in the scalp. Research on gonadotropin secretion in PCOS-afflicted women have found that these women produce more LH in response to gonadotropin-releasing hormone (GnRH) challenge when FSH secretion is at the proper levels (Rebar et al., 1976). Obesity reduces the average LH level and GnRH stimulated level in PCOS-affected women, however, their response is still higher when compared to healthy women with the same age and weight (Morales et al., 1996).

### 2.2. Primary Ovarian and Adrenal Hyperandrogenism

Women suffering from PCOS have abnormal ovarian steroidogenesis due to elevated amounts of androgen in the blood. Antral follicles had increased intrafollicular androgen levels, which is evidence that the granulosa aromatase activity is insufficient (Schneyer et al., 2000). Long-term culture of thecal cells from PCOS patients reveals abnormal steroidogenesis along with elevated androgen synthesis, suggesting that the cells may have a genetic abnormality (Nelson et al., 1999). Increased level of dehydroepiandrosterone (DHEAS), an androgen marker for adrenal function, is the primary cause of adrenal hyperandrogenism in 20–30% of women suffering from PCOS, indicating that the ovary and consequently the adrenal is also affected by the primary steroidogenesis defect.

### 2.3. Primary Disorder of IR

Insulin action exhibits different abnormalities in women with PCOS. Dynamic research of insulin action, insulin clamps, and recurrently collected intravenous sugar tolerance evaluations have revealed that women with PCOS exhibit greater IR than weight-matched healthy ones. The main site of the defect appears to be skeletal muscle (Dunaif & Finegood, 1996; Dunaif et al., 1989). The theca cells derived from individuals having PCOS has been shown to produce increased amounts of hormone androgens in laboratory settings when subjected to insulin treatment. A variety of genetic IR disorders, such as leprechaunism, Rabson Mendenhall syndrome, and lipodystrophies, are linked to compensatory hyperinsulinemia, ovarian hyperandrogenism, and adrenal hyperandrogenism (Dunaif, 1997). The occurrences of glucose intolerance and T2D are most commonly known to be predicted by IR and beta-cell malfunction (Reaven, 1988). Hence, it is assumed that PCOS women have an increased chance of getting T2D. Using WHO standards, it was first stated that 40% of obese females having PCOS had poor sugar tolerance or open T2D (Dunaif et al., 1987). Using WHO criteria, these PCOS prevalence percentages are noticeably greater than the 10.3% discovered in significant population-based studies of women from related age groups (Harris et al., 1987). Compromised glucose tolerance and T2D (Reaven, 1988), high blood pressure (Ferrannini et al., 1987), abdominal obesity, and adverse lipid profiles (Orchard et al., 1983), which is referred to as "metabolic syndrome X," which is preceded by IR and is viewed as a risk factor for heart disease (Wild et al., 1990).

While the presentation of symptoms may vary, PCOS commonly manifests with hyperandrogenism, and ovulatory dysfunction, and is linked with conditions such as obesity, IR, and sub-fertility (Dunaif et al., 1992). About 65-70% of women suffering from PCOS exhibit IR and compensatory hyperinsulinemia (DeUgarte et al., 2005). Around 20-25% of women with a lean body mass index (BMI<25) and 70-80% of those with obesity (BMI>30) exhibit comparable characteristics. Research has indicated that some of the IR noted in women having PCOS is not solely a result of obesity, but rather related to PCOS itself, as anomalies in insulin receptor function and cellular insulin action have been identified (Ciaraldi et al., 1992; Dunaif et al., 1995). Hyperinsulinemia serves as a co-gonadotropin, enhancing the impacts of the high LH activation observed in most of PCOS patients, as well as working directly to promote increased androgen production by theca cells (Nestler et al., 1998). As the higher insulin was linked to the central androgen actions that impaired progesterone's regulation of the GnRH pulse generator, it may have further effects (Blank et al., 2009). Insulin raised the mRNAs for adrenal steroidogenic enzymes in vitro and rapidly boosted the secretory responses of the adrenal glands to ACTH (Moghetti et al., 1996).

Women having PCOS are much more susceptible to developing hyperglycemia, T2D, dyslipidemia, and other inflammatory signs and symptoms, which is consistent with the high prevalence of IR and obesity (Mathur & Alexander, 2008). Similar to how many men do, many women also exhibit symptoms of metabolic syndrome, including high triglycerides, increased LDL, and decreased HDL (Ehrmann et al., 2006).

Measuring IR is a complex process that can be challenging to carry out accurately. Several assays have been developed to measure this biochemical process, with some being more complex but highly reliable, and others being less accurate but more straightforward and less invasive, making them more suitable for clinical research. The golden standard for directly analyzing metabolic insulin sensitivity is the hyperinsulinemic-euglycemic glucose clamp, which involves continuous insulin infusion to achieve a novel stable insulin level higher than the fasted level. This results in improved glucose clearance in skeletal muscle and fat tissue and reduced liver glucose synthesis. To maintain euglycemia, 20% dextrose is administered. While the method accurately monitors the entire body's glucose elimination under stable insulin parameters, it is slow, costly, labor-intensive, and technically challenging (Ralph A DeFronzo et al., 1979).

The HOMA-IR is a method that utilizes a simple nonlinear equation, derived from mathematical principles, to calculate IR and pancreatic β-cell function on the basis of basal levels of sugar and insulin (or C-peptide). The equation used for calculating HOMA-IR is as follows: (concentration of insulin during the fast (mU/ml) × concentration of glucose during the fast (mmol/l))/22.5 (normalizing-factor) (David R Matthews et al., 1985).

The quantitative insulin sensitivity check index (QUICKI) is a straightforward adaptation of the HOMA equation which offers an accurate and reliable insulin sensitivity index (ISI) with favorable predictive value and a markedly higher correlation to measurements of insulin sensitivity obtained using a glucose clamp than other straightforward surrogates (Chen et al., 2005). It is frequently utilized in clinical research investigations since it is simple, affordable, and minimally intrusive. The oral glucose tolerance test (OGTT) is a simple analysis method that is frequently employed in clinical studies to test T2D or glucose intolerance. Blood sugar and insulin levels are measured at initial, 1/2, 1, and 2 hours following an oral glucose load (75 g). OGTT is a useful tool for evaluating glucose tolerance, although it does not directly assess insulin sensitivity or resistance (Dalla Man et al., 2005).

## 3. Mechanism of Action of Insulin Hormone

The anabolic peptide hormone insulin is released by pancreatic cells and develops into its mature form over the course of two stages (Banting & Best, 2007). By severing the signal fragment, preproinsulin is first processed to create proinsulin (Steiner et al., 1967). The center fragment (C chain—35 aa) is then removed, resulting in a dipeptide composed of 2 chains (A-21 aa, B- 30 aa) linked by 2 di-sulfide links (Dodson & Steiner, 1998). A protein with multiple functions, insulin controls the metabolism of lipids and carbohydrates. The post-prandial increase in blood sugar level is the primary stimulus for insulin generation. The amount of glucose transported into the cells is raised while the blood sugar level is decreased by boosting insulin synthesis and their influence on effector cells (muscle cells, lipocytes, and liver cells). The insulin-dependent glucose transporters (GLUT), of which GLUT-4 is present in skeletal muscle, liver cells, and adipocytes, are translocated more frequently to do this (Olson & Pessin, 1996).

When the small intestine's glucose concentration rises over 30mM, GLUT2 starts to transport glucose insulin independently to the pancreatic cells' interior. With the help of a concentration gradient, GLUT2 aids transport. The internal transformation of glucose to glucose-6-phosphate stops glucose levels from equilibrating and hinders sustained transport to the cell. Entering glycolysis, which produces ATP molecules, is glucose-6-phosphate. The level of ATP is always rising as a result of an ongoing glucose supply. As a result, the potassium channel is inhibited, preventing $K^+$ ions from leaving the cell. The cell's $K^+$ ion concentration rises, making the cell electro-positive till the membrane's charges line up and cause the cell membrane to depolarize. The voltage-dependent $Ca^{2+}$ channels is opened by depolarization, which encourages the entrance of calcium ions into the cell. The ryanodine channel, which is present in the membrane of insulin-accumulating vesicles, is opened up by $Ca^{2+}$ ions, causing the vesicles to move into the plasma membrane and release their contents (Kellett et al., 2008).

## 4. Insulin Signaling Pathway

Insulin that is secreted plays a vital function in a wide range of metabolic processes, such as the storage of glycogen in the hepatic and skeletal muscles, the promotion of adipogenesis and the suppression of lipolysis, and the inhibition of gluconeogenesis in the liver. However, the primary metabolic effect of secreted insulin is an enhancement in glucose uptake via the insulin receptor pathway (Newsholme & Dimitriadis, 2001). The process of transmitting signals from the bloodstream into the cell is complex and tightly incorporated. It commences with the binding of the hormone to its receptor, which results in the formation of a large protein signaling complex surrounding the cytoplasmic domains of the insulin receptors, located just beneath the cell membrane (Ullrich & Schlessinger, 1990). Insulin receptors are heterotetrameric glycoproteins that have two subunits that are external and two subunits that are intracellular. They mainly appear on the cell surfaces of tissues with active metabolism, such as muscles, the liver, and fat. Extracellular subunits interact to insulin, which causes insulin receptor dimerization and enables ATP binding to subunits (Perlman et al., 1989). As a result of which the cytoplasmic catalytic domains of tyrosine kinases become active (Baron et al., 1992). Many substrate proteins are phosphorylated in the first stage, with IRS (insulin receptor substrate) proteins appearing to be the most crucial ones. This is followed by the autophosphorylation of the receptor. The site of phosphorylation is the tyrosine residues, and once IRS proteins are phosphorylated, they can activate two significant signaling pathways. The first step in a pathway that leads to mitogen-activated protein kinases (MAPK), which are implicated in regulating the genetic expression involved in growth and differentiation of cell, is Ras. The next pathway, known as the phosphoinositide 3-kinase (PI3K) route, results to the phosphorylation of AKT/PKB kinase and is concerned for insulin's metabolic activity.

## 4.1. PI3K/AKT Pathway

The binding of the IRS protein to the regulatory subunits of PI3-kinase via SH2 domains is the first step in the stimulation of the PI3K/AKT signaling pathway. Once stimulated, PI3K phosphorylates phosphatidylinositol 4,5-bisphosphate (PIP2) to create phosphatidylinositol (3,4,5)-trisphosphate (PIP3). The activation of PDK-1 and PDK-2 (PIP3-dependent kinases), is triggered by PIP3, ultimately resulting in the stimulation of the AKT/PKB kinase pathway and atypical PKCs (Manna & Jain, 2013). AKT kinase phosphorylates the AS160 (AKT-substrate protein), which in turn facilitates the movement of GLUT from cytoplasmic vesicles to the surface of the plasma membrane, leading to a rise in the insulin-dependent transportation of sugar into the cell. Under normal conditions, GLUT4 is primarily found inside the cell due to a balance between slow exocytosis and fast endocytosis. However, in adipocytes, AS160 promotes GLUT4 exocytosis and inhibits endocytosis via its downstream target, Rab10, which leads to the accumulation of GLUT4 at the cell membrane (Sano et al., 2007). Besides activating insulin-dependent glucose uptake, AKT has various intracellular targets and modulates a range of metabolic implications. For instance AKT phosphorylates glycogen synthase kinase 3 (GSK3), which stimulates glycogen production in the liver and skeletal muscle (Friedrichsen et al., 2013).

### *4.1.1. PI3K/AKT Pathway Regulation*

The PI3K/AKT signaling pathway is tightly regulated, and disruptions to it are the root of multiple disorders, most notably IR. One of the most significant issues facing modern research is the need for more understanding of the systems controlling this signaling. Three distinct signaling nodes have so far been identified: IRS proteins, regulatory-PI3K kinase subunits, and kinase isoform Akt/PKB are only a few examples (Cullen M Taniguchi et al., 2006). The decrease in signal transmission efficiency and disorders associated with it are mostly caused by disturbances of any of these nodes.

#### *4.1.1.1. IRS Protein Node*

Six proteins make up the IRS family (IRS1-6), of which IRS1 and IRS2 are essential for the transduction of the insulin signal. Tissue-specific expression and activity of IRS proteins are observed (Cai et al., 2003). In order to bind to insulin receptors, they have 3 distinctive domains: (i) a pleckstrin homology domain at the N-terminal (ii) a phosphotyrosine-binding domain in the middle, and (iii) many phosphorylation sites on tyrosine and serine residues at the C-terminus. Tyrosine residues that have been phosphorylated cause IRS to attach to molecules with an Src-homology-2 domain via their C-terminus domain (SH2)(Gustafson et al., 1995). Muscle, fat, liver, and pancreatic islets are just a few of the tissues that have high levels of IRS-1 and IRS-2 expression and play significant parts in the regulatory function of energy balance. IRS2 appears to be important in hepatocytes and islet cells, whereas IRS1 appears to be the primary actor in myocytes and adipose tissue (Thirone et al., 2006)

In general, there are three avenues via which IRS regulation is possible . Several ser/thr residues that can undergo phosphorylation by kinases plays a major role in crucial regulation. Tyrosine phosphorylation, required for signal transduction, is blocked by the phosphorylation of serine residues, which may prevent insulin signaling. Yet, it is still unclear exactly how this inhibitory mechanism works. In fact, there is a direct connection between defects in the PI3K pathway and serine phosphorylation, reduced tyrosine phosphorylation, and IR. Stress inducing kinases including extracellular signal-regulated kinases (ERK), c-Jun N-terminal *kinases*(JNK), and 5' AMP-activated protein kinase(AMPK), as well as inflammatory kinase IKK and other downstream kinases like AKT, atypical PKC isoforms, mTOR, or S6K, are the most important enzymes capable of phosphorylating IRS in serine residue(Nandipati et al., 2017). IR, the primary stage in the growth of diabetes, is formed when the IRS is blocked, which results in a decreased cell responsiveness to insulin stimulation. Low-grade inflammation, brought on by fat buildup, is the primary cause of this inhibitory phosphorylation (Engin, 2017). According to research, palmitate dramatically reduced the insulin-stimulated Ser phosphorylation of Akt and Tyrosine phosphorylation of IRS-1 (Ajuwon & Spurlock, 2005). A number of drugs have been found to have similar effects on insulin signaling. One instance is simvastatin, which is frequently prescribed for preventing and treating cardiovascular diseases. Simvastatin has been observed to hinder insulin-induced phosphorylation of insulin receptors at tyrosine, IRS-1 at tyrosine, and AKT at Thr (Li et al., 2016). As a result, the use of simvastatin or other statin medications may enhance the risk of developing IR or diabetes. However, there are certain organic compounds, such as silibinin, that could potentially mitigate this effect. Silibinin, which is the primary flavonoid in silymarin, a combination of flavonolignans obtained from Silybum marianum seeds, can reduce IRS1 phosphorylation at Tyr and prevent inhibition of the PI3K/AKT pathway (Li et al., 2015). Overexpression of PTP1B (protein-tyrosine phosphatase 1B) can deactivate the entire PI3K signaling pathway through a similar mechanism (Goldstein et al., 2000). The identification of PTP1B inhibitors has emerged as a significant research domain for the treatment of disruptions in the signaling pathway of insulin as this was revealed to be upregulated in insulin-sensitive peripheral tissues (such as fats and muscles) as well as in liver cells during an insulin-resistant state. FYGL (Fudan-Yueyang G. lucidum extract) is a potentially appealing compound with limited cell permeability and bioavailability but has shown inhibitory activity against PTP1B (Yang et al., 2018).

Proteins with phosphotyrosine-binding (PTB) domains can regulate IRS activity by competitively restricting insulin receptors binding to IRS. One of these PTB domain-containing proteins is NYGGF4, whose expression levels are higher in obese people. Research on skeletal myotubes have shown that NYGGF4 can reduce insulin-induced phosphorylation of IRS1 at Tyrosine and Akt at Serine residue. However, the tyrosine phosphorylation of insulin receptors following insulin stimulation remained unaffected (Wu et al., 2011).

In addition to other IRS modulatory pathways, the regulatory expression of insulin receptor substrate facilitated by hyperinsulinemia and other hormones is noteworthy (Hirashima et al., 2003). FSH promotes expression of IRS2 in granulosa cells (Anjali et al., 2015). Additionally, some herbal remedies, such as the combination of five herbs known as Tangzhiqing formula, alter the degree of IRS expression in HEPG2 cells (IRS1 and IRS2) and L-6 myotubes (IRS1) (Gao et al., 2014).

#### *4.1.1.2. PI3K Kinase Subunits*

The family of proteins known as PI3 kinases is active in the phosphorylation of proteins and lipids. In accordance with their structural characteristics and preferred substrates, they are split into three classes. The most important components of the insulin signaling pathway are I class members. PI3K-1 consists of regulatory and catalytic subunit heterodimers. Generally speaking, the regulatory component is known as p85. They all share the same domain architecture: Breakpoint cluster area homology (BH), the iSH2 (interSH2) domain, two SH2 domains, and the SH3 domain (Fruman, 2011). The IRS phosphotyrosine motif and p85 engage via the SH2 domain to start the signaling process. After that, the adapter-binding domains (ABD) of the catalytic subunit p110 is connected to p85 via its iSH2 domain. Together with ABD, p110 also has a Ras-binding domain (RBD), which interacts with the Ras protein superfamily, C2, and helical scaffolding domains, as well as a kinase domain involved in the production of PIP3 (Jiménez et al., 2002).p85 forms a heterodimer with p110 to shield it against deterioration. The catalytic subunit of p110 can convey a signal by phosphorylating PIP2 to PIP3, a lipid secondary messenger, thanks to its interaction, which also enables p110 translocation to the plasma membrane. Surprisingly, the most noticeable PI3K catalytic subunit in the insulin-dependent pathway is p110 (Bi et al., 1999). Cells lacking this show hyperglycemia and glucose intolerance (Nelson et al., 2014). Although p110 appears to have a supporting role, its existence is required for p110 activity, which maintains the basal threshold of PIP3 (Yu et al., 1998). AKT and PDK1, two proteins having PH domains, bind to PIP3. Further signal transduction to downstream proteins is made possible by this crucial process.

Many factors are taken into consideration in this control node. First off, the PI3K regulatory subunit, p85, mediates either the restriction or encouragement of PI3K signaling, which is critically dependent upon it. P85 lessens the activity of p110 in cells that aren't receiving upstream inputs. It is carried out by the C2 and helical scaffolding domains, which interact with p85 to block it. Moreover, monomeric p85 blocks the p85-p110 heterodimer bound to IRS by binding to phosphorylated regions of IRS (Mauvais-Jarvis et al., 2002). In some kinds of human cancer, the spatial control of p110, another important regulatory protein, occurs. Research on HepG2 cells showed that PAQR3, or the progestin and adipoQ receptor family member 3, binds to p110 by drawing it to the Golgi apparatus, which is the only location where PAQR3 is found. The interaction between p85a and p110 is inhibited by this event (Wang et al., 2013).

Two additional PI3K activation mechanisms exist, both of which rely on ligand membrane receptor interaction. The primary method relies on RTK's interaction with the adaptor protein GRB2 (Growth factor receptor-bound *protein* 2). GRB2 is permitted to bind p85 when it is already bound to the GAB protein. Another method of PI3K activation, in contrast, is independent of the p85 subunit. In such circumstances, GRB2 binds with SOS, activating RAS and the p110 subunit in the process. Furthermore, G protein-coupled receptors may be used to excite the p110 catalytic subunit in a manner similar to but independent of the p85 (Castellano & Downward, 2011).

The regulation of the PIP3 level involves another important regulatory mechanism. Phosphatase and tensin homolog (PTEN) is the most common inhibitor that dephosphorylates PIP3, however, there are other well-known inhibitors as well. PTEN is unquestionably a fascinating protein for studies related to the field of illnesses with impaired PI3K signaling. For example, H2S or its precursor, L-cysteine, can inhibit it in adipose tissue. L-cysteine supplementation improves glucose metabolism by raising PIP3 levels and mediating the activation of PI3K (Manna & Jain, 2011). Moreover, adipocytes' ability to express PTEN is controlled epigenetically by a number of miRNAs, including miRNA-21, miRNA-26a, miRNA-26b, miRNA-23a-3p, and miRNA-181a-5p (Ling et al., 2012; Seeger et al., 2014; Xu et al., 2015). The PIP3 inhibitor SHIP (SH2-containing inositol 5′-phosphatase) is another well-known enzyme. PTEN targets the 3′-inositol position, whereas SHIP targets the 5′-inositol position, and inhibits AKT largely by controlling its cellular location (Carver et al., 2000).

Last but not least, genetic mutation of the p110 and p85 subunits or PI3K catabolic regulators may potentially contribute to PI3K dysregulation. For instance, it is known that PTEN can lose its function or be deleted in a variety of cancers. The hunt for molecules that target PI3K is therefore pursued with great effort. The most popular PI3K regulators are LY294002 and Wortmannin (a steroid fungal metabolite) (morpholine-containing chemical compound) (Ui et al., 1995). However, a number of compounds from a new generation that are much more stable, such as SF-1126, GSK615, XL147, CAL101, and PF-4989216, cause the inhibition of excessive PI3K signaling, especially during malignancies (Maira et al., 2009).

#### *4.1.1.3. Kinase Isoform AKT/PKB*

Mammalian AKT, also known as PKB, has 3 iso-forms (AKT1, AKT2, and AKT3). AKT isoforms have distinctive roles and display target specificity despite having comparable domain structures (N-terminal PH domain, central kinase domain, and C-terminal domain). The most crucial factor in glucose absorption is AKT2 (Hanada et al., 2004).

AKT can be drawn to PIP3 by the PH domain, just as PDK1. AKT undergoes structural changes after binding to PIP3 that make the phosphorylation site visible. PDK can phosphorylate AKT on Thr308 while they are close by. However, a second phosphorylation on the Serine residue is required for complete activation of AKT (other than AKT3) (AKT1-Ser473 and Ser-474 AKT2). PDK-2/mTORC2 modifies Ser473 (mammalian target for rapamycin complex 2) (Guertin et al., 2006).

Thr308 and Ser473 are dephosphorylated by the enzymes PP2 (protein phosphatase 2) and PHLPP (PH domain leucine-rich repeat phosphatase), respectively, to stop AKT activation. (Chen et al., 2001). Although the phosphorylation condition of each of the mentioned sites is crucial for the activity of AKT, a variety of additional post-translational changes also have an impact on its functionality (Risso et al., 2015). For instance, PDGF-induced (platelet-derived growth factor) ROS cause oxidation of Cys124, which results in the blocking of AKT2 function

(Wani et al., 2011). Other modulators may activate AKT in addition to PI3K-dependent activation. In particular, tyrosine kinases (such as ACK1, SRC, and PTK6) and serine/threonine kinases are recognized as two types of rare AKT activators (e.g., TBK1, IKBKE). Because AKT is phosphorylated on Tyr176 and preferentially binds to phosphatidic acid, a membrane phospholipid, this phosphorylation allows ACK1, a non-receptor tyrosine kinase, to control the recruitment of AKT to the plasma membrane. This causes AKT adhesion to the plasma membrane even when certain PI3K inhibitors are present. Several malignancies exhibit an increase in AKT2 activity, which might be caused by ACK1 self-activating mutations. Src is yet another non-receptor kinase that controls AKT. Tyrs 315 and 326 are the locations of its activity. Contrarily, the Epidermal Growth Factor (EGF), the overexpression of which is common in malignancies, is responded to by PTK6 through phosphorylation of Tyr215 and 326. Src and PTK6-induced modifications are resilient to a few well-known PI3K inhibitors. Ser/Thr kinases, the second class of AKT activators, modify Ser137, Thr308, and Ser473 (TBK1) as well as Thr195, Ser378, and Ser473 (TBK1) (IKBKE). These different activation mechanisms may indicate that cells can quickly activate AKT signaling in response to certain circumstances (Mahajan & Mahajan, 2012).

### 4.2. PI3K/AKT Pathway Impairment

IR and various malignancies are among the most prevalent and important disorders associated with PI3K pathway dysfunction. A maladjusted glucose response to endogenous and/or exogenous insulin is one way to identify IR. The hormone does not cause peripheral tissues to increase circulation glucose uptake in response. Pancreatic beta-cells are initially unharmed and react to high glucose concentrations by generating more and more insulin. However, if this condition persists for an extended period of time, islet cells begin to overgrow, which results in the decline of their activity and/or a reduction in the mass of -cells. Since the level of glucose does not return to normal, cells become increasingly insulin resistant, creating a vicious cycle of IR. The most metabolically active tissues, such as the liver, muscles, and fat, are those that are most impacted. The specific process is still unclear, despite advances in our knowledge of the etiology of IR. While aberrant insulin synthesis may be a contributing factor, post-receptor signaling issues and alterations to insulin receptors and their substrates are more often to blame.

One of the signaling pathways that is most frequently dysregulated in human malignancies is the PI3K pathway. Its dysregulation may lead to cancer since it is crucial for various biological processes, such as cell survival, proliferation, migration, and differentiation. The most frequent alterations are mutation in the PIK3CA gene, AKT1gene, and PTEN genes, PIK3CA, AKT1, and AKT2 gene amplifications, and loss of expression or deletion in tumor suppressor PTEN (Li et al., 2017). Lung, breast, endometrial, neck, and head cancer, and glioblastoma have the highest rates of PI3K pathway mutations (Faes & Dormond, 2015).

## 5. Melatonin and PI3K/AKT Signaling Pathway

A crucial endogenous hormone known as melatonin (N-acetyl-5-methoxytryptamine) controls the circadian rhythm, biological clock, and reproductive physiology (J. Chen et al., 2019; Heo et al., 2018). Melatonin is also called the darkness hormone because daytime levels are low and night time levels are higher. Two receptor types, MT1 and MT2, that are located in the pineal gland as well as other body components like granulosa cells, are responsible for its effects (El-Raey et al., 2011; Kang et al., 2009). In vitro, cultured cells and animal research have demonstrated that melatonin is beneficial for female reproductive stages like follicular growth, embryogenesis, and oocyte maturation (Z. Chen et al., 2019). The melatonin's impact on its receptors causes a phase difference in the cells, which is what causes insulin generation by the islets of Langerhans to occur in a circadian fashion both in vivo and in vitro. Melatonin receptors act as a mediator for melatonin's effects on insulin secretion (MT1 and MT2). It increases the secretion of insulin by turning on the phospholipase C/IP3 pathway, which mobilizes $Ca^{2+}$ from organelles and decreases insulin secretion by blocking the cAMP and cGMP pathways. Melatonin affects pancreatic islets to control energy metabolism. Melatonin concentrations were found to be reduced and there was evidence of a functional interaction between melatonin and insulin in diabetics, suggesting that melatonin may be involved in the onset of diabetes. Melatonin causes the creation of insulin growth factor and encourages the tyrosine phosphorylation of the insulin receptor, according to evidence from scientific data. IR and glucose intolerance are brought on by internal circadian system disruption, which can be remedied by melatonin supplementation. Consequently, T2D medication may be impacted by the presence of melatonin receptors in human pancreatic islets.

Melatonin regulates the expression of glucose transporter type-4 (GLUT4) and/or stimulates insulin receptors to initiate the insulin signaling cascade (Cipolla-Neto et al., 2014). It has been discovered that melatonin reduces IR in rat models with metabolic syndrome (Ewida & Al-Sharaky, 2016). In diabetic type 2 rats, melatonin dramatically increases GLUT4 expression and reduces IR (Rahman et al., 2017). In PCOS individuals, melatonin improved mental health metrics and decreased serum insulin levels (Shabani et al., 2019). Melatonin enhanced insulin-mediated glucose uptake and the pathological alterations linked to PCOS in rats, according to a different study (Pai & Majumdar, 2014).

The connection between the melatonin, pineal gland, and metabolism of energy was first suggested in both humans (Alcozer et al., 1956) and rats (Milcu et al., 1965) about a decade ago. After conducting preliminary research, it was found that the separation of the pineal gland tends to result in a decrease in the body's potential to tolerate glucose and a reduction in the production of glycogen in both the liver and muscles. Conversely, administering pineal extracts caused a drop in blood sugar levels, a rise in glucose tolerance, and a rise in glycogen production in the liver and muscles following glucose intake (Csaba & Barãth, 1971; Diaz & Blázquez, 1986; Milcu et al., 1963). More recently, a diabetogenic syndrome characterized by intolerance of glucose and peripheral (liver, fat, and skeletal muscle) and central (hypothalamus) IR was identified as the disruption of metabolism brought on by the lack of melatonin in the animal that had its pinealectomized gland (Lima et al., 1998; Nogueira et al., 2011). Melatonin replacement therapy or reduced eating can reverse this alarming pathological picture (Mendes et al., 2013; Nogueira et al., 2011; Zanquetta et al., 2003), but not by physical exercise (Borges-Silva et al., 2007; Borges-Silva, Alonso-Vale, et al., 2005; Borges-Silva, Fonseca-Alaniz, et al., 2005). Additionally, some physiological or pathophysiological conditions linked to decreases in blood melatonin levels, such as aging, diabetes, shift work, and environments with higher levels of night time lightning, can be seen to cause IR, glucose intolerance, and various changes in other metabolic parameters (Karlsson et al., 2001; Nishida et al., 2003; Rasmussen et al., 1999). It is underlined that in these circumstances, appropriate melatonin replacement therapy relieves the majority of the metabolic changes mentioned. Furthermore, MT1-knockout animals exhibit a similar metabolic condition (Contreras-Alcantara et al., 2010).

The absence of melatonin can lead to several biological consequences such as impaired insulin-signaling pathways and reduced levels of both the gene expression and protein content of GLUT4. These effects have been linked to IR and glucose intolerance development following pinealectomy. However, adequate melatonin replacement therapy has been observed to increase the decrease in the levels of GLUT4 messenger RNA, as well as microsomal and membrane protein levels in tissues with insulin-sensitivity, including white and brown adipose tissue, as well as the skeletal and heart muscles, of pinealectomized rats (Lima et al., 1998; Seraphim et al., 1997; Zanquetta et al., 2003). Further studies have demonstrated that melatonin and insulin functionally complement each other. Specifically, melatonin alone can activate the subunit of tyr kinase of the insulin receptors and initiate various intracellular signal transduction stages of the insulin signaling pathway such as the tyr phosphorylation of IRS-1 gene, IRS-1/PI(3)-kinase, and IRS-1/S. This suggests that there is a functional synergism between melatonin and insulin (Anhê et al., 2004; Ha et al., 2006).

Two decades ago, Lima and co-workers published one of the earliest clear examples of the functional complementarity among melatonin and insulin (Lima et al., 1994). This group demonstrated that the dose/response curve for [14C] 2-deoxyglucose (2DG) up-take driven by insulin was shifted towards the left when isolated visceral white adipocytes were incubated in vitro with melatonin. It was also the first instance of melatonin acting directly on adipocytes, proving for the first time that the hormone potentiated the peripheral effect of insulin. Research demonstrated that melatonin's peripheral target for the control of metabolism as a whole is adipose tissue. Additionally, Brydon et al. showed that human adipocytes' MT2 receptors' activation by melatonin modifies these cells' uptake of glucose (Brydon et al., 2001). It was feasible to show that melatonin has a synergistic effect on a number of additional insulin activities in addition to glucose uptake with regard to the physiology of adipose tissue. Alonso-Vale et al. showed in a number of studies that the MT1-mediated melatonin effect potentiates insulin and stimulates leptin production and release in isolated lipocytes (Alonso-Vale et al., 2004; Alonso-Vale et al., 2006). This potentiating effect was attained by interchanging the melatonin-added medium for the first 12 hours (in-vitro and induced at night) without containing melatonin medium for the next remaining hours (in-vitro and induced at day) for 3 to 5 cycles. When the in-vitro incubation with melatonin resembles its typical 24-hour cycle, the potentiating effect is increased by 100%. There is evidence demonstrating that melatonin controls additional adipocyte biological processes, such as lipolysis, lipogenesis, adipocyte differentiation, and fatty acids intake, that affect energy metabolism, hyperlipidemia, and body mass (Dauchy et al., 2003; Zalatan et al., 2001).

The islets of Langerhans, where melatonin affects glucagon and insulin synthesis and release, are another important site of the hormone's activity in relation to the control of energy metabolism. In isolated islets of Langerhans (rat model) and rat's insulinoma β-cells, melatonin activity reduces glucose-stimulated insulin production. The suppression of glucose- and forskolin-induced insulin release by activating these receptors demonstrates melatonin works via blocking the adenylyl cyclase/cAMP pathway as well as decreasing the concentration of PKA while leaving the concentration of PKC-subunit unaffected, in addition to a decrease in cGMP. Melatonin also triggers the phosphorylation of the insulin receptor, insulin receptor substrate 1 (IRS-1), AKT kinase, STAT3, and ERK1/2, which regulates the islets B cells' ability to generate and release insulin through the activation of MT1 (Burks & White, 2001; Kulkarni, 2002; Kulkarni et al., 1999).

Moreover, this indolamine triggers phosphorylation of the IGF-1 receptor, which contributes to the stability and trophism of islet cells (Lima et al., 2001). Also, studies have demonstrated that melatonin enhanced the synthesis and secretion of glucagon in both vivo and in one specific line of glucagon-producing alpha-cells (Bähr et al., 2011; Kosa et al., 2001). The daily peak of insulin secretion is kept to the early half of the active period of the day by these melatonin-induced actions, which is crucial for constructing the circadian profiles of insulin production. Additionally, these effects help to synchronize the pancreatic metabolic rhythmic patterns with the circadian cycle of activity-feeding/rest-fasting (Picinato et al., 2002).

Last, but not least, it's been hypothesized with the help of GWAS (genome-wide association studies), typical non-coding forms in MTNR1B protein (encodes for melatonin receptor 1B, referred as MT2) raise the incidence probability of T2D. This happens due to the pathophysiological as well as physiological significance of the regulatory function of melatonin on the islets of Langerhans function (Bouatia-Naji et al., 2009; Prokopenko et al., 2009). This results in morning hyperglycemia as an outcome of a putatively insufficient pancreatic β-cell reaction to the effect of melatonin on the release of insulin. It should be emphasized that at two critical times during the night, soon after lights out and just before lights on, insulin can potentiate norepinephrine-stimulated melatonin production and hence regulate pineal melatonin synthesis (Garcia et al., 2008; Peliciari-Garcia et al., 2010).

Furthermore, regarding the significance of melatonin in the control of energy metabolism, current research has shown that a lack of melatonin in a pregnant woman will change the intrauterine metabolic programming (Ferreira et al., 2012). Adult off-springs of melatonin-lacking dams exhibit IR, glucose intolerance, and a severe alteration in the glucose-induced insulin production by isolated islets of Langerhans. With the proper timing of melatonin replacement therapy administered to the moms during pregnancy, these programming effects vanish.

## Conclusion

To summarize, IR and the melatonin PI3/AKT signaling pathway have a great impact on the function of granulosa cells. IR disrupts the normal insulin signaling pathway and impairs the ability of granulosa cells to react to insulin, potentially leading to infertility and related disorders. Conversely, melatonin has been found to modulate the PI3/AKT signaling pathway and reduce IR, thus playing a protective factor in granulosa cells. These findings demonstrate the intricate interplay between IR and the melatonin PI3/AKT signaling pathway in granulosa cells, providing a better insight of the underlying mechanisms that regulate reproductive health.

## Future Scope

Given the significance of IR in the context of PCOS, it is crucial to establish additional biochemical parameters which can aid in identifying IR in both research and clinical settings.

Further studies are required to explore the potential therapeutic applications of melatonin in treating disorders related to IR in granulosa cells.

## References


Ajuwon, K. M., & Spurlock, M. E. (2005). Palmitate activates the NF-κB transcription factor and induces IL-6 and TNFα expression in 3T3-L1 adipocytes. *The Journal of nutrition*, *135*(8), 1841-1846.

Alcozer, G., Giordano, G., & Masciocco, D. (1956). [Studies on the epiphysis; influence of aqueous pineal extract on some aspects of carbohydrate metabolism in healthy and eucrine subjects]. *Arch Maragliano Patol Clin*, *12*(6), 1105-1113. (Studi sull'epifisi; influenze dell'estratto acquoso di pineale su alcuni aspetti del metabolismo glicidico in soggetti sani ed eucrinici.).

Alonso-Vale, M. I. C., Anhê, G. F., das Neves Borges-Silva, C., Andreotti, S., Peres, S. B., Cipolla-Neto, J., & Lima, F. B. (2004). Pinealectomy alters adipose tissue adaptability to fasting in rats. *Metabolism*, *53*(4), 500-506.

Alonso-Vale, M. I. C., Andreotti, S., Borges-Silva, C. d. N., Mukai, P. Y., Cipolla-Neto, J., & Lima, F. B. (2006). Intermittent and rhythmic exposure to melatonin in primary cultured adipocytes enhances the insulin and dexamethasone effects on leptin expression. *Journal of pineal research*, *41*(1), 28-34.

Amato, M. C., Vesco, R., Vigneri, E., Ciresi, A., & Giordano, C. (2015). Hyperinsulinism and polycystic ovary syndrome (PCOS): role of insulin clearance. *J Endocrinol Invest*, *38*(12), 1319-1326. https://doi.org/10.1007/s40618-015-0372-x

Anhê, G. F., Caperuto, L. C., Pereira-Da-Silva, M., Souza, L. C., Hirata, A. E., Velloso, L. A., Cipolla-Neto, J., & Carvalho, C. R. (2004). In vivo activation of insulin receptor tyrosine kinase by melatonin in the rat hypothalamus. *Journal of neurochemistry*, *90*(3), 559-566.

Anjali, G., Kaur, S., Lakra, R., Taneja, J., Kalsey, G. S., Nagendra, A., Shrivastav, T., Devi, M. G., Malhotra, N., & Kriplani, A. (2015). FSH stimulates IRS-2 expression in human granulosa cells through cAMP/SP1, an inoperative FSH action in PCOS patients. *Cellular signalling*, *27*(12), 2452-2466.

Artunc, F., Schleicher, E., Weigert, C., Fritsche, A., Stefan, N., & Häring, H. U. (2016). The impact of insulin resistance on the kidney and vasculature. *Nat Rev Nephrol*, *12*(12), 721-737. https://doi.org/10.1038/nrneph.2016.145

Asunción, M., Calvo, R. M., San Millán, J. L., Sancho, J., Avila, S., & Escobar-Morreale, H. F. (2000). A prospective study of the prevalence of the polycystic ovary syndrome in unselected Caucasian women from Spain. *J Clin Endocrinol Metab*, *85*(7), 2434-2438. https://doi.org/10.1210/jcem.85.7.6682

Bähr, I., Mühlbauer, E., Schucht, H., & Peschke, E. (2011). Melatonin stimulates glucagon secretion in vitro and in vivo. *Journal of pineal research*, *50*(3), 336-344.

Banting, F. G., & Best, C. H. (2007). The internal secretion of the pancreas. *Indian Journal of Medical Research*, *125*(3), L251.

Baron, V., Kaliman, P., Gautier, N., & Van Obberghen, E. (1992). The insulin receptor activation process involves localized conformational changes. *Journal of Biological Chemistry*, *267*(32), 23290-23294.

Bi, L., Okabe, I., Bernard, D. J., Wynshaw-Boris, A., & Nussbaum, R. L. (1999). Proliferative defect and embryonic lethality in mice homozygous for a deletion in the p110α subunit of phosphoinositide 3-kinase. *Journal of Biological Chemistry*, *274*(16), 10963-10968.

Blank, S., McCartney, C., Chhabra, S., Helm, K., Eagleson, C., Chang, R., & Marshall, J. (2009). Modulation of GnRH pulse generator sensitivity to progesterone inhibition in hyperandrogenic adolescent girls-Implications for regulation of pubertal maturation. *J Clin Endocrinol Metab*, *94*(7), 2360-2366.

Borges-Silva, C., Takada, J., Alonso-Vale, M. I., Peres, S. B., Fonseca-Alaniz, M. H., Andreotti, S., Cipolla-Neto, J., Pithon-Curi, T. C., & Lima, F. B. (2007). Pinealectomy reduces hepatic and muscular glycogen content and attenuates aerobic power adaptability in trained rats. *J Pineal Res*, *43*(1), 96-103. https://doi.org/10.1111/j.1600-079X.2007.00450.x

Borges-Silva, C. N., Alonso-Vale, M. I., Franzói-De-Moraes, S. M., Takada, J., Peres, S. B., Andreotti, S., Skorupa, A. L., Cipolla-Neto, J., Pithon-Curi, T. C., & Lima, F. B. (2005). Pinealectomy impairs adipose tissue adaptability to exercise in rats. *J Pineal Res*, *38*(4), 278-283. https://doi.org/10.1111/j.1600-079X.2004.00203.x

Borges-Silva, C. N., Fonseca-Alaniz, M. H., Alonso-Vale, M. I., Takada, J., Andreotti, S., Peres, S. B., Cipolla-Neto, J., Pithon-Curi, T. C., & Lima, F. B. (2005). Reduced lipolysis and increased lipogenesis in adipose tissue from pinealectomized rats adapted to training. *J Pineal Res*, *39*(2), 178-184. https://doi.org/10.1111/j.1600-079X.2005.00241.x

Bouatia-Naji, N., Bonnefond, A., Cavalcanti-Proença, C., Sparsø, T., Holmkvist, J., Marchand, M., Delplanque, J., Lobbens, S., Rocheleau, G., & Durand, E. (2009). A variant near MTNR1B is associated with increased fasting plasma glucose levels and type 2 diabetes risk. *Nature genetics*, *41*(1), 89-94.

Brydon, L., Petit, L., Delagrange, P., Strosberg, A. D., & Jockers, R. (2001). Functional expression of MT2 (Mel1b) melatonin receptors in human PAZ6 adipocytes. *Endocrinology*, *142*(10), 4264-4271.

Burks, D. J., & White, M. F. (2001). IRS proteins and beta-cell function. *Diabetes*, *50*(suppl_1), S140.

Cai, D., Dhe-Paganon, S., Melendez, P. A., Lee, J., & Shoelson, S. E. (2003). Two new substrates in insulin signaling, IRS5/DOK4 and IRS6/DOK5. *Journal of Biological Chemistry*, *278*(28), 25323-25330.

Carver, D. J., Aman, M. J., & Ravichandran, K. S. (2000). SHIP inhibits Akt activation in B cells through regulation of Akt membrane localization. *Blood, The Journal of the American Society of Hematology*, *96*(4), 1449-1456.

Castellano, E., & Downward, J. (2011). RAS interaction with PI3K: more than just another effector pathway. *Genes & cancer*, *2*(3), 261-274.

Chen, H., Sullivan, G., & Quon, M. J. (2005). Assessing the predictive accuracy of QUICKI as a surrogate index for insulin sensitivity using a calibration model. *Diabetes*, *54*(7), 1914-1925.

Chen, J., Hou, H., Chen, H., Luo, Y., He, Y., Zhang, L., Zhang, Y., Liu, H., Zhang, F., Liu, Y., Wang, A., & Hu, Q. (2019). Identification of β-hydroxybutyrate as a potential biomarker for female papillary thyroid cancer. *Bioanalysis*, *11*(6), 461-470. https://doi.org/10.4155/bio-2018-0273

Chen, R., Kim, O., Yang, J., Sato, K., Eisenmann, K. M., McCarthy, J., Chen, H., & Qiu, Y. (2001). Regulation of Akt/PKB activation by tyrosine phosphorylation. *J Biol Chem*, *276*(34), 31858-31862. https://doi.org/10.1074/jbc.C100271200.

Chen, Z., Lei, L., Wen, D., & Yang, L. (2019). Melatonin attenuates palmitic acid-induced mouse granulosa cells apoptosis via endoplasmic reticulum stress. *J Ovarian Res*, *12*(1), 43. https://doi.org/10.1186/s13048-019-0519-z.

Ciaraldi, T. P., el-Roeiy, A., Madar, Z., Reichart, D., Olefsky, J. M., & Yen, S. (1992). Cellular mechanisms of insulin resistance in polycystic ovarian syndrome. *The Journal of Clinical Endocrinology & Metabolism*, *75*(2), 577-583.

Cipolla-Neto, J., Amaral, F. G., Afeche, S. C., Tan, D. X., & Reiter, R. J. (2014). Melatonin, energy metabolism, and obesity: a review. *J Pineal Res*, *56*(4), 371-381. https://doi.org/10.1111/jpi.12137.

Contreras-Alcantara, S., Baba, K., & Tosini, G. (2010). Removal of melatonin receptor type 1 induces insulin resistance in the mouse. *Obesity (Silver Spring)*, *18*(9), 1861-1863. https://doi.org/10.1038/oby.2010.24.

Csaba, G., & Barãth, P. (1971). Are Langerhan's islets influenced by the pineal body? *Experientia*, *27*(8), 962. https://doi.org/10.1007/bf02135774.

Dalla Man, C., Campioni, M., Polonsky, K. S., Basu, R., Rizza, R. A., Toffolo, G., & Cobelli, C. (2005). Two-hour seven-sample oral glucose tolerance test and meal protocol: minimal model assessment of β-cell responsivity and insulin sensitivity in nondiabetic individuals. *Diabetes*, *54*(11), 3265-3273.

Dauchy, R. T., Blask, D. E., Sauer, L. A., Davidson, L. K., Krause, J. A., Smith, L. C., & Dauchy, E. M. (2003). Physiologic melatonin concentration, omega-3 fatty acids, and conjugated linoleic acid inhibit fatty acid transport in rodent hind limb skeletal muscle in vivo. *Comparative medicine*, *53*(2), 186-190.

DeFronzo, R. A., Tobin, J. D., & Andres, R. (1979). Glucose clamp technique: a method for quantifying insulin secretion and resistance. *Am J Physiol*, *237*(3), E214-223. https://doi.org/10.1152/ajpendo.1979.237.3.E214.

DeFronzo, R. A., Tobin, J. D., & Andres, R. (1979). Glucose clamp technique: a method for quantifying insulin secretion and resistance. *American Journal of Physiology-Endocrinology And Metabolism*, *237*(3), E214.

DeUgarte, C. M., Bartolucci, A. A., & Azziz, R. (2005). Prevalence of insulin resistance in the polycystic ovary syndrome using the homeostasis model assessment. *Fertility and sterility*, *83*(5), 1454-1460.

Diaz, B., & Blázquez, E. (1986). Effect of pinealectomy on plasma glucose, insulin and glucagon levels in the rat. *Horm Metab Res*, *18*(4), 225-229. https://doi.org/10.1055/s-2007-1012279.

Dodson, G., & Steiner, D. (1998). The role of assembly in insulin's biosynthesis. *Current opinion in structural biology*, *8*(2), 189-194.

Dunaif, A. (1997). Insulin resistance and the polycystic ovary syndrome: mechanism and implications for pathogenesis. *Endocr Rev*, *18*(6), 774-800. https://doi.org/10.1210/edrv.18.6.0318.

Dunaif, A., & Finegood, D. T. (1996). Beta-cell dysfunction independent of obesity and glucose intolerance in the polycystic ovary syndrome. *J Clin Endocrinol Metab*, *81*(3), 942-947. https://doi.org/10.1210/jcem.81.3.8772555.

Dunaif, A., Given, J., & Haseltine, F. (1992). Diagnostic criteria for Polycystic ovary syndrome: towards a rational apporoach. *polycystic ovary syndrome, Boston*, 377-384.

Dunaif, A., Graf, M., Mandeli, J., Laumas, V., & Dobrjansky, A. (1987). Characterization of groups of hyperandrogenic women with acanthosis nigricans, impaired glucose tolerance, and/or hyperinsulinemia. *J Clin Endocrinol Metab*, *65*(3), 499-507. https://doi.org/10.1210/jcem-65-3-499.

Dunaif, A., Segal, K. R., Futterweit, W., & Dobrjansky, A. (1989). Profound peripheral insulin resistance, independent of obesity, in polycystic ovary syndrome. *Diabetes*, *38*(9), 1165-1174. https://doi.org/10.2337/diab.38.9.1165.

Dunaif, A., Xia, J., Book, C.-B., Schenker, E., & Tang, Z. (1995). Excessive insulin receptor serine phosphorylation in cultured fibroblasts and in skeletal muscle. A potential mechanism for insulin resistance in the polycystic ovary syndrome. *The Journal of clinical investigation*, *96*(2), 801-810.

Ehrmann, D. A., Liljenquist, D. R., Kasza, K., Azziz, R., Legro, R. S., Ghazzi, M. N., & Group, P. T. S. (2006). Prevalence and predictors of the metabolic syndrome in women with polycystic ovary syndrome. *The Journal of Clinical Endocrinology & Metabolism*, *91*(1), 48-53.

El-Raey, M., Geshi, M., Somfai, T., Kaneda, M., Hirako, M., Abdel-Ghaffar, A. E., Sosa, G. A., El-Roos, M. E., & Nagai, T. (2011). Evidence of melatonin synthesis in the cumulus oocyte complexes and its role in enhancing oocyte maturation in vitro in cattle. *Mol Reprod Dev*, *78*(4), 250-262. https://doi.org/10.1002/mrd.21295

Engin, A. (2017). The pathogenesis of obesity-associated adipose tissue inflammation. *Obesity and lipotoxicity*, 221-245.

Ewida, S. F., & Al-Sharaky, D. R. (2016). Implication of Renal Aquaporin-3 in Fructose-Induced Metabolic Syndrome and Melatonin Protection. *J Clin Diagn Res*, *10*(4), Cf06-11. https://doi.org/10.7860/jcdr/2016/18362.7656.

Faes, S., & Dormond, O. (2015). PI3K and AKT: Unfaithful Partners in Cancer. *Int J Mol Sci*, *16*(9), 21138-21152. https://doi.org/10.3390/ijms160921138.

Ferrannini, E., Buzzigoli, G., Bonadonna, R., Giorico, M. A., Oleggini, M., Graziadei, L., Pedrinelli, R., Brandi, L., & Bevilacqua, S. (1987). Insulin resistance in essential hypertension. *N Engl J Med*, *317*(6), 350-357. https://doi.org/10.1056/nejm198708063170605.

Ferreira, D. S., Amaral, F. G., Mesquita, C. C., Barbosa, A. P. L., Lellis-Santos, C., Turati, A. O., Santos, L. R., Sollon, C. S., Gomes, P. R., & Faria, J. A. (2012). Maternal melatonin programs the daily pattern of energy metabolism in adult offspring. *PloS one*, *7*(6), e38795.

Friedrichsen, M., Birk, J. B., Richter, E. A., Ribel-Madsen, R., Pehmøller, C., Hansen, B. F., Beck-Nielsen, H., Hirshman, M. F., Goodyear, L. J., & Vaag, A. (2013). Akt2 influences glycogen synthase activity in human skeletal muscle through regulation of NH2-terminal (sites 2+ 2a) phosphorylation. *American Journal of Physiology-Endocrinology and Metabolism*, *304*(6), E631-E639.

Fruman, D. A. (2011). Regulatory subunits of class IA PI3K. *Phosphoinositide 3-kinase in Health and Disease: Volume 1*, 225-244.

Gao, J., Li, J., An, Y., Liu, X., Qian, Q., Wu, Y., Zhang, Y., & Wang, T. (2014). Increasing effect of Tangzhiqing formula on IRS-1-dependent PI3K/AKT signaling in muscle. *BMC complementary and alternative medicine*, *14*, 1-8.

Garcia, R. A. P., Afeche, S. C., Scialfa, J. H., do Amaral, F. G., dos Santos, S. H. J., Lima, F. B., Young, M. E., & Cipolla-Neto, J. (2008). Insulin modulates norepinephrine-mediated melatonin synthesis in cultured rat pineal gland. *Life sciences*, *82*(1-2), 108-114.

Goldstein, B. J., Bittner-Kowalczyk, A., White, M. F., & Harbeck, M. (2000). Tyrosine dephosphorylation and deactivation of insulin receptor substrate-1 by protein-tyrosine phosphatase 1B: possible facilitation by the formation of a ternary complex with the Grb2 adaptor protein. *Journal of Biological Chemistry*, *275*(6), 4283-4289.

Guertin, D. A., Stevens, D. M., Thoreen, C. C., Burds, A. A., Kalaany, N. Y., Moffat, J., Brown, M., Fitzgerald, K. J., & Sabatini, D. M. (2006). Ablation in mice of the mTORC components raptor, rictor, or mLST8 reveals that mTORC2 is required for signaling to Akt-FOXO and PKCα, but not S6K1. *Developmental cell*, *11*(6), 859-871.

Gustafson, T. A., He, W., Craparo, A., Schaub, C. D., & O'Neill, T. J. (1995). Phosphotyrosine-dependent interaction of SHC and insulin receptor substrate 1 with the NPEY motif of the insulin receptor via a novel non-SH2 domain. *Molecular and cellular biology*, *15*(5), 2500-2508.

Ha, E., Yim, S. V., Chung, J. H., Yoon, K. S., Kang, I., Cho, Y. H., & Baik, H. H. (2006). Melatonin stimulates glucose transport via insulin receptor substrate-1/phosphatidylinositol 3-kinase pathway in C2C12 murine skeletal muscle cells. *Journal of pineal research*, *41*(1), 67-72.

Hanada, M., Feng, J., & Hemmings, B. A. (2004). Structure, regulation and function of PKB/AKT—a major therapeutic target. *Biochimica et Biophysica Acta (BBA)-Proteins and Proteomics*, *1697*(1-2), 3-16.

Harris, M. I., Hadden, W. C., Knowler, W. C., & Bennett, P. H. (1987). Prevalence of diabetes and impaired glucose tolerance and plasma glucose levels in U.S. population aged 20-74 yr. *Diabetes*, *36*(4), 523-534. https://doi.org/10.2337/diab.36.4.523.

Heo, J. I., Yoon, D. W., Yu, J. H., Kim, N. H., Yoo, H. J., Seo, J. A., Kim, S. G., Choi, K. M., Baik, S. H., Choi, D. S., & Kim, N. H. (2018). Melatonin improves insulin resistance and hepatic steatosis through attenuation of alpha-2-HS-glycoprotein. *J Pineal Res*, *65*(2), e12493. https://doi.org/10.1111/jpi.12493.

Himsworth, H. P. (2013). Diabetes mellitus: its differentiation into insulin-sensitive and insulin-insensitive types. 1936. *Int J Epidemiol*, *42*(6), 1594-1598. https://doi.org/10.1093/ije/dyt203.

Hirashima, Y., Tsuruzoe, K., Kodama, S., Igata, M., Toyonaga, T., Ueki, K., Kahn, C., & Araki, E. (2003). Insulin down-regulates insulin receptor substrate-2 expression through the phosphatidylinositol 3-kinase/Akt pathway. *Journal of endocrinology*, *179*(2), 253-266.

Jiménez, C., Hernández, C., Pimentel, B., & Carrera, A. C. (2002). The p85 regulatory subunit controls sequential activation of phosphoinositide 3-kinase by Tyr kinases and Ras. *Journal of Biological Chemistry*, *277*(44), 41556-41562.

Kang, J. T., Koo, O. J., Kwon, D. K., Park, H. J., Jang, G., Kang, S. K., & Lee, B. C. (2009). Effects of melatonin on in vitro maturation of porcine oocyte and expression of melatonin receptor RNA in cumulus and granulosa cells. *J Pineal Res*, *46*(1), 22-28. https://doi.org/10.1111/j.1600-079X.2008.00602.x.

Karlsson, B., Knutsson, A., & Lindahl, B. (2001). Is there an association between shift work and having a metabolic syndrome? Results from a population based study of 27,485 people. *Occup Environ Med*, *58*(11), 747-752. https://doi.org/10.1136/oem.58.11.747.

Kellett, G. L., Brot-Laroche, E., Mace, O. J., & Leturque, A. (2008). Sugar absorption in the intestine: the role of GLUT2. *Annu. Rev. Nutr.*, *28*, 35-54.

King, G. L., Park, K., & Li, Q. (2016). Selective Insulin Resistance and the Development of Cardiovascular Diseases in Diabetes: The 2015 Edwin Bierman Award Lecture. *Diabetes*, *65*(6), 1462-1471. https://doi.org/10.2337/db16-0152.

Kosa, E., Maurel, D., & Siaud, P. (2001). Effects of pinealectomy on glucagon responsiveness to hypoglycaemia induced by insulin injections in fed rats. *Experimental Physiology*, *86*(5), 617-620.

Kulkarni, R. N. (2002). Receptors for insulin and insulin-like growth factor-1 and insulin receptor substrate-1 mediate pathways that regulate islet function. *Biochemical Society Transactions*, *30*(2), 317-322.

Kulkarni, R. N., Brüning, J. C., Winnay, J. N., Postic, C., Magnuson, M. A., & Kahn, C. R. (1999). Tissue-specific knockout of the insulin receptor in pancreatic β cells creates an insulin secretory defect similar to that in type 2 diabetes. *Cell*, *96*(3), 329-339.

Li, A., Qiu, M., Zhou, H., Wang, T., & Guo, W. (2017). PTEN, Insulin Resistance and Cancer. *Curr Pharm Des*, *23*(25), 3667-3676. https://doi.org/10.2174/1381612823666170704124611.

Li, H., Yang, Y., Mo, Z., Ding, Y., & Jiang, W. (2015). Silibinin improves palmitate-induced insulin resistance in C2C12 myotubes by attenuating IRS-1/PI3K/Akt pathway inhibition. *Brazilian Journal of Medical and Biological Research*, *48*, 440-446.

Li, W., Liang, X., Zeng, Z., Yu, K., Zhan, S., Su, Q., Yan, Y., Mansai, H., Qiao, W., & Yang, Q. (2016). Simvastatin inhibits glucose uptake activity and GLUT4 translocation through suppression of the IR/IRS-1/Akt signaling in C2C12 myotubes. *Biomedicine & Pharmacotherapy*, *83*, 194-200.

Lima, F. B., Machado, U. F., Bartol, I., Seraphim, P. M., Sumida, D. H., Moraes, S. M., Hell, N. S., Okamoto, M. M., Saad, M. J., Carvalho, C. R., & Cipolla-Neto, J. (1998). Pinealectomy causes glucose intolerance and decreases adipose cell responsiveness to insulin in rats. *Am J Physiol*, *275*(6), E934-941. https://doi.org/10.1152/ajpendo.1998.275.6.E934

Lima, F. B., Matsushita, D., Hell, N. S., Dolnikoff, M. S., & Okamoto, M. (1994). The regulation of insulin action in isolated adipocytes. Role of the periodicity of food intake, time of day and melatonin. *Brazilian Journal of Medical and Biological Research= Revista Brasileira de Pesquisas Medicas e Biologicas*, *27*(4), 995-1000.

Lima, L. D., Reis, L. D., & Lima, M. D. (2001). Influence of the pineal gland on the physiology, morphometry and morphology of pancreatic islets in rats. *Revista Brasileira de Biologia*, *61*, 333-340.

Ling, H. Y., Hu, B., Hu, X. B., Zhong, J., Qin, L., Liu, G., Wen, G. B., & Liao, D. F. (2012). MiRNA-21 reverses high glucose and high insulin induced insulin resistance in 3T3-L1 adipocytes through targeting phosphatase and tensin homologue. *Experimental and clinical endocrinology & diabetes*, *120*(09), 553-559.

Mahajan, K., & Mahajan, N. P. (2012). PI3K-independent AKT activation in cancers: a treasure trove for novel therapeutics. *J Cell Physiol*, *227*(9), 3178-3184. https://doi.org/10.1002/jcp.24065

Maira, S. M., Stauffer, F., Schnell, C., & García-Echeverría, C. (2009). PI3K inhibitors for cancer treatment: where do we stand? *Biochemical Society Transactions*, *37*(1), 265-272.

Manna, P., & Jain, S. K. (2011). Hydrogen sulfide and L-cysteine increase phosphatidylinositol 3, 4, 5-trisphosphate (PIP3) and glucose utilization by inhibiting phosphatase and tensin homolog (PTEN) protein and activating phosphoinositide 3-kinase (PI3K)/serine/threonine protein kinase (AKT)/protein kinase Cζ/λ (PKCζ/λ) in 3T311 adipocytes. *Journal of Biological Chemistry*, *286*(46), 39848-39859.

Manna, P., & Jain, S. K. (2013). PIP3 but not PIP2 increases GLUT4 surface expression and glucose metabolism mediated by AKT/PKCζ/λ phosphorylation in 3T3L1 adipocytes. *Molecular and cellular biochemistry*, *381*, 291-299.

Mathur, R., & Alexander, C. (2008). Yano J, tRivax B, azziz R. Use of metformin in polycystic ovary syndrome. *Am J Obstet Gynecol*, *199*, 596-609.

Matthews, D. R., Hosker, J. P., Rudenski, A. S., Naylor, B., Treacher, D. F., & Turner, R. C. (1985). Homeostasis model assessment: insulin resistance and β-cell function from fasting plasma glucose and insulin concentrations in man. *Diabetologia*, *28*, 412-419.

Matthews, D. R., Hosker, J. P., Rudenski, A. S., Naylor, B. A., Treacher, D. F., & Turner, R. C. (1985). Homeostasis model assessment: insulin resistance and beta-cell function from fasting plasma glucose and insulin concentrations in man. *Diabetologia*, *28*(7), 412-419. https://doi.org/10.1007/bf00280883.

Mauvais-Jarvis, F., Ueki, K., Fruman, D. A., Hirshman, M. F., Sakamoto, K., Goodyear, L. J., Iannacone, M., Accili, D., Cantley, L. C., & Kahn, C. R. (2002). Reduced expression of the murine p85α subunit of phosphoinositide 3-kinase improves insulin signaling and ameliorates diabetes. *The Journal of clinical investigation*, *109*(1), 141-149.

Mendes, C., Lopes, A. M., do Amaral, F. G., Peliciari-Garcia, R. A., Turati Ade, O., Hirabara, S. M., Scialfa Falcão, J. H., & Cipolla-Neto, J. (2013). Adaptations of the aging animal to exercise: role of daily supplementation with melatonin. *J Pineal Res*, *55*(3), 229-239. https://doi.org/10.1111/jpi.12065.

Milcu, I., Nanu, L., Marcean, R., & Ionescu, V. (1965). [THE EFFECT OF EPIPHYSECTOMY ON THE METABOLISM OF CARBOHYDRATES. STUDIES WITH RATS]. *Stud Cercet Endocrinol*, *16*, 17-23. (Efectul epifizectomiei asupra metabolismului glucidic. Studii pe sobolan.)

Milcu, I., Nanu, L., Marcean, R., & Sitaru, S. (1963). [THE ACTION OF PINEAL EXTRACT AND EPIPHYSECTOMY ON HEPATIC AND MUSCULAR GLYCOGEN AFTER PROLONGED INFUSION OF GLUCOSE]. *Stud Cercet Endocrinol*, *14*, 651-655. (Ac tiunea extractului epifizar si a epifizectomiei asupra glicogenului hepatic si muscular dup a influzia prelungit a de glucoz a.).

Moghetti, P., Castello, R., Negri, C., Tosi, F., Spiazzi, G. G., Brun, E., Balducci, R., Toscano, V., & Muggeo, M. (1996). Insulin infusion amplifies 17 alpha-hydroxycorticosteroid intermediates response to adrenocorticotropin in hyperandrogenic women: apparent relative impairment of 17, 20-lyase activity. *The Journal of Clinical Endocrinology & Metabolism*, *81*(3), 881-886.

Morales, A. J., Laughlin, G. A., Bützow, T., Maheshwari, H., Baumann, G., & Yen, S. S. (1996). Insulin, somatotropic, and luteinizing hormone axes in lean and obese women with polycystic ovary syndrome: common and distinct features. *J Clin Endocrinol Metab*, *81*(8), 2854-2864. https://doi.org/10.1210/jcem.81.8.8768842.

Nandipati, K. C., Subramanian, S., & Agrawal, D. K. (2017). Protein kinases: mechanisms and downstream targets in inflammation-mediated obesity and insulin resistance. *Molecular and cellular biochemistry*, *426*, 27-45.

Nelson, V. L., Jiang, Y. P., Dickman, K. G., Ballou, L. M., & Lin, R. Z. (2014). Adipose tissue insulin resistance due to loss of PI3K p110α leads to decreased energy expenditure and obesity. *American Journal of Physiology-Endocrinology and Metabolism*, *306*(10), E1205-E1216.

Nelson, V. L., Legro, R. S., Strauss, J. F., 3rd, & McAllister, J. M. (1999). Augmented androgen production is a stable steroidogenic phenotype of propagated theca cells from polycystic ovaries. *Mol Endocrinol*, *13*(6), 946-957. https://doi.org/10.1210/mend.13.6.0311.

Nestler, J. E., Jakubowicz, D. J., Falcon de Vargas, A., Brik, C., Quintero, N., & Medina, F. (1998). Insulin stimulates testosterone biosynthesis by human thecal cells from women with polycystic ovary syndrome by activating its own receptor and using inositolglycan mediators as the signal transduction system. *The Journal of Clinical Endocrinology & Metabolism*, *83*(6), 2001-2005.

Newsholme, E., & Dimitriadis, G. (2001). Integration of biochemical and physiologic effects of insulin on glucose metabolism. *Experimental and Clinical Endocrinology & Diabetes*, *109*(Suppl 2), S122-S134.

Nishida, S., Sato, R., Murai, I., & Nakagawa, S. (2003). Effect of pinealectomy on plasma levels of insulin and leptin and on hepatic lipids in type 2 diabetic rats. *J Pineal Res*, *35*(4), 251-256. https://doi.org/10.1034/j.1600-079x.2003.00083.x.

Nogueira, T. C., Lellis-Santos, C., Jesus, D. S., Taneda, M., Rodrigues, S. C., Amaral, F. G., Lopes, A. M., Cipolla-Neto, J., Bordin, S., & Anhê, G. F. (2011). Absence of melatonin induces night-time hepatic insulin resistance and increased gluconeogenesis due to stimulation of nocturnal unfolded protein response. *Endocrinology*, *152*(4), 1253-1263. https://doi.org/10.1210/en.2010-1088.

Olson, A. L., & Pessin, J. E. (1996). Structure, function, and regulation of the mammalian facilitative glucose transporter gene family. *Annual review of nutrition*, *16*(1), 235-256.

Orchard, T. J., Becker, D. J., Bates, M., Kuller, L. H., & Drash, A. L. (1983). Plasma insulin and lipoprotein concentrations: an atherogenic association? *Am J Epidemiol*, *118*(3), 326-337. https://doi.org/10.1093/oxfordjournals.aje.a113639.

Pai, S. A., & Majumdar, A. S. (2014). Protective effects of melatonin against metabolic and reproductive disturbances in polycystic ovary syndrome in rats. *J Pharm Pharmacol*, *66*(12), 1710-1721. https://doi.org/10.1111/jphp.12297

Peliciari-Garcia, R. A., Marçal, A. C., Silva, J. A., Carmo-Buonfiglio, D., Amaral, F. G., Afeche, S. C., Cipolla-Neto, J., & Carvalho, C. R. (2010). Insulin temporal sensitivity and its signaling pathway in the rat pineal gland. *Life sciences*, *87*(5-6), 169-174.

Perlman, R., Bottaro, D., White, M., & Kahn, C. (1989). Conformational changes in the α-and β-subunits of the insulin receptor identified by anti-peptide antibodies. *Journal of Biological Chemistry*, *264*(15), 8946-8950.

Picinato, M. C., Haber, E. P., Carpinelli, A. R., & Cipolla-Neto, J. (2002). Daily rhythm of glucose-induced insulin secretion by isolated islets from intact and pinealectomized rat. *Journal of Pineal Research*, *33*(3), 172-177.

Prokopenko, I., Langenberg, C., Florez, J. C., Saxena, R., Soranzo, N., Thorleifsson, G., Loos, R. J., Manning, A. K., Jackson, A. U., & Aulchenko, Y. (2009). Variants in MTNR1B influence fasting glucose levels. *Nature genetics*, *41*(1), 77-81.

Rahman, M. M., Kwon, H. S., Kim, M. J., Go, H. K., Oak, M. H., & Kim, D. H. (2017). Melatonin supplementation plus exercise behavior ameliorate insulin resistance, hypertension and fatigue in a rat model of type 2 diabetes mellitus. *Biomed Pharmacother*, *92*, 606-614. https://doi.org/10.1016/j.biopha.2017.05.035.

Rasmussen, D. D., Boldt, B. M., Wilkinson, C. W., Yellon, S. M., & Matsumoto, A. M. (1999). Daily melatonin administration at middle age suppresses male rat visceral fat, plasma leptin, and plasma insulin to youthful levels. *Endocrinology*, *140*(2), 1009-1012. https://doi.org/10.1210/endo.140.2.6674.

Reaven, G. M. (1988). Banting lecture 1988. Role of insulin resistance in human disease. *Diabetes*, *37*(12), 1595-1607. https://doi.org/10.2337/diab.37.12.1595.

Rebar, R., Judd, H. L., Yen, S. S., Rakoff, J., Vandenberg, G., & Naftolin, F. (1976). Characterization of the inappropriate gonadotropin secretion in polycystic ovary syndrome. *J Clin Invest*, *57*(5), 1320-1329. https://doi.org/10.1172/jci108400.

Risso, G., Blaustein, M., Pozzi, B., Mammi, P., & Srebrow, A. (2015). Akt/PKB: one kinase, many modifications. *Biochem J*, *468*(2), 203-214. https://doi.org/10.1042/bj20150041.

Sano, H., Eguez, L., Teruel, M. N., Fukuda, M., Chuang, T. D., Chavez, J. A., Lienhard, G. E., & McGraw, T. E. (2007). Rab10, a target of the AS160 Rab GAP, is required for insulin-stimulated translocation of GLUT4 to the adipocyte plasma membrane. *Cell metabolism*, *5*(4), 293-303.

Santoleri, D., & Titchenell, P. M. (2019). Resolving the Paradox of Hepatic Insulin Resistance. *Cell Mol Gastroenterol Hepatol*, *7*(2), 447-456. https://doi.org/10.1016/j.jcmgh.2018.10.016.

Schneyer, A. L., Fujiwara, T., Fox, J., Welt, C. K., Adams, J., Messerlian, G. M., & Taylor, A. E. (2000). Dynamic changes in the intrafollicular inhibin/activin/follistatin axis during human follicular development: relationship to circulating hormone concentrations. *J Clin Endocrinol Metab*, *85*(9), 3319-3330. https://doi.org/10.1210/jcem.85.9.6767.

Seeger, T., Fischer, A., Muhly-Reinholz, M., Zeiher, A. M., & Dimmeler, S. (2014). Long-term inhibition of miR-21 leads to reduction of obesity in db/db mice. *Obesity*, *22*(11), 2352-2360.

Seraphim, P., Bartol, I., Cipolla Neto, J., & Machado, U. F. (1997). Quantification of GLUT 4 transporter in insulin-sensitive tissues from pinealectomized rats. *Pineal update from molecular mechanisms to clinical implications*.

Shabani, A., Foroozanfard, F., Kavossian, E., Aghadavod, E., Ostadmohammadi, V., Reiter, R. J., Eftekhar, T., & Asemi, Z. (2019). Effects of melatonin administration on mental health parameters, metabolic and genetic profiles in women with polycystic ovary syndrome: A randomized, double-blind, placebo-controlled trial. *J Affect Disord*, *250*, 51-56. https://doi.org/10.1016/j.jad.2019.02.066.

Steiner, D. F., Cunningham, D., Spigelman, L., & Aten, B. (1967). Insulin biosynthesis: evidence for a precursor. *Science*, *157*(3789), 697-700.

Taniguchi, C. M., Emanuelli, B., & Kahn, C. R. (2006). Critical nodes in signalling pathways: insights into insulin action. *Nature reviews Molecular cell biology*, *7*(2), 85-96.

Taniguchi, C. M., Emanuelli, B., & Kahn, C. R. (2006). Critical nodes in signalling pathways: insights into insulin action. *Nat Rev Mol Cell Biol*, *7*(2), 85-96. https://doi.org/10.1038/nrm1837.

Thirone, A. C., Huang, C., & Klip, A. (2006). Tissue-specific roles of IRS proteins in insulin signaling and glucose transport. *Trends in Endocrinology & Metabolism*, *17*(2), 72-78.

Titchenell, P. M., Lazar, M. A., & Birnbaum, M. J. (2017). Unraveling the Regulation of Hepatic Metabolism by Insulin. *Trends Endocrinol Metab*, *28*(7), 497-505. https://doi.org/10.1016/j.tem.2017.03.003.

Ui, M., Okada, T., Hazeki, K., & Hazeki, O. (1995). Wortmannin as a unique probe for an intracellular signalling protein, phosphoinositide 3-kinase. *Trends in biochemical sciences*, *20*(8), 303-307.

Ullrich, A., & Schlessinger, J. (1990). Signal transduction by receptors with tyrosine kinase activity. *Cell*, *61*(2), 203-212.

Wang, X., Wang, L., Zhu, L., Pan, Y., Xiao, F., Liu, W., Wang, Z., Guo, F., Liu, Y., & Thomas, W. G. (2013). PAQR3 modulates insulin signaling by shunting phosphoinositide 3-kinase p110α to the Golgi apparatus. *Diabetes*, *62*(2), 444-456.

Wani, R., Qian, J., Yin, L., Bechtold, E., King, S. B., Poole, L. B., Paek, E., Tsang, A. W., & Furdui, C. M. (2011). Isoform-specific regulation of Akt by PDGF-induced reactive oxygen species. *Proc Natl Acad Sci U S A*, *108*(26), 10550-10555. https://doi.org/10.1073/pnas.1011665108.

Wild, R. A., Grubb, B., Hartz, A., Van Nort, J. J., Bachman, W., & Bartholomew, M. (1990). Clinical signs of androgen excess as risk factors for coronary artery disease. *Fertil Steril*, *54*(2), 255-259. https://doi.org/10.1016/s0015-0282(16)53699-1.

Wu, W., Gan, W., Tong, M., Li, X., Dai, J., Zhang, C., & Guo, X. (2011). Over-expression of NYGGF4 (PID1) inhibits glucose transport in skeletal myotubes by blocking the IRS1/PI3K/AKT insulin pathway. *Molecular genetics and metabolism*, *102*(3), 374-377.

Xu, G., Ji, C., Song, G., Zhao, C., Shi, C., Song, L., Chen, L., Yang, L., Huang, F., & Pang, L. (2015). MiR-26b modulates insulin sensitivity in adipocytes by interrupting the PTEN/PI3K/AKT pathway. *International journal of obesity*, *39*(10), 1523-1530.

Yang, Z., Wu, F., He, Y., Zhang, Q., Zhang, Y., Zhou, G., Yang, H., & Zhou, P. (2018). A novel PTP1B inhibitor extracted from Ganoderma lucidum ameliorates insulin resistance by regulating IRS1-GLUT4 cascades in the insulin signaling pathway. *Food & function*, *9*(1), 397-406.

Yu, J., Zhang, Y., McIlroy, J., Rordorf-Nikolic, T., Orr, G. A., & Backer, J. M. (1998). Regulation of the p85/p110 phosphatidylinositol 3′-kinase: stabilization and inhibition of the p110α catalytic subunit by the p85 regulatory subunit. *Molecular and cellular biology*, *18*(3), 1379-1387.

Zalatan, F., Krause, J. A., & Blask, D. E. (2001). Inhibition of isoproterenol-induced lipolysis in rat inguinal adipocytes in vitro by physiological melatonin via a receptor-mediated mechanism. *Endocrinology*, *142*(9), 3783-3790.

Zanquetta, M. M., Seraphim, P. M., Sumida, D. H., Cipolla-Neto, J., & Machado, U. F. (2003). Calorie restriction reduces pinealectomy-induced insulin resistance by improving GLUT4 gene expression and its translocation to the plasma membrane. *J Pineal Res*, *35*(3), 141-148. https://doi.org/10.1034/j.1600-079x.2003.00067.x.

## Chapter 8

# PCOS and Osteoporosis: The Correlation Between Hormonal Alterations and Vitamin D Levels

**Shalini Sharma[1,*]**
**and Subhrojyoti Ghosh[2]**
[1]Department of Biosciences, Faculty of Natural Sciences, Jamia Millia Islamia, New Delhi, India
[2]Department of Biotechnology, Indian Institute of Technology, Madras, India

## Abstract

PCOS is the most prevalent condition of the endocrine system of the female which affects around 4 -18% of women of child bearing age. Vitamin D deficiency (VDD) is frequent in females who are in their reproductive ages, not necessarily having polycystic ovarian syndrome (PCOS). Problems with metabolic and endocrine function are connected to PCOS. Women with PCOS may be more susceptible to vitamin D insufficiency which is commonly abbreviated as VDD. According to research, PCOS increases a woman's risk of developing osteoporosis, a chronic condition with serious health effects and well-being. Patients with PCOS may have an improvement in their menstrual cycle and folliculogenesis if they take vitamin D supplements, which may reduce the levels of androgen in blood, anti-Müllerian hormone (AMH), and endometrial thickness. Furthermore, concentrations of Vitamin D have a negative relationship with measurements of body fat mass and IR. Supplementing with Vitamin D has been demonstrated to enhance IR and lipid metabolism. Furthermore, according to theory, the mental health of PCOS patients may benefit by taking vitamin D. Comprehension of the connection between vitamin D level and PCOS symptoms is critical for treating and preventing the advancement of PCOS and osteoporosis, which can have major consequences for a healthy living and improving the quality of life.

**Keywords:** polycystic ovarian syndrome, insulin resistance, Vitamin D, 25-hydroxyvitamin D, androgen, infertility

---

* Corresponding Author's Email: shalini2002371@st.jmi.ac.in.

In: Polycystic Ovarian Syndrome (PCOS) and Our Biological Clock
Editors: Arpita Roy, Gowhar Rashid and Nihad Ashraf Khan
ISBN: 979-8-89113-100-2
© 2023 Nova Science Publishers, Inc.

## 1. Introduction

The most prevalent endocrine and metabolic issue in premenopausal women is polycystic ovarian syndrome (PCOS), which affects more than 20% of women of reproductive age group. Stein et al., 1935 suggested that by combining hirsutism (the growth of male-like terminal hair in females), enlarged cystic ovaries, amenorrhea, chronic anovulation, insulin resistance (IR), infertility, and obesity. It is known that PCOS is a complex multigene syndrome that is impacted by factors like epigenetics and lifestyle, still, the cause of PCOS is unclear (Escobar-Morreale 2018). *In vivo* studies done in human and animal models demonstrated the significance of Vitamin D3 in the secretion of insulin and its sensitivity. Low levels of vitamin D have been linked to decreased insulin secretion and glucose clearance. The amount of 25-hydroxyvitamin D (25[OH]D3) in the blood is considered a useful indicator of the body's vitamin D status (Zeitz et al. 2003).

IR is viewed as a usual symptom of PCOS and recent research indicates the function of vitamin D in the occurrence of IR as well as glucose metabolism (Selimoglu et al. 2010). It is possible that vitamin D contributes to the pathogenesis of diabetes mellitus (Type-2) because of the existence of vitamin D-binding proteins (DBP) and vitamin D receptors (VDR) in pancreatic islets as well as the connecting link between particular allelic variants in the DBP and VDR genes; and insulin secretion and glucose tolerance(Thys-Jacobs et al. 1999). Several research has been shown that IGF-1 (Insulin-like growth factor) and vitamin D interact, and the most recent study showed that vitamin D affected steroidogenesis and IGFBP-1 (IGF-binding proteins) synthesis in cultured ovarian cells of humans (Parikh et al. 2010; Ameri et al. 2013). However, follicular maturation and menstrual cycle regulation differed in PCOS patients taking supplements of calcium and vitamin D whether they contain metformin or not (Tehrani, Mostajeran, and Shahsavari 2014), and no prior studies examined how these supplements influenced the IGF-1 system in the general population (Mostajeran, and Shahsavari 2014). It is yet unclear how many endocrine alterations in PCOS women would affect their bone health (Tehrani, Mostajeran, and Shahsavari 2014). PCOS women have hormonal imbalances in many areas, including gonadotrophin-releasing hormone (GnRH), insulin, and the ratio of luteinizing/follicle-stimulating hormone (LH/FSH), cortisol, androgens, parathyroid hormone (PTH), estrogens, growth hormones (GH), and calcitonin. All of these hormones have an indirect and direct impact on how bones are metabolized in humans. As a result of this hormonal imbalance, PCOS women have a higher risk of osteoporosis. There is little proof that medications used to treat PCOS patients' endocrine disorders actually raise the risk of bone fractures.

## 2. Vitamin D

Glisson provided the earliest clinical report of the vitamin D-related illness known as rickets in 1651. Given that rickets were extremely prevalent in England at the time. Early in the 20th century, a link was discovered between rickets and avoiding sunshine, and solar therapy for rickets was first documented around 1920 (Holick 1994). Vitamin D exists in two different forms: 1) Vitamin D2 (also known as ergocalciferol), obtained by irradiating plants, plant-derived products, or food, and 2) Vitamin D3 (also known as cholecalciferol), formed beneath the skin when exposed to sunlight or UV light.

The side chain may show variances. In the summer, vitamin D3 is either created in the skin or consumed through food, notably fatty fish like herring and mackerel, mushrooms that have been exposed to sunshine, and egg yolk. Age, skin tone, sunscreen use, and the number of layers and colors of clothing worn are all restrictions. In liver, vitamin D3 is converted to 25-hydroxyvitamin D3 (25(OH)D3) whereas 1,25-dihydroxyvitamin D3 (1,25$(OH)_2$D) in the kidney through the process of hydroxylation. It is the substance that increases calcium absorption in the intestine. The kidney produces 24,25-dihydroxyvitamin D (24,25(OH)2D), which is then catabolized, when 1,25(OH)2D is in excess (Figure 1). Vitamin D metabolites bind to receptor protein of Vitamin D in the blood, which shows more affinity for 25(OH)D, 24,25(OH)2D, and 1,25(OH)2D and shows similarity with albumin. As vitamin D enters a cell, its active metabolite, 1,25(OH)2D, attaches to the receptor of Vitamin D. This complex depends on vitamin D sensitive element on a gene, like osteocalcin, a calcium-binding protein, or 24-hydroxylase to form a heterodimer with a retinoid receptor. It is true that transcription and translation take place, leading to the synthesis of proteins like osteocalcin, a protein that binds calcium. Intestinal cells, where 1,25(OH)2D has its impact on the active transport of calcium. The membrane protein allows the calcium to enter the cell and the calcium-binding protein regulates the active transport throughout the cell when 1,25(OH)2D interacts with vitamin D.

ATP is essential for the process of calcium transport to the extracellular fluid. Paracellular diffusion is another passive method of calcium transport. Calcium absorption dependent on vitamin D is at its peak. There is no maximum amount of calcium that can be absorbed through passive diffusion without the presence of vitamin D; instead, the calcium intake, or calcium gradient, controls this. The 1,25(OH)2D works by boosting the transport of calcium from the tissues to the blood in the traditional target organs of bone, gut, and kidney. 1,25(OH) 2D production is boosted by PTH. There is direct negative feedback from 1,25(OH)2D to PTH as well as calcium to PTH. It is widely believed that the amount of 25[OH]D in serum serves as a functional marker of vitamin D status (Couchman and Moniz 2017). The optimal 25(OH)D serum level for human well-being is presently unknown. An inadequate amount of vitamin D is indicated by a blood 25(OH)D level lower than the 50 nmol/L (20 ng/mL), whereas vitamin D sufficiency is indicated by a serum 25(OH)D level between 50 and 74 nmol/L (20-30 ng/mL) (Thys-Jacobs et al. 1999). Clinical symptoms are not related to 25(OH)D concentrations of serum ranging from 30 and 50 nmol/L (12–20 ng/mL), which are linked to metabolic issues such as high PTH levels. A blood 25(OH)D level of 50 to 80 nmol/L (20-32 ng/mL) is necessary for ideal bone health, as suggested by vitamin-D experts. According to a recent study, exceeding the current vitamin D amount may be linked with better health results. For mineral density, lower extremity function, oral health, fractures, and incident hypertension, the blood levels of 25-OH-D3 should be at least 75 nmol/L (30 ng/mL), and 90 to 120 nmol/L (36-48 ng/mL) for cancer prevention, as demonstrated by researchers (Bischoff-Ferrari 2014). A lack of vitamin D encourages increased PTH release, which has the effect of speeding up bone resorption and turnover. This results in bone loss, primarily from cortical bone, and may cause osteoporosis. Hence, a severe vitamin D deficit results in problems with mineralization and osteomalacia, whereas high PTH levels encourage rapid bone turnover, resorption of bone, and the development of osteoporosis, all of which can result in fractures, particularly hip fractures. Consequently, serum 25(OH)D and PTH show inverse relations with respect to each other. Longitudinal Aging Study Amsterdam conducted on 1320 men and women of old-age. The bulk of the trabecular and cortical bone surfaces have thick osteoid seams in osteomalacia. It differs from osteoporosis, in which only minute levels of osteoid are present. As 25(OH)D serum levels rise, serum PTH level decreases, and as levels of 25(OH)D climb, serum PTH stabilizes (Paul Lips 2001). This peak was reached at approximately 75 nmol/l, which was far higher than expected.

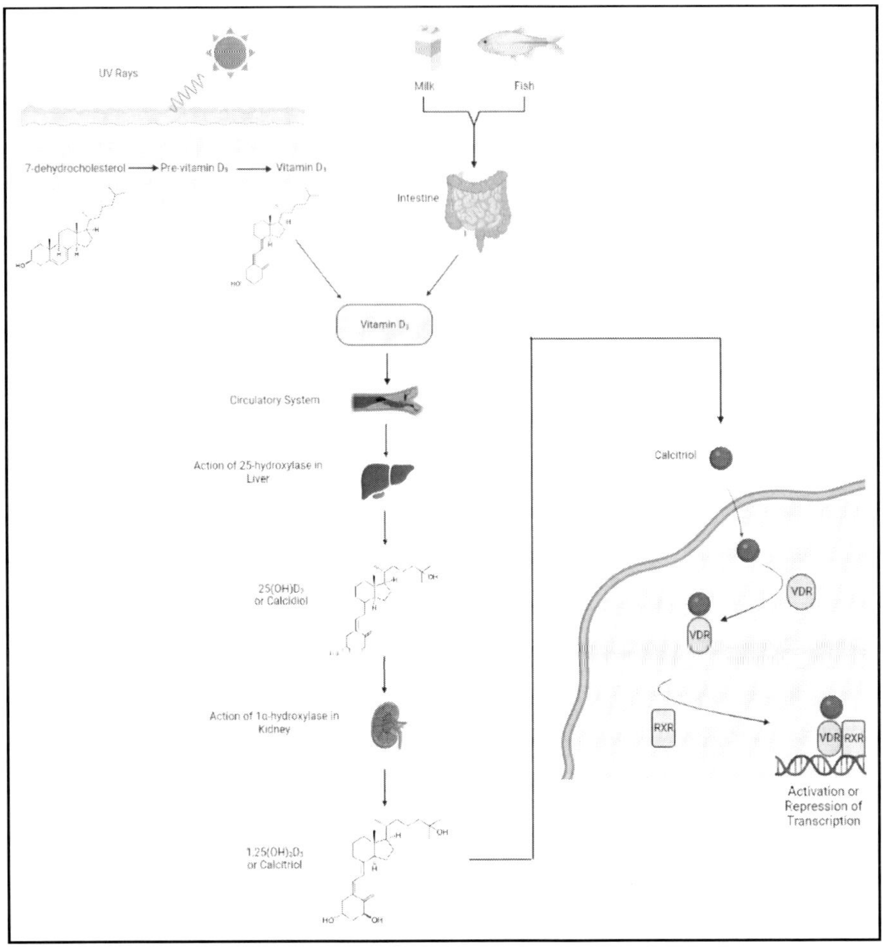


**Figure 1**. Biosynthesis and Function of Vit D3. The skin produces VD3 (cholecalciferol) from 7-dehydrocholesterol which is converted by 25-hydroxylases to 25-hydroxyvitamin D3 (25(OH)D3) or calcidiol in the liver. The ultimate bioactivation of calcidiol occurs in the kidney where it is either transformed to calcitriol by 1-hydroxylase or 1,25-dihydroxy vitamin D3 (1,25(OH)2D3). Once in the bloodstream, calcitriol acts biologically on its intended target tissues.

France and the US have both found findings that are similar. The population of old-age people who are deficient in vitamin D, decreased serum PTH levels, and increased bone mineral density, when treated with vitamin D showed increased levels of 25(OH)D (P. Lips 2006).

In light of a wealth of evidence, vitamin D is no longer thought to be the primary regulator of bone metabolism and maintainer of calcium homeostasis. Instead, it is now believed to affect cell proliferation, differentiation, apoptosis, immunological modulation, genome integrity, and neurogenesis (Hanmin Wang et al. 2017). The female reproductive system contains numerous organs, including the ovary (especially granulosa cells), uterus, and placenta. This implies that vitamin D may be involved in female reproductive disorders (Irani and Merhi 2014). According to an animal study, female VDR null mice had poor folliculogenesis and uterine hypoplasia, rendering them infertile (Yoshizawa et al. 1997). Moreover, 300 genes, including those involved in lipid and glucose metabolism, are under the control of vitamin D. A deficiency in vitamin D may be the connection between IR and PCOS that has been missing (Krul-Poel et al. 2013).

## 3. PCOS Pathophysiology

PCOS has been linked to Cushing's disease, adrenal hyperplasia, hypothyroidism, ovarian and adrenal cancers, as well as several genetic disorders (Insler and Lunenfeld 1991). The pathophysiological mechanism behind the disease is currently being researched. A comprehensive explanation of PCOS etiology was developed through meticulous analysis of historical data, appraisal of new studies about the potential role of insulin, growth hormones, and their binding proteins, and extrapolation of neuro endocrinological research. This point of view claims that PCOS is a complex disorder. The LH/FSH ratio is increased in the majority of PCOS patients due to unusually high LH release and normal or low FSH production (De Leo et al. 2016). The fact that the etiology of the condition is complex and no single fault is known to be its cause, IR is thought to be a crucial contributor.

### 3.1. Excess of Ovarian, Adrenal, Androgens

PCOS is marked by a rise in ovarian or adrenal androgen production. Elevated levels of adrenal androgens, notably dehydroepiandrosterone sulfate, were seen in more than half of those with PCOS (DHS). Yet, it is still unknown what causes the excess of adrenal androgen.

### 3.2. Insulin Resistance (IR)

IR is the primary contributor to PCOS. Women with PCOS frequently have both IR and hyperinsulinemia. A post-binding decrease in the insulin receptor-mediated signal transduction in skeletal muscle has been used to show PCOS insulin resistance in adipocytes (Kousta, Tolis, and Franks 2005). This is related to a rise in testosterone, which makes peripheral tissues more resistant to insulin. Both independently and by worsening IR in PCOS, obesity aggravates the problems related to hyperandrogenism, hirsutism, infertility, and irregular menstrual cycle. Hyperinsulinemia is associated with obesity, which impacts 30–60% of PCOS patients with a BMI of greater than 30 kg/m$^2$. With PCOS, even thin women develop IR, which gets worse as BMI increases (Figure 2).

### 3.3. Neuroendocrine Factors

According to reports, the most common reason for infertility affects 5 to 20% of women of childbearing age. Women with PCOS had higher levels of LH as well as higher ratios of LH to FSH. The most likely cause of increased LH pulse amplitude and frequency in PCOS is high pulsatile GnRH production. Progesterone receptor-related AR is not present in GnRH neurons, only estrogen receptor-related AR (androgen receptor). The hypothalamic neuronal network, which is upstream of the GnRH neuron, receives indirect negative input from steroids (Ibáñez et al. 2017; George et al. 2016).

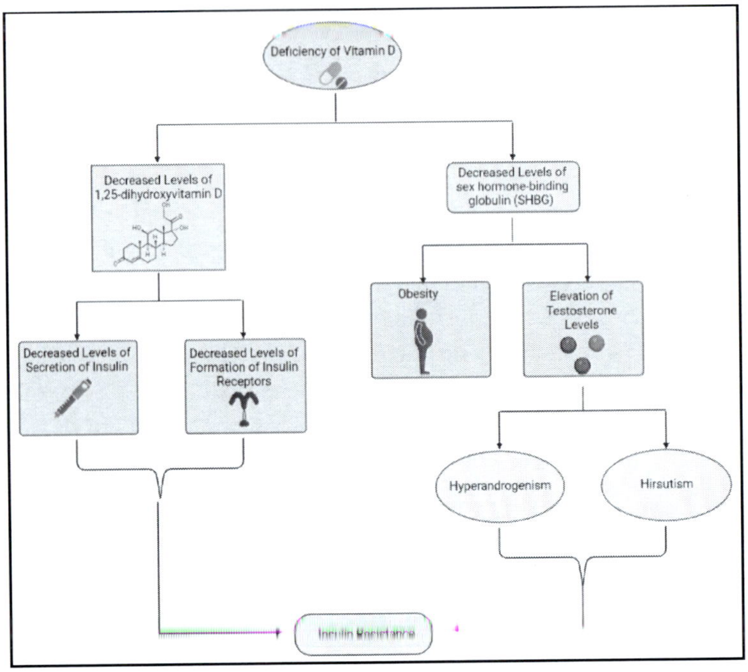


**Figure 2.** The role of vitamin D in the emergence of PCOS. Vitamin D appears to be able to affect glucose-insulin homeostasis by interacting with its own unique receptors (VDR) in skeletal muscle and pancreatic beta cells. These receptors *in vitro* directly activate insulin-mediated glucose transport, the human insulin receptor gene, peroxisome proliferator activator receptor, and insulin receptor expression.

### 3.4. Gonadotropin Release and Hyperandrogenism

To reduce the frequency of GnRH pulse release, which results in insufficient FSH synthesis and persistent LH activation of ovarian androgens, women with PCOS need more progesterone. The onset of PCOS during puberty may be explained by the GnRH pulse generator's reduced sensitivity. 60 to 80% of PCOS sufferers exhibited elevated testosterone levels (Blank, McCartney, and Marshall 2006; Shetty et al. 2017).

### 3.5. Ovulatory Dysfunction

In PCOS, follicular disruption in the ovaries encourages granulose cells to produce AMH (Anti-Mullerian Hormone). By decreasing progesterone release and boosting estrogen release, endometrial hyperplasia brought on by anovulation increases the risk of developing endometrial cancer. Follicular development is hindered by low levels of FSH in the ovary, which causes amenorrhea and anovulation. LH hypersecretion is the main factor in infertility and miscarriage in women with PCOS (Kim et al. 2018).

### 3.6. PCOS Etiology

PCOS has no identified etiology yet. However, there are correlations between high insulin levels, low-grade inflammation, and hereditary. Scientists are baffled as to what are the causative factors of PCOS. It has been said that high levels of male hormones hinder the ovaries' capacity to create hormones and normal eggs (Kaygusuz et al. 2013).

- *Genes:* PCOS appears to run in families, according to a study. The sickness is likely to be caused by several genes, not just one (Ibáñez et al. 2004).
- *Insulin Resistance*: It has been seen that IR impacts almost 70% of women with PCOS condition, which means their cells are unable to use insulin adequately. So, the body's requirement for insulin increases. To compensate for the extra insulin, the pancreas generates more insulin, causing the ovaries to release more male hormones (Salvesen, Vanky, and Carlsen 2007).
- *Inflammation:* Women suffering from PCOS have been seen to have increased levels of inflammation in their bodies. Exceeding the normal weight range can also be a factor to inflammation. Furthermore, numerous studies have linked excess inflammation to increased androgen levels in the body (Salvesen, Vanky, and Carlsen 2007).

### 3.7. Aetiological Theories of PCOS

Odunsi and Kidd summarized the main ideas for the etiology of PCOS proposed in previous studies (Odunsi and Kidd 1999). As per the luteinizing hormone - theca interstitial cell (LHTIC) hypothesis, PCOS is caused by pathophysiologic mechanisms that result in high LH levels abnormally. As per the theory, an excess level of circulating LH stimulates the proliferation of TIC in growing follicles which results in the overproduction of androgen and follicular atresia.

As per the follicle-stimulating hormone-granulosa cell (FSH-GC) theory, low FSH encourages subnormal stimulation of cytochrome P450 aromatase of granulosa cells which leads to the rise in the levels of androgen. This might be caused by a lack of bioactive FSH in the follicular milieu, a broken signal transduction route for the FSH receptor, or the presence of inhibitors (such as epidermal growth factor and IGF-binding protein 3), which restrict the expression of the normal activity of P450 aromatase (Diamanti-Kandarakis and Dunaif 2012).

## 4. Role of Vitamin D and PCOS

Females with PCOS frequently have dyslipidemia and IR, both of which are metabolic diseases (PCOS). According to recent studies, IR is a key player in the pathophysiology of PCOS, which causes problems with both metabolism and reproduction

To understand the mechanism of metabolic abnormalities, particularly IR, in PCOS women, numerous studies have been conducted. Obesity could play a part in IR. However regardless of BMI, a sizable proportion of thin women with PCOS also experience IR (Dunaif et al. 1989; Ketel et al. 2011). An insufficient amount of vitamin D has recently been identified as a potential missing link between IR and PCOS. The discovery that the vitamin D-receptor (VDR) active complex controls 300 genes, including those involved in the metabolism of glucose and lipid and blood pressure regulation, supports this hypothesis (Bouillon et al. 2008). In addition, type 2 diabetics with low vitamin D levels have been related to IR (Ashraf and Alvarez 2010; Chiu et al. 2004; Ford et al. 2005; Pittas et al. 2007; Scragg, Sowers, and Bell 2004). It is still not clear whether IR and vitamin D are two distinct characteristics or whether they are physically related in women with PCOS. Thomson et al. found a relationship between the level of vitamin D, PCOS hormonal level, and metabolic dysfunctions. Furthermore, Poor evidence on the connection between PCOS-affected women's metabolic and hormonal disorders, and vitamin D status, and these concerns have led the scientific community to draw conflicting conclusions. (Thomson, Spedding, and Buckley 2012).

### 4.1. The Role of Vitamin D in Insulin Resistance

In both *in vivo* animal models and in humans, vitamin D3 has been found to affect the secretion and sensitivity of insulin. Reduced glucose clearance and insulin secretion have been linked to insufficient vitamin D levels (Zeitz et al. 2003). The mechanism, which has not yet been fully explained, is thought to involve both direct and indirect activities of vitamin D3. The insulin response to secretagogues is affected differently by the calcium and vitamin D endocrine systems and intracellular calcium homeostasis as suggested by studies (Kotsa et al. 2009).

According to a recent study, the insulin hormone controls the activity of the renal 1-hydroxylase enzyme and serum levels in response to PTH, while 1,25(OH)2D3 acts as a genomic activator of the insulin response to govern the transport of glucose (Kochupillai 2008). There is a chance that vitamin D may contribute to the pathogenesis of diabetes mellitus due to the presence of vitamin-D receptors (VDR) and vitamin D-binding proteins (DBP) in the pancreatic islets and the correlation between particular allelic variations in the DBP and VDR genes, glucose tolerance, and insulin secretion (Type-2).

According to recent research, taking calcium and vitamin D3 supplements together may help type 2 diabetic individuals manage their glucose metabolism. Although calcium and vitamin D replacement medication has been demonstrated to help PCOS women with menstrual cycle management (Thys-Jacobs et al. 1999). The VDR nuclear receptor functions in DNA transcription as a member of the family (Pike and Meyer 2012; Kato 2000). Despite the VDR's basic function as a nuclear transcription factor, there have been speculations about non-genomic vitamin D activities, such as the fast binding of 1,25(OH)2D to cytosolic and membrane VDR, which activates a number of second messenger systems (Norman 2008). The presence of a vitamin D response element region in the insulin receptor gene's promoter raises the possibility that vitamin D regulates the transcription of the insulin gene (Maestro et al. 2003).

Retinoid X receptors (RXRs) are ligand-inducible transcription factors that belong to the superfamily of nuclear receptors that can assemble into homo- or heterodimers with other receptors, such as VDR, to control vital genes which are involved in energy balancing (Yamada and Kakuta 2014; Mangelsdorf et al. 1995; Haussler et al. 1998). A vitamin A molecule known as 9-cis retinoic acid, which functions as an RXR ligand, has been identified as a pancreas-specific autacoid capable of regulating blood glucose levels. Elevated 9-cis retinoic acid levels have been connected to obesity in animal models in several studies. In light of this, the development of IR may be influenced by the interaction between the RXR, the vitamin D receptor, and their ligands (Cione et al. 2016; Shaffer and Gewirth 2004). Also essential to the control of vitamin D are glutathione levels. Supplied vitamin D is converted into active vitamin D metabolites in the presence of glutathione. According to research on both animals and people, it has a positive impact on the bioavailability of 25(OH)D and 1,25(OH)2D (Parsanathan and Jain 2019; Jain et al. 2018). Moreover, it has been demonstrated that vitamin D raises glutathione, which lowers oxidative stress (Jain and Micinski 2013). IR, according to these studies, may be connected to glutathione depletion, which is found in many illnesses such as obesity and diabetes (Ballatori et al. 2009). Vitamin D may be crucial for the regulation and function of pancreatic cells in T2D patients because calcitriol (1,25(OH)2D-3) interacts with calcium flux-regulating receptors to act as a chemical messenger on cells (Bland et al. 2004; Upreti et al. 2018; Mirhosseini et al. 2017; Reusch et al. 1991).

Vitamin D can also reduce renin-angiotensin system hyperactivity and enhance cell function. Vitamin D, on the other hand, may affect the secretion of insulin by opening and closing calcium channels, and 1,25(OH)2D may improve sensitivity to insulin by increasing the expression of insulin receptors and by stimulating the peroxisome proliferator-activated receptor delta (PPAR-δ) (Leung 2016).

Finally, vitamin D has been shown to deactivate the inflammatory cytokines linked to IR and to boost the production of calbindin, which protects cells from apoptosis, suggesting that it may minimize the effects of chronic inflammation (Chun et al. 2014). It has been demonstrated that insulin stimulates osteoblast differentiation, enhancing the production of the peptide produced by osteoblasts called osteocalcin, which can encourage pancreatic cell growth and increase insulin sensitivity in skeletal muscle. Nonetheless, women with PCOS have greater insulin levels, which leads to IR and BMD deterioration (Klein 2014).

### 4.2. Vitamin D and Infertility

Infertility is a complicated medical, behavioral, and economic condition that affects roughly 15% of couples (Benyamini, Gozlan, and Kokia 2005). Most cases of infertile females are brought on by PCOS. PCOS is typically linked to oligo- or anovulation in female patients, correlated with obesity and IR. There is substantial data that Vitamin D regulates female reproductive processes in addition to the traditional reproductive regulators, sex steroid hormones; its nuclear receptors have been located in the uterus, ovary, oviduct, placenta, and fetal membranes (Du et al. 2005).

Insufficient vitamin D has been connected to reduced fertility and mated success in female rats. Still, the overall fertility and litter size in female rats fed a diet low in vitamin D are reduced by 75% and 10%, respectively (Halloran and Deluca 1980). Lack of VDR or 1-hydroxylase causes infertility in female mice with uterine hypoplasia, poor folliculogenesis, and anovulation. Yet, a wide range of methods may be used to account for vitamin D's role in human reproduction. One potential mechanism is the direct stimulation of aromatase gene expression in reproductive organs by 1,25(OH)2D3, which has been shown in female mice (Du et al. 2005; Yoshizawa et al. 1997; Kovacs et al. 2005). The importance of vitamin D in human reproduction, however, may be demonstrated via a variety of techniques. The direct stimulatory effect of 1,25(OH)2D3 has been illustrated as one of the possible explanations for the expression of the aromatase gene in reproductive organs, which has been demonstrated in female mice.

Nevertheless, uterine and endometrial development—which enables uterine response to implantation—requires HOXA10 gene expression (Taylor, Vanden Heuvel, and Igarashi 1997). Aberrant HOXA10 gene expression in infertile patients reveals the protein's importance for human implantation. (Cermik, Selam, and Taylor 2003). Vitamin D itself is the main hormone that supports the homeostasis of calcium. It has been also found that calcium plays a part in the activation and maturation of oocytes, which results in the advancement of follicular development (De Felici, Dolci, and Siracusa 1991). In this case, vitamin D and calcium therapy may help PCOS patients' ovulation restoration and stabilize their menstrual cycles (Kinuta et al. 2000). While using IVF, women with sufficient levels of vitamin D had a greater rate of success than those with insufficient levels of vitamin D (Ozkan et al. 2010). Patients with high (>75 nmol/l) vitamin D levels in follicular fluid had a lower pregnancy rate and poorer embryo quality. Individuals with low (50 nmol/l) and intermediate (50-75 nmol/l) 25OHD3 follicular fluid levels did not show any significant changes in pregnancy rates or the quality of the embryo (Anifandis et al. 2010).

### 4.3. Vitamin D and AMH

Female granulosa cells produce the gonadal-specific glycoprotein AMH as the follicle grows. AMH level has shown to be a fairly accurate prognostic marker in assisted reproductive technology (ART), as it is produced by growing ovarian follicles and does not dramatically change throughout the menstrual cycle. While vitamin D insufficiency and other environmental factors, such as AMH expression and serum levels, have been shown to affect ovarian reserve, despite the fact that AMH is notably a reliable diagnostic indicator of ovarian reserve. Researchers found a dose-dependent decrease in AMH mRNA levels in the granulosa cells after vitamin D therapy in a study to determine whether 1, 25(OH) 2D3 affects AMH mRNA expression. Cell proliferation and the expression of the hormone FSH increased in comparison (Dennis et al. 2012). A second study examining the impact of 1,25(OH)2D3 on ovarian follicular development observed altered AMH signaling in granulosa cells treated with the compound. It has been demonstrated that the expression of the AMH receptor-II (AMHR-II) mRNA gene is inversely correlated with the levels of 25-hydroxyvitamin D (25(OH) D) in follicular fluid. It was discovered that females with low 25(OH) D levels (25(OH) D 30 ng/mL) had twice the amount of AMHR-II mRNA expressed. According to the researchers, it also decreased the nuclear localization of phosphor-Smad 1/5/8, which in turn decreased the action of AMH. By inhibiting the expression of AMHRII, vitamin D therapy may reduce the impact of AMH on granulosa cells and advance follicle growth. Female granulosa cells produce the gonadal-specific glycoprotein AMH as the follicle grows. AMH is currently regarded as one of the most accurate diagnostic markers of ovarian reserve, despite research showing that environmental factors like vitamin D deficiency can change AMH expression and blood levels. [82–84] Researchers found a dose-dependent decrease in AMH mRNA levels in granulosa cells after vitamin D therapy in a study to determine whether 1, 25(OH) 2D3 affects the expression of AMH mRNA (Malloy et al. 2009; Dennis et al. 2012; Merhi et al. 2014).

Cell proliferation and the expression of the hormone FSH increased in comparison. The AMH levels in winter may be 18% lower than the summertime ones. Vitamin D levels have remained low throughout the season (Dennis et al. 2012). Low vitamin D levels are thought to reduce ovarian reserve and cause early menopause in delicate individuals. To maintain bone health, early ovarian insufficiency sufferers should also take calcium and vitamin D supplements. The synthesis of sex hormones is controlled by several enzymes. According to a recent study, the expression, and function of some of these enzymes may be altered by vitamin D (Lundqvist 2014).

### 4.4. Vitamin D Deficiency and PCOS Phenotypes

A surprising finding is that PCOS symptoms worsen when serum VD levels are low and that there is an inverse correlation between PCOS metabolic and hormonal abnormalities and serum VD levels (He et al. 2015). The link between VD insufficiency and PCOS features has been the subject of numerous investigations. Using Rotterdam criteria, Davis et al. evaluated females with PCOS condition who fell into one of three diagnostic phenotypes:

1. Those women who have polycystic ovaries as well as ovulatory dysfunction;
2. Those women having ovulatory dysfunction as well as excess androgen levels; and
3. Women who suffer from ovulatory dysfunction, polycystic ovaries, and an excess of testosterone in their blood (Maktabi, Chamani, and Asemi 2017).

### 4.5. Hypothalamic-Pituitary-Gonadal Axis, Androgen Levels, and Vitamin D

We still have a limited grasp of how VD affects reproductive physiology despite several investigations on the influence of VD on gonadal hormone production and reproductive function. Mini-puberty, which occurs in the first few months of life when the hypothalamic-pituitary-gonadal (HPG) axis is momentarily activated and gonadal hormone production is briefly stimulated (Kuiri-Hänninen, Sankilampi, and Dunkel 2014), offers an intriguing window into the effect of VD on the HPG axis. The future gonadal function requires HPG activation. Klnç et al. discovered a link between gonadal hormones and the levels of 25-OH-D during mini-puberty. In 25-OH-D deficient females compared to sufficient females, total testosterone levels were greater and inhibin B levels were lower, but 25-OH-D had no effect on these levels. Thus, 25-OH-D seems to affect gonadal function in fetal development (Kılınç et al. 2019). One study found an association between serum VD levels, total testosterone, and the free androgen index in terms of androgen levels. This finding led us to the hypothesis that VD might increase female fertility by altering androgenic activity (Chang et al. 2014). This is understandable considering VD's capacity to control the expression and activity of a number of enzymes involved in the synthesis of sex hormones (Hahn et al. 2006; Lundqvist 2014).

**Table 1.** Clinical investigations examining how vitamin D3 ($VD_3$) supplementation affects the hormonal and metabolic parameters in women with PCOS

| S. No. | Type of Population | Size of Sample Studied | Vitamin D Dosage | Duration of Study | Results | References |
|---|---|---|---|---|---|---|
| 1. | PCOS patients from New Delhi, India | 50 | Patients received 12,000 IU VD3 weekly vs placebo | 12 weeks | The quantitative control of insulin sensitivity (QUICK1), insulin levels, and the homeostasis model assessment of insulin resistance (HOMA-IR) were all decreased by VD3 supplementation in comparison to the placebo. | Garg G, Kachhawa G, Ramot R, et al. Effect of supplementation of Vitamin D on PCOS- related insulin kinetics and cardiovascular risk factors: a pilot study. Endocr Connect 2015; 4: 108-116. |
| 2. | PCOS patients with infertility were also candidates for IVF from Kashan, Iran | 40 | Patients received 50,000 IU VD3 weekly vs. placebo | 8 weeks | Supplementing with VD3 substantially reduced blood, anti-Müllerian hormone (AMH), insulin levels, HOMA-IR, total cholesterol, and LDL levels and improved QUICKI when compared to placebo. | Dastorani M, Aghadavod E, Mirhosseini N, et al. The effects of vitamin D supplementation on insulin and lipid metabolism gene expression and metabolic profiles in infertile candidates for *in vitro* fertilization with polycystic ovarian syndrome. Reprod Biol Endocrinol 2018; 16: 94. doi: 10.1186/s12958-018-0413-3 |
| 3. | Obese PCOS patients from Bursa, Turkey | 11 | Patients received 300,000 IU VD3 vs. controls | 3 weeks | In contrast to HOMA-IR, glucose and insulin levels did not significantly drop after a single dosage of VD3 was administered. | Selimoglu H, Duran C, Kiyici S, et al. The impact of vitamin D replacement therapy on IR and testosterone levels in PCOS sufferers. J Endocrinol Invest 2010; 33: 234-238. |
| 4. | PCOS patients from Graz, Austria | 57 | Patients received 20,000 IU cholecalciferol weekly vs. controls | 24 weeks | While total cholesterol and LDL levels considerably rose, fasting glucose, C-peptide, triglyceride, and estradiol levels decreased as a result of VD3 treatment. The amount of androgen did not alter. | Wehr E, Pieber T, Obermayer-Pietsch B. Efficacy of vitamin D3 therapy on women with PCOS's glucose metabolism and menstruation frequency: a pilot study. J Endocrinol Invest 2011; 34: 757-763 |

### 4.6. Deficiency of Vitamin D and Fertility Outcomes in PCOS Women

Vitamin D is linked to monthly irregularities, changes in follicular development, dysfunctional ovulation, metabolic abnormalities, and a lower conception rate in women with PCOS. When infertile PCOS women were administered clomiphene citrate stimulation, PTH, 1,25OH-active D3's form, and testosterone levels were assessed (Ott et al. 2012). Although high PTH was connected to a high BMI and greater testosterone serum levels, high PTH was linked to low blood calcium and 1,25OH-D3 as well. Blood levels of 1,25OH-D3 were lower in women who produced a follicle following 50 mg of clomiphene citrate stimulation than in those who did not. Also, the likelihood of conception was noticeably higher among women with more BMIs and lower 1,25OH-D3 levels in their blood. Finally, 1,25OH-well-known D3's involvement in ovarian activity may be connected to the strong link between lower 1,25OH-D3 blood levels and decreased follicle development after 50 mg of clomiphene citrate stimulation. In a randomized clinical experiment with 60 infertile PCOS patients, the menstrual cycle and ovulation were evaluated in relation to the effects of calcium-VD and metformin administration (Rashidi et al. 2009). Over the period of 2-3 months of follow-up, menstrual regularity, and the number of conspicuous follicles (14 mm) were more in the calcium-vitamin D plus metformin group than in any of the other two groups (Table 1). Fang et al. explored the consequences of vitamin D supplementation on PCOS patients. Based on this study, VD supplementation increases the number of dominant follicles, which in turn drives follicular expansion. Metformin and VD together also enhance the regularity of the menstrual cycle (Fang et al. 2017).

## 5. Vitamin D and the Risk of Fractures in PCOS

The health of PCOS patients' bones and their risk of fracture have not been the subject of numerous research. The study, which was also conducted in Denmark, included women with PCOS and hirsutism, which may have increased the study's heterogeneity. With 19,199 women (aged 12 to 60) participating, the largest cohort study yet conducted in Denmark found a decreased risk of fracture (Noyan, Yucel, and Sagsoz 2004). In contrast, a population-based observational study of 11,106 women with PCOS (aged 15 to 80) in Taiwan found that they had a more incidence of fractures overall than non-PCOS women (Rubin et al. 2016; Yang et al. 2018).

The inclusion of women with PCOS and hirsutism in the Danish study (Rubin et al. 2016) may have increased the study's heterogeneity. Furthermore, Chinese women with PCOS showed higher rates of polycystic ovary morphology, milder hyperandrogenism, and lower prevalence of impaired glucose tolerance and IR compared to Caucasian women, suggesting that there may be distinctions between European and Asian PCOS patients (Yang et al. 2018). Nevertheless, neither of these two studies looked at how confounding factors like body weight or BMI, physical activity, lifestyle decisions, or the pathophysiology of bone loss later in life would affect peak bone mass. Compared to matched healthy controls, PCOS women showed significantly greater rates of osteoporotic fractures, fractures of the spine, and fractures of the forearm, but comparable rates of femur or hip, wrist, humerus, and non-osteoporotic fractures (Rubin et al. 2016). Results from BMD measurements in PCOS women were also inconclusive.

Although bone mineral density (BMD) is the primary factor influencing bone strength, fragility fractures in females with normal or slightly reduced BMD have been documented (Siris et al. 2004). While some studies (Yüksel et al. 2001; Katulski et al. 2014; Kalyan et al. 2017; Karadağ, Yoldemir, and Gogas Yavuz 2017; Attlee et al. 2014) found no change in BMD when compared to healthy controls, others found lower BMD values in PCOS women (Kirchengast and Huber 2001; Adami et al. 1998; Noyan, Yucel, and Sagsoz 2004; Good et al. 1999; D. Glintborg et al. 2013; Gao et al. 2016; McBreairty et al. 2018; Schmidt et al. 2012) (Kassanos et al. 2010; Berberoglu et al. 2015; Carmina et al. 2009; Dorte Glintborg et al. 2008), possibly due to differences in participant ages and selection methods. According to a thorough review and meta-analysis, women with PCOS and a BMI of 27 kg/m$^2$ exhibited lower spinal and femoral BMD than women without PCOS and a BMI of 27 kg/m$^2$, which supports the idea that obesity affects certain bone metrics(Reusch et al. 1991). Studies on surrogate indicators of bone turnover, notably osteocalcin and procollagen type 1 N-terminal propeptide, markers for bone production, and carboxy-terminal collagen type 1 telopeptide, a marker for bone resorption, show that women with PCOS have impaired bone metabolism (Diamanti-Kandarakis et al. 2011; Lingaiah et al. 2017; Pepene 2013; Damone et al. 2019; Lerner, Sharony, and Miodownik 2018). Overall, blood levels of bone formation indicators were lower in PCOS women, which may have an adverse effect on BMD (bone metabolic density) and raise the risk of fractures (Figure 3).

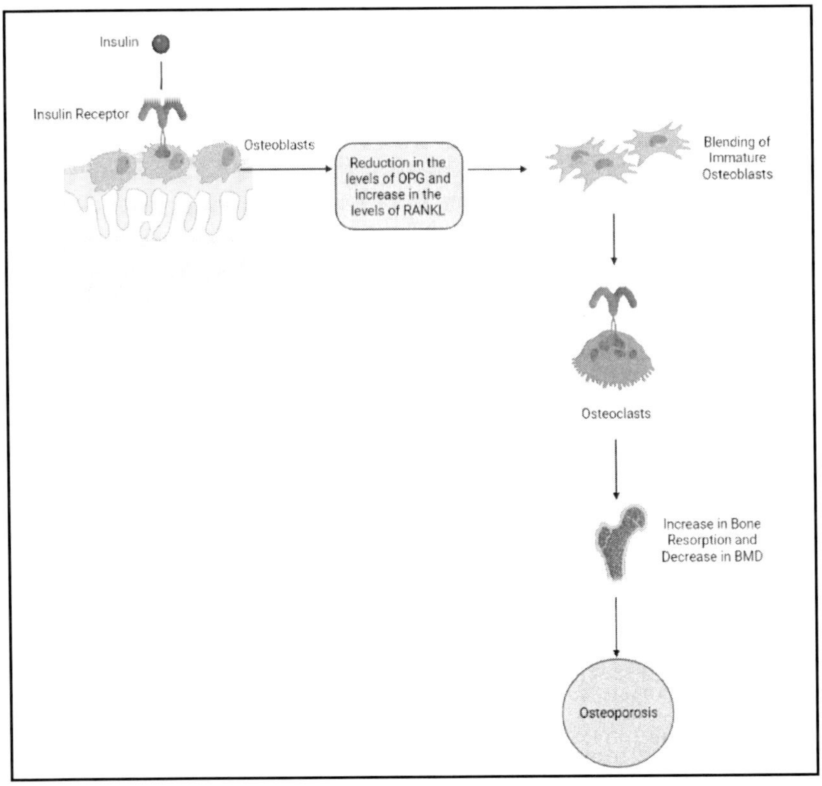


**Figure 3.** Schematic illustration illustrating the potential consequences of elevated circulating insulin levels and its resistance in PCOS-afflicted females.

## 6. Impact of Insulin Resistance on Bone in Women with PCOS Condition

Expression of osteoprotegerin (OPG) is reduced by insulin signaling, which limits the production of bone (Clemens and Karsenty 2011). Because osteoprotegerin is a receptor activator of nuclear factor kappa beta ligand which might encourage bone resorption (RANKL). Insulin influences osteoclastogenesis and increases RANKL expression in MG63 osteoblasts, according to research by Wang and colleagues (Huixin Wang and Zhong 2013). These behaviors seem to be related to PTH activity. The osteoblast protein tyrosine phosphatase (OST-PTP) is a substrate of the insulin receptor, according to a substrate-trapping assay. In osteoblasts, expression of osteoprotegerin expression is reduced by insulin signaling. A decline in OPG/RANKL can increase the expression of the Tcirg1 gene in osteoclasts, which encodes for a proton pump and adds to the acidity of the resorption lacunae. The osteocalcin molecule can be activated and decarboxylated with this acidic pH level alone. On the other hand, undercarboxylated molecules have been shown to enhance/modify insulin expression, insulin sensitivity, insulin secretion, and expenditure of energy in pancreatic cells (Clemens and Karsenty 2011). Thomas and colleagues did the in-vitro studies in mature mononucleated and multinucleated murine osteoclast-like cells and in mouse osteoclasts as well which demonstrated the expression of insulin receptor (Thomas et al. 1998).

## 7. Food and Nutrition in Relation to PCOS

The osteocalcin moiety or molecule can be activated and decarboxylated at this acidic pH level alone. Furthermore, it has been shown that undercarboxylated molecules can influence or increase pancreatic cell proliferation, expression of insulin, secretion of insulin, insulin sensitivity, and energy expenditure (Clemens and Karsenty 2011). Thomas and colleagues investigated the immunochemical proof of insulin receptor expression in mature mononucleated and multinucleated murine osteoclast-like cells cultivated *in vitro*, as well as in primary neonatal and mouse osteoclasts (Thomas et al. 1998). It is therefore likely that a diet low in fiber and rich in lipids may have a negative impact on the metabolism of sex hormones in specific subgroups of PCOS women by increasing the availability of androgen and favoring obesity development.

In women suffering from PCOS, obesity is a common trait, and research shows that obesity leads to the etiology of PCOS by exacerbating these women's inherent IR (Thomson et al. 2015).

There are numerous opinions on how to treat PCOS; many believe it can't be addressed because it is a long-term illness, while others believe that modifying one's lifestyle and hormone medication may help with PCOS (Escobar-Morreale 2018). There are many health issues of PCOS which may include non-functioning or dysfunction of certain organs, that's why it gets the treatment of this illness or reduce the stress in one's life. For instance, if a woman is fat, she may have a vitamin D deficit since obesity is directly connected to a drop in vitamin D levels, and that person is more prone to develop osteoporosis or rickettsia (Nestler 2000). As a result, the very first step in therapy is a change in lifestyle. Some lifestyle management measures are effective in PCOS:

- Prevent becoming obese or overweight (management of weight is really important)

- Change in meals by eating a low-carbohydrate diet
- Inculcation an activity or an exercise routine
- Focusing on mental health
- Reducing stress
- Reducing consumption of fast food
- Limiting the intake of processed food
- Reducing the consumption of alcoholic beverages (Escobar-Morreale 2018)

As a result of the higher risk of cancers like breast and endometrial cancer brought on by the IR prevalent in PCOS-affected women, including type 2 diabetes, hypertension, abnormal lipid levels in the body, cardiovascular disease, and other chronic diseases. Although there is no known cause for this illness, environmental factors including dietary habits are crucial for prevention and therapy, and for PCOS patients, lifestyle changes are the most effective therapeutic therapies. The approach to diet therapy in these patients must be used to achieve specific targeted objectives by following a low-calorie diet to achieve weight loss or the maintenance of a healthy weight, limiting the intake of refined foods like carbs and simple sugars, and consuming foods with a low glycemic index, reducing consumption of saturated and trans fats, and improving IR, metabolic and reproductive functions. Every food group has its own glycaemic index, and it is advantageous for females to consume foods with low glycaemic index because they release energy slowly in the body, resulting in a non-abrupt sugar spike in the blood. The glycaemic index measures how quickly each food has an impact on blood sugar (glucose) levels when that food is eaten. A 5% weight loss can help these women overcome problems including IR, high levels of androgens, dysfunctional reproductive systems, and fertility because overweight and obesity are common as is IR (Faghfoori et al. 2017).

## 7. Possible Treatment of PCOS

A well-known traditional herb from Malaysia is called *Labisia pumila*. It is used to treat PCOS because it has phytoestrogenic characteristics that can increase the production of estrogen. As a result, PCOS rats are given *Labisia pumila* aqueous solution in doses such as LP25 (25 mg/kg) to LP50 (50 mg/kg). It has been discovered that in rats with PCOS, it reduced the expression of inflammatory cytokines such as c-reactive protein and TNF-alpha, which are linked to the development of osteoporosis. In PCOS rats, it also improved insulin sensitivity without changing body weight, reduced hormonal imbalances, and osteoporosis, and boosted skin elasticity without any obvious toxicities. In PCOS patients, lignin-rich flaxseed (*Linum usitatissimum*) has been reported to significantly lower BMI and promote weight loss, and Cinnamon (*Cinnamomum verum*) supplementation was also reported to reduce insulin resistance.

Liquorice (*Glycyrrhiza glabra*) root has been reported to assist PCOS-affected women lower their serum testosterone levels. Furthermore, glycyrrhizin, the active ingredient in liquorice, can be utilized as an adjuvant treatment for hirsutism (Rashid et al. 2022).

## Conclusion

It is crucial to use therapeutic diets in PCOS patients in order to achieve specific objectives like improving metabolic, IR, and reproductive system functions. This can be done by designing a low-calorie diet to attain the loss of weight or maintenance of a healthy weight, limiting the consumption of simple sugars and consumption of refined carbohydrates and intake of foods that have a low glycemic index, reducing satiety, and more. This has been seen in PCOS females, if overweight or obese and suffering from IR can reduce their weight by at least 5% can get over issues such as out-of-whack levels of androgen in the body, reproductive functioning, boosting fertility, and IR and in many cases. Regarding vitamin D's multiple functions throughout a PCOS woman's life, it is critical to determine the appropriate 25-OH-D levels during the reproductive period, as well as the amount of vitamin D supplementation needed to achieve those levels. Even though the causes of this impairment are still unknown, PCOS women generally have lower 25-OH-D levels than healthy controls. In addition, vitamin D levels and obesity are related.

A thorough understanding of these vitamin D mechanisms could result in the use of this oral, comparatively safe, and affordable vitamin as adjuvant therapy for PCOS. In this context, it should always be recommended that PCOS patients receive clinical care that includes monitoring their vitamin D blood levels, along with other endocrine indicators and their phospho-calcium metabolism. The doctor will be prompted by this to determine the proper oral VD dosage in conjunction with other, more focused medications. Both PCOS patients with IR and obese women may benefit from this approach. Findings from the literature indicate that a dosage of 1000 IU per day, equivalent to 25 mcg, appears to be the most successful for raising 25-OH-D levels to acceptable levels over the course of three months of therapy in PCOS women with Vitamin D deficiency, barring kidney, liver, or internal illness that alters absorption. Patients with PCOS have been discovered to have abnormal levels of several hormones, including estrogens, androgens, insulin, cortisol, GH, GnRH, ratio of LH/FSH, vitamin D, and parathyroid hormone. IR, which is related to hyperinsulinemia, is a key factor in the emergence of PCOS. By raising testosterone levels, insulinemia can result in IR. By lowering osteoprotegerin expression and raising RANKL expression, insulin signaling has been shown to enhance bone resorption. Hence, it is expected that the eater insulin levels in PCOS patients will bind to insulin receptors in osteoblasts, reducing bone production and increasing bone resorption (Faghfoori et al. 2017).

## References


Adami, S., N. Zamberlan, R. Castello, F. Tosi, D. Gatti, and P. Moghetti. 1998. "Effect of Hyperandrogenism and Menstrual Cycle Abnormalities on Bone Mass and Bone Turnover in Young Women." *Clinical Endocrinology* 48 (2). https://doi.org/10.1046/j.1365-2265.1998.3691182.x.

Ameri, Pietro, Andrea Giusti, Mara Boschetti, Giovanni Murialdo, Francesco Minuto, and Diego Ferone. 2013. "Interactions between Vitamin D and IGF-I: From Physiology to Clinical Practice." *Clinical Endocrinology*. https://doi.org/10.1111/cen.12268.

Anifandis, Georgios M., Konstantinos Dafopoulos, Christina I. Messini, Nektarios Chalvatzas, Nikolaos Liakos, Spyros Pournaras, and Ioannis E. Messinis. 2010. "Prognostic Value of Follicular Fluid 25-OH Vitamin D and Glucose Levels in the IVF Outcome." *Reproductive Biology and Endocrinology* 8. https://doi.org/10.1186/1477-7827-8-91.

Ashraf, Ambika, and Jessica A. Alvarez. 2010. “Role of Vitamin D in Insulin Secretion and Insulin Sensitivity for Glucose Homeostasis.” *International Journal of Endocrinology*. https://doi.org/10.1155/2010/351385.

Attlee, Amita, Asma Nusralla, Rashida Eqbal, Hanaa Said, Mona Hashim, and Reyad Shaker Obaid. 2014. “Polycystic Ovary Syndrome in University Students: Occurrence and Associated Factors.” *International Journal of Fertility and Sterility* 8 (3).

Ballatori, Nazzareno, Suzanne M. Krance, Sylvia Notenboom, Shujie Shi, Kim Tieu, and Christine L. Hammond. 2009. “Glutathione Dysregulation and the Etiology and Progression of Human Diseases.” *Biological Chemistry*. https://doi.org/10.1515/BC.2009.033.

Benyamini, Yael, Miri Gozlan, and Ehud Kokia. 2005. “Variability in the Difficulties Experienced by Women Undergoing Infertility Treatments.” *Fertility and Sterility* 83 (2). https://doi.org/10.1016/j.fertnstert.2004.10.014.

Berberoglu, Zehra, Aynur Aktas, Yasemin Fidan, Ayse Canan Yazici, and Yalcin Aral. 2015. “Association of Plasma GDF-9 or GDF-15 Levels with Bone Parameters in Polycystic Ovary Syndrome.” *Journal of Bone and Mineral Metabolism* 33 (1). https://doi.org/10.1007/s00774-013-0560-8.

Bischoff-Ferrari, Heike A. 2014. “Optimal Serum 25-Hydroxyvitamin D Levels for Multiple Health Outcomes.” *Advances in Experimental Medicine and Biology*. https://doi.org/10.1007/978-1-4939-0437-2_28.

Bland, Rosemary, Danijela Markovic, Claire E. Hills, Susan V. Hughes, Susan L.F. Chan, Paul E. Squires, and Martin Hewison. 2004. “Expression of 25-Hydroxyvitamin D3-1α-Hydroxylase in Pancreatic Islets.” In *Journal of Steroid Biochemistry and Molecular Biology*. Vol. 89–90. https://doi.org/10.1016/j.jsbmb.2004.03.115.

Blank, S. K., C. R. McCartney, and J. C. Marshall. 2006. “The Origins and Sequelae of Abnormal Neuroendocrine Function in Polycystic Ovary Syndrome.” *Human Reproduction Update*. https://doi.org/10.1093/humupd/dml017.

Bouillon, Roger, Geert Carmeliet, Lieve Verlinden, Evelyne Van Etten, Annemieke Verstuyf, Hilary F. Luderer, Liesbet Lieben, Chantal Mathieu, and Marie Demay. 2008. “Vitamin D and Human Health: Lessons from Vitamin D Receptor Null Mice.” *Endocrine Reviews*. https://doi.org/10.1210/er.2008-0004.

Carmina, E., E. Guastella, R. A. Longo, G. B. Rini, and R. A. Lobo. 2009. “Correlates of Increased Lean Muscle Mass in Women with Polycystic Ovary Syndrome.” *European Journal of Endocrinology* 161 (4). https://doi.org/10.1530/EJE-09-0398.

Cermik, Dilek, Belgin Selam, and Hugh S. Taylor. 2003. “Regulation of HOXA-10 Expression by Testosterone *in Vitro* and in the Endometrium of Patients with Polycystic Ovary Syndrome.” *Journal of Clinical Endocrinology and Metabolism* 88 (1). https://doi.org/10.1210/jc.2002-021072.

Chang, Eun Mi, You Shin Kim, Hyung Jae Won, Tae Ki Yoon, and Woo Sik Lee. 2014. “Association between Sex Steroids, Ovarian Reserve, and Vitamin D Levels in Healthy Nonobese Women.” *Journal of Clinical Endocrinology and Metabolism* 99 (7). https://doi.org/10.1210/jc.2013-3873.

Chiu, Ken C., Audrey Chu, Vay Liang W. Go, and Mohammed F. Saad. 2004. “Hypovitaminosis D Is Associated with Insulin Resistance and β Cell Dysfunction.” *American Journal of Clinical Nutrition* 79 (5). https://doi.org/10.1093/ajcn/79.5.820.

Chun, Rene F., Philip T. Liu, Robert L. Modlin, John S. Adams, and Martin Hewison. 2014. “Impact of Vitamin D on Immune Function: Lessons Learned from Genome-Wide Analysis.” *Frontiers in Physiology*. https://doi.org/10.3389/fphys.2014.00151.

Cione, Erika, Maria Cristina Caroleo, Roberto Cannataro, Mariarita Perri, Attilio Pingitore, and Giuseppe Genchi. 2016. “Vitamin A and Diabesity: New Insight for Drug Discovery.” *Mini-Reviews in Medicinal Chemistry* 16 (9). https://doi.org/10.2174/1389557515666150709112822.

Clemens, Thomas L., and Gerard Karsenty. 2011. “The Osteoblast: An Insulin Target Cell Controlling Glucose Homeostasis.” *Journal of Bone and Mineral Research* 26 (4). https://doi.org/10.1002/jbmr.321.

Couchman, Lewis, and Cajetan F. Moniz. 2017. “Analytical Considerations for the Biochemical Assessment of Vitamin D Status.” *Therapeutic Advances in Musculoskeletal Disease*. https://doi.org/10.1177/1759720X17692500.

Damone, Anna L., Anju E. Joham, Deborah Loxton, Arul Earnest, Helena J. Teede, and Lisa J. Moran. 2019. "Depression, Anxiety and Perceived Stress in Women with and without PCOS: A Community-Based Study." *Psychological Medicine* 49 (9). https://doi.org/10.1017/S0033291718002076.

Dennis, Nicola A., Lisa A. Houghton, Gregory T. Jones, Andre M. Van Rij, Kirstie Morgan, and Ian S. McLennan. 2012. "The Level of Serum Anti-Müllerian Hormone Correlates with Vitamin D Status in Men and Women but Not in Boys." *Journal of Clinical Endocrinology and Metabolism* 97 (7). https://doi.org/10.1210/jc.2012-1213.

Diamanti-Kandarakis, Evanthia, and Andrea Dunaif. 2012. "Insulin Resistance and the Polycystic Ovary Syndrome Revisited: An Update on Mechanisms and Implications." *Endocrine Reviews* 33 (6). https://doi.org/10.1210/er.2011-1034.

Diamanti-Kandarakis, Evanthia, Sarantis Livadas, Ilias Katsikis, Christine Piperi, Mantziou Aimilia, Athanasios G. Papavassiliou, and Dimitrios Panidis. 2011. "Serum Concentrations of Carboxylated Osteocalcin Are Increased and Associated with Several Components of the Polycystic Ovarian Syndrome." *Journal of Bone and Mineral Metabolism* 29 (2). https://doi.org/10.1007/s00774-010-0211-2.

Du, Hongling, Gaurang S. Daftary, Sasmira I. Lalwani, and Hugh S. Taylor. 2005. "Direct Regulation of HOXA10 by 1,25-(OH)2D3 in Human Myelomonocytic Cells and Human Endometrial Stromal Cells." *Molecular Endocrinology* 19 (9). https://doi.org/10.1210/me.2004-0336.

Dunaif, A., K. R. Segal, W. Futterweit, and A. Dobrjansky. 1989. "Profound Peripheral Insulin Resistance, Independent of Obesity, in Polycystic Ovary Syndrome." *Diabetes* 38 (9). https://doi.org/10.2337/diabetes.38.9.1165.

Escobar-Morreale, Héctor F. 2018. "Polycystic Ovary Syndrome: Definition, Aetiology, Diagnosis and Treatment." *Nature Reviews Endocrinology*. https://doi.org/10.1038/nrendo.2018.24.

Faghfoori, Zeinab, Siavash Fazelian, Mahdi Shadnoush, and Reza Goodarzi. 2017. "Nutritional Management in Women with Polycystic Ovary Syndrome: A Review Study." *Diabetes and Metabolic Syndrome: Clinical Research and Reviews*. https://doi.org/10.1016/j.dsx.2017.03.030.

Fang, Fang, Ke Ni, Yiting Cai, Jin Shang, Xiaoke Zhang, and Chengliang Xiong. 2017. "Effect of Vitamin D Supplementation on Polycystic Ovary Syndrome: A Systematic Review and Meta-Analysis of Randomized Controlled Trials." *Complementary Therapies in Clinical Practice*. https://doi.org/10.1016/j.ctcp.2016.11.008.

Felici, Massimo De, Susanna Dolci, and Gregorio Siracusa. 1991. "An Increase of Intracellular Free Ca2+ Is Essential for Spontaneous Meiotic Resumption by Mouse Oocytes." *Journal of Experimental Zoology* 260 (3). https://doi.org/10.1002/jez.1402600314.

Ford, Earl S., Umed A. Ajani, Lisa C. McGuire, and Simin Liu. 2005. "Concentrations of Serum Vitamin D and the Metabolic Syndrome among U.S. Adults." *Diabetes Care* 28 (5). https://doi.org/10.2337/diacare.28.5.1228.

Gao, Shanshan, Yan Cheng, Lingling Zhao, Yuxin Chen, and Yu Liu. 2016. "The Relationships of Irisin with Bone Mineral Density and Body Composition in PCOS Patients." *Diabetes/Metabolism Research and Reviews* 32 (4). https://doi.org/10.1002/dmrr.2767.

George, Jyothis T., Rahul Kakkar, Jayne Marshall, Martin L. Scott, Richard D. Finkelman, Tony W. Ho, Johannes Veldhuis, et al. 2016. "Neurokinin B Receptor Antagonism in Women with Polycystic Ovary Syndrome: A Randomized, Placebo-Controlled Trial." *Journal of Clinical Endocrinology and Metabolism* 101 (11). https://doi.org/10.1210/jc.2016-1202.

Glintborg, D., A. P. Hermann, L. M. Rasmussen, and M. Andersen. 2013. "Plasma Osteoprotegerin Is Associated with Testosterone Levels but Unaffected by Pioglitazone Treatment in Patients with Polycystic Ovary Syndrome." *Journal of Endocrinological Investigation* 36 (7). https://doi.org/10.3275/8767.

Glintborg, Dorte, Marianne Andersen, Claus Hagen, Lene Heickendorff, and Anne Pernille Hermann. 2008. "Association of Pioglitazone Treatment with Decreased Bone Mineral Density in Obese Premenopausal Patients with Polycystic Ovary Syndrome: A Randomized, Placebo-Controlled Trial." *Journal of Clinical Endocrinology and Metabolism* 93 (5). https://doi.org/10.1210/jc.2007-2249.

Good, Candace, Mark Tulchinsky, David Mauger, Laurence M. Demers, and Richard S. Legro. 1999. "Bone Mineral Density and Body Composition in Lean Women with Polycystic Ovary Syndrome." *Fertility and Sterility* 72 (1). https://doi.org/10.1016/S0015-0282(99)00203-4.

Hahn, Susanne, U. Haselhorst, S. Tan, B. Quadbeck, M. Schmidt, S. Roesler, R. Kimmig, K. Mann, and O. E. Janssen. 2006. "Low Serum 25-Hydroxyvitamin D Concentrations Are Associated with Insulin Resistance and Obesity in Women with Polycystic Ovary Syndrome." *Experimental and Clinical Endocrinology and Diabetes* 114 (10). https://doi.org/10.1055/s-2006-948308.

Halloran, B. P., and H. F. Deluca. 1980. "Effect of Vitamin D Deficiency on Fertility and Reproductive Capacity in the Female Rat." *Journal of Nutrition* 110 (8). https://doi.org/10.1093/jn/110.8.1573.

Haussler, M. R., G. K. Whitfield, C. A. Haussler, J. C. Hsieh, P. D. Thompson, S. H. Selznick, C. E. Dominguez, and P. W. Jurutka. 1998. "The Nuclear Vitamin D Receptor: Biological and Molecular Regulatory Properties Revealed." *Journal of Bone and Mineral Research*. https://doi.org/10.1359/jbmr.1998.13.3.325.

He, Chunla, Zhoumeng Lin, Sara Wagner Robb, and Amara E. Ezeamama. 2015. "Serum Vitamin d Levels and Polycystic Ovary Syndrome: A Systematic Review and Meta-Analysis." *Nutrients*. https://doi.org/10.3390/nu7064555.

Holick, M F. 1994. "Vitamin D-New Horizons for the 21st Century." *The American Journal of Clinical Nutrition* 60 (4).

Ibáñez, Lourdes, Angela Ferrer, Ken Ong, Rakesh Amin, David Dunger, and Francis De Zegher. 2004. "Insulin Sensitization Early after Menarche Prevents Progression from Precocious Pubarche to Polycystic Ovary Syndrome." *Journal of Pediatrics* 144 (1). https://doi.org/10.1016/j.jpeds.2003.08.015.

Ibáñez, Lourdes, Sharon E. Oberfield, Selma Witchel, Richard J. Auchus, R. Jeffrey Chang, Ethel Codner, Preeti Dabadghao, Feyza Darendeliler, Nancy Samir Elbarbary, Alessandra Gambineri, Cecilia Garcia Rudaz, Kathleen M Hoeger, Abel López-Bermejo, Ken Ong, Alexia S Peña, Thomas Reinehr, Nicola Santoro, Manuel Tena-Sempere, Rachel Tao, Bulent O Yildiz, Haya Alkhayyat, Asma Deeb, Dipesalema Joel, Reiko Horikawa, Francis de Zegher, Peter A Lee. 2017. "An International Consortium Update: Pathophysiology, Diagnosis, and Treatment of Polycystic Ovarian Syndrome in Adolescence." *Hormone Research in Paediatrics*. https://doi.org/10.1159/000479371.

Insler, Vaclav, and Bruno Lunenfeld. 1991. "Opinion: Pathophysiology of Polycystic Ovarian Disease: New Insights." *Human Reproduction* 6 (8). https://doi.org/10.1093/oxfordjournals.humrep.a137478.

Irani, Mohamad, and Zaher Merhi. 2014. "Role of Vitamin D in Ovarian Physiology and Its Implication in Reproduction: A Systematic Review." *Fertility and Sterility* 102 (2). https://doi.org/10.1016/j.fertnstert.2014.04.046.

Jain, Sushil K., and David Micinski. 2013. "Vitamin D Upregulates Glutamate Cysteine Ligase and Glutathione Reductase, and GSH Formation, and Decreases ROS and MCP-1 and IL-8 Secretion in High-Glucose Exposed U937 Monocytes." *Biochemical and Biophysical Research Communications* 437 (1). https://doi.org/10.1016/j.bbrc.2013.06.004.

Jain, Sushil K., Rajesh Parsanathan, Arunkumar E. Achari, Preeti Kanikarla-Marie, and Joseph A. Bocchini. 2018. "Glutathione Stimulates Vitamin D Regulatory and Glucose-Metabolism Genes, Lowers Oxidative Stress and Inflammation, and Increases 25-Hydroxy-Vitamin D Levels in Blood: A Novel Approach to Treat 25-Hydroxyvitamin D Deficiency." *Antioxidants and Redox Signaling* 29 (17). https://doi.org/10.1089/ars.2017.7462.

Kalyan, Shirin, Millan S. Patel, Elaine Kingwell, Hélène C.F. Côté, Danmei Liu, and Jerilynn C. Prior. 2017. "Competing Factors Link to Bone Health in Polycystic Ovary Syndrome: Chronic Low-Grade Inflammation Takes a Toll." *Scientific Reports* 7 (1). https://doi.org/10.1038/s41598-017-03685-x.

Karadağ, Cihan, Tevfik Yoldemir, and Dilek Gogas Yavuz. 2017. "Determinants of Low Bone Mineral Density in Premenopausal Polycystic Ovary Syndrome Patients." *Gynecological Endocrinology* 33 (3). https://doi.org/10.1080/09513590.2016.1250256.

Kassanos, D., E. Trakakis, C. S. Baltas, O. Papakonstantinou, G. Simeonidis, G. Salamalekis, I. Grammatikakis, Basios, G., Labos, G., Skarantavos, G., Balanika, A. 2010. "Augmentation of Cortical Bone Mineral Density in Women with Polycystic Ovary Syndrome: A Peripheral Quantitative Computed Tomography (PQCT) Study." *Human Reproduction* 25 (8). https://doi.org/10.1093/humrep/deq149.

Kato, Shigeaki. 2000. "The Function of Vitamin D Receptor in Vitamin D Action." *Journal of Biochemistry*. https://doi.org/10.1093/oxfordjournals.jbchem.a022662.

Katulski, K., S. Slawek, A. Czyzyk, A. Podfigurna-Stopa, K. Paczkowska, N. Ignaszak, N. Podkowa, and B. Meczekalski. 2014. "Bone Mineral Density in Women with Polycystic Ovary Syndrome." *Molecular Diagnosis and Therapy* 37 (12). https://doi.org/10.1007/s40618-014-0175-5.

Kaygusuz, Ikbal, Omer Faruk Karatas, Hasan Kafali, Ersin Cimentepe, and Dogan Unal. 2013. "Is Polycystic Ovarian Syndrome a Risk Factor for Urolithiasis." *Urological Research* 41 (4). https://doi.org/10.1007/s00240-013-0564-9.

Ketel, I. J.G., E. H. Sern, R. G. Ijzerman, T. J.M. Korsen, J. W. Twisk, P. G.A. Hompes, Y. M. Smulders, et al. 2011. "Insulin-Induced Capillary Recruitment Is Impaired in Both Lean and Obese Women with PCOS." *Human Reproduction* 26 (11). https://doi.org/10.1093/humrep/der296.

Kim, Joon Young, Hala Tfayli, Sara F. Michaliszyn, and Silva Arslanian. 2018. "Impaired Lipolysis, Diminished Fat Oxidation, and Metabolic Inflexibility in Obese Girls with Polycystic Ovary Syndrome." *Journal of Clinical Endocrinology and Metabolism* 103 (2). https://doi.org/10.1210/jc.2017-01958.

Kinuta, K., H. Tanaka, T. Moriwake, K. Aya, S. Kato, and Y. Seino. 2000. "Vitamin D Is an Important Factor in Estrogen Biosynthesis of Both Female and Male Gonads." *Endocrinology* 141 (4). https://doi.org/10.1210/endo.141.4.7403.

Kirchengast, S., and J. Huber. 2001. "Body Composition Characteristics and Body Fat Distribution in Lean Women with Polycystic Ovary Syndrome." *Human Reproduction* 16 (6). https://doi.org/10.1093/humrep/16.6.1255.

Kılınç, Suna, Enver Atay, Ömer Ceran, and Zeynep Atay. 2019. "Evaluation of Vitamin D Status and Its Correlation with Gonadal Function in Children at Mini-Puberty." *Clinical Endocrinology* 90 (1). https://doi.org/10.1111/cen.13856.

Klein, Gordon L. 2014. "Insulin and Bone: Recent Developments." *World J Diabetes* 5 (1). https://doi.org/10.4239/wjd.v5.i1.14.

Kochupillai, N. 2008. "The Physiology of Vitamin D: Current Concepts." *Indian Journal of Medical Research*.

Kotsa, Kalliopi, Maria P. Yavropoulou, Olympia Anastasiou, and John G. Yovos. 2009. "Role of Vitamin D Treatment in Glucose Metabolism in Polycystic Ovary Syndrome." *Fertility and Sterility* 92 (3). https://doi.org/10.1016/j.fertnstert.2008.07.1757.

Kousta, Eleni, George Tolis, and Stephen Franks. 2005. "Polycystic Ovary Syndrome. Revised Diagnostic Criteria and Long-Term Health Consequences." *Hormones (Athens, Greece)*. https://doi.org/10.14310/horm.2002.11151.

Kovacs, Christopher S., Mandy L. Woodland, Neva J. Fudge, and James K. Friel. 2005. "The Vitamin D Receptor Is Not Required for Fetal Mineral Homeostasis or for the Regulation of Placental Calcium Transfer in Mice." *American Journal of Physiology - Endocrinology and Metabolism* 289 (1 52-1). https://doi.org/10.1152/ajpendo.00354.2004.

Krul-Poel, Y. H. M., C. Snackey, Y. Louwers, P. Lips, C. B. Lambalk, J. S. E. Laven, and S. Simsek. 2013. "The Role of Vitamin D in Metabolic Disturbances in Polycystic Ovary Syndrome: A Systematic Review." *European Journal of Endocrinology* 169 (6). https://doi.org/10.1530/EJE-13-0617.

Kuiri-Hänninen, Tanja, Ulla Sankilampi, and Leo Dunkel. 2014. "Activation of the Hypothalamic-Pituitary-Gonadal Axis in Infancy: Minipuberty." *Hormone Research in Paediatrics*. https://doi.org/10.1159/000362414.

Leo, V. De, M. C. Musacchio, V. Cappelli, M. G. Massaro, G. Morgante, and F. Petraglia. 2016. "Genetic, Hormonal and Metabolic Aspects of PCOS: An Update." *Reproductive Biology and Endocrinology*. https://doi.org/10.1186/s12958-016-0173-x.

Lerner, Paul P., Laura Sharony, and Chanoch Miodownik. 2018. "Association between Mental Disorders, Cognitive Disturbances and Vitamin D Serum Level: Current State." *Clinical Nutrition ESPEN* 23. https://doi.org/10.1016/j.clnesp.2017.11.011.

Leung, Po Sing. 2016. "The Potential Protective Action of Vitamin D in Hepatic Insulin Resistance and Pancreatic Islet Dysfunction in Type 2 Diabetes Mellitus." *Nutrients*. https://doi.org/10.3390/nu8030147.

Lingaiah, Shilpa, Laure Morin-Papunen, Terhi Piltonen, Johanna Puurunen, Inger Sundström-Poromaa, Elisabet Stener-Victorin, Risto Bloigu, Juha Risteli, and Juha S. Tapanainen. 2017. "Bone Markers in

Polycystic Ovary Syndrome: A Multicentre Study." *Clinical Endocrinology* 87 (6). https://doi.org/10.1111/cen.13456.

Lips, P. 2006. "Vitamin D Physiology." *Progress in Biophysics and Molecular Biology*. https://doi.org/10.1016/j.pbiomolbio.2006.02.016.

Lips, Paul. 2001. "Vitamin D Deficiency and Secondary Hyperparathyroidism in the Elderly: Consequences for Bone Loss and Fractures and Therapeutic Implications." *Endocrine Reviews*. https://doi.org/10.1210/edrv.22.4.0437.

Lundqvist, Johan. 2014. "Vitamin D as a Regulator of Steroidogenic Enzymes." *F1000Research* 3. https://doi.org/10.12688/f1000research.4714.1.

Maestro, Begoña, Norma Dávila, M. Carmen Carranza, and Consuelo Calle. 2003. "Identification of a Vitamin D Response Element in the Human Insulin Receptor Gene Promoter." In *Journal of Steroid Biochemistry and Molecular Biology*. Vol. 84. https://doi.org/10.1016/S0960-0760(03)00032-3.

Maktabi, Maryam, Maryam Chamani, and Zatollah Asemi. 2017. "The Effects of Vitamin D Supplementation on Metabolic Status of Patients with Polycystic Ovary Syndrome: A Randomized, Double-Blind, Placebo-Controlled Trial." *Hormone and Metabolic Research* 49 (7). https://doi.org/10.1055/s-0043-107242.

Malloy, Peter J., Lihong Peng, Jining Wang, and David Feldman. 2009. "Interaction of the Vitamin D Receptor with a Vitamin D Response Element in the Müllerian-Inhibiting Substance (MIS) Promoter: Regulation of MIS Expression by Calcitriol in Prostate Cancer Cells." *Endocrinology* 150 (4). https://doi.org/10.1210/en.2008-1555.

Mangelsdorf, David J., Carl Thummel, Miguel Beato, Peter Herrlich, Günther Schütz, Kazuhiko Umesono, Bruce Blumberg, Kastner, P., Mark, M., Chambon, P., & Evans, R. M. 1995. "The Nuclear Receptor Superfamily: The Second Decade." *Cell* 83 (6). https://doi.org/10.1016/0092-8674(95)90199-X.

McBreairty, Laura E., Gordon A. Zello, Julianne J. Gordon, Shani B. Serrao, Roger A. Pierson, Donna R. Chizen, and Philip D. Chilibeck. 2018. "Women With Polycystic Ovary Syndrome Have Comparable Hip Bone Geometry to Age-Matched Control Women." *Journal of Clinical Densitometry* 21 (1). https://doi.org/10.1016/j.jocd.2016.10.007.

Merhi, Zaher, Angela Doswell, Kendall Krebs, and Marilyn Cipolla. 2014. "Vitamin D Alters Genes Involved in Follicular Development and Steroidogenesis in Human Cumulus Granulosa Cells." *Journal of Clinical Endocrinology and Metabolism* 99 (6). https://doi.org/10.1210/jc.2013-4161.

Mirhosseini, Naghmeh, Hassanali Vatanparast, Mohsen Mazidi, and Samantha M. Kimball. 2017. "The Effect of Improved Serum 25-Hydroxyvitamin D Status on Glycemic Control in Diabetic Patients: A Meta-Analysis." *Journal of Clinical Endocrinology and Metabolism* 102 (9). https://doi.org/10.1210/jc.2017-01024.

Nestler, J. E. 2000. "Obesity, Insulin, Sex Steroids and Ovulation." In *International Journal of Obesity*. Vol. 24. https://doi.org/10.1038/sj.ijo.0801282.

Norman, Anthony W. 2008. "From Vitamin D to Hormone D: Fundamentals of the Vitamin D Endocrine System Essential for Good Health." *American Journal of Clinical Nutrition*. https://doi.org/10.1093/ajcn/88.2.491s.

Noyan, Volkan, Aykan Yucel, and Nevin Sagsoz. 2004. "The Association of Bone Mineral Density with Insulin Resistance in Patients with Polycystic Ovary Syndrome." *European Journal of Obstetrics and Gynecology and Reproductive Biology* 115 (2). https://doi.org/10.1016/j.ejogrb.2004.01.031.

Odunsi, K., and K. K. Kidd. 1999. "A Paradigm for Finding Genes for a Complex Human Trait: Polycystic Ovary Syndrome and Follistatin." *Proceedings of the National Academy of Sciences of the United States of America*. https://doi.org/10.1073/pnas.96.15.8315.

Ott, J., L. Wattar, C. Kurz, R. Seemann, J. C. Huber, K. Mayerhofer, and E. Vytiska-Binstorfer. 2012. "Parameters for Calcium Metabolism in Women with Polycystic Ovary Syndrome Who Undergo Clomiphene Citrate Stimulation: A Prospective Cohort Study." *European Journal of Endocrinology* 166 (5). https://doi.org/10.1530/EJE-11-1070.

Ozkan, Sebiha, Sangita Jindal, Keri Greenseid, Jun Shu, Gohar Zeitlian, Cheryl Hickmon, and Lubna Pal. 2010. "Replete Vitamin D Stores Predict Reproductive Success Following *in Vitro* Fertilization." *Fertility and Sterility* 94 (4). https://doi.org/10.1016/j.fertnstert.2009.05.019.

Parikh, G., M. Varadinova, P. Suwandhi, T. Araki, Z. Rosenwaks, L. Poretsky, and D. Seto-Young. 2010. "Vitamin D Regulates Steroidogenesis and Insulin-like Growth Factor Binding Protein-1 (IGFBP-1)

Production in Human Ovarian Cells." *Hormone and Metabolic Research* 42 (10). https://doi.org/10.1055/s-0030-1262837.

Parsanathan, Rajesh, and Sushil K. Jain. 2019. "Glutathione Deficiency Alters the Vitamin D-Metabolizing Enzymes CYP27B1 and CYP24A1 in Human Renal Proximal Tubule Epithelial Cells and Kidney of HFD-Fed Mice." *Free Radical Biology and Medicine* 131. https://doi.org/10.1016/j.freeradbiomed.2018.12.017.

Pepene, Carmen E. 2013. "Serum Under-Carboxylated Osteocalcin Levels in Women with Polycystic Ovary Syndrome: Weight-Dependent Relationships with Endocrine and Metabolic Traits." *Journal of Ovarian Research* 6 (1). https://doi.org/10.1186/1757-2215-6-4.

Pike, J. Wesley, and Mark B. Meyer. 2012. "The Vitamin D Receptor: New Paradigms for the Regulation of Gene Expression by 1,25-Dihydroxyvitamin D 3." *Rheumatic Disease Clinics of North America.* https://doi.org/10.1016/j.rdc.2012.03.004.

Pittas, Anastassios G., Joseph Lau, Frank B. Hu, and Bess Dawson-Hughes. 2007. "Review: The Role of Vitamin D and Calcium in Type 2 Diabetes. A Systematic Review and Meta-Analysis." *Journal of Clinical Endocrinology and Metabolism.* https://doi.org/10.1210/jc.2007-0298.

Rashid, Rumaisa, Suhail Ahmad Mir, Ozaifa Kareem, Tabassum Ali, Rifat Ara, Anjum Malik, Fiza Amin, and G. N. Bader. 2022. "Polycystic Ovarian Syndrome-Current Pharmacotherapy and Clinical Implications." *Taiwanese Journal of Obstetrics and Gynecology.* https://doi.org/10.1016/j.tjog.2021.11.009.

Rashidi, Batool, Fedieh Haghollahi, Mamak Shariat, and Farid Zayerii. 2009. "The Effects of Calcium-Vitamin D and Metformin on Polycystic Ovary Syndrome: A Pilot Study." *Taiwanese Journal of Obstetrics and Gynecology* 48 (2). https://doi.org/10.1016/S1028-4559(09)60275-8.

Reusch, Jane E. B., Najma Begum, Karl E. Sussman, and Boris Draznin. 1991. "Regulation of GLUT-4 Phosphorylation by Intracellular Calcium in Adipocytes." *Endocrinology* 129 (6). https://doi.org/10.1210/endo-129-6-3269.

Rubin, Katrine Hass, Dorte Glintborg, Mads Nybo, Marianne Andersen, and Bo Abrahamsen. 2016. "Fracture Risk Is Decreased in Women with Polycystic Ovary Syndrome: A Register-Based and Population-Based Cohort Study." *Journal of Bone and Mineral Research* 31 (4). https://doi.org/10.1002/jbmr.2737.

Salvesen, K. Å, E. Vanky, and S. M. Carlsen. 2007. "Metformin Treatment in Pregnant Women with Polycystic Ovary Syndrome - Is Reduced Complication Rate Mediated by Changes in the Uteroplacental Circulation?" *Ultrasound in Obstetrics and Gynecology* 29 (4). https://doi.org/10.1002/uog.3965.

Schmidt, Johanna, Eva Dahlgren, Mats Brännström, and Kerstin Landin-Wilhelmsen. 2012. "Body Composition, Bone Mineral Density and Fractures in Late Postmenopausal Women with Polycystic Ovary Syndrome - A Long-Term Follow-up Study." *Clinical Endocrinology* 77 (2). https://doi.org/10.1111/j.1365-2265.2012.04378.x.

Scragg, Robert, Mary Fran Sowers, and Colin Bell. 2004. "Serum 25-Hydroxyvitamin D, Diabetes, and Ethnicity in the Third National Health and Nutrition Examination Survey." *Diabetes Care.* https://doi.org/10.2337/diacare.27.12.2813.

Selimoglu, H., C. Duran, S. Kiyici, C. Ersoy, M. Guclu, G. Ozkaya, E. Tuncel, E. Erturk, and S. Imamoglu. 2010. "The Effect of Vitamin D Replacement Therapy on Insulin Resistance and Androgen Levels in Women with Polycystic Ovary Syndrome." *Journal of Endocrinological Investigation* 33 (4). https://doi.org/10.3275/6560.

Shaffer, Paul L., and Daniel T. Gewirth. 2004. "Vitamin D Receptor-DNA Interactions." *Vitamins and Hormones* 68. https://doi.org/10.1016/S0083-6729(04)68009-5.

Shetty, Disha, Baskaran Chandrasekaran, ArulWatson Singh, and Joseph Oliverraj. 2017. "Exercise in Polycystic Ovarian Syndrome: An Evidence-Based Review." *Saudi Journal of Sports Medicine* 17 (3). https://doi.org/10.4103/sjsm.sjsm_10_17.

Siris, Ethel S., Ya Ting Chen, Thomas A. Abbott, Elizabeth Barrett-Connor, Paul D. Miller, Lois E. Wehren, and Marc L. Berger. 2004. "Bone Mineral Density Thresholds for Pharmacological Intervention to Prevent Fractures." *Archives of Internal Medicine* 164 (10). https://doi.org/10.1001/archinte.164.10.1108.

Taylor, Hugh S., Gregory B. Vanden Heuvel, and Peter Igarashi. 1997. "A Conserved Hox Axis in the Mouse and Human Female Reproductive System: Late Establishment and Persistent Adult Expression of the Hoxa Cluster Genes." *Biology of Reproduction* 57 (6). https://doi.org/10.1095/biolreprod57.6.1338.

Tehrani, Hatav Ghasemi, Fatemeh Mostajeran, and Somayeh Shahsavari. 2014. "The Effect of Calcium and Vitamin D Supplementation on Menstrual Cycle, Body Mass Index and Hyperandrogenism State of Women with Poly Cystic Ovarian Syndrome." *Journal of Research in Medical Sciences : The Official Journal of Isfahan University of Medical Sciences* 19 (9).

Thomas, D. M., N. Udagawa, D. K. Hards, J. M. W. Quinn, J. M. Moseley, D. M. Findlay, and J. D. Best. 1998. "Insulin Receptor Expression in Primary and Cultured Osteoclast-like Cells." *Bone* 23 (3). https://doi.org/10.1016/S8756-3282(98)00095-7.

Thomson, Rebecca L., Simon Spedding, and Jonathan D. Buckley. 2012. "Vitamin D in the Aetiology and Management of Polycystic Ovary Syndrome." *Clinical Endocrinology*. https://doi.org/10.1111/j.1365-2265.2012.04434.x.

Thomson, Rebecca L., Helena J. Teede, Nigel K. Stepto, Lauren K. Banting, and Lisa J. Moran. 2015. "The Role of Diet and Lifestyle Modification in the Treatment of Polycystic Ovary Syndrome." In *Nutrition, Fertility, and Human Reproductive Function*. https://doi.org/10.1201/b18190-3.

Thys-Jacobs, Susan, Daniel Donovan, Anatasio Papadopoulos, Philip Sarrel, and John P. Bilezikian. 1999. "Vitamin D and Calcium Dysregulation in the Polycystic Ovarian Syndrome." *Steroids* 64 (6). https://doi.org/10.1016/S0039-128X(99)00012-4.

Upreti, Vimal, Vijay Maitri, Pawan Dhull, Ajay Handa, M. S. Prakash, and Anil Behl. 2018. "Effect of Oral Vitamin D Supplementation on Glycemic Control in Patients with Type 2 Diabetes Mellitus with Coexisting Hypovitaminosis D: A Parellel Group Placebo Controlled Randomized Controlled Pilot Study." *Diabetes and Metabolic Syndrome: Clinical Research and Reviews* 12 (4). https://doi.org/10.1016/j.dsx.2018.03.008.

Wang, Hanmin, Weiwen Chen, Dongqing Li, Xiaoe Yin, Xiaode Zhang, Nancy Olsen, and Song Guo Zheng. 2017. "Vitamin D and Chronic Diseases." *Aging and Disease* 8 (3). https://doi.org/10.14336/AD.2016.1021.

Wang, Huixin, and Xiaohuan Zhong. 2013. "Insulin Effect on RANKL and OPG Expression in Human Osteoblast-like MG63 Cells." *Turkish Journal of Medical Sciences* 43 (4). https://doi.org/10.3906/sag-1203-108.

Yamada, Shoya, and Hiroki Kakuta. 2014. "Retinoid X Receptor Ligands: A Patent Review (2007-2013)." *Expert Opinion on Therapeutic Patents*. https://doi.org/10.1517/13543776.2014.880692.

Yang, Hsin Yi, Herng Sheng Lee, Wan Ting Huang, Ming Jer Chen, Solomon Chih Cheng Chen, and Yueh Han Hsu. 2018. "Increased Risk of Fractures in Patients with Polycystic Ovary Syndrome: A Nationwide Population-Based Retrospective Cohort Study." *Journal of Bone and Mineral Metabolism* 36 (6). https://doi.org/10.1007/s00774-017-0894-8.

Yoshizawa, T., Y. Handa, Y. Uematsu, S. Takeda, K. Sekine, Y. Yoshihara, T. Kawakami, Arioka, K., Sato, H., Uchiyama, Y., Masushige, S., Fukamizu, A., Matsumoto, T., Kato, S. 1997. "Mice Lacking the Vitamin D Receptor Exhibit Impaired Bone Formation, Uterine Hypoplasia and Growth Retardation after Weaning." *Nature Genetics* 16 (4). https://doi.org/10.1038/ng0897-391.

Yüksel, Osman, Hatice Sebila Dökmetaş, Saniye Topcu, Taner Erselcan, and Mehmet Şencan. 2001. "Relationship between Bone Mineral Density and Insulin Resistance in Polycystic Ovary Syndrome." *Journal of Bone and Mineral Metabolism* 19 (4). https://doi.org/10.1007/s007740170029.

Zeitz, Ute, Karin Weber, Desi W. Soegiarto, Eckhard Wolf, Rudi Balling, and Reinhold G. Erben. 2003. "Impaired Insulin Secretory Capacity in Mice Lacking a Functional Vitamin D Receptor." *The FASEB Journal : Official Publication of the Federation of American Societies for Experimental Biology* 17 (3). https://doi.org/10.1096/fj.02-0424fje.

# Chapter 9

# PCOS and the Anti-Mullerian Hormone: Reprogramming the Female Fetus and Increased Chances of PCOS in Adulthood

**Subhrojyoti Ghosh[1,*]**
**Anuvab Dey[2]**
**Debasmita Sarma Chaudhuri[3]**
**Nainika Srivastava[4]**
**Tiyasa Malik[4]**
**Shreya Jha[4]**
**and Rijula Batabyal[4]**
[1]Department of Biotechnology, IIT Madras, Chennai, Tamil Nadu, Tamil Nadu, India
[2]Department of Biological Sciences and Bioengineering, IIT Guwahati, North Guwahati, Assam, India
[3]Department of Biotechnology, IIT Kharagpur, Kharagpur, West Bengal, India
[4]Department of Biotechnology, Heritage Institute of Technology, Kolkata, West Bengal, India

## Abstract

Polycystic Ovary Syndrome (PCOS) occurs to be a prevalent endocrine condition among women of reproductive age group, causing hyperandrogenism and oligo-anovulation which leads to infertility. The increased production of AMH (Anti-Müllerian Hormone) in pre-antral and small antral follicles is a hallmark of PCOS, with higher levels observed in pregnant women with PCOS compared to healthy controls. The quantifiable detection of AMH in serum has made way for the development of sensitive assays, with levels found to be two to four-fold overexpressed among women with PCOS. AMH is released by the granulosa cells of antral follicles and tends to be inversely correlated with the number of actively growing follicles in the ovaries. The difficulties associated with observing Polycystic ovarian morphology (PCOM) on ultrasound suggest quantifying AMH as a substitute. The effectiveness of serum AMH in managing infertility has been established; however, the lack of a global standard for the test of serum AMH poses challenges in its

[*] Corresponding Author's Email: subhrojyotighosh8@gmail.com.

In: Polycystic Ovarian Syndrome (PCOS) and Our Biological Clock
Editors: Arpita Roy, Gowhar Rashid and Nihad Ashraf Khan
ISBN: 979-8-89113-100-2
© 2023 Nova Science Publishers, Inc.

application. This book chapter explores the significance of AMH as a potential detection tool for PCOS and its therapeutic effect in reprogramming the fetus.

**Keywords:** Polycystic ovarian syndrome (PCOS), Anti-Mullerian hormone (AMH), Hyperandrogenism (HA), Oligo-anovulation (OA), infertility, diagnostic assay

## 1. Introduction to PCOS (Diagnostic Standards, Characteristics, and Pathophysiology of PCOS*)*

PCOS is observed to be one of the leading hormonal threats to women of reproductive age all over the world (Bozdag et al., 2016). This problem usually starts in the early teenage when the ovarian system doesn't function properly, followed by hyperandrogenism, which finally results in reduced ovulation (Teede et al., 2018). PCOS does not affect fertility only, it also hampers several other metabolisms in the human body, which makes it a clinically heterogeneous syndrome (di Clemento et al., 2022). In PCOS, the affected women show comorbidities, where they become highly resistant to insulin, also their blood cholesterol and sugar levels elevate. Moreover, it escalates the occurrence of type 2 diabetes Mellitus and circulatory systems disorders (Escobar & Hector, 2018). Along with these effects, PCOS hampers the mental health of the patients so badly that they slowly become anxious, depressed, and insomniac day by day (Stener et al., 2019). Also, women have a high chance to be diabetic during their pregnancy period, followed by various problems during their delivery (Palomba et al., 2018). Even in an extreme case, it can lead to developing endometrial cancer the ultimate life threat (Azziz & Ricardo, 2018).

In this syndrome, the number of preantral and antral follicles is considerably increased and consequently, the level of serum AMH and leutinizing hormone (LH) is also increased 2-4 folds more in affected patients (Teede et al., 2019; Pellatt et al., 2007; Lie eta al., 2012; Villarroel et al., 2011). Earlier, scientists thought that this escalation of AMH amount in serum happened because of the elevated number of pre-antral as well as antral follicles (Dumont et al., 2015). But in the laboratory, other experiments showed that granulosa cells synthesize AMH seventy-five-fold more in the case of PCOS women than any fit woman (Pellatt et al., 2007). This result indicates that the upregulated level of serum AMH in PCOS can be a reflection of the inherent hyperexcitability of the granulosa cells, followed by the participation of AMH itself in this process because the AMH receptor type 2 has been highly expressed (Catteau et al., 2008; Alebic et al., 2015). Though several researchers are simultaneously working on this syndrome, the proper reason for that much large amount of AMH in antral follicles in PCOS is still not found (Laven et al., 2004; Pigny et al., 2003; Gilling et al., 1994; Carlsen et al., 2009; Eldar et al., 2005). However, scientists suspect that sex hormones take an important part in this large production (Laven et al., 2004; Pigny et al., 2003; Gilling et al., 1994; Carlsen et al., 2009; Eldar et al., 2005). Also, several studies have demonstrated that the sex hormones present in the serum and the AMH production are directly correlated with each other and help in the identification of PCOS as well as its extremity (Baarends et al., 1995). Besides this, due to an innate problem of thecal cells, in PCOS, sex hormones are produced in a high amount (Baarends et al., 1995; Panidis et al., 2011). So, in the diagnosis of this disease, hyperandrogenism and oligo-anovulation could be preliminary considered as reliable methods (Teede et al., 2019). In our quest to understand the disease, ultrasonic sound may not be enough to reveal its pathophysiology. However, there's a glimmer of hope! A high concentration of AFC/AMH in the serum can act as a beacon, guiding us toward a diagnosis. Join us on a thrilling journey as we explore the intricacies of disease detection and unlock the secrets hidden within our bodies (Dumont et al., 2015).

Unlocking the mysteries of hormone production and regulation can be a daunting task, but fear not! Recent studies have shed light on the complex interplay between androgens, FSH, E2, and AMH levels. While some studies have shown a negative correlation between androgens and AMH production, new research has revealed that the picture is more nuanced than we once thought (Baarends et al., 1995; Panidis et al., 2011). E2 can inhibit AMH production in the absence of aromatase, while FSH stimulates it in small follicles. But the plot thickens! In larger follicles, E2 becomes a negative regulator, stimulating FSH and indirectly halting AMH production. Join us on an exciting journey of discovery as we delve into the fascinating world of hormone regulation and uncover the latest research in the field (Pierre et al., 2013; Grynberg et al., 2012). The intricate dance of hormone regulation in small follicles is a fascinating topic, and recent research has emerged as an alternative including the complexities. It turns out that AMH plays a crucial role in preventing pre-aromatase expression by reducing FSH receptor and aromatase expression. However, when AMH levels become too elevated, it can lead to an excess of follicles and ultimately result in "follicular arrest" and PCOS. And that's not all! LH also plays a role in the synthesis of AMH, acting as a positive regulator of AMHR2 expression. This excess AMH can then trigger anovulation and contribute to the development of PCOS (Teede et al., 2019; Pellat et al., 2011). Researchers are trying hard to explore this intricate web of hormone interactions and unlock the secrets of small follicle regulation (Teede et al., 2019; Pellatt et al., 2007; Willis et al., 1998; Pellatt et al., 2010). Recent medical research has uncovered the critical role that insulin plays in PCOS, in addition to sex hormones. One study found that in women with the condition, the placental enzyme 3-3β-hydroxysteroid dehydrogenase (3β-HSD) is reduced, leading to an increase in anogenital length. These findings shed new light on the intricate mechanisms at play in PCOS and highlight the importance of considering insulin levels in its diagnosis and treatment (Di Clemente et al., 2022; Barrett et al., 2018). Recent studies report that, due to the increased level of AMH during pregnancy, PCOS tends to be genetically inherited from the affected mother, during the androgenization of the fetus, in the placenta (Silva et al., 2021). One experiment has shown that, in the case of hereditary PCOS, it is found to have a five-fold higher risk to be PCOS affected from their teenage, than normal PCOS (Dumesic et al., 2020; Crisosto et al., 2019).

## 2. Pathophysiology of AMH

The PCOS condition is diverse, and women with this condition may exhibit metabolic, reproductive, and/or endocrine symptoms that can change over their lifetimes. According to the Rotterdam Criteria, a woman must meet two of the three following criteria to be diagnosed- (a) oligo- or anovulation, (b) clinical and/or biochemical signs of hyperandrogenism, and/or (b) polycystic ovaries by ultrasound, excluding other related conditions (ESHRE 2004).

AMH, also addressed as Müllerian- inhibiting hormone (MIH), is a major type of glycoprotein hormone structurally related to the inhibins and activins of the transforming growth factor beta superfamily and is important in growth differentiation and folliculogenesis

(Rzeszowska et al., 2016). PCOS means an increased number of follicles at all stages of development. Elevated serum AMH, reflecting anterior follicular reserve and cavernous cysts, is 2–4 times more prone in women with PCOS compared to healthy women (Fong et al., 2011; Pellat et al., 2007; Azziz et al., 2009; Villarroel et al., 2011; Laven et al., 2004; Pigny et al., 2003).

Initially, it was believed that the rise in serum AMH levels in women with PCOS was solely due to a change in the amount of small and developing follicles. Though, in vitro studies found out that the generation of AMH by granulosa cells was 75 times higher in non-ovulatory PCOS and 20 times higher in normal PCOS compared to healthy ovaries (Pellat et al., 2007).

According to some recent findings, E2 inhibits the expression of AMH through the estrogen β receptor (Grynbaer et al., 2012). In small follicles, FSH can directly stimulate AMH, but by elevating E2 production in larger follicles, FSH can also block AMH expression by negative E2 feedback (Grynbaer et al., 2012). This pathway is disrupted in women with PCOS, who do not have a concomitant increase in E2 levels. That is why, AMH expression and follicular fluid AMH levels are decreased in gonadotropin-dependent follicles in normally ovulating women, but not in PCOS patients (Jakimiuk et al., 2001).

Numerous research has shown conflicting results regarding AMH regulation by gonadotropins. Gonadotropins (particularly her FSH) inhibit normal ovarian serum AMH production in vivo (Baarends et al., 1995; Panidis et al., 2011). Recent studies have shown that FSH can directly influence one's AMH in small antral follicles unless it expresses aromatase (Pierre et al., 2013). However, in larger follicles, FSH has an indirect suppressive ability on AMH expression by the negative feedback of E2 and by means of increasing E2 production upon recruitment of dominant follicles (Figure 1) (Pellatt et al., 2007; Grynbaer et al., 2012; Pierre et al., 2013).

AMH is observed to positively influence the decrease of the FSH receptor expression but also ovarian aromatase expression (Pellatt et al., 2011). This can protect small follicles from premature aromatase expression. However, if this protective effect outweighs its pathophysiological role due to excess AMH and/or due to their persistence longer than it should in larger follicles, the selection of the dominant follicle becomes defective, leading to the so-called " It can lead to follicular arrest. Premature action of LH may also lead to 'follicular arrest' via mechanisms involving the AMH system (Willis et al., 1998; Jakimuki et al., 2001).

## 3. Assays for AMH

AMH is a hormone, part of the transforming growth factor beta family, and is produced exclusively in gonads. It is expressed by the granulosa cells of follicles growing independently of gonadotropins in the ovary (Cate et al., 1986; Weenen et al., 2004). AMH is usually released as a 140 kDa disulfide-linked homodimer (proAMH) (Cate et al., 1986). The activation of proAMH is generally done by proteolytic cleavage, resulting in a stable complex ($AMH_{N, C}$) composed of the N-terminal pro region ($AMH_N$) and the C-terminal mature region ($AMH_C$) (Nachtigal et al., 1996). $AMH_{N, C}$, and $AMH_C$ isoforms can bind to the AMH-specific type II receptor (AMHRII) and activate downstream SMAD signaling after binding to the AMH type I receptor (Mishina et al., 1999; Mullen et al., 2014). A second cleavage site, located at aa229 in the N-terminal pro region, further divides the $AMH_N$ region into two isoforms, the pro region, and the middle region ($AMH_{N,229}$ and $AMH_M$, respectively) (Pepinsky et al., 1988). Dimerization of $AMH_M$ and $AMH_C$ may lead to another potential isoform ($AMH_{M,\ C}$). Therefore, there are theoretically at least seven potential AMH isoforms that may be circulating (Moolhuijsen et al., 2020).

Simultaneously manual as well as automated tests were developed to assess serum AMH profiles, and different tests are utilized in therapeutic settings. These tests employ antibodies that target particular sites of AMH. The overall concentration of AMH in circulation is determined by the existence of particular AMH isoforms and the capacity of the antibodies used to identify these isoforms. Since there is no established standard for measuring AMH, there can be variations between tests. Nevertheless, AMH measurement is frequently used in clinical practice to keep track of ovarian reserve and predict ovarian response to stimulate during in vitro fertilization (IVF) treatment (Broer et al., 2014; Broer et al., 2009). PCOS is a type of heterogeneous disorder mostly observed in women of reproductive age and characterized by a combination of hyperandrogenism, ovulatory dysfunction, and PCOM (Bozdag et al., 2016; Naven et al., 2018; ESHRE 2004). AMH profiles are correlated with the follicular number and in PCOS this allows a significant increase in serum AMH levels (Laven et al., 2004; Pigny et al., 2003). Studies investigating the AMH threshold for the diagnosis of PCOS have established a wide range of values because of the heterogeneous diagnostic criteria, differences between tests, and the use of multiple AMH tests (Fraissinet et al., 2017).

Unlocking the secrets of female fertility just got easier! By determining the levels of the AMH, doctors can now assess a woman's ovarian egg reserves at any time during her menstrual cycle. What's more, AMH levels remain stable throughout the cycle, making it a reliable indicator. This test is particularly useful for women in their 40s or older, as AMH levels naturally decline with age. Conversely, women with PCOS tend to exhibit higher AMH levels. To diagnose PCOS, doctors usually rely on one of three commonly used AMH assays: the Gen II AMH Enzyme-Linked Immunosorbent Assay (ELISA) from Beckman Coulter, the picoAMH Assay from Ansh Labs, or the Elecsys AMH Plus Assay from Roche (Moolhuijsen et al., 2022).

### 3.1. Gen II AMH ELISA (Beckman Coulter)

The Human AMH Gen II ELISA Kit is a reliable and quantitative method for measuring anti-Müllerian hormone (AMH, AMH Gen II) in human serum and lithium plasma samples. The minimum sensitivity detection limit for this assay is 0.08 ng/mL. The dynamic range of this assay is 0.14–22.0 ng/mL. All reagents included in the kit should be stored at 2°C to 8°C. Unopened reagents retain reactivity until the expiration date. "Kit Contents – Micro-titer wells 12 x 8 (break apart) strips: Wells coated with AMH antigen; Standard 0-5: Lyophilized; Concentrations 0-22.0 ng/ml; Control Low and Control High; Enzyme Conjugate: Consisting of an antibody conjugated to horseradish peroxidase; Substrate Solution: Tetramethylbenzidine (TMB); Stop Solution: 0.5 M $H_2SO_4$; Avoid contact with the stop solution, It may cause skin irritations and burns; Wash Solution (40x Concentrated)" (Fraissinet et al., 2017).

### 3.2. PicoAMH Assay (Ansh Labs)

The pico AMH is a protein released by reproductive tissues. Its role and amount present vary by gender and age (Cate et al., 1986). The picoAMH ELISA, a quantitative 3-step sandwich immunoassay, uses the material for measuring ultra-low levels of her AMH in human serum. Low-end detection of AMH is necessary for many research applications such as the detection of AMH level reduction in gonadotoxicity, premature ovarian aging, carcinogenicity, primary ovarian failure, and menopause studies. The 96-well microplate is used and the sensitivity of the picoAMH assay is 2 pg/mL. The detection range is 7, 3.8 to 1091 pg/mL and the test time is 4.5 hours (Weenen et al., 2004).

### 3.3. Elecsys AMH Plus Assay (Roche)

The Elecsys AMH assay is an automatic test that measures the levels of AMH in human serum/plasma. This test, when combined with other clinical and laboratory results, can aid in the assessment of ovarian reserve. The test has high accuracy and sensitivity, a broad range of detection, and demonstrates a strong correlation with manual AMH testing and transvaginal ultrasound assessment of follicle count, with the added benefit of lower variability. Moreover, it has a shorter test time of 18 minutes, which is faster compared to other AMH tests (Deeks & Emma, 2015).

The Elecsys AMH assay uses monoclonal antibodies specific to AMH to perform a sandwich test. The test produces a pairing complex by binding endogenous AMH with both biotinylated and ruthenium complex-labeled AMH-specific monoclonal antibodies. The test results are determined by a specific instrument-generated calibration curve using two-point calibration, and a master curve is provided via the reagent bar code (Demirdjian et al., 2016).

## 4. Overexpression of AMH in PCOS Women

AMH overexpression in women with PCOS favors escalation of follicular grouping and androgen levels, causing follicular arrest and anovulation. In the ovaries of all species tested till date, AMH expression begins in the primary follicles, is maximum in the small and pre-cavernous follicles, decreases in the large, and becomes almost undetectable except in the cytoskeleton (reviewed in (Di Clemente et al., 2021)). Manifestations of AMH were not detected in the corpus luteum and atrial cyst.

High serum AMH levels in women with PCOS are because of an escalated number of small follicles, AMH expression – the main AMHR2-expressing organelle – and the effect of AMH in the gonads, mainly AMH produced by the gonads (big blue arrows). Organs that express AMHR2 (thin arrows) are placenta, mammary glands, uterus and ovaries in women, and Müller's ducts, prostate and testes in men. In the ovary, AMH inhibits aromatase, FSH-sensitive follicles, and follicular atrophy. In the testes, AMH inhibits steroid synthesis.

The altered responsiveness of GC to some hormones dysregulated in PCOS may lead to the overexpression of AMH and AMHR2. Thus, up-regulating androgens AMH mRNA profiles in vitro were only present in GCs from women with overexpressing PCOS androgen receptors, and there is widespread consensus that androgen and AMH profiles are correlated positively in people suffering from this disease except in ovulatory women (review in (Di Clemente et al., 2021)). Since AMH has proven to increase gonadotropin-releasing hormone (GnRH) -dependent on the volatility and secretion of LH (Cimino et al., 2016), its overexpression may add to this vicious circle (Refer to Figure 1).

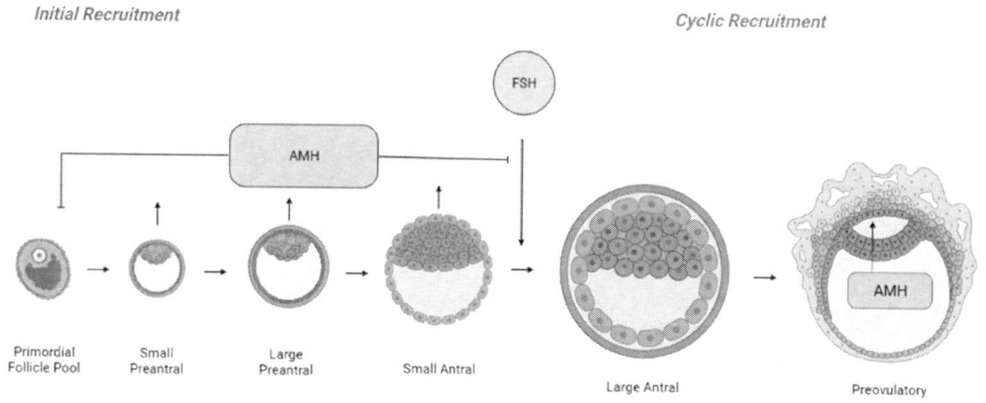


**Figure 1.** The role of AMH in the diagnosis of PCOS. Increased levels of AMH in women with PCOS are responsible for ovarian defects by affecting both the ovary and the hypothalamic-pituitary complex. Moreover, increased levels of AMH in pregnant women with PCOS may contribute to fetal hyperandrogenism by interfering with placental steroidogenesis.

## 5. The Function of AMH in Assessing the Ovarian Reserve and Follicular Development

There is a general consensus that AMH plays a critical function in selecting dominant follicles and promoting ovulation by regulating different phases of follicle development and influencing various cell types in the hypothalamic-pituitary-ovarian system. While AMH has been observed to inhibit primordial follicles in rodents, its effect on women remains controversial (as reviewed in (Di Clemente et al., 2021)). However, it is clear that AMH inhibits the differentiation of developing follicles at all stages of follicular formation by decreasing the expression of aromatase and LH receptor, two markers of GC, both in vitro and in vivo (Hayes et al., 2016). AMH downregulates FSH receptor expression, which may be responsible for its inhibitory role on GC sensitivity to FSH (Pellatt et al., 2011). AMH can also induce the expression of miR-181b, targeting adenylate cyclase 9, thereby reducing cAMP levels and leading to decreased FSH sensitivity and/or suppression of FSH signaling (Hayes et al., 2016).

Moreover, AMH protects follicles from atrophy by preventing GC apoptosis. This effect is incorporated by the fact that stenosis follicles lack AMH expression (Bezard et al., 1988) and mice without AMH have been proven to elevate the number of oocytes and atrial cysts (Visser et al., 2007). AMH treatment has been shown to reduce follicle counts in vivo and ex vivo (Hayes et al., 2016, Racine et al., 2021; Kong et al., 2016; Detti et al., 2018). In contrast, decreased AMH expression in monkey pre-cavernous follicles has a negative effect on follicular survival (Xu et al., 2018). At the physiological level concentrations, AMH has an anti-apoptotic effect on primary culture and cancer GC lines of mouse and human GCs (Racine et al., 2021; Dilaver et al., 2019). Research has demonstrated that AMH has the ability to control steroid production by cortical cells, as it can suppress androgen production in ovarian cortical cells in small developing follicles that have been stimulated by LH (Campbell et al., 2012).

Enhancing the result of AMH on follicular maturation could lead to an increase in its inhibitory effects on aromatase and FSH-related effects on the development of follicular dominance and selection, ultimately leading to follicular cessation. Additionally, the enhanced protective effect of AMH on cystic atrophy may contribute to an increased number of follicles in the cohort as well as AMH levels, followed by an exacerbation of the dominant follicle selection process. Simultaneously, an increased effect of AMH on follicle maturation and aromatase expression and on the other hand, GnRH and LH neuronal oscillations production may improve androgen levels in women with PCOS. Increased levels of androgen in these types of patients stimulate the growth of primordial and protective follicles, thus participating in the proliferation of the follicular cohort suitable for these effects of male hormones. All models of male hormone-induced PCOS show an increase in the number of developing follicles (Stener et al., 2020). In women with PCOS, the inhibitory effect of AMH on primordial follicle recruitment and androgen production by cortical cells (as reviewed in (Di Clemente et al., 2021)), if confirmed in humans, could be counterbalanced by the effects of androgens and LHs, respectively. Additionally, increased AMH levels can affect other reproductive organs in women with PCOS. Recent evidence shows that AMH may regulate sexual behavior through an impaired nitric oxide hypothalamic pathway in an AMH-treated rats PCOS model (Silva et al., 2022). Furthermore, the expression of AMHR2 in utero (Wang et al., 2009) and placenta (Tata et al., 2018) suggests that AMH may be associated with the observed pregnancy complications in women with PCOS, leading to abnormal gestational age and shoot up preterm birth delivery (Palomba et al., 2018).

There are 3 hypotheses to enumerate the role of AMH in ovarian reserve and follicular growth.

*Hypothesis 1:*

The decline in AMH at the end of the reproductive period stimulates an increase in the relative activation rate of primordial follicles. The increased activation rate results in a more rapidly depleted ovarian reserve but may allow the growing pool of follicles to remain large enough to support fertility for longer.

*Hypothesis 2:*

Recent studies suggest that women with low AMH levels at puberty have a greater chance of primordial follicle activation throughout their lives. Although the overall rate of activation remains low, the reduction in AMH levels may help these women maintain a healthy follicular source despite having a small ovarian reserve. These findings shed new light on the role of AMH in female reproductive health and offer hope to women with low AMH levels.

*Hypothesis 3:*

Women having more ovarian reserve during puberty possess extreme AMH levels and a correspondingly low rate of primordial follicle activation during the primary stages of reproductive life. Above a certain size, larger groups of growing follicles can produce diminishing returns on fertility. In these cases, females with large ovarian reserves can afford to inhibit the activation of primordial follicles to prolong their reproductive life while also producing large numbers of follicles. Eggs are developing enough to maintain high fertility.

## 6. Use of Serum AMH in the Diagnosis of PCOS

Age plays a crucial role in determining the risk of DOR and PCOS. As we age, the risk of PCOS drops while the risk of DOR increases. But why? The answer lies in the aging process that leads to a decrease in the number of follicles and AMH levels while increasing basal FSH levels. It's possible that PCOS may not be diagnosed in the elderly, leading to a reduced incidence (Practice Committee, 2015; No Committee Opinion, 2014).

Did you know that AMH and FSH levels are inversely correlated in PCOS? AMH can inhibit aromatase, decrease FSH levels, and reduce follicular sensitivity to FSH. This study highlights the link between high FSH levels and DOR risk, which is widely accepted. On the other hand, high LH levels are associated with an increased risk of PCOS, as AMH and LH work together in suppressing follicles (Pigny et al., 2003; Pellatt et al., 2010).

Age isn't just a number when it comes to fertility. Oocyte quantity and quality decrease as we age, making age a dominant factor in DOR. Aging leads to decreased follicles, AMH levels, and increased basal FSH levels, affecting follicular development and ovulation. The difficulty in diagnosing PCOS in the elderly could be why the risk of PCOS drops with increasing age (Cimino et al., 2016; Practice committee, 2015; Beltadze et al., 2015).

The relationship between AMH levels and follicle count has been a hot topic in medicine, and recent studies have delved into the correlation across different assay methods. The results showed a strong positive correlation between AMH levels and follicle count, with correlation values ranging from 0.57 to 0.62. While the correlation coefficients decreased from moderate to low values, the percentage of women without polycystic ovary syndrome (PCOM) was still remarkably low, especially in the high AMH level subgroup.

Aging also plays a significant role in AMH levels and follicle count, and it's been investigated whether the correlation between the two factors depends on age. The findings were astounding, as the overall correlation between AMH levels and follicle count remained similar across all age groups, regardless of the assay method used. This highlights the crucial role that AMH levels play in assessing fertility potential, as they get lower with age and eventually become undetectable after menopause.

Serum AMH assays have become a highly scrutinized topic in medicine due to their remarkable accuracy in indicating the number of antral follicles present in the ovaries. These assays are often conducted as a comparative study, revealing a significant difference in follicle types that contribute to PCOM within the PCOS population, despite a relatively narrow range in serum AMH levels. The subgroups within this population exhibit an altered expression of AMH, which correlates directly with the follicle count. For women with PCOS, knowledge of the exact number of follicles and AMH expression per follicle is critical, as these individuals are at a heightened risk for ovarian hyperstimulation syndrome (OHSS). Recent studies suggest that a high AMH level may indicate the presence of PCOM, but it does not necessarily reflect the total number of follicles in PCOS. Therefore, the standardization of AMH measurement is crucial to ensure the accurate interpretation of AMH values in medical practice (Mourad et al., 2017).

## 7. Function of AMH in PCOS-Related Gonadotropin Dysregulation

In the context of polycystic ovary syndrome (PCOS), the rise of anti-Müllerian hormone (AMH) levels is a hallmark feature. Multiple factors contribute to this phenomenon, including a higher count of small antral follicles in the ovaries, the simultaneous activation of multiple antral follicles, and increased AMH production per follicle. In fact, the production of AMH by granulosa cells in the polycystic ovary is a whopping 75 times higher than in healthy women. As a result, plasma AMH levels in PCOS patients soar to two to three times the average levels observed in healthy individuals. Additionally, it's noteworthy that the decline in AMH levels typically seen in healthy women after five years is delayed in those with PCOS (Wiweko et al., 2014).

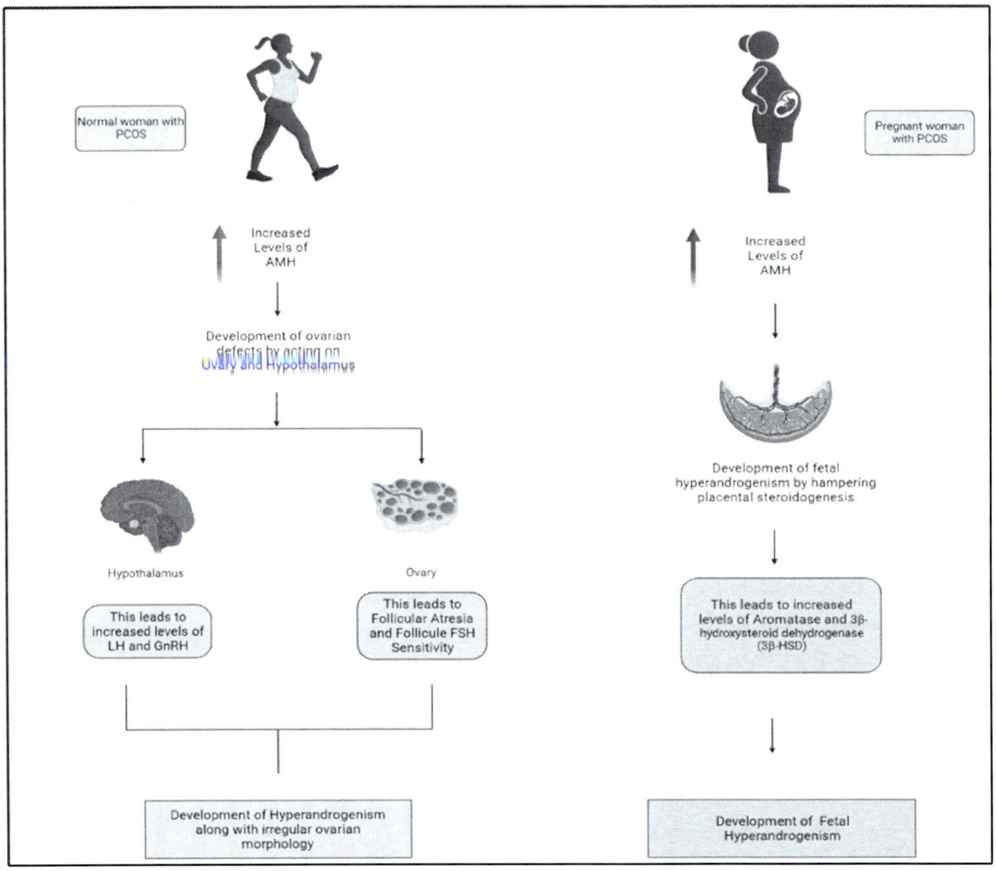


**Figure 2.** A schematic illustration of the actions of AMH in the ovary is presented. The granulosa cells of small growing follicles produce AMH, which inhibits follicle recruitment, as well as the growth and selection of preantral and small antral follicles that are dependent on FSH. Additionally, mature follicle cumulus cells maintain a high expression of AMH.

Gonadotropins (LH and FSH) are hormones released by the pituitary gland that stimulate the ovaries to produce oestrogen and progesterone. In PCOS, there is an imbalance in the gonadotropin feedback loop, which leads to overproduction of androgens (male sex hormones) by the ovaries. This leads to characteristic symptoms of PCOS such as irregular menstruation, hirsutism (excessive hair growth), and acne. AMH is thought to contribute to this dysregulation by suppressing follicle-stimulating hormone (FSH) production in the pituitary. FSH is essential for ovarian follicle development, and suppression of FSH by AMH leads to the accumulation of small immature follicles that are unable to mature or ovulate. This further increases AMH levels and sustains the cycle of gonadotropin dysregulation. AMH expression occurs after the follicle unfolds and continues through the antral phase of follicular development. It affects follicle growth by suppressing follicle-stimulating hormone (FSH) production and inhibiting aromatase-dependent FSH and luteinizing hormone (LH) receptor expression.

Patients with PCOS have barriers that prevent follicles from becoming dominant follicles. In addition to very low FSH levels, high AMH levels make follicles less sensitive to FSH (Refer to Figure 2). Therefore, follicles fail to develop into dominant follicles, and small antral follicles, 2–9 mm in diameter, accumulate. AMH also inhibited the activity of the aromatase enzyme, indicating that AMH contributed to the severity of PCOS (Wiweko et al., 2014).

Numerous studies have consistently suggested that AMH levels are positively correlated with luteinizing hormone (LH) levels in patients suffering from polycystic ovary syndrome (PCOS), independent of androgen and follicle-stimulating hormone (FSH) levels. However, some disagreement persists regarding this association. While in vitro studies have shown that LH can stimulate both AMH release and expression in luteinizing granulosa cells (GCs), in vivo studies indicate that AMH synthesis initiates in primary follicles before LHR release. Additionally, elevated GC expression slows down the luteinizing hormone receptor (LHR). Empirical research has also shown that AMH has extragonadal effects and stimulates GnRH neurons, as 50% of GnRH neurons in mice and adult humans have AMH type 2 receptors. Both in vivo and in vitro studies suggest that AMH stimulates the pulsatile release of GnRH-dependent LH through central action. Electrophysiological studies have demonstrated that exogenous AMH potentiates neural activity in GnRH neurons. Furthermore, AMHR2 is expressed in the hypothalamic region and is thought to synergistically regulate the synthesis and secretion of GnRH from neurons in the hypothalamus, which in turn controls the release of LH and FSH from the anterior pituitary.

Evidence also suggests that AMH affects pituitary levels and regulates gonadotropin function. The AMHR2 gene is activated by GnRH in both human and mouse gonadotropic cells. Aggregated data indicate that high frequency (1 pulse every 30 min) release of GnRH increases AMHR2 expression by gonadotropic cells, whereas low frequency (1 pulse every 2 h) does not appear to affect species like primates. However, the relationship between GnRH pulsatility and pituitary AMHR2 activation in humans, particularly in those with PCOS, remains unclear. Thus, it is challenging to establish a connection between the extragonadal effects of AMH and the pathophysiological development of PCOS.

Furthermore, individuals with PCOS often exhibit low levels of circulating FSH, alongside high LH levels, and this is often accompanied by certain changes in body composition, such as a high body mass index (BMI), low waist-to-height ratio (WHtR), and high waist circumference (WC) or waist-to-hip ratio (WHR). Another common characteristic observed in PCOS patients is the presence of small-diameter follicles in the ovaries. Although AMH is known to be related to PCOS, the association between AMH and FSH levels has not been established conclusively. Nevertheless, some studies have been conducted in this area. Congenital gonadotrophins can lead to decreased AMH levels, but these levels increase under the influence of exogenous FSH. Thus, the relationship between AMH and FSH is unclear and may vary depending on the disease state.

Overall, it is still uncertain whether AMH is responsible for the neuronal and hormonal dysregulation observed in PCOS. No human experiments have yet provided conclusive evidence to support this claim. However, GnRH pulse rate activation and elevated AMH levels have been associated with increased release of LH and decreased release of FSH, suggesting that AMH may contribute to hormonal dysregulation in PCOS. (Bhattacharya et al., 2022).

## 8. Role of Elevated AMH Levels in Reprogramming Fetus

The transforming growth factor (TGF) superfamily member, anti-Müllerian hormone (AMH), is employed in clinical settings as a marker for assessing ovarian reserve. Serum AMH levels were shown to be significantly 2-4-fold higher in PCOS patients, reflecting the increased stock of preantral and tiny antral follicles, and were positively correlated with total testosterone and free androgen index levels. Peripubertal daughters of PCOS women showed greater amounts of AMH, according to earlier research, corroborating the theory that the follicular changes that led to adult PCOS may have occurred early in the course of development. Also, compared to healthy controls, pregnant women with PCOS had greater serum AMH levels in the first trimester and during delivery, according to a small number of studies. Experiments on rodents, sheep, and primates supported the idea that a PCOS-like phenotype in children could be caused by excessive steroid exposure or AMH. A significant number of research findings have shown that the female ovary is "programmed" throughout fetal development and may subsequently result in PCOS. This vulnerability occurs during the differentiation of organs and systems (Zhou et al., 2022).

Initially, it was believed that AMH levels during pregnancy were consistently low in women without fertility issues, leading to the assumption that the same would hold true for those with PCOS. However, it was later discovered that lean pregnant women with PCOS actually exhibit markedly higher levels of circulating AMH compared to pregnant women with normal fertility. Further research comparing neonates born to healthy mothers with those born to mothers with PCOS also showed that AMH levels were significantly higher in the former group (Detti et al., 2019).

Laura et al. (2018) revealed fascinating insights into the impact of AMH serum levels on fetal development. Their research found non-significant increases in AMH serum levels in the umbilical artery across both genders. However, in female fetuses from PCOS mothers, higher AMH levels were discovered, potentially impeding Müllerian duct development and contributing to the emergence of milder forms of Müllerian anomalies, such as sub-septate uteri. This finding was combined with a heightened incidence of PCOS in women with sub-septate uteri, lending credibility to the notion that PCOS women with PCOS mothers are at greater risk of developing Müllerian anomalies. Elevated AMH concentrations could therefore delay or halt Müllerian duct fusion and inner wall reabsorption, influencing the final uterine fundus' shape and resulting in a bicornuate or sub-septate uterus. This ground-breaking research sheds new light on the intricate interplay between AMH and fetal development (Detti & Laura, 2014; Detti et al., 2017). The inheritance of PCOS and its effects on fetal development have been the subject of extensive research in recent years. Notably, Vanky et al. uncovered potential evidence that sheds new light on the genetic inheritance of PCOS and its impact on fetal development. Their research demonstrated that AMH can be detected in cord blood as early as

21 weeks of gestation, coinciding with the completion of Müllerian structure development. This finding was especially significant because it showed that women with PCOS have higher levels of AMH at delivery than those without the condition, with the female fetus being particularly susceptible to elevated AMH levels (Detti et al., 2017, Vanky et al., 2012).

The study conducted by Vanky et al. highlights the potential correlation between elevated levels of AMH in female fetuses and the development of Müllerian abnormalities in the uterine fundus. This finding sheds new light on the genetic inheritance of PCOS and the developmental differences observed in the offspring of PCOS women. Surprisingly, the research suggests that these differences may be attributed to genetic inheritance rather than the hormonal environment of the mother. These important insights could have significant implications for the future diagnosis and treatment of PCOS (Vanky et al., 2012).

Vanky et al.'s findings provide a new perspective on the underlying mechanisms of PCOS and fetal development, shedding light on a previously unexplored facet of this complex condition. These findings will be of significant interest to researchers, clinicians, and patients alike, as they deepen our understanding of PCOS and could potentially lead to new treatments and interventions (Vanky et al., 2012).

In a study, Tata et al. suggested that gestational hyperandrogenism, which is basically driven by MH, has significant implications for female offspring. Their research showed, "this condition triggers a masculinization of both the neonatal T and LH surge, leading to marked masculinization of the sexually dimorphic brain regions that regulate reproduction in female offspring" (Tata et al., 2018).

It turns out that by administering prenatal GnRH antagonists, the neonatal T and LH surges of PAMH female pups can be corrected, even before birth! This ground-breaking finding highlights the crucial role of in-utero programming in the development of PCOS and underscores the importance of early intervention.

Tata et al.'s findings have significant implications for our understanding of how gestational hyperandrogenism impacts the sexual development and reproductive health of female offspring. These insights may also pave the way for new interventions and treatments that can mitigate the effects of this condition and improve the health outcomes of affected individuals (Tata et al., 2018).

Exciting new research has shed light on the critical role of GnRH in the prenatal programming of polycystic ovary syndrome (PCOS). In a recent study, researchers found that co-treatment of AMH with the GnRH antagonist prevented the appearance of PCOS-like neuroendocrine traits in offspring. This discovery has significant implications for the development of new interventions and treatments for this debilitating condition.

The latest cutting-edge Nano-HPLC-HRMS analyses have revealed that peripherally-injected Cetrorelix (1.4 kDa) can effectively penetrate both maternal and fetal brains, opening up the exciting possibility of precisely targeting key neuroendocrine pathways. This breakthrough discovery has significant implications for the development of new treatments for a range of conditions, including PCOS.

Fascinatingly, the researchers made an intriguing discovery - recombinant AMH is unable to pass through the placental barrier. This suggests that the prenatal GnRH antagonist treatment's effectiveness in preventing PCOS-like traits in offspring is likely due to the normalization of the maternal HPG axis, rather than the direct effects of AMH. This finding underscores the intricate relationship between prenatal programming and maternal health and has important implications for the development of new PCOS treatments.

## 9. Future Prospects

There are several potential future research directions that could improve our understanding of the relationship between prenatal androgen exposure, AMH, and the development of PCOS in adulthood (Sloboda et al., 2011).

First, researchers could explore the epigenetic mechanisms by which prenatal androgen exposure leads to altered gene expression patterns in female fetuses. Epigenetic modifications can be passed down from generation to generation, and understanding how these modifications contribute to the development of PCOS could provide new avenues for prevention and treatment (Abbott et al., 1998).

Second, studies could investigate potential interventions to reduce the risk of PCOS in women who were exposed to high levels of androgens during fetal development. For example, researchers could explore the efficacy of anti-androgen medications in reducing the risk of PCOS in at-risk populations (Dumestic et al., 1997).

Third, researchers could investigate potential sex-specific differences in the programming effects of prenatal androgen exposure. While PCOS is a female-specific disorder, males may also be at risk of developing metabolic and reproductive abnormalities as a result of prenatal androgen exposure (Wu et al., 2014).

Fourth, researchers could explore potential biomarkers other than AMH that may be predictive of the development of PCOS in adulthood. Identifying other biomarkers could help identify individuals at high risk of developing PCOS and could aid in the development of targeted prevention and treatment strategies (Chen et al., 2016).

Overall, continued research into the programming effects of prenatal androgen exposure on the development of PCOS could have significant implications for preventing and treating this common endocrine disorder (Rosenfield & Robert, 2007).

## Conclusion

The potential association between PCOS and the anti-Mullerian hormone represents an intriguing field of study that sheds light on the origins of this multifaceted hormonal disorder. Although the exact mechanisms behind this connection are not yet fully understood, recent research has suggested that exposure to elevated levels of AMH during fetal development may increase the risk of developing PCOS in adulthood. By targeting the fetal environment through innovative interventions, such as reducing exposure to environmental toxins or providing maternal hormonal interventions, we may mitigate this risk and reduce the incidence of PCOS in women. Moreover, this chapter has highlighted the effectiveness of serum AMH in managing infertility, a common complication of PCOS. By measuring the levels of AMH, clinicians can monitor the number of actively growing follicles in the ovaries and adjust treatment plans accordingly. However, the lack of a global standard for the test of serum AMH poses challenges in its application. The book chapter has also explored the therapeutic effect of AMH in reprogramming the fetus, which suggests that this hormone may have a broader impact on reproductive medicine beyond the diagnosis and management of PCOS. The potential use of AMH in fetal development and the implications of this for reproductive medicine are exciting areas of research that require further exploration. As scientists continue to explore this topic, we can anticipate new and innovative approaches for preventing and treating PCOS, offering a promising outlook for millions of women affected by this condition. By unraveling the complex interplay between hormones and development, we may be able to uncover new treatment options that address the root causes of PCOS and improve the quality of life for those affected by this disorder.

## References

Abbott, David H., Daniel A. Dumesic, Joel R. Eisner, Ricki J. Colman, and Joseph W. Kemnitz. "Insights into the development of polycystic ovary syndrome (PCOS) from studies of prenatally androgenized female rhesus monkeys." *Trends in Endocrinology & Metabolism* 9, no. 2 (1998): 62-67.

Alebić, M. Š., N. Stojanović, A. Duhamel, and D. Dewailly. "The phenotypic diversity in per-follicle anti-Müllerian hormone production in polycystic ovary syndrome." *Human Reproduction* 30, no. 8 (2015): 1927-1933.

Azziz, Ricardo, Enrico Carmina, Didier Dewailly, Evanthia Diamanti-Kandarakis, Héctor F. Escobar-Morreale, Walter Futterweit, Onno E. Janssen, Richard S. Legro, Robert J. Norman, Ann E. Taylor, Selma F. Witchel;. "The Androgen Excess and PCOS Society criteria for the polycystic ovary syndrome: the complete task force report." *Fertility and sterility* 91, no. 2 (2009): 456-488.

Azziz, Ricardo. "Polycystic ovary syndrome." *Obstetrics & Gynecology* 132, no. 2 (2018): 321-336.

Baarends, Willy M., J. T. Uilenbroek, P. I. E. T. Kramer, J. W. Hoogerbrugge, E. C. Van Leeuwen, A. P. Themmen, and J. Anton Grootegoed. "Anti-müllerian hormone and anti-müllerian hormone type II receptor messenger ribonucleic acid expression in rat ovaries during postnatal development, the estrous cycle, and gonadotropin-induced follicle growth." *Endocrinology* 136, no. 11 (1995): 4951-4962.

Barrett, Emily S., Kathleen M. Hoeger, Sheela Sathyanarayana, David H. Abbott, J. Bruce Redmon, Ruby HN Nguyen, and Shanna H. Swan. "Anogenital distance in newborn daughters of women with polycystic ovary syndrome indicates fetal testosterone exposure." *Journal of developmental origins of health and disease* 9, no. 3 (2018): 307-314.

Beltadze, Ketevan, and Ludmila Barbakadze. "Ovarian reserve in women of late reproductive age by the method of treatment of PCOS." *Iranian Journal of Reproductive Medicine* 13, no. 5 (2015): 263.

Bézard, J., Vigier, B., Dien, T. R. A. N., Mauleon, P., & Josso, N. (1988). Anti-Müllerian hormone in sheep follicles. *Reproduction Nutrition Developpement*, *28*(4B), 1105-1112.

Bhattacharya, Koushik, Ishita Saha, Debanjana Sen, Chaitali Bose, Gargi Ray Chaudhuri, Sulagna Dutta, Pallav Sengupta, Soumita Bhattacharya, Sharit Shekhar Barman, and Alak Kumar Syamal. "Role of anti-Mullerian hormone in polycystic ovary syndrome." *Middle East Fertility Society Journal* 27, no. 1 (2022): 1-10.

Bozdag, Gurkan, Sezcan Mumusoglu, Dila Zengin, Erdem Karabulut, and Bulent Okan Yildiz. "The prevalence and phenotypic features of polycystic ovary syndrome: a systematic review and meta-analysis." *Human reproduction* 31, no. 12 (2016): 2841-2855.

Broer, Simone L., Ben Willem J. Mol, Dave Hendriks, and Frank JM Broekmans. "The role of antimullerian hormone in prediction of outcome after IVF: comparison with the antral follicle count." *Fertility and sterility* 91, no. 3 (2009): 705-714.

Broer, Simone L., Frank JM Broekmans, Joop SE Laven, and Bart CJM Fauser. "Anti-Müllerian hormone: ovarian reserve testing and its potential clinical implications." *Human reproduction update* 20, no. 5 (2014): 688-701.

Campbell, Bruce K., M. Clinton, and R. Webb. "The role of anti-Müllerian hormone (AMH) during follicle development in a monovulatory species (sheep)." *Endocrinology* 153, no. 9 (2012): 4533-4543.

Carlsen, SM1, E. Vanky, and R. Fleming. "Anti-Müllerian hormone concentrations in androgen-suppressed women with polycystic ovary syndrome." *Human Reproduction* 24, no. 7 (2009): 1732-1738.

Cate, R. L., R. J. Mattaliano, C. Hession, R. Tizard, N. M. Farber, A Cheung, E. G. Ninfa, A. Z. Frey, D. J. Gash, E. P. Chow, et al. "Isolation of the bovine and human genes for Müllerian inhibiting substance and expression of the human gene in animal cells." *Cell* 45, no. 5 (1986): 685-698.

Catteau-Jonard, Sophie, Soazik P. Jamin, Arnaud Leclerc, Jacques Gonzalès, Didier Dewailly, and Nathalie Di Clemente. "Anti-Mullerian hormone, its receptor, FSH receptor, and androgen receptor genes are overexpressed by granulosa cells from stimulated follicles in women with polycystic ovary syndrome." *The Journal of Clinical Endocrinology & Metabolism* 93, no. 11 (2008): 4456-4461.

Chen, Zi-Jiang, Yuhua Shi, Yun Sun, Bo Zhang, Xiaoyan Liang, Yunxia Cao, Jing Yang, Jiayin Liu, Daimin Wei, Ning Weng, Lifeng Tian, Cuifang Hao, Dongzi Yang, Feng Zhou, Juanzi Shi, Yongle Xu, Jing Li, Junhao Yan, Yingying Qin, Han Zhao, Heping Zhang and Richard S. Legro. "Fresh versus frozen embryos for infertility in the polycystic ovary syndrome." *N engl j med* 375 (2016): 523-533.

Cimino, Irene, Filippo Casoni, Xinhuai Liu, Andrea Messina, Jyoti Parkash, Soazik P Jamin, Sophie Catteau-Jonard, Francis Collier, Marc Baroncini, Didier Dewailly, Pascal Pigny, Mel Prescott, Rebecca Campbell, Allan E Herbison, Vincent Prevot, Paolo Giacobini. "Novel role for anti-Müllerian hormone in the regulation of GnRH neuron excitability and hormone secretion." *Nature communications* 7, no. 1 (2016): 10055.

Crisosto, Nicolás, Amanda Ladrón de Guevara, Bárbara Echiburú, Manuel Maliqueo, Gabriel Cavada, Ethel Codner, Francisco Paez, and Teresa Sir-Petermann. "Higher luteinizing hormone levels associated with antimüllerian hormone in postmenarchal daughters of women with polycystic ovary syndrome." *Fertility and sterility* 111, no. 2 (2019): 381-388.

Deeks, Emma D. "Elecsys® AMH assay: a review in anti-Müllerian hormone quantification and assessment of ovarian reserve." *Molecular diagnosis & therapy* 19 (2015): 245-249.

Demirdjian, Gaiane, Stephanie Bord, Caroline Lejeune, Ryan Masica, Dominique Rivière, Lucie Nicouleau, Philippe Denizot, and Pierre-Yves Marquet. "Performance characteristics of the Access AMH assay for the quantitative determination of anti-Müllerian hormone (AMH) levels on the Access* family of automated immunoassay systems." *Clinical Biochemistry* 49, no. 16-17 (2016): 1267-1273.

Detti, Laura, Holly Hickman, Roberto Levi D'Ancona, Alicia W. Wright, and Mary E. Christiansen. "Relevance of uterine subseptations: what length should warrant hysteroscopic resection?." *Journal of Ultrasound in Medicine* 36, no. 4 (2017): 757-765.

Detti, Laura, Mary E. Christiansen, Ludwig Francillon, Gini Ikuwezunma, Michael P. Diamond, Giancarlo Mari, and Ana M. Tobiasz. "Serum Anti-Müllerian hormone (AMH) in mothers with polycystic ovary syndrome (PCOS) and their term fetuses." *Systems biology in reproductive medicine* 65, no. 2 (2019): 147-154.

Detti, Laura, Nicole M. Fletcher, Ghassan M. Saed, Trevor W. Sweatman, Rebecca A. Uhlmann, Alberto Pappo, and Irene Peregrin-Alvarez. "Xenotransplantation of pre-pubertal ovarian cortex and prevention of follicle depletion with anti-Müllerian hormone (AMH)." *Journal of assisted reproduction and genetics* 35 (2018): 1831-1841.

Detti, Laura. "Ultrasound assessment of uterine cavity remodeling after surgical correction of subseptations." *American Journal of Obstetrics and Gynecology* 210, no. 3 (2014): 262-e1.

Di Clemente, Nathalie, Chrystèle Racine, Alice Pierre, and Joëlle Taieb. "Anti-Müllerian hormone in female reproduction." *Endocrine reviews* 42, no. 6 (2021): 753-782.

Di Clemente, Nathalie, Chrystèle Racine, and Rodolfo A. Rey. "Anti-Müllerian Hormone and Polycystic Ovary Syndrome in Women and Its Male Equivalent." *Biomedicines* 10, no. 10 (2022): 2506.

Dilaver, Nafi, Laura Pellatt, Ella Jameson, Michael Ogunjimi, Gul Bano, Roy Homburg, Helen D Mason, and Suman Rice. "The regulation and signalling of anti-Müllerian hormone in human granulosa cells: relevance to polycystic ovary syndrome." *Human Reproduction* 34, no. 12 (2019): 2467-2479.

Dumesic, Daniel A., David H. Abbott, Joel R. Eisner, and Robert W. Goy. "Prenatal exposure of female rhesus monkeys to testosterone propionate increases serum luteinizing hormone levels in adulthood." *Fertility and sterility* 67, no. 1 (1997): 155-163.

Dumesic, Daniel A., Luis R. Hoyos, Gregorio D. Chazenbalk, Rajanigandha Naik, Vasantha Padmanabhan, and David H. Abbott. "Mechanisms of intergenerational transmission of polycystic ovary syndrome." *Reproduction* (Cambridge, England) 159, no. 1 (2020): R1.

Dumont, Agathe, Geoffroy Robin, Sophie Catteau-Jonard, and Didier Dewailly. "Role of Anti-Müllerian Hormone in pathophysiology, diagnosis and treatment of Polycystic Ovary Syndrome: a review." *Reproductive Biology and Endocrinology* 13 (2015): 1-10.

Durlinger, A. L., M. J. Gruijters, P. Kramer, B. Karels, T. R. Kumar, M. M. Matzuk, U. M. Rose, F. H. de Jong, J. T. Uilenbroek, J. A. Grootegoed, A. P. Themmen. "Anti-Mullerian hormone attenuates the effects of FSH on follicle development in the mouse ovary." *Endocrinology* 142, no. 11 (2001): 4891-4899.

Eldar-Geva, Talia, Ehud J. Margalioth, Michael Gal, Avraham Ben-Chetrit, Nurit Algur, Edit Zylber-Haran, Baruch Brooks, Michael Huerta, and Irving M. Spitz. "Serum anti-Mullerian hormone levels during controlled ovarian hyperstimulation in women with polycystic ovaries with and without hyperandrogenism." *Human Reproduction* 20, no. 7 (2005): 1814-1819.

Escobar-Morreale, Héctor F. "Polycystic ovary syndrome: definition, aetiology, diagnosis and treatment." *Nature Reviews Endocrinology* 14, no. 5 (2018): 270-284.

ESHRE, The Rotterdam, and ASRM-Sponsored PCOS Consensus Workshop Group. "Revised 2003 consensus on diagnostic criteria and long-term health risks related to polycystic ovary syndrome." *Fertility and sterility* 81, no. 1 (2004): 19-25.

Fong, Sharon Lie, Izaäk Schipper, Frank H. de Jong, Axel PN Themmen, Jenny A. Visser, and Joop SE Laven. "Serum anti-Müllerian hormone and inhibin B concentrations are not useful predictors of ovarian response during ovulation induction treatment with recombinant follicle-stimulating hormone in women with polycystic ovary syndrome." *Fertility and sterility* 96, no. 2 (2011): 459-463.

Fraissinet, Alice, Geoffroy Robin, Pascal Pigny, Tiphaine Lefebvre, Sophie Catteau-Jonard, and Didier Dewailly. "Use of the serum anti-Müllerian hormone assay as a surrogate for polycystic ovarian morphology: impact on diagnosis and phenotypic classification of polycystic ovary syndrome." *Human Reproduction* 32, no. 8 (2017): 1716-1722.

Gilling-Smith, Carole, Debbie S. Willis, Richard W. Beard, and Stephen Franks. "Hypersecretion of androstenedione by isolated thecal cells from polycystic ovaries." *The Journal of Clinical Endocrinology & Metabolism* 79, no. 4 (1994): 1158-1165.

Grynberg, Michaël, Alice Pierre, Rodolfo Rey, Arnaud Leclerc, Nassim Arouche, Laetitia Hesters, Sophie Catteau-Jonard, René Frydman, Jean-Yves Picard, Renato Fanchin, Reiner Veitia, Nathalie di Clemente, Joëlle Taieb. "Differential regulation of ovarian anti-müllerian hormone (AMH) by estradiol through α- and β-estrogen receptors." *The Journal of Clinical Endocrinology & Metabolism* 97, no. 9 (2012): E1649-E1657.

Hayes, Emily, Vitaly Kushnir, Xiaoting Ma, Anindita Biswas, Hen Prizant, Norbert Gleicher, and Aritro Sen. "Intra-cellular mechanism of Anti-Müllerian hormone (AMH) in regulation of follicular development." *Molecular and cellular endocrinology* 433 (2016): 56-65.

Jakimiuk, Artur J., Stacy R. Weitsman, Alireza Navab, and Denis A. Magoffin. "Luteinizing hormone receptor, steroidogenesis acute regulatory protein, and steroidogenic enzyme messenger ribonucleic acids are overexpressed in thecal and granulosa cells from polycystic ovaries." *The Journal of Clinical Endocrinology & Metabolism* 86, no. 3 (2001): 1318-1323.

Kong, Hyun Sun, Seul Ki Kim, Jaewang Lee, Hye Won Youm, Jung Ryeol Lee, Chang Suk Suh, and Seok Hyun Kim. "Effect of exogenous anti-Müllerian hormone treatment on cryopreserved and transplanted mouse ovaries." *Reproductive sciences* 23, no. 1 (2016): 51-60.

Laven, Joop SE, Annemarie GMGJ Mulders, Jenny A. Visser, Axel P. Themmen, Frank H. De Jong, and Bart CJM Fauser. "Anti-Mullerian hormone serum concentrations in normoovulatory and anovulatory women of reproductive age." *The Journal of Clinical Endocrinology & Metabolism* 89, no. 1 (2004): 318-323.

Lie Fong, Sharon, J. A. Visser, C. K. Welt, Y. B. De Rijke, M. J. C. Eijkemans, F. J. Broekmans, Eva Maria Roes, W. H. M. Peters, A. C. S. Hokken-Koelega, B. C. J. M Fauser, A. P. N. Themmen, F. H. de Jong, I. Schipper, J. S. E. Laven. "Serum anti-müllerian hormone levels in healthy females: a nomogram ranging from infancy to adulthood." *The Journal of Clinical Endocrinology & Metabolism* 97, no. 12 (2012): 4650-4655.

Mishina, Yuji, Deanne J. Whitworth, Chrystèle Racine, and Richard R. Behringer. "High specificity of Mullerian-inhibiting substance signaling in vivo." *Endocrinology* 140, no. 5 (1999): 2084-2088.

Moolhuijsen, Loes ME, and Jenny A. Visser. "Anti-Müllerian hormone and ovarian reserve: update on assessing ovarian function." *The Journal of Clinical Endocrinology & Metabolism* 105, no. 11 (2020): 3361-3373.

Moolhuijsen, Loes ME, Yvonne V. Louwers, Joop SE Laven, and Jenny A. Visser. "Comparison of 3 Different AMH Assays With AMH Levels and Follicle Count in Women With Polycystic Ovary Syndrome." *The Journal of Clinical Endocrinology & Metabolism* 107, no. 9 (2022): e3714-e3722.

Mourad, Selma, Julie Brown, and Cindy Farquhar. "Interventions for the prevention of OHSS in ART cycles: an overview of Cochrane reviews." *Cochrane Database of Systematic Reviews* 1 (2017).

Mullen, Rachel D., and Richard R. Behringer. "Molecular genetics of Müllerian duct formation, regression and differentiation." *Sexual Development* 8, no. 5 (2014): 281-296.

Nachtigal, Mark W., and Holly A. Ingraham. "Bioactivation of Müllerian inhibiting substance during gonadal development by a kex2/subtilisin-like endoprotease." *Proceedings of the National Academy of Sciences* 93, no. 15 (1996): 7711-7716.

Neven, Adriana Catharina Helena, Joop Laven, Helena J. Teede, and Jacqueline A. Boyle. "A summary on polycystic ovary syndrome: diagnostic criteria, prevalence, clinical manifestations, and management according to the latest international guidelines." In *Seminars in reproductive medicine*, vol. 36, no. 01, pp. 005-012. Thieme Medical Publishers, 2018.

No, Committee Opinion. "Female age-related fertility decline." *Fertility and Sterility* 101, no. 3 (2014): 633-634.

Palomba, Stefano, Angela Falbo, Jessica Daolio, Francesco A. Battaglia, and Giovanni B. La Sala. "Pregnancy complications in infertile patients with polycystic ovary syndrome: updated evidence." *Minerva ginecologica* 70, no. 6 (2018): 754-760.

Palomba, Stefano, Angela Falbo, Jessica Daolio, Francesco A. Battaglia, and Giovanni B. La Sala. "Pregnancy complications in infertile patients with polycystic ovary syndrome: updated evidence." *Minerva ginecologica* 70, no. 6 (2018): 754-760.

Panidis, Dimitrios, Ilias Katsikis, Artemis Karkanaki, Athanasia Piouka, Anastasia K. Armeni, and Neoklis A. Georgopoulos. "Serum anti-Müllerian hormone (AMH) levels are differentially modulated by both serum gonadotropins and not only by serum follicle stimulating hormone (FSH) levels." *Medical Hypotheses* 77, no. 4 (2011): 649-653.

Pellatt, Laura, Laurine Hanna, Mark Brincat, Ray Galea, Henrietta Brain, Saffron Whitehead, and Helen Mason. "Granulosa cell production of anti-Mullerian hormone is increased in polycystic ovaries." *The Journal of Clinical Endocrinology & Metabolism* 92, no. 1 (2007): 240-245.

Pellatt, Laura, Laurine Hanna, Mark Brincat, Ray Galea, Henrietta Brain, Saffron Whitehead, and Helen Mason. "Granulosa cell production of anti-Mullerian hormone is increased in polycystic ovaries." *The Journal of Clinical Endocrinology & Metabolism* 92, no. 1 (2007): 240-245.

Pellatt, Laura, Suman Rice, and Helen D. Mason. "Anti-Müllerian hormone and polycystic ovary syndrome: a mountain too high?." *Reproduction* 139, no. 5 (2010): 825.

Pellatt, Laura, Suman Rice, Nafi Dilaver, Amira Heshri, Raymond Galea, Mark Brincat, Kristy Brown, Evan R. Simpson, and Helen D. Mason. "Anti-Müllerian hormone reduces follicle sensitivity to follicle-stimulating hormone in human granulosa cells." *Fertility and sterility* 96, no. 5 (2011): 1246-1251.

Pepinsky, R. Blake, Lesley K. Sinclair, E. Pingchang Chow, Robert J. Mattaliano, T. F. Manganaro, Patricia K. Donahoe, and Richard L. Cate. "Proteolytic processing of mullerian inhibiting substance produces a transforming growth factor-beta-like fragment." *Journal of Biological Chemistry* 263, no. 35 (1988): 18961-18964.

Pierre, Alice, Maëliss Peigné, Michaël Grynberg, Nassim Arouche, Joëlle Taieb, Laetitia Hesters, Jacques Gonzalès, Jean-Yves Picard, Didier Dewailly, Renato Fanchin, Sophie Catteau-Jonard, Nathalie di Clemente. "Loss of LH-induced down-regulation of anti-Müllerian hormone receptor expression may contribute to anovulation in women with polycystic ovary syndrome." *Human reproduction* 28, no. 3 (2013): 762-769.

Pigny, Pascal, Emilie Merlen, Yann Robert, Christine Cortet-Rudelli, Christine Decanter, Sophie Jonard, and Didier Dewailly. "Elevated serum level of anti-mullerian hormone in patients with polycystic ovary syndrome: relationship to the ovarian follicle excess and to the follicular arrest." *The Journal of Clinical Endocrinology & Metabolism* 88, no. 12 (2003): 5957-5962.

Practice Committee of the American Society for Reproductive Medicine. "Testing and interpreting measures of ovarian reserve: a committee opinion." *Fertility and sterility* 103, no. 3 (2015): e9-e17.

Racine, Chrystèle, Carine Genêt, Camille Bourgneuf, Charlotte Dupont, Florence Plisson-Petit, Julien Sarry, Christelle Hennequet-Antier, Corinne Vigouroux, Emmanuelle Mathieu d'Argent, Alice Pierre, Danielle Monniaux, Stéphane Fabre, Nathalie di Clemente. "New anti-Müllerian hormone target genes involved in granulosa cell survival in women with polycystic ovary syndrome." *The Journal of Clinical Endocrinology & Metabolism* 106, no. 3 (2021): e1271-e1289.

Rosenfield, Robert L. "Identifying children at risk for polycystic ovary syndrome." *The Journal of Clinical Endocrinology & Metabolism* 92, no. 3 (2007): 787-796.

Rzeszowska, Marzena, Agnieszka Leszcz, Lechosław Putowski, Magdalena Hałabiś, Joanna Tkaczuk-Włach, Jan Kotarski, and Grzegorz Polak. "Anti-Müllerian hormone: structure, properties and appliance." *Ginekologia polska* 87, no. 9 (2016).

Silva, Mauro SB, and Paolo Giacobini. "New insights into anti-Müllerian hormone role in the hypothalamic–pituitary–gonadal axis and neuroendocrine development." *Cellular and Molecular Life Sciences* 78, no. 1 (2021): 1-16.

Silva, Mauro SB, Laurine Decoster, Sara Trova, Nour EH Mimouni, Virginia Delli, Konstantina Chachlaki, Qiang Yu, Ulrich Boehm, Vincent Prevot, and Paolo Giacobini. "Female sexual behavior is disrupted in a preclinical mouse model of PCOS via an attenuated hypothalamic nitric oxide pathway." *Proceedings of the National Academy of Sciences* 119, no. 30 (2022): e2203503119.

Sloboda, Deborah M., Martha Hickey, and Roger Hart. "Reproduction in females: the role of the early life environment." *Human Reproduction Update* 17, no. 2 (2011): 210-227.

Stener-Victorin, Elisabet, Maria Manti, Romina Fornes, Sanjiv Risal, Haojiang Lu, and Anna Benrick. "Origins and impact of psychological traits in polycystic ovary syndrome." *Medical sciences* 7, no. 8 (2019): 86.

Stener-Victorin, Elisabet, Vasantha Padmanabhan, Kirsty A. Walters, Rebecca E. Campbell, Anna Benrick, Paolo Giacobini, Daniel A. Dumesic, and David H. Abbott. "Animal models to understand the etiology and pathophysiology of polycystic ovary syndrome." *Endocrine reviews* 41, no. 4 (2020): bnaa010.

Tata, Brooke, Nour El Houda Mimouni, Anne-Laure Barbotin, Samuel A. Malone, Anne Loyens, Pascal Pigny, Didier Dewailly, Sophie Catteau-Jonard, Inger Sundström-Poromaa, Terhi T. Piltonen, Federica Dal Bello, Claudio Medana, Vincent Prevot, Jerome Clasadonte, Paolo Giacobini. "Elevated prenatal anti-Müllerian hormone reprograms the fetus and induces polycystic ovary syndrome in adulthood." *Nature medicine* 24, no. 6 (2018): 834-846.

Teede, Helena J., Marie L. Misso, Michael F. Costello, Anuja Dokras, Joop Laven, Lisa Moran, Terhi Piltonen, and Robert J. Norman. "Recommendations from the international evidence-based guideline for the assessment and management of polycystic ovary syndrome." *Human reproduction* 33, no. 9 (2018): 1602-1618.

Teede, H., Misso, M., Tassone, E. C., Dewailly, D., Ng, E. H., Azziz, R., Norman, R. J., Andersen, M., Franks, S., Hoeger, K., Hutchison, S., Oberfield, S., Shah, D., Hohmann, F., Ottey, S., Dabadghao, P., & Laven, J. S. E. "Anti-Müllerian hormone in PCOS: a review informing international guidelines." *Trends in Endocrinology & Metabolism* 30, no. 7 (2019): 467-478.

Vanky, Eszter, and Sven Magnus Carlsen. "Androgens and antimüllerian hormone in mothers with polycystic ovary syndrome and their newborns." *Fertility and sterility* 97, no. 2 (2012): 509-515.

Villarroel, C., P. M. Merino, P. Lopez, F. C. Eyzaguirre, A. Van Velzen, G. Iniguez, and E. Codner. "Polycystic ovarian morphology in adolescents with regular menstrual cycles is associated with elevated anti-Müllerian hormone." *Human reproduction* 26, no. 10 (2011): 2861-2868.

Visser, Jenny A., Alexandra L. L. Durlinger, Isolde J. J. Peters, Edwin R. van den Heuvel, Ursula M. Rose, Piet Kramer, Frank H. de Jong, and Axel PN Themmen. "Increased oocyte degeneration and follicular atresia during the estrous cycle in anti-Mullerian hormone null mice." *Endocrinology* 148, no. 5 (2007): 2301-2308.

Wang, Jeff, Cary Dicken, Joyce W. Lustbader, and Drew V. Tortoriello. "Evidence for a Müllerian-inhibiting substance autocrine/paracrine system in adult human endometrium." *Fertility and sterility* 91, no. 4 (2009): 1195-1203.

Weenen, Christien, Joop S. E. Laven, Anne R. M. Von Bergh, Mark Cranfield, Nigel P. Groome, Jenny A. Visser, Piet Kramer, Bart C. J. M. Fauser, and Axel P. N. Themmen. "Anti-Müllerian hormone expression pattern in the human ovary: potential implications for initial and cyclic follicle recruitment." *MHR: Basic science of reproductive medicine* 10, no. 2 (2004): 77-83.

Willis, Debbie S., Hazel Watson, Helen D. Mason, Ray Galea, Mark Brincat, and Stephen Franks. "Premature response to luteinizing hormone of granulosa cells from anovulatory women with polycystic ovary syndrome: relevance to mechanism of anovulation." *The Journal of Clinical Endocrinology & Metabolism* 83, no. 11 (1998): 3984-3991.

Wiweko, Budi, Mila Maidarti, M. Dwi Priangga, Nadia Shafira, Darrell Fernando, Kanadi Sumapraja, Muharam Natadisastra, and Andon Hestiantoro. "Anti-mullerian hormone as a diagnostic and prognostic tool for PCOS patients." *Journal of assisted reproduction and genetics* 31 (2014): 1311-1316.

Wu, Sheng, Sara Divall, Amanda Nwaopara, Sally Radovick, Fredric Wondisford, CheMyong Ko, and Andrew Wolfe. "Obesity-induced infertility and hyperandrogenism are corrected by deletion of the insulin receptor in the ovarian theca cell." *Diabetes* 63, no. 4 (2014): 1270-1282.

Xu, Jing, Fuhua Xu, Maralee S. Lawson, Olena Y. Tkachenko, Alison Y. Ting, Christoph A. Kahl, Byung S. Park, Richard R. Stouffer, and Cecily V. Bishop. "Anti-Müllerian hormone is a survival factor and promotes the growth of rhesus macaque preantral follicles during matrix-free culture." *Biology of Reproduction* 98, no. 2 (2018): 197-207.

Zhou, Siyu, Danhua Lu, Shu Wen, Yongcheng Sheng, Deying Kang, and Liangzhi Xu. "Elevated Anti-Müllerian Hormone Levels in Newborns of Women with Polycystic Ovary Syndrome: a Systematic Review and Meta-analysis Based on Observational Studies." *Reproductive Sciences* 29, no. 1 (2022): 301-311.

# Chapter 10

# PCOS and Polymorphisms: The Role of Various Potential Genes

**Syed Douhath Yousuf**[1]
**Humira Jeelani**[2]
**and Mohammad Ashraf Ganie**[3,*]

[1]Department of Clinical Biochemistry, Sher-i-Kashmir Institute of Medical Sciences, SKIMS, Soura, Srinagar, Jammu and Kashmir, India
[2]Department of Biochemistry, Government Medical College, Srinagar, Jammu and Kashmir, India
[3]Department of Endocrinology, Sher-i-Kashmir Institute of Medical Sciences, SKIMS, Soura, Srinagar, Jammu and Kashmir, India

## Abstract

Polycystic ovary syndrome (PCOS) exhibits symptoms of hyperandrogenism, oligo anovulation, and polycystic ovarian morphology. Many aspects of this syndrome have significant long-term health effects that include obesity, insulin resistance (IR), glucose intolerance, infertility, and cardiovascular disease (CVD). PCOS is highly prevalent in females of reproductive age. PCOS has a multifactorial etiology, which has vital genetic and environmental components and has been proven to run in families. Many candidate genes have been identified, and polymorphisms in these have been implicated as predispositions to this disorder. In addition, genome-wide association studies (GWAS) were conducted to discover the genetic determinants of this disease. Genetic profiling could assist in determining which community inhabitants need to be assessed and treated with eradication therapy before permanent outcomes like infertility, type 2 diabetes (T2D), and CVD occur. A promising treatment for this disorder seems to be individualized medicine combined with targeted therapy. Studying the molecular causes of any disease's development ultimately aims to develop individualized treatments. The present chapter aims to provide updated information on the genetic changes studied in PCOS.

**Keywords:** genetics, single nucleotide polymorphism, GWAS, candidate genes, polycystic ovary syndrome

* Corresponding Author's Email: ashraf.endo@gmail.com.

In: Polycystic Ovarian Syndrome (PCOS) and Our Biological Clock
Editors: Arpita Roy, Gowhar Rashid and Nihad Ashraf Khan
ISBN: 979-8-89113-100-2
© 2023 Nova Science Publishers, Inc.

## 1. Introduction

The most prevalent hormonal disorder Polycystic ovary syndrome (PCOS) is affecting premenopausal women globally between 2-26%, i.e., 18 and 45 years of age (Jalilian et al., 2015; Teede et al., 2010). PCOS was initially identified by Stein and Leventhal in 1935 as a disease marked by obesity, hirsutism, and infertility and was named Stein Leventhal Syndrome after American gynecologist Irving F Stein, SR and Michael L. Leventhal (RS, 2009). However, due to its wide range of clinical and metabolic implications, PCOS has recently gained significant attention from various specialties.

### 1.1. Clinical Features/Signs and Symptoms

PCOS is a hypothalamic-pituitary condition characterized by abnormal gonadotropin [Follicle-stimulating hormone (FSH) and Luteinizing hormone (LH)] and androgen release, which disrupts normal hormonal signaling (Hall et al., 1998). Excess of androgens in PCOS is related to symptoms of oligo-amenorrhea, hirsutism, acne, and alopecia (Somani et al., 2008). Multiple follicles (cysts) grow on the ovaries due to abnormal gonadotrophin production, which is unable to mature and hence fails to stimulate ovulation. Polycystic ovaries (PCO) result from a buildup of tiny follicles with a diameter of 4 to 9 mm in the ovary. None of these small follicles can cause ovulation, resulting in oligomenorrhea or amenorrhea, which makes it difficult for PCOS women to conceive (Rebar et al., 1976). The development of cysts during an ultrasound scan cannot diagnose PCOS without the clinical symptoms of hyperandrogenism (Guzick, 2004). Due to the metabolic disorders connected with PCOS, such as hyperinsulinemia, dyslipidemia, obesity, and IR, and these women may be more susceptible to cardiovascular disease (CVD) (Apridonidze et al., 2005) (Figure 1). Hyperandrogenism caused by insulin resistance (IR) and hyperinsulinemic compensatory mechanisms stimulates ovarian androgen release and prevent the synthesis of sex hormone binding globulin (SHBG) (Diamanti-Kandarakis & Dunaif, 2012).

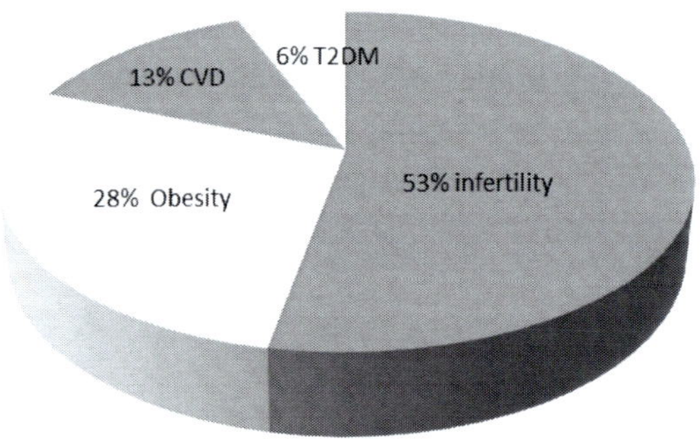


**Figure 1.** The long-term implications of PCOS are depicted in the Pie Chart.

### 1.2. Diagnosis

So far, to establish a PCOS diagnosis, numerous consensus conferences have been held. None of them have been able to resist a variety of validation methods. Table 1 shows three of the most common criteria for diagnosis of PCOS.

**Table 1.** Diagnostic criteria used to diagnose PCOS

| NIH /NICHD 1990 (Zawadzki, 1992) | Rotterdam 2004 ("Revised 2003 consensus on diagnostic criteria and long-term health risks related to polycystic ovary syndrome," 2004) | Androgen Excess Society 2006 (Azziz et al., 2006) |
|---|---|---|
| It consists of the following criteria<br>• Long-lasting anovulation.<br>• Hyperandrogenism | Includes two of the following criteria<br>• Oligo or anovulation<br>• Hyperandrogenism<br>• Polycystic ovarian morphology (PCOM) | It consists of the following criteria<br>• Biochemical and clinical evidence of hyperandrogenism.<br>• Dysfunction ovaries.<br>• Polycystic ovary morphology (PCOM). |

## 2. Etiology of PCOS

The PCOS etiology is a result of both environmental and genetic factors, including poor lifestyle and nutrition (Diamanti-Kandarakis et al., 2006) (Figure 2). Single nucleotide polymorphisms (SNPs) in candidate genes are among the genetic factors that contribute to PCOS etiology. Databases show that 241 gene variations contribute to the etiology of PCOS (Joseph et al., 2016). A polymorphism or other nucleotide alteration in a gene results in a deficiency in the transcriptional activity of that gene, which causes PCOS (Strachan & Read, 1999).

Ovarian dysfunction is caused by a metabolic disorder triggered by a gene mutation. All of the following polymorphisms have been connected to PCOS. These include FSHR, StAR, VDR, GnRHR, FTO, IR and IRS, and AR polymorphisms (Chen & Fang, 2018; Xita et al., 2002). When insulin and androgen levels increase, PCOS severity and progression worsen. Hyperinsulinemia damages theca cells of the ovary and elevates androgen levels. This condition causes the liver's production of SHBG and IGFBP-1 to decrease. Conversely, increased testosterone levels cause the visceral adipose tissue (VAT) to produce more free fatty acids (FFAs), which adds to IR (Shaikh et al., 2014).

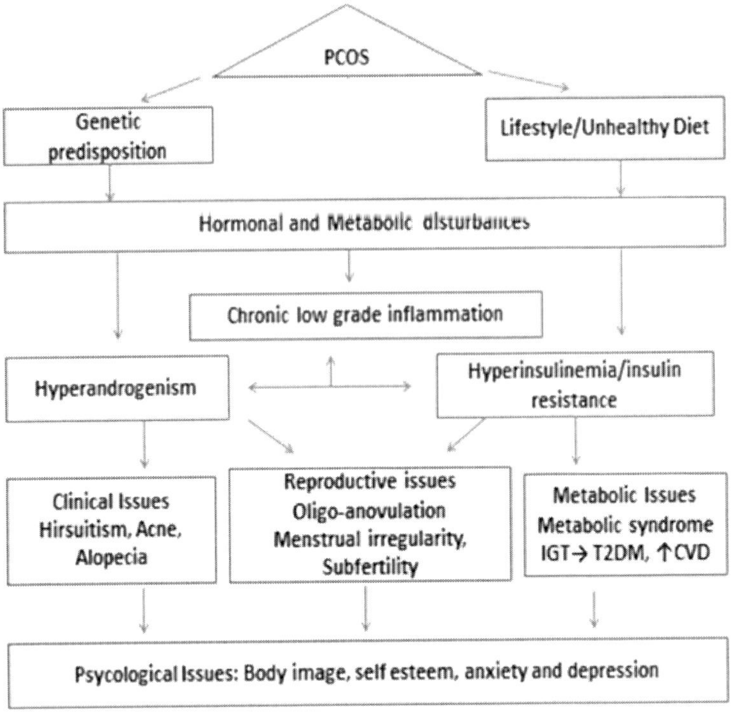


**Figure 2.** Possible mechanisms connected with the appearance of PCOS.

## 3. Candidate Gene Systematic Reviews and Genome-Wide Association Studies (GWAS): An Overview

PCOS has a high heritability factor. Relatives of PCOS females, both genders, are more likely to develop PCOS-related reproductive and metabolic diseases. The heredity of PCOS has been estimated to be 70% in monozygotic twins. As a result, some genetic changes appear to be involved in PCOS etiology. However, the heritability of human PCOS susceptibility loci discovered by GWAS is lower than 10%. Two types of genetic studies, GWAS and candidate gene investigations, complement each other. In this chapter, information on PCOS genetics from candidate gene systematic reviews and GWAS will be discussed in an organized manner.

### 3.1. Candidate Gene Systematic Reviews

For a better understanding of clinical implications, candidate gene studies are helpful in validating and elucidating the potential relevance of gene loci identified using GWAS. These findings suggest a method for discovering genetic variations that are causative or belong to a common causative haplotype.

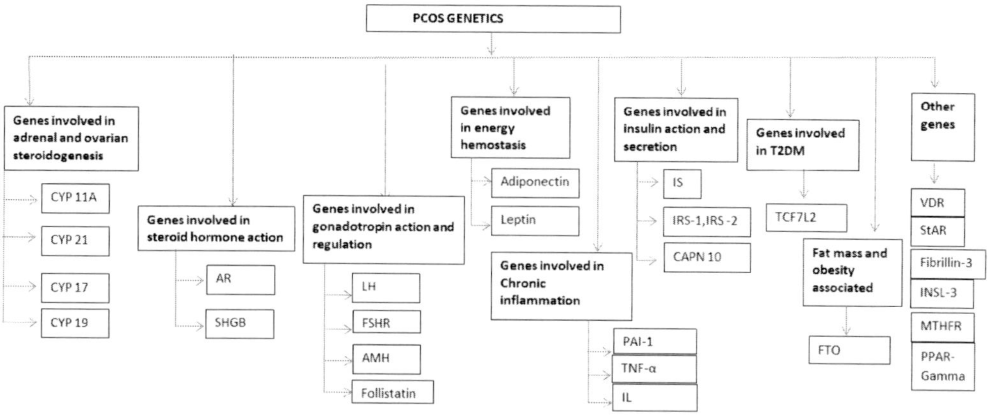


**Figure 3.** Key genes associated with PCOS.

Candidate gene studies do, however, have a number of basic drawbacks, like selection bias and sample size due to confounding factors like diagnostic criteria, ancestry, body mass index (BMI), and participant source. These can reduce statistical power and lead to inconsistent results. Hereditary and environmental factors contribute to PCOS. Many genes presented with altered expression, suggesting that the genetic mutations influence the signal transduction regulating pathway of steroidogenesis, gonadotrophin hormone control and action, action of steroidogenic hormones, energy balance, chronic inflammation, insulin action, and secretion, and other processes in PCOS (Figure 3).

## 3.2. Ovarian and Adrenal Gland Genes Involved in Steroidogenesis

### *3.2.1. CYP11A*

The CYP11a gene on 15q24 produces the P450 cytochrome side chain cleavage enzyme that promotes the formation of progesterone from cholesterol, the initial step in the process of steroidogenesis (Franks et al., 2000). Blood testosterone levels were observed to significantly correlate with the CYP11a gene alleles with a five untranslated region (UTR) made up of repeats of a (tttta) n pentanucleotide, known as a variable number tandem repeat (VNTR) polymorphism (Gharani et al., 1997). The results obtained were confirmed by two other case-control studies (Diamanti-Kandarakis et al., 2000; Wang et al., 2005) adding to the expanding body of evidence connecting CYP11a to PCOS. Further investigation, however, failed to uncover any proof of a connection between the VNTR alleles at this gene locus and PCOS. More investigation is required in order to establish that this gene is involved in causing PCOS in light of these contradictory results (Gaasenbeek et al., 2004; Tan & Zhu, 2005).

### *3.2.2. CYP21*

Another stage of steroidogenesis involves the 21-hydroxylase enzyme, which is produced by the CYP21 gene. It promotes the conversion of 17-hydroxyprogesterone (17 OHP) to 11-deoxycortisol. Congenital adrenal hyperplasia (CAH) mostly results due to a deficiency in this enzyme, and raised 17-OHP serum levels are connected with it (Azziz et al., 1995; Escobar-Morreale et al., 1994). A pattern resembling PCOS is present in patients with heterozygote

CYP21 mutations with clinical symptoms. CYP21 mutations have consequently been looked at as possible genes in PCOS patients. Children with early pubertal development and adolescent girls with hyperandrogenism were shown to have CYP21 heterozygous mutations in two studies (Witchel & Aston, 2000; Witchel et al., 1997). However, other studies found no evidence of a connection between the androgen excess and the CYP21 genotype (Escobar-Morreale et al., 1999; Glintborg et al., 2005). The onset of PCOS does not seem to be significantly influenced by CYP21 or its mutations.

#### *3.2.3. CYP17*

Pregnenolone and progesterone are converted by the P450c17 enzyme into 17-hydroxypregnenolone and 17-OHP, respectively, as well as dehydroepiandrosterone (DHEA) and 4-androstenedione. This enzyme, which is represented by CYP17 on chromosome 10q24, is active as both a 17,20-lyase and a 17-hydroxylase (Picado-Leonard & Miller, 1987). Increased P450c17 expression and enzymatic activity, as well as CYP17 promoter greater transactivation, was observed in ovarian theca cells of PCOS women (Escobar-Morreale et al., 1997). Additionally, the stability of CYP17 mRNA is dysregulated in PCOS theca cells (Wickenheisser et al., 2000). The promoter region of CYP17 rare T/C SNP was discovered to enhance the chance of developing PCOS (Carey et al., 1994). Since then, larger studies have not been able to definitively link connecting CYP17 to PCOS (Gharani et al., 1996; Techatraisak et al., 1997; Witchel et al., 1998). The post-translational regulation of the CYP17 gene product wasn't observed to be involved in PCOS pathophysiology, this gene product may have a function in the pathogenesis of the condition.

#### *3.2.4. CYP19*

The aromatase enzyme complex promotes the synthesis of estrogens from androgens. The cytochrome P450 aromatase and the NADPH cytochrome P450 reductase make up this enzyme complex (Simpson et al., 1994), and the CYP19 gene encodes P450 aromatase on chromosome 15p21.1 (Chen et al., 1988). Hyperandrogenic patients have been shown to have aromatase deficiency (Harada et al., 1992; Ito et al., 1993). Granulosa cells from follicles of PCOS-affected women were reported to exhibit low aromatase activity (Erickson et al., 1979). Likewise, it was discovered that compared to control follicles, follicles from PCOS women had lower P450 aromatase mRNA concentration, estrogen, and aromatase-stimulating bioactivity (Jakimiuk et al., 1998). These results suggest that the androgen excess that results from decreased aromatase activity in PCOS follicles may be a factor in abnormal follicle growth. PCOS symptoms and blood testosterone levels were linked by SNPs and haplotypes in association studies (Petry et al., 2005, 2006).

### 3.3. Genes Involved in Steroid Hormone Actions

#### *3.3.1. Androgen Receptor(AR) Gene*

All androgens interact with the androgen receptor, a member of the nuclear transcription factor family. The AR gene located at Xq11–12 codes for the three functional domains of the androgen receptor: the DNA-binding domain, the ligand–binding domain, and the transactivation domain (Lubahn et al., 1988). The repeats of CAG located on the exon-1 of AR have a VNTR polymorphism that produces a polyglutamine chain present in the N-terminal transactivation region (Carson-Jurica et al., 1990). The quantity of CAG repeats is negatively related to androgen receptor transcriptional activity (Chamberlain et al., 1994). Variations of these repeats have been connected to numerous disorders connected to low- or high-androgenic activity even within the usual polymorphism range (Dowsing et al., 1999; Prapas et al., 2009; Tut et al., 1997). Therefore, a decrease in CAG repeats along with an increase in androgen receptor function may help to understand some of the PCOS symptoms, including hyperandrogenism and normal serum testosterone levels (Mifsud et al., 2000).

However, focused investigations have not discovered a connection between this VNTR and PCOS. On the other hand, infertile PCOS women showed a considerably higher presence of alleles with longer CAG repeats than fertile PCOS women (Hickey et al., 2002; Mifsud et al., 2000; Urbanek et al., 1999). Finally, the AR gene couldn't act as a promising factor for the pathophysiology of PCOS.

### *3.3.2. Serum Sex Hormone-Binding Globulin (SHBG)*

Serum levels of SHBG are decreased in women with hyperandrogenism, mainly when PCOS is present (Pugeat et al., 1996). SHBG is a hepatocyte-produced homodimeric glycoprotein transcribed by a 4-kb gene located on chromosome 17p12-p13 (Selby, 1990). A pentanucleotide repeat polymorphism at the SHBG gene's promoter region affects the transcriptional activity of this gene. Researchers have therefore looked into the relationship between this polymorphism and PCOS as well as the relationship between polymorphic forms of the gene and blood SHBG levels in PCOS patients. According to reports, this polymorphism has a crucial connection to PCOS (Bérubé et al., 1990; Hogeveen et al., 2001; Xita et al., 2003).

SHBG levels were reduced in PCOS patients with more extended allele genotypes. Cousin et al., recently revealed that longer alleles were linked with reduced serum SHBG levels in women with hirsutism in comparison to six repeat alleles (Cousin et al., 2004). Even though Urbanek et al., reported no linkage or correlation between the PCOS and the marker around the locus. It is feasible to draw the conclusion that the SHBG gene may act as an important determinant in PCOS pathogenesis (Urbanek et al., 1999).

## 3.4. Genes Involved In Gonadotropin Action and Regulation

### *3.4.1. LH Receptor Gene*

The gene encoding the LH β-subunit is crucial for the specificity of LH and is thoroughly investigated in PCOS patients. At first, two-point mutations of LH-subunit genes namely Ilg15Thr and Trp8Arg were found to produce an aberrant type of LH (Furui et al., 1994). Moreover, these point mutations created structural changes in variant molecules of LH (v-LH)(Okuda et al., 1994), generating v-LH with higher *in-vitro* activity and a shorter half-life *in-vivo* than the nonmutant form (Haavisto et al., 1995). However, the *in-vivo* activity of v-LH couldn't be accounted for. After examining the function of v-LH, it was determined that there is a similar frequency of LH-subunit gene mutations between PCOS patients and healthy women (Rajkhowa et al., 1995). Further analysis within the subgroups demonstrated that obese PCOS women had raised incidence of v-LH heterozygous compared to obese healthy women (Rajkhowa et al., 1995). Further investigations, on the other hand, found no link between PCOS and the condition (Elter et al., 1999; Nilsson et al., 1997; Ramanujam et al., 1999). It was disproved that individuals with PCOS and normal serum LH levels but excessive androgen levels might develop hyperandrogenism due to an activating mutation in the LH receptor gene. Overall, it is unclear what purpose the v-LHs provide. In the case of female infertility or the etiology of PCOS, it doesn't seem to be necessary.

### *3.4.2. Follistatin*

The monomeric glycoprotein follistatin, which is generated by a single gene, functions as a high-affinity binding protein and is associated with activation. A transforming growth factor (TGF) family dimeric glycoprotein called activin promotes the release of the hormones FSH and insulin as well as the growth of ovarian follicles while inhibiting the ovarian androgen synthesis that is triggered by LH (Knight & Glister, 2001). Follistatin overexpression in transgenic mice decreased serum levels of FSH and stopped folliculogenesis in ovaries (Guo et al., 1998). As a result, increased follistatin neutralizes activin, lowering levels of FSH, delaying the maturation of follicles, increasing the production of androgen, and impairing the release of insulin. The gene encoding follistatin has been found as a possible important candidate gene in PCOS (Urbanek et al., 1999) given that each of these modifications is indicative of PCOS. Numerous studies have produced inconsistent results, and no clear association has yet been found (Calvo et al., 2001; Legro et al., 1998; Urbanek et al., 2000).

### *3.4.3. AMH*

The gene for AMH is positioned on chromosome 19 long arm at cytogenetic position 13.3. Five exons make up the gene, which produces a protein that contributes to infertility (Cate et al., 1986). AMH gene variants are related to PCOS. GWAS and whole exome sequencing have found several AMH gene variants as potent PCOS predictors (Gorsic et al., 2017).

### *3.4.4. Follicular Stimulating Hormone Receptor (FSHR)*

The FSHR plays a part in steroidogenesis, oocyte maturation, and follicle creation and is found on the granulosa cell's surface of ovarian tissue (Kim et al., 2017). A transmembrane, intracellular, and extracellular G-protein-coupled receptor with these three domains is known as the FSHR. The FSHR gene has a total of 9 introns and 10 exons and is found on chromosome 2p21 (Kim et al., 2017). There are only two known FSHR polymorphisms, both of which are present in exon 10 (p.Thr307Ala and p.Asn680Ser) (Layman et al., 1998; Simoni et al., 1997). Due to the altered receptor sensitivity, the variant allele p.Asn680Ser is linked to greater basal levels of FSH, prolonged menstrual cycles, and an increased threshold for induction of ovarian ovulation (Perez Mayorga et al., 2000). Several studies observed the connection between the FSHR genetic p.Thr307Ala and p.Asn680Ser polymorphisms and PCOS because disruption of follicular growth is the characteristic feature of PCOS. Results were frequently disputed and ambiguous. The TaqMan allelic discrimination test was utilized to genotype of 377 people with PCOS and 388 women without the condition. They found significant correlations between p.Thr307Ala and p.Asn680Ser polymorphisms and PCOS. Variable homozygote genetics may raise the risk of PCOS (Kim et al., 2017). However, these connections were not verified in two more studies using the same genotyping method (Fu et al., 2013; Perez Mayorga et al., 2000). To completely understand the FSHR gene variation effects on PCOS, more study is required.

## 3.5. Genes Involved in Insulin Action and Secretion

### *3.5.1. The Insulin Gene*

Through the use of receptors on theca cells, insulin also contributes to the synthesis of androgen (Nardo et al., 2008). The phosphoinositide 3-kinase/protein kinase B pathway, active in theca cells of PCOS women, causes this insulin action (Munir et al., 2004). A high insulin dose, like LH, boosts androgen production (Baillargeon & Carpentier, 2007). At 11p15.5, the INS is sandwiched between tyrosine hydroxylase and IGF-II (Kennedy et al., 1995). VNTR tandem repeat (Paquette et al., 1998) occupies the 5′ untranslated regions. The VNTR gene polymorphism controls the transcription rate of INS and IGF-II (Waterworth et al., 1997). There are between 26 and 200 VNTR repetitions. PCOS and this VNTR polymorphism are related (Goldfine, 1987).

### *3.5.2. INSR*

This gene codes for the two alpha and two beta chains that make up the turmeric protein. Numerous studies were conducted to determine whether there was a connection between obesity and infertility in obese PCOS women, but none were successful (Sorbara et al., 1994). Kashima et al., examined the INSR-associated tyrosine kinase domain-encoding area in women with PCOS (Kashima et al., 2013). The whole gene in PCOS women was studied to understand the molecular mechanism of insulin resistance (Diamanti-Kandarakis & Papavassiliou, 2006). In neither of these investigations, a relationship between PCOS and INSR was found. After searching the chromosome 19p13.2 region, D19S884 was found to have the highest relationship with PCOS (Urbanek et al., 2005). The INSR gene also belongs to this region of the chromosomal area.

### *3.5.3. Insulin Receptor Substrate Proteins*

The insulin binds to the receptor. When insulin attaches to the receptor, the receptor undergoes autophosphorylation and turns active. The INS receptor's tyrosine kinase activity then promotes IRS-1 and IRS-2 and promotes phosphorylation. The subsequent phase of the procedure uses these activated substrates. The association between PCOS and genes of IRS-2 and IRS-1 has been investigated in several ways. According to Petermann et al., PCOS women present with greater Arg972 IRS-1 frequency (Sir-Petermann et al., 2001). However, El Mkadem et al. observed no significant difference between PCOS women and controls (El Mkadem et al., 2001). Turkish PCOS women had a noticeably higher frequency of Gly972Arg IRS-1 polymorphism, reported by Dilek et al. (Dilek et al., 2005). Both connections and a lack of a relationship have been reported in reports. These distinctions highlight how the importance of racial and environmental factors.

### *3.5.4. Calpain-10*

The gene CAPN10, which contains 12 exons, is situated on the "q" arm of chromosome 2. This gene produces the heterodimeric protein calcium-dependent cysteine protease. This gene is related to type 1 diabetes mellitus (Sáez et al., 2008). A protein called Calpain 10 obstructs insulin synthesis and metabolism. Since PCOS is brought on by an insufficient insulin level, a Calpain 10 mutation also contributes to PCOS. CAPN10 is therefore a possible gene for PCOS (Ajmal et al., 2019).

### 3.6. Genes Involved in Energy Homeostasis

Adipocytokines are secretory chemicals produced by the adipose tissue which is an endocrine organ and a connective tissue, according to recent studies (Kershaw & Flier, 2004). Numerous genes linked to the most prevalent adipocytokines have been investigated as potential PCOS pathogens for the reason that many PCOS women are overweight, obese, or morbidly obese. Leptin gene sequencing was performed on a PCOS women group with a small number of participants, but no coding exon changes were discovered (Oksanen et al., 2000). The leptin receptor gene was also sequenced in this work. This showed exons 2, 4, and 12 had previously unidentified amino acid variants, as well as the 3-untranslated region had a pentanucleotide insertion (Oksanen et al., 2000). However, the allele frequencies of these polymorphisms were similar to those found in the general population.

Recent research has concentrated on G276T in intron two and in exon two of T45G. These polymorphisms were connected with the risk of obesity, diabetes mellitus, and IR (Hu et al., 2004; Menzaghi et al., 2002; Stumvoll et al., 2002). No correlation was reported between two frequent adiponectin gene polymorphisms and PCOS, in a study looking at the connection between PCOS and 15 chromosomal variants known to affect obesity, hyperinsulinemia, IR, and diabetes mellitus (San Millán et al., 2004). Panidis et al. investigated if PCOS might be associated with T45G adiponectin gene polymorphisms (Panidis et al., 2004). When the genotypes GG and TG were compared, a significant distinction between the groups was discovered (Xita et al., 2005). Also, it was discovered that in the PCOS group, G allele carriers had lower serum adiponectin levels (Xita et al., 2005). Recently, the possibility that the adiponectin gene's T45G and G276T polymorphisms are related to PCOS was disputed by two investigations (Escobar-Morreale et al., 2006). Finally, they appear to reflect PCOS severity in terms of heterogeneity of PCOS and metabolic abnormalities defects to PCOS. The adiponectin gene does not contribute directly to the etiology of PCOS.

### 3.7. Genes Involved in Chronic Inflammation

#### *3.7.1. Tumour Necrosis Factor (TNF)*

Adipose tissue produces tumor necrosis factor (TNF), a cytokine that contributes to insulin resistance (Hotamisligil et al., 1996). There is no evidence that the TNF-gene polymorphisms contribute to PCOS development. In one study, testosterone and 17-OHP levels were greater in carriers of the 308A allele both before and after GnRH stimulation (Escobar-Morreale et al., 2001). These results provide credence to the idea that the TNF gene polymorphism modifies phenotypes. It has been investigated whether other chronic inflammatory genes, such as IL-6, TNFR2 (type-2 TNF receptor) gene (Peral et al., 2002), IL-6 signal transducer glycoprotein (GP) 130, and IL-6 receptor genes, are related to PCOS. However, no notable outcomes have been discovered (Escobar-Morreale et al., 2003; Villuendas et al., 2002).

#### *3.7.2. Plasminogen Activator Inhibitor-1 (PAI-1)*

CVD in PCOS individuals is influenced by anomalies in pro-coagulation mechanisms and fibrinolytic pathways (Yildiz et al., 2002). Increased levels of PAI-1 are connected with a higher risk of thrombogenicity and CVD. Increased PAI-1 activity is observed in women with

PCOS (Legro, 2003). Greek PCOS women were studied to observe PAI-1 polymorphism significance in women with PCOS. 4G/5G polymorphism is connected with raised levels of PAI-1 and was found to be significant. It was reported that there is a greater frequency of 4G/5G polymorphism in PCOS than did controls. Furthermore, it has been found that PAI-1 concentration is greater in PCOS patients, and is further increased when 4G allele is present in the PAI-1 gene's promoter region (Diamanti-Kandarakis et al., 2004).

HSD3B2 (Nayak et al., 1998), 17-hydroxysteroid dehydrogenases (Moghrabi et al., 1998), dopamine receptor (Legro et al., 1995), IGF107, aldosterone synthetase (Zhao et al., 2003), glycogen synthetase (Rajkhowa et al., 1996), resistin (Urbanek et al., 2003), apoprotein E126 (Heinonen et al., 2001) have all been examined together with the above-stated genes. These findings were either debatable or lacked unambiguous conclusions.

### *3.7.3. IL-1β/IL-1Ra Gene Polymorphisms*

PCOS is a known inflammatory condition (Shorakae et al., 2015). Increased levels of inflammatory mediators in circulation, including chemokines, white blood cells, pro-inflammatory cytokines, and other endothelial inflammation markers, have been associated with PCOS(Jatzko & Ott, 2011; Papalou et al., 2015). Cytokines are thought to contribute to PCOS and are involved in inflammatory processes (Ebejer & Calleja-Agius, 2013). The pro-inflammatory cytokine IL-1, belonging to the IL-1 family of cytokines, has a profound effect on reproductive physiology. The regulation of fertilization, ovulation, tissue remodeling, and embryo implantation have all been linked to IL-1 (Prutsch et al., 2012). Another crucial IL-1 family member, IL-1RA, has the potential to lessen inflammation. There have been shown to be six distinct alleles of the IL-1Ra gene polymorphisms (Prutsch et al., 2012).

## 3.8. T2D-Related Genes

T2D and PCOS share many traits, including intricate genetic aspects with IR and compensatory hyperinsulinemia. PCOS is a risk factor for T2DM. The TCF7L2 gene plays a part in embryogenesis, cell proliferation, pancreatic islet formation, and optimal pancreas function. TCF7L2 SNPs rs12255372 and rs7903146 are associated with the onset of developing T2D (Grant et al., 2006; Groves et al., 2006). A small over-representation of the T allele of the TCF7L2 rs7903146 SNP was found in early studies of PCOS patients in Greece (Christopoulos et al., 2008). Later studies attempted to correlate these SNPs to PCOS but were unsuccessful (Barber et al., 2007; Liu et al., 2010; Tan et al., 2010).

The TCF7L2 rs7903146 C > T polymorphism, however, was strongly connected with an enhanced PCOS risk in Asian and Caucasian women, according to a meta-analysis study that included 2458 PCOS patients and 5109 control individuals (dominant model, OR = 1.40, 95% CI = 1.12-1.75, P = 0.003; allele model, OR = 1.33, 95% CI = 1.15-1.54, P=0.001) (Ben-Salem et al., 2014). Biyasheva et al. reported that two additional TCF7L2 sites, rs11196229, and rs11196236, migrated more than 100kb downstream, suggesting a high correlation with PCOS despite the fact that they did not identify a connection between these SNPs and PCOS. It is uncertain how much TCF7L2 contributes to the emergence of PCOS (Biyasheva et al., 2009).

#### *3.8.1. Fat Mass And Obesity-Associated (FTO) Genes*

In humans, chromosome 16q12.2 contains the FTO gene. This gene synthesizes a 2-oxoglutarate-dependent nucleic acid demethylase that is found in almost all tissues and is taking part in energy metabolism (Frayling et al., 2007; Hubacek et al., 2010; Willer et al., 2009). In 2007, a genome-wide association analysis linked the FTO gene to obesity and BMI (Demirci et al., 2010). Overweight or obesity affects more than half of PCOS patients, making it a common sign of the condition (Shi et al., 2007). Therefore, it is logical to believe that the FTO gene contributes to PCOS pathogenesis via BMI and/or obesity. A T-to-A alteration in PCOS women has been connected to a frequent SNP (rs9939609) in the FTO gene first intron, according to current research.

It is still unclear, nevertheless, whether PCOS is caused by FTO gene polymorphisms. A meta-analysis recently found that East Asians, not the overall population, are having a greater incidence of PCOS due to the FTO rs9939609 polymorphism (Cai et al., 2014). The FTO gene polymorphism namely rs9939609 A/T is connected with PCOS risk, and an allele may be an attributing factor to PCOS pathology, according to another meta-analysis of five studies encompassing 5010 PCOS women and 5300 healthy controls (Liu et al., 2017). Finding out the effects of the FTO gene polymorphism on PCOS development will be made easier with more participants in the study and the inclusion of various ethnic and geographical groups.

### 3.9. Other Genes

#### *3.9.1. StAR Polymorphisms*

Hyperandrogenism, which can impede the process of steroidogenesis, accounts for the majority of PCOS's etiology. The StAR protein controls the mitochondrial membrane's transport of cholesterol during the first stage of androgen synthesis (Barbar et al., 2009; Miller, 2007). According to evidence, androgen production may be an issue for PCOS patients, with StAR being a potential target. According to Kashar-Miller et al., raised StAR production or concentration may be the reason why some PCOS patients have greater levels of ovarian and adrenal androgen (Kahsar-Miller et al., 2001).

According to the researchers, StAR may be involved in the initial phases of androgen synthesis in PCOS. The gene for StAR is recognized as a potential gene for PCOS on the basis of the findings of this and other investigations (Jakubowski, 2005). The relationship between genetic variants of StAR and PCOS pathophysiology is still unclear. In a study involving 80 controls and 45 PCOS patients, seven polymorphisms in the StAR gene were reported using the polymerase chain reaction-restriction fragment length polymorphism (PCR-RFLP) method. The majority of the StAR gene polymorphisms were not connected to PCOS (Nazouri et al., 2015). According to the researchers, additional research into changes in active sites of amino acids and their effects on the biosynthesis of steroids might help to pinpoint the connection between StAR and PCOS. It may also be possible to pinpoint the precise roles played by StAR genetic variations in PCOS by using larger study populations.

#### *3.9.2. VDR Polymorphisms*

Nearly all tissues contain the DNA-binding transcription factor VDR (Reis et al., 2017). Many vitamin D-regulated genes are transcribed due to vitamin D's enhanced interaction with the retinoid X receptor and VDR (Haussler et al., 2011). Vitamin D levels are connected with PCOS severity and have a considerable impact on the metabolic pathways impacted by PCOS (Ogunkolade et al., 2002). Additionally, a number of PCOS symptoms have been associated with VDR polymorphisms. The PCR-RFLP method has been employed by numerous studies to investigate potential connections between these polymorphisms and the PCOS phenotype.

Mahmoudi et al., investigated the genetic frequency of the FokI, BsmI, TaqI VDR, and ApaI polymorphisms in Iranian women in good health and Iranian women with PCOS (Mahmoudi, 2009). The CC genotype in ApaI was linked to a greater incidence of PCOS risk. The greater prevalence of the C and CC TaqI genotypes in PCOS women was corroborated by El-Shal et al., (El-Shal et al., 2013).

However, Ranjzad et al., reported no significant change in ApaI between PCOS women and controls statistically (Ranjzad et al., 2012). Jedrzejuk et al., discovered no differences in the pattern of those polymorphisms between PCOS women and healthy women significantly using PCR and mini sequencing (Jedrzejuk et al., 2015). The disparities in data could be explained by ethnicity and the number of women with classic PCOS, but more research is needed.

### *3.9.3. MTHFR C677T Polymorphism*

Homocysteine is converted to methionine by MTHFR, which changes 5,10-methylenetetrahydrofolate to 5-methyltetrahydrofolate (Yamada et al., 2001). In young, superovulated rats, high folate consumption suppresses ovulation (Willmott et al., 1968). Insufficient folate caused the destruction of Graffian follicles in monkeys, and enhance in cystic and atretic follicles (Mohanty & Das, 1982). Clinical data demonstrate that PCOS women have greater than normal levels of homocysteine in humans, which can be reduced by taking folic acid supplements (Badawy et al., 2007).

According to the data, MTHFR is a promising candidate gene for PCOS. Acute leukemia, PCOS, neural tube abnormalities, Alzheimer's disease, and MTHFR polymorphisms have all been connected (Trimmer, 2013). Additionally, they influence the regulation pathway of homocysteine or reduced activity of the folate pathway. According to research, the MTHFR gene's variation C677T decreases the folate pathway's functionality by 50% (Cortese & Motti, 2001; McQuillan et al., 1999). However, few clinical studies produced equivalent findings, pointing to a connection between MTHFR and PCOS (Glueck et al., 1999; Sills et al., 2001).

Wang et al. reported a meta-analysis wherein C677T polymorphism of MTHFR and the risk of PCOS were studied. According to an analysis of 14 research that included 1478 PCOS cases from 16 different racial and ethnic groups, the MTHFR C667T variant had a variety of functions in PCOS risk in different racial and ethnic groups. The T allele was discovered to have a protective effect in Caucasians, a higher incidence of PCOS in Asians, and no significant associations in Middle Easterners (Wang et al., 2017).

### *3.9.4. Peroxisome Proliferator-Activated Receptor Gamma (PPAR-γ) Polymorphism*

IR is one of the most common metabolic problems, and there are some links between PCOS and hormonal and metabolic ailments (Farrell & Antoni, 2010). The PPAR-γ gene controls lipid metabolism and insulin sensitivity (Auwerx, 1999). The gene product PPAR-γ is essential for managing insulin sensitivity and energy storage due to its functions in lipid metabolism and glucose regulation (Auwerx, 1999).

Wang et al., observed the relationship between PPARγ-1 alpha and PPAR γ gene polymorphisms and PCOS in 201 PCOS women belonging to the Chinese Han population and 147 healthy women (Wang et al., 2007). The data reported no association between these gene variations and the PCOS risk. In 2010, a meta-analysis examined the association between PCOS and the Pro12Ala polymorphism of PPAR γ (Tang et al., 2012).

There was no proof of a connection between Pro12Ala gene polymorphism and PCOS, as per the findings of 13 meta-analysis studies encompassing 1598 PCOS women and 1881 healthy controls. Polymorphic allele genetic frequency was reported to be significantly greater in PCOS women than controls in a recent research study wherein PPARG Pro12Ala polymorphism was studied in PCOS, indicating that the polymorphism may have a role in predisposing to PCOS risk (Zaki et al., 2017).

### *3.9.5. SRD5A2 and SRD5A1*

On chromosome 2p23.1, there is a gene called SRD5A2. In 1999, Jakimiuk et al. reported that PCOS-affected women had raised SRD5A activity than non-PCOS-affected individuals (Jakimiuk et al., 1999). Later in 2006, the PCOS susceptibility of hirsutism patients was compared between SRD5A2 and SRD5A1, and it was found that the SRD5A2 variant is connected with PCOS protection, whereas SRD5A1 variants were connected with the development of hirsutism and consequently with PCOS risk (Goodarzi et al., 2006).

### *3.9.6. HSD17B5 gene*

The 17 b-hydroxysteroid dehydrogenase type 5 enzyme is encoded by HSD17B5 (HSD17B5). The enzyme helps to produce testosterone from androstenedione in theca cells, adrenal glands, and ovarian cells, which are the sites of testosterone production in women. It also lowers androstenedione in theca cells, adrenals, and ovarian cells (Goodarzi et al., 2008; Ju et al., 2015). It is an important gene for the investigation of PCOS-related hyperandrogenemia. When Qin et al., looked at the prevalence of the polymorphism in the promoter area in a group of PCOS-afflicted women from various ethnic backgrounds, they found it. Qin et al., claim that the gene modifies testosterone synthesis, which has a significant effect on plasma testosterone levels. Despite having an impact on testosterone levels, the intronic polymorphism rs12529 has no association with PCOS risk (Qin et al., 2006). On the other side, rs1937845 enhances predisposition to PCOS by increasing the concentration of testosterone and the HOMA index, which measures b-cell activity in a homeostasis model (Ju et al., 2015). The Aldo-keto reductase superfamily consists of several multifunctional enzymes with various substrate specializations and tissue-specific expression profiles, including HSD17B5 as a member (Qin et al., 2006).

### *3.9.7. INSL3 Gene*

An important peptide hormone from the relaxin-insulin family that moves through the bloodstream is called insulin-like factor 3 (INSL3). In males, it is synthesized by the Leydig cells in the testes. The corpus luteum and thecal cells of the ovary contain insulin-like factor 3. INSL3-RXFP2 role in sustaining androgen synthesis by ovarian theca cells was documented by Glister et al. There have been reports of increased INSL3 levels in PCOS women (Glister et al., 2013). An important character in the etiology of PCOS is played by ovarian steroidogenesis, which is tightly regulated by INSL3 polymorphisms. Region polymorphisms and the rs6543

SNP affect hyperandrogenemia traits and metabolic disorders in both controls and women with PCOS, depending on the physiological state (Shaikh et al., 2016).

**Table 2.** Genome-Wide Association Studies (GWAS) identified SNPs in Polycystic Ovary Syndrome (PCOS). NIH, National Institute of Health

| Study | Diagnostic Criteria | Gene Locus | SNPs | Nearest Gene |
|---|---|---|---|---|
| Chen et al., 2011 | Rotterdam | 2p16.3 | rs13405728<br>rs12468394 | LHCGR, STON1-GTF2A1L |
| | | 2p21 | rs13429458<br>rs12478601 | THADA |
| | | 9q33.3 | rs10818854<br>rs2479106<br>rs10986105 | DENND1A |
| | | 2p16.3 | rs13405728 | LHCGR, STON1-GTF2A1L |
| Shi et al., 2012 | Rotterdam | 2p16.3 | rs2268361<br>rs2349415 | FSHR |
| | | 2p21 | rs12468394<br>rs13429458<br>rs12478601 | THADA |
| | | 9q33.3 | rs10818854<br>rs2479106<br>rs10986105 | DENND1A |
| | | 9q22.32 | rs4385527<br>rs3802457 | C9orf3 |
| | | 11q22.1 | rs18974116 | YAP1 |
| | | 12q13.2 | rs705702 | RAB5B, SUOX |
| | | 12q14.3 | rs2272046 | HMGA2 |
| | | 16q12.1 | rs4784165 | TOX3 |
| | | 19p13.3 | rs2059807 | INSR |
| | | 20q13.2 | rs6022786 | SUMO1P1 |
| Lee et al., 2015 | Rotterdam | 8q24.2 | rs10505648 | KHDRBS3, LINC02055 |
| Hwang et al., 2012 | Rotterdam | 12p12.2 | rs10841843<br>rs6487237<br>rs7485509 | GYS2 |
| Hayes et al., 2015 | NIH | 8p32.1 | rs804279 | GATA4, NEIL2 |
| | | 9q22.32 | rs10993397 | C9orf3 |
| | | 11p14.1 | rs11031006 | ARL14EP, FSHB |
| Day et al., 2015 | NIH | 2q.34 | rs1351592 | ERBB4 |
| | | 11q22.1 | rs11225154 | YAP1 |
| | | 2q21 2q21 | rs7563201 | THADA |
| | | 11p14.1 | rs11031006 | FSHB |
| | | 5q31.1 | rs13164856 | RAD50 |
| | | 12q21.2 | rs1275468 | KRR1 |

### 3.9.8. Fibrillin-3 (FBN3) Genes

D19S884 the microsatellite marker found in the FBN3 gene at the intron 55 has been previously connected to PCOS and INS (Ewens et al., 2010). Fibrillins regulate TGF bioactivity, which promotes collagen production and fibroblast replication. Enlargement in the ovarian cortex and raised stromal collagen in PCOS could be explained by a fibrillin deficit. Contrarily, Prodoehl, et al., reported no appreciable variation between 173 PCOS women and 194 healthy controls in the frequency of the microsatellite D19S884 (Prodoehl et al., 2009). The microsatellite

D19S884 allele 7 distribution was found to be significantly correlated in a case-control study with PCOS in Han Chinese women with PCOS and healthy controls, whereas allele 8 was connected with increased susceptibility to PCOS (Xie et al., 2013). The relationship between FBN3 and PCOS is still unknown.

### 3.10. Genome-Wide Association Studies (GWAS)

GWAS investigates relationships between widespread genetic variations and the trait or disease in the absence of a preconceived hypothesis regarding the potential role of genetic variants in pathophysiology. The idea that GWAS pinpoints particular genes is a common misunderstanding. They offer information on a part of the genome (gene loci) that is closely related to the trait. If the identified gene loci are located in or close to a gene, they may directly affect how that gene functions. Alternatively, they may act as a regulator for genes upstream or downstream. Therefore, GWAS-identified genomic regions offer great a priori candidate genes to investigate.

To identify gene loci connected with the risk of PCOS, six GWAS were conducted. 19 different genetic loci in or close to known PCOS genes were identified by GWAS investigations in Korean, European, and Chinese populations (Chen et al., 2011; Day et al., 2018; Day et al., 2015; Hayes et al., 2015; Shi et al., 2012). According to local ancestry genetic analysis, two GWAS were conducted on women from both North and South Han Chinese ancestry, (Chen et al., 2011; Shi et al., 2012), two on women of Korean ancestry (Hwang et al., 2012; Lee et al., 2015), and two in women of European ancestry (Day et al., 2018, Hayes et al., 2015).

In women of European heritage, just one GWAS meta-analysis has been conducted (Day et al., 2018). Three biogeographical ancestries—Han Chinese, European, and Korean —have each had one or more genetic loci that have been related with enhanced risk of PCOS. People of European and Han Chinese ancestry share eleven of the 19 loci. Table 2 provides a summary of the findings from the six GWAS. The SNPs observed in the meta-analysis, which included three analyses and three unique loci, are summarized in Table 3 (Day et al., 2018).

**Table 3.** SNPs were identified from a GWAS meta-analysis in women of European biogeographical ancestry

| Study | Diagnostic Criteria | Gene Locus | SNPs | Nearest Gene |
|---|---|---|---|---|
| Day et al., 2018 | Rotterdam | 2q21 | rs7563201 | THADA * |
| | | 2q.34 | rs2178575 | ERBB4 |
| | | 5q31.1 | rs13164856 | IRF1/RAD50 |
| | | 8p32.1 | rs804279 | GATA4/NEIL2 |
| | | 9p24.1 | rs10739076 | PLGRKT |
| | | 9q22.32 | rs7864171 | C9orf3 * |
| | | 9q33.3 | rs9696009 | DENND1A * |
| | NIH | 11p14.1 | rs11031005 | ARL14EP/FSHB |
| | | 11q22.1 | rs11225154 | YAP1 * |
| | | 11q23.2 | rs1784692 | ZBTB16 |
| | | 12q13.2 | rs2271194 | ERBB3/RAB5B |
| | | 12q21.2 | rs1795379 | KRR1 |
| | | 16q12.1 | rs8043701 | TOX3 * |
| | | 20q11.21 | rs853854 | MAPRE1 |

* Gene loci that have been found in common in women of Han Chinese ancestry.

## Conclusion

PCOS is a multifactorial, heterogeneous, and complex disorder. It is difficult to understand the underlying pathophysiological mechanisms of this syndrome and to tackle the consequences of female fertility is very challenging. The clinical manifestations seen in PCOS are diverse which indicates that multiple factors are involved in the etiology of this syndrome. A number of genetic factors (candidate genes) together with environmental factors like lifestyle changes, obesity, and disruptors of hormonal and metabolic parameters lead to PCOS development throughout life. Recent genetic studies, particularly the GWAS together with the confirmatory studies, are being carried to document the association of candidate genes in causing PCOS. These studies are aimed to improve the diagnostics of PCOS and develop treatment strategies for PCOS women. The wider genetic landscape in PCOS was explained in this chapter, and the most relevant candidate genes associated with the risk of PCOS have been discussed. The findings obtained from the recent GWAS on PCOS have been reported. A clear description of many genetic studies and susceptibility towards PCOS is provided in detail.

## Future Perspective

Individualized medicine combined with targeted therapy seems to be a viable option for the treatment of this disorder. Molecular profiling could help identify the populations needed to be evaluated and treated before permanent effects like infertility, T2D, and CVD occur. The ultimate aim of studying the genetics of any disease is to develop individualized treatments. Nevertheless, more research is warranted in the future to elucidate the role of genetic changes in the pathogenesis of PCOS.

## References

Ajmal, N., Khan, S. Z., & Shaikh, R. (2019). Polycystic ovary syndrome (PCOS) and genetic predisposition: A review article. *Eur J Obstet Gynecol Reprod Biol X*, *3*, 100060. https://doi.org/10.1016/j.eurox.2019.100060.

Apridonidze, T., Essah, P. A., Iuorno, M. J., & Nestler, J. E. (2005). Prevalence and characteristics of the metabolic syndrome in women with polycystic ovary syndrome. *J Clin Endocrinol Metab*, *90*(4), 1929-1935. https://doi.org/10.1210/jc.2004-104

Auwerx, J. (1999). PPARgamma, the ultimate thrifty gene. *Diabetologia*, *42*(9), 1033-1049. https://doi.org/10.1007/s001250051268.

Azziz, R., Bradley, E. L., Jr., Potter, H. D., & Boots, L. R. (1995). Adrenal androgen excess in women: lack of a role for 17-hydroxylase and 17,20-lyase dysregulation. *J Clin Endocrinol Metab*, *80*(2), 400-405. https://doi.org/10.1210/jcem.80.2.7852496.

Azziz, R., Carmina, E., Dewailly, D., Diamanti-Kandarakis, E., Escobar-Morreale, H. F., Futterweit, W., Janssen, O. E., Legro, R. S., Norman, R. J., Taylor, A. E., & Witchel, S. F. (2006). Positions statement: criteria for defining polycystic ovary syndrome as a predominantly hyperandrogenic syndrome: an Androgen Excess Society guideline. *J Clin Endocrinol Metab*, *91*(11), 4237-4245. https://doi.org/10.1210/jc.2006-0178.

Badawy, A., State, O., El Gawad, S. S. A., & El Aziz, O. A. (2007). Plasma homocysteine and polycystic ovary syndrome: the missed link. *Eur J Obstet Gynecol Reprod Biol*, *131*(1), 68-72. https://doi.org/10.1016/j.ejogrb.2006.10.015.

Baillargeon, J. P., & Carpentier, A. (2007). Role of insulin in the hyperandrogenemia of lean women with polycystic ovary syndrome and normal insulin sensitivity. *Fertil Steril*, *88*(4), 886-893. https://doi.org/10.1016/j.fertnstert.2006.12.055.

Barbar, E., Lehoux, J. G., & Lavigne, P. (2009). Toward the NMR structure of StAR. *Mol Cell Endocrinol*, *300*(1-2), 89-93. https://doi.org/10.1016/j.mce.2008.12.007.

Barber, T. M., Bennett, A. J., Groves, C. J., Sovio, U., Ruokonen, A., Martikainen, H., Pouta, A., Hartikainen, A. L., Elliott, P., Wass, J. A., Järvelin, M. R., Zeggini, E., Franks, S., & McCarthy, M. I. (2007). Disparate genetic influences on polycystic ovary syndrome (PCOS) and type 2 diabetes revealed by a lack of association between common variants within the TCF7L2 gene and PCOS. *Diabetologia*, *50*(11), 2318-2322. https://doi.org/10.1007/s00125-007-0804-z.

Ben-Salem, A., Ajina, M., Suissi, M., Daher, H. S., Almawi, W. Y., & Mahjoub, T. (2014). Polymorphisms of transcription factor-7-like 2 (TCF7L2) gene in Tunisian women with polycystic ovary syndrome (PCOS). *Gene*, *533*(2), 554-557. https://doi.org/10.1016/j.gene.2013.09.104.

Bérubé, D., Séralini, G. E., Gagné, R., & Hammond, G. L. (1990). Localization of the human sex hormone-binding globulin gene (SHBG) to the short arm of chromosome 17 (17p12----p13). *Cytogenet Cell Genet*, *54*(1-2), 65-67. https://doi.org/10.1159/000132958.

Biyasheva, A., Legro, R. S., Dunaif, A., & Urbanek, M. (2009). Evidence for association between polycystic ovary syndrome (PCOS) and TCF7L2 and glucose intolerance in women with PCOS and TCF7L2. *J Clin Endocrinol Metab*, *94*(7), 2617-2625. https://doi.org/10.1210/jc.2008-1664.

Cai, X., Liu, C., & Mou, S. (2014). Association between fat mass- and obesity-associated (FTO) gene polymorphism and polycystic ovary syndrome: a meta-analysis. *PLoS One*, *9*(1), e86972. https://doi.org/10.1371/journal.pone.0086972.

Calvo, R. M., Villuendas, G., Sancho, J., San Millán, J. L., & Escobar-Morreale, H. F. (2001). Role of the follistatin gene in women with polycystic ovary syndrome. *Fertil Steril*, *75*(5), 1020-1023. https://doi.org/10.1016/s0015-0282(01)01697-1.

Carey, A. H., Waterworth, D., Patel, K., White, D., Little, J., Novelli, P., Franks, S., & Williamson, R. (1994). Polycystic ovaries and premature male pattern baldness are associated with one allele of the steroid metabolism gene CYP17. *Hum Mol Genet*, *3*(10), 1873-1876. https://doi.org/10.1093/hmg/3.10.1873.

Carson-Jurica, M. A., Schrader, W. T., & O'Malley, B. W. (1990). Steroid receptor family: structure and functions. *Endocr Rev*, *11*(2), 201-220. https://doi.org/10.1210/edrv-11-2-201.

Cate, R. L., Mattaliano, R. J., Hession, C., Tizard, R., Farber, N. M., Cheung, A., Ninfa, E. G., Frey, A. Z., Gash, D. J., Chow, E. P., (1986). Isolation of the bovine and human genes for Müllerian inhibiting substance and expression of the human gene in animal cells. *Cell*, *45*(5), 685-698. https://doi.org/10.1016/0092-8674(86)90783-x.

Chamberlain, N. L., Driver, E. D., & Miesfeld, R. L. (1994). The length and location of CAG trinucleotide repeats in the androgen receptor N-terminal domain affect transactivation function. *Nucleic Acids Res*, *22*(15), 3181-3186. https://doi.org/10.1093/nar/22.15.3181.

Chen, S. A., Besman, M. J., Sparkes, R. S., Zollman, S., Klisak, I., Mohandas, T., Hall, P. F., & Shively, J. E. (1988). Human aromatase: cDNA cloning, Southern blot analysis, and assignment of the gene to chromosome 15. *DNA*, *7*(1), 27-38. https://doi.org/10.1089/dna.1988.7.27.

Chen, Y., & Fang, S. Y. (2018). Potential genetic polymorphisms predicting polycystic ovary syndrome. *Endocr Connect*, *7*(5), R187-r195. https://doi.org/10.1530/ec-18-0121.

Chen, Z. J., Zhao, H., He, L., Shi, Y., Qin, Y., Shi, Y., Li, Z., You, L., Zhao, J., Liu, J., Liang, X., Zhao, X., Zhao, J., Sun, Y., Zhang, B., Jiang, H., Zhao, D., Bian, Y., Gao, X., Geng, L., Li, Y., Zhu, D., Sun, X., Xu, J. E., Hao, C., Ren, C. E., Zhang, Y., Chen, S., Zhang, W., Yang, A., Yan, J., Li, Y., Ma, J., & Zhao, Y. (2011). Genome-wide association study identifies susceptibility loci for polycystic ovary syndrome on chromosome 2p16.3, 2p21 and 9q33.3. *Nat Genet*, *43*(1), 55-59. https://doi.org/10.1038/ng.732.

Christopoulos, P., Mastorakos, G., Gazouli, M., Panidis, D., Deligeoroglou, E., Katsikis, I., Papadias, K., Diamandi-Kandarakis, E., & Creatsas, G. (2008). Genetic variants in TCF7L2 and KCNJ11 genes in a Greek population with polycystic ovary syndrome. *Gynecol Endocrinol*, *24*(9), 486-490. https://doi.org/10.1080/09513590802196379.

Cortese, C., & Motti, C. (2001). MTHFR gene polymorphism, homocysteine and cardiovascular disease. *Public Health Nutr*, *4*(2b), 493-497. https://doi.org/10.1079/phn2001159.

Cousin, P., Calemard-Michel, L., Lejeune, H., Raverot, G., Yessaad, N., Emptoz-Bonneton, A., Morel, Y., & Pugeat, M. (2004). Influence of SHBG gene pentanucleotide TAAAA repeat and D327N polymorphism on serum sex hormone-binding globulin concentration in hirsute women. *J Clin Endocrinol Metab*, *89*(2), 917-924. https://doi.org/10.1210/jc.2002-021553.

Day, F., Karaderi, T., Jones, M. R., Meun, C., He, C., Drong, A., Kraft, P., Lin, N., Huang, H., Broer, L., Magi, R., Saxena, R., Laisk, T., Urbanek, M., Hayes, M. G., Thorleifsson, G., Fernandez-Tajes, J., Mahajan, A., Mullin, B. H., Stuckey, B. G. A., Spector, T. D., Wilson, S. G., Goodarzi, M. O., Davis, L., Obermayer-Pietsch, B., Uitterlinden, A. G., Anttila, V., Neale, B. M., Jarvelin, M. R., Fauser, B., Kowalska, I., Visser, J. A., Andersen, M., Ong, K., Stener-Victorin, E., Ehrmann, D., Legro, R. S., Salumets, A., McCarthy, M. I., Morin-Papunen, L., Thorsteinsdottir, U., Stefansson, K., Styrkarsdottir, U., Perry, J. R. B., Dunaif, A., Laven, J., Franks, S., Lindgren, C. M., & Welt, C. K. (2018). Large-scale genome-wide meta-analysis of polycystic ovary syndrome suggests shared genetic architecture for different diagnosis criteria. *PLoS Genet*, *14*(12), e1007813. https://doi.org/10.1371/journal. pgen.1007813.

Day, F. R., Hinds, D. A., Tung, J. Y., Stolk, L., Styrkarsdottir, U., Saxena, R., Bjonnes, A., Broer, L., Dunger, D. B., Halldorsson, B. V., Lawlor, D. A., Laval, G., Mathieson, I., McCardle, W. L., Louwers, Y., Meun, C., Ring, S., Scott, R. A., Sulem, P., Uitterlinden, A. G., Wareham, N. J., Thorsteinsdottir, U., Welt, C., Stefansson, K., Laven, J. S. E., Ong, K. K., & Perry, J. R. B. (2015). Causal mechanisms and balancing selection inferred from genetic associations with polycystic ovary syndrome. *Nat Commun*, *6*, 8464. https://doi.org/10.1038/ncomms9464.

Demirci, H., Yilmaz, M., Ergun, M. A., Yurtcu, E., Bukan, N., & Ayvaz, G. (2010). Frequency of adiponectin gene polymorphisms in polycystic ovary syndrome and the association with serum adiponectin, androgen levels, insulin resistance and clinical parameters. *Gynecol Endocrinol*, *26*(5), 348-355. https://doi.org/10.3109/09513590903367051.

Diamanti-Kandarakis, E., Bartzis, M. I., Bergiele, A. T., Tsianateli, T. C., & Kouli, C. R. (2000). Microsatellite polymorphism (tttta)(n) at -528 base pairs of gene CYP11alpha influences hyperandrogenemia in patients with polycystic ovary syndrome. *Fertil Steril*, *73*(4), 735-741. https://doi.org/10.1016/s0015-0282(99)00628-7.

Diamanti-Kandarakis, E., & Dunaif, A. (2012). Insulin resistance and the polycystic ovary syndrome revisited: an update on mechanisms and implications. *Endocr Rev*, *33*(6), 981-1030. https://doi.org/10.1210/er.2011-1034.

Diamanti-Kandarakis, E., Kandarakis, H., & Legro, R. S. (2006). The role of genes and environment in the etiology of PCOS. *Endocrine*, *30*(1), 19-26. https://doi.org/10.1385/endo:30:1:19.

Diamanti-Kandarakis, E., Palioniko, G., Alexandraki, K., Bergiele, A., Koutsouba, T., & Bartzis, M. (2004). The prevalence of 4G5G polymorphism of plasminogen activator inhibitor-1 (PAI-1) gene in polycystic ovarian syndrome and its association with plasma PAI-1 levels. *Eur J Endocrinol*, *150*(6), 793-798. https://doi.org/10.1530/eje.0.1500793

Diamanti-Kandarakis, E., & Papavassiliou, A. G. (2006). Molecular mechanisms of insulin resistance in polycystic ovary syndrome. *Trends Mol Med*, *12*(7), 324-332. https://doi.org/10.1016/ j.molmed.2006.05.006.

Dilek, S., Ertunc, D., Tok, E. C., Erdal, E. M., & Aktas, A. (2005). Association of Gly972Arg variant of insulin receptor substrate-1 with metabolic features in women with polycystic ovary syndrome. *Fertil Steril*, *84*(2), 407-412. https://doi.org/10.1016/j.fertnstert.2005.01.133.

Dowsing, A. T., Yong, E. L., Clark, M., McLachlan, R. I., de Kretser, D. M., & Trounson, A. O. (1999). Linkage between male infertility and trinucleotide repeat expansion in the androgen-receptor gene. *Lancet*, *354*(9179), 640-643. https://doi.org/10.1016/s0140-6736(98)08413-x.

Ebejer, K., & Calleja-Agius, J. (2013). The role of cytokines in polycystic ovarian syndrome. *Gynecol Endocrinol*, *29*(6), 536-540. https://doi.org/10.3109/09513590.2012.760195.

El-Shal, A. S., Shalaby, S. M., Aly, N. M., Rashad, N. M., & Abdelaziz, A. M. (2013). Genetic variation in the vitamin D receptor gene and vitamin D serum levels in Egyptian women with polycystic ovary syndrome. *Mol Biol Rep*, *40*(11), 6063-6073. https://doi.org/10.1007/s11033-013-2716-y.

El Mkadem, S. A., Lautier, C., Macari, F., Molinari, N., Lefèbvre, P., Renard, E., Gris, J. C., Cros, G., Daurès, J. P., Bringer, J., White, M. F., & Grigorescu, F. (2001). Role of allelic variants Gly972Arg of IRS-1 and

Gly1057Asp of IRS-2 in moderate-to-severe insulin resistance of women with polycystic ovary syndrome. *Diabetes*, *50*(9), 2164-2168. https://doi.org/10.2337/diabetes.50.9.2164.

Elter, K., Erel, C. T., Cine, N., Ozbek, U., Hacihanefioglu, B., & Ertungealp, E. (1999). Role of the mutations Trp8 => Arg and Ile15 => Thr of the human luteinizing hormone beta-subunit in women with polycystic ovary syndrome. *Fertil Steril*, *71*(3), 425-430. https://doi.org/10.1016/s0015-0282(98)00491-9.

Erickson, G. F., Hsueh, A. J., Quigley, M. E., Rebar, R. W., & Yen, S. S. (1979). Functional studies of aromatase activity in human granulosa cells from normal and polycystic ovaries. *J Clin Endocrinol Metab*, *49*(4), 514-519. https://doi.org/10.1210/jcem-49-4-514.

Escobar-Morreale, H., Pazos, F., Potau, N., García-Robles, R., Sancho, J. M., & Varela, C. (1994). Ovarian suppression with triptorelin and adrenal stimulation with adrenocorticotropin in functional hyperadrogenism: role of adrenal and ovarian cytochrome P450c17 alpha. *Fertil Steril*, *62*(3), 521-530. https://doi.org/10.1016/s0015-0282(16)56940-4.

Escobar-Morreale, H. F., Calvo, R. M., Sancho, J., & San Millán, J. L. (2001). TNF-alpha and hyperandrogenism: a clinical, biochemical, and molecular genetic study. *J Clin Endocrinol Metab*, *86*(8), 3761-3767. https://doi.org/10.1210/jcem.86.8.7770.

Escobar-Morreale, H. F., Calvo, R. M., Villuendas, G., Sancho, J., & San Millán, J. L. (2003). Association of polymorphisms in the interleukin 6 receptor complex with obesity and hyperandrogenism. *Obes Res*, *11*(8), 987-996. https://doi.org/10.1038/oby.2003.136.

Escobar-Morreale, H. F., San Millán, J. L., Smith, R. R., Sancho, J., & Witchel, S. F. (1999). The presence of the 21-hydroxylase deficiency carrier status in hirsute women: phenotype-genotype correlations. *Fertil Steril*, *72*(4), 629-638. https://doi.org/10.1016/s0015-0282(99)00317-9.

Escobar-Morreale, H. F., Serrano-Gotarredona, J., García-Robles, R., Sancho, J. M., & Varela, C. (1997). Lack of an ovarian function influence on the increased adrenal androgen secretion present in women with functional ovarian hyperandrogenism. *Fertil Steril*, *67*(4), 654-662. https://doi.org/10.1016/s0015-0282(97)81362-3.

Escobar-Morreale, H. F., Villuendas, G., Botella-Carretero, J. I., Alvarez-Blasco, F., Sanchón, R., Luque-Ramírez, M., & San Millán, J. L. (2006). Adiponectin and resistin in PCOS: a clinical, biochemical and molecular genetic study. *Hum Reprod*, *21*(9), 2257-2265. https://doi.org/10.1093/humrep/del146

Ewens, K. G., Stewart, D. R., Ankener, W., Urbanek, M., McAllister, J. M., Chen, C., Baig, K. M., Parker, S. C., Margulies, E. H., Legro, R. S., Dunaif, A., Strauss, J. F., 3rd, & Spielman, R. S. (2010). Family-based analysis of candidate genes for polycystic ovary syndrome. *J Clin Endocrinol Metab*, *95*(5), 2306-2315. https://doi.org/10.1210/jc.2009-2703.

Farrell, K., & Antoni, M. H. (2010). Insulin resistance, obesity, inflammation, and depression in polycystic ovary syndrome: biobehavioral mechanisms and interventions. *Fertil Steril*, *94*(5), 1565-1574. https://doi.org/10.1016/j.fertnstert.2010.03.081.

Franks, S., Gilling-Smith, C., Gharani, N., & McCarthy, M. (2000). Pathogenesis of polycystic ovary syndrome: evidence for a genetically determined disorder of ovarian androgen production. *Hum Fertil (Camb)*, *3*(2), 77-79. https://doi.org/10.1080/1464727002000198731.

Frayling, T. M., Timpson, N. J., Weedon, M. N., Zeggini, E., Freathy, R. M., Lindgren, C. M., Perry, J. R., Elliott, K. S., Lango, H., Rayner, N. W., Shields, B., Harries, L. W., Barrett, J. C., Ellard, S., Groves, C. J., Knight, B., Patch, A. M., Ness, A. R., Ebrahim, S., Lawlor, D. A., Ring, S. M., Ben-Shlomo, Y., Jarvelin, M. R., Sovio, U., Bennett, A. J., Melzer, D., Ferrucci, L., Loos, R. J., Barroso, I., Wareham, N. J., Karpe, F., Owen, K. R., Cardon, L. R., Walker, M., Hitman, G. A., Palmer, C. N., Doney, A. S., Morris, A. D., Smith, G. D., Hattersley, A. T., & McCarthy, M. I. (2007). A common variant in the FTO gene is associated with body mass index and predisposes to childhood and adult obesity. *Science*, *316*(5826), 889-894. https://doi.org/10.1126/science.1141634.

Fu, L., Zhang, Z., Zhang, A., Xu, J., Huang, X., Zheng, Q., Cao, Y., Wang, L., & Du, J. (2013). Association study between FSHR Ala307Thr and Ser680Asn variants and polycystic ovary syndrome (PCOS) in Northern Chinese Han women. *J Assist Reprod Genet*, *30*(5), 717-721. https://doi.org/10.1007/s10815-013-9979-z.

Furui, K., Suganuma, N., Tsukahara, S., Asada, Y., Kikkawa, F., Tanaka, M., Ozawa, T., & Tomoda, Y. (1994). Identification of two point mutations in the gene coding luteinizing hormone (LH) beta-subunit, associated with immunologically anomalous LH variants. *J Clin Endocrinol Metab*, *78*(1), 107-113. https://doi.org/10.1210/jcem.78.1.7904610.

Gaasenbeek, M., Powell, B. L., Sovio, U., Haddad, L., Gharani, N., Bennett, A., Groves, C. J., Rush, K., Goh, M. J., Conway, G. S., Ruokonen, A., Martikainen, H., Pouta, A., Taponen, S., Hartikainen, A. L., Halford, S., Järvelin, M. R., Franks, S., & McCarthy, M. I. (2004). Large-scale analysis of the relationship between CYP11A promoter variation, polycystic ovarian syndrome, and serum testosterone. *J Clin Endocrinol Metab*, *89*(5), 2408-2413. https://doi.org/10.1210/jc.2003-031640.

Gharani, N., Waterworth, D. M., Batty, S., White, D., Gilling-Smith, C., Conway, G. S., McCarthy, M., Franks, S., & Williamson, R. (1997). Association of the steroid synthesis gene CYP11a with polycystic ovary syndrome and hyperandrogenism. *Hum Mol Genet*, *6*(3), 397-402. https://doi.org/10.1093/hmg/6.3.397.

Gharani, N., Waterworth, D. M., Williamson, R., & Franks, S. (1996). 5' polymorphism of the CYP17 gene is not associated with serum testosterone levels in women with polycystic ovaries. *J Clin Endocrinol Metab*, *81*(11), 4174. https://doi.org/10.1210/jcem.81.11.8923880.

Glintborg, D., Hermann, A. P., Brusgaard, K., Hangaard, J., Hagen, C., & Andersen, M. (2005). Significantly higher adrenocorticotropin-stimulated cortisol and 17-hydroxyprogesterone levels in 337 consecutive, premenopausal, caucasian, hirsute patients compared with healthy controls. *J Clin Endocrinol Metab*, *90*(3), 1347-1353. https://doi.org/10.1210/jc.2004-1214.

Glister, C., Satchell, L., Bathgate, R. A., Wade, J. D., Dai, Y., Ivell, R., Anand-Ivell, R., Rodgers, R. J., & Knight, P. G. (2013). Functional link between bone morphogenetic proteins and insulin-like peptide 3 signaling in modulating ovarian androgen production. *Proc Natl Acad Sci USA*, *110*(15), E1426-1435. https://doi.org/10.1073/pnas.1222216110.

Glueck, C. J., Wang, P., Fontaine, R. N., Sieve-Smith, L., Tracy, T., & Moore, S. K. (1999). Plasminogen activator inhibitor activity: an independent risk factor for the high miscarriage rate during pregnancy in women with polycystic ovary syndrome. *Metabolism*, *48*(12), 1589-1595. https://doi.org/10.1016/s0026-0495(99)90250-0.

Goldfine, I. D. (1987). The insulin receptor: molecular biology and transmembrane signaling. *Endocr Rev*, *8*(3), 235-255. https://doi.org/10.1210/edrv-8-3-235.

Goodarzi, M. O., Jones, M. R., Antoine, H. J., Pall, M., Chen, Y. D., & Azziz, R. (2008). Nonreplication of the type 5 17beta-hydroxysteroid dehydrogenase gene association with polycystic ovary syndrome. *J Clin Endocrinol Metab*, *93*(1), 300-303. https://doi.org/10.1210/jc.2007-1712.

Goodarzi, M. O., Shah, N. A., Antoine, H. J., Pall, M., Guo, X., & Azziz, R. (2006). Variants in the 5alpha-reductase type 1 and type 2 genes are associated with polycystic ovary syndrome and the severity of hirsutism in affected women. *J Clin Endocrinol Metab*, *91*(10), 4085-4091. https://doi.org/10.1210/jc.2006-0227.

Gorsic, L. K., Kosova, G., Werstein, B., Sisk, R., Legro, R. S., Hayes, M. G., Teixeira, J. M., Dunaif, A., & Urbanek, M. (2017). Pathogenic Anti-Müllerian Hormone Variants in Polycystic Ovary Syndrome. *J Clin Endocrinol Metab*, *102*(8), 2862-2872. https://doi.org/10.1210/jc.2017-00612.

Grant, S. F., Thorleifsson, G., Reynisdottir, I., Benediktsson, R., Manolescu, A., Sainz, J., Helgason, A., Stefansson, H., Emilsson, V., Helgadottir, A., Styrkarsdottir, U., Magnusson, K. P., Walters, G. B., Palsdottir, E., Jonsdottir, T., Gudmundsdottir, T., Gylfason, A., Saemundsdottir, J., Wilensky, R. L., Reilly, M. P., Rader, D. J., Bagger, Y., Christiansen, C., Gudnason, V., Sigurdsson, G., Thorsteinsdottir, U., Gulcher, J. R., Kong, A., & Stefansson, K. (2006). Variant of transcription factor 7-like 2 (TCF7L2) gene confers risk of type 2 diabetes. *Nat Genet*, *38*(3), 320-323. https://doi.org/10.1038/ng1732.

Groves, C. J., Zeggini, E., Minton, J., Frayling, T. M., Weedon, M. N., Rayner, N. W., Hitman, G. A., Walker, M., Wiltshire, S., Hattersley, A. T., & McCarthy, M. I. (2006). Association analysis of 6,736 U.K. subjects provides replication and confirms TCF7L2 as a type 2 diabetes susceptibility gene with a substantial effect on individual risk. *Diabetes*, *55*(9), 2640-2644. https://doi.org/10.2337/db06-0355.

Guo, Q., Kumar, T. R., Woodruff, T., Hadsell, L. A., DeMayo, F. J., & Matzuk, M. M. (1998). Overexpression of mouse follistatin causes reproductive defects in transgenic mice. *Mol Endocrinol*, *12*(1), 96-106. https://doi.org/10.1210/mend.12.1.0053.

Guzick, D. S. (2004). Polycystic ovary syndrome. *Obstet Gynecol*, *103*(1), 181-193. https://doi.org/10.1097/01.Aog.0000104485.44999.C6.

Haavisto, A. M., Pettersson, K., Bergendahl, M., Virkamäki, A., & Huhtaniemi, I. (1995). Occurrence and biological properties of a common genetic variant of luteinizing hormone. *J Clin Endocrinol Metab*, *80*(4), 1257-1263. https://doi.org/10.1210/jcem.80.4.7714098.

Hall, J. E., Taylor, A. E., Hayes, F. J., & Crowley, W. F., Jr. (1998). Insights into hypothalamic-pituitary dysfunction in polycystic ovary syndrome. *J Endocrinol Invest*, *21*(9), 602-611. https://doi.org/10.1007/bf03350785.

Harada, N., Ogawa, H., Shozu, M., & Yamada, K. (1992). Genetic studies to characterize the origin of the mutation in placental aromatase deficiency. *Am J Hum Genet*, *51*(3), 666-672..

Haussler, M. R., Jurutka, P. W., Mizwicki, M., & Norman, A. W. (2011). Vitamin D receptor (VDR)-mediated actions of 1α,25(OH)$_2$vitamin D$_3$: genomic and non-genomic mechanisms. *Best Pract Res Clin Endocrinol Metab*, *25*(4), 543-559. https://doi.org/10.1016/j.beem.2011.05.010.

Hayes, M. G., Urbanek, M., Ehrmann, D. A., Armstrong, L. L., Lee, J. Y., Sisk, R., Karaderi, T., Barber, T. M., McCarthy, M. I., Franks, S., Lindgren, C. M., Welt, C. K., Diamanti-Kandarakis, E., Panidis, D., Goodarzi, M. O., Azziz, R., Zhang, Y., James, R. G., Olivier, M., Kissebah, A. H., Stener-Victorin, E., Legro, R. S., & Dunaif, A. (2015). Genome-wide association of polycystic ovary syndrome implicates alterations in gonadotropin secretion in European ancestry populations. *Nat Commun*, *6*, 7502. https://doi.org/10.1038/ncomms8502.

Heinonen, S., Korhonen, S., Hippeläinen, M., Hiltunen, M., Mannermaa, A., & Saarikoski, S. (2001). Apolipoprotein E alleles in women with polycystic ovary syndrome. *Fertil Steril*, *75*(5), 878-880. https://doi.org/10.1016/s0015-0282(01)01691-0.

Hickey, T., Chandy, A., & Norman, R. J. (2002). The androgen receptor CAG repeat polymorphism and X-chromosome inactivation in Australian Caucasian women with infertility related to polycystic ovary syndrome. *J Clin Endocrinol Metab*, *87*(1), 161-165. https://doi.org/10.1210/jcem.87.1.8137.

Hogeveen, K. N., Talikka, M., & Hammond, G. L. (2001). Human sex hormone-binding globulin promoter activity is influenced by a (TAAAA)n repeat element within an Alu sequence. *J Biol Chem*, *276*(39), 36383-36390. https://doi.org/10.1074/jbc.M104681200.

Hotamisligil, G. S., Peraldi, P., Budavari, A., Ellis, R., White, M. F., & Spiegelman, B. M. (1996). IRS-1-mediated inhibition of insulin receptor tyrosine kinase activity in TNF-alpha- and obesity-induced insulin resistance. *Science*, *271*(5249), 665-668. https://doi.org/10.1126/science.271.5249.665.

Hu, F. B., Doria, A., Li, T., Meigs, J. B., Liu, S., Memisoglu, A., Hunter, D., & Manson, J. E. (2004). Genetic variation at the adiponectin locus and risk of type 2 diabetes in women. *Diabetes*, *53*(1), 209-213. https://doi.org/10.2337/diabetes.53.1.209.

Hubacek, J. A., Stanek, V., Gebauerová, M., Pilipcincová, A., Dlouhá, D., Poledne, R., Aschermann, M., Skalická, H., Matousková, J., Kruger, A., Penicka, M., Hrabáková, H., Veselka, J., Hájek, P., Lánská, V., Adámková, V., & Pitha, J. (2010). A FTO variant and risk of acute coronary syndrome. *Clin Chim Acta*, *411*(15-16), 1069-1072. https://doi.org/10.1016/j.cca.2010.03.037.

Hwang, J. Y., Lee, E. J., Jin Go, M., Sung, Y. A., Lee, H. J., Heon Kwak, S., Jang, H. C., Soo Park, K., Lee, H. J., Byul Jang, H., Song, J., Park, K. H., Kim, H. L., Cho, M. C., & Lee, J. Y. (2012). Genome-wide association study identifies GYS2 as a novel genetic factor for polycystic ovary syndrome through obesity-related condition. *J Hum Genet*, *57*(10), 660-664. https://doi.org/10.1038/jhg.2012.92.

Ito, Y., Fisher, C. R., Conte, F. A., Grumbach, M. M., & Simpson, E. R. (1993). Molecular basis of aromatase deficiency in an adult female with sexual infantilism and polycystic ovaries. *Proc Natl Acad Sci U S A*, *90*(24), 11673-11677. https://doi.org/10.1073/pnas.90.24.11673.

Jakimiuk, A. J., Weitsman, S. R., Brzechffa, P. R., & Magoffin, D. A. (1998). Aromatase mRNA expression in individual follicles from polycystic ovaries. *Mol Hum Reprod*, *4*(1), 1-8. https://doi.org/10.1093/molehr/4.1.1.

Jakimiuk, A. J., Weitsman, S. R., & Magoffin, D. A. (1999). 5alpha-reductase activity in women with polycystic ovary syndrome. *J Clin Endocrinol Metab*, *84*(7), 2414-2418. https://doi.org/10.1210/jcem.84.7.5863.

Jakubowski, L. (2005). [Genetic aspects of polycystic ovary syndrome]. *Endokrynol Pol*, *56*(3), 285-293. (Aspekty genetyczne zespołu policystycznych jajników.).

Jalilian, A., Kiani, F., Sayehmiri, F., Sayehmiri, K., Khodaee, Z., & Akbari, M. (2015). Prevalence of polycystic ovary syndrome and its associated complications in Iranian women: A meta-analysis. *Iran J Reprod Med*, *13*(10), 591-604.

Jatzko, B., & Ott, J. (2011). Circulating inflammatory markers in polycystic ovary syndrome: a systematic review and meta-analysis. *Fertil Steril*, *96*(4), e158. https://doi.org/10.1016/j.fertnstert.2011.07.1098.

Jedrzejuk, D., Łaczmański, Ł., Milewicz, A., Kuliczkowska-Płaksej, J., Lenarcik-Kabza, A., Hirnle, L., Zaleska-Dorobisz, U., & Lwow, F. (2015). Classic PCOS phenotype is not associated with deficiency of endogenous vitamin D and VDR gene polymorphisms rs731236 (TaqI), rs7975232 (ApaI), rs1544410 (BsmI), rs10735810 (FokI): a case-control study of lower Silesian women. *Gynecol Endocrinol*, *31*(12), 976-979. https://doi.org/10.3109/09513590.2015.1062865.

Joseph, S., Barai, R. S., Bhujbalrao, R., & Idicula-Thomas, S. (2016). PCOSKB: A KnowledgeBase on genes, diseases, ontology terms and biochemical pathways associated with PolyCystic Ovary Syndrome. *Nucleic Acids Res*, *44*(D1), D1032-1035. https://doi.org/10.1093/nar/gkv1146.

Ju, R., Wu, W., Fei, J., Qin, Y., Tang, Q., Wu, D., Xia, Y., Wu, J., & Wang, X. (2015). Association analysis between the polymorphisms of HSD17B5 and HSD17B6 and risk of polycystic ovary syndrome in Chinese population. *Eur J Endocrinol*, *172*(3), 227-233. https://doi.org/10.1530/eje-14-0615.

Kahsar-Miller, M. D., Conway-Myers, B. A., Boots, L. R., & Azziz, R. (2001). Steroidogenic acute regulatory protein (StAR) in the ovaries of healthy women and those with polycystic ovary syndrome. *Am J Obstet Gynecol*, *185*(6), 1381-1387. https://doi.org/10.1067/mob.2001.118656.

Kashima, K., Yahata, T., Fujita, K., & Tanaka, K. (2013). Polycystic ovary syndrome: association of a C/T single nucleotide polymorphism at tyrosine kinase domain of insulin receptor gene with pathogenesis among lean Japanese women. *J Reprod Med*, *58*(11-12), 491-496..

Kennedy, G. C., German, M. S., & Rutter, W. J. (1995). The minisatellite in the diabetes susceptibility locus IDDM2 regulates insulin transcription. *Nat Genet*, *9*(3), 293-298. https://doi.org/10.1038/ng0395-293.

Kershaw, E. E., & Flier, J. S. (2004). Adipose tissue as an endocrine organ. *J Clin Endocrinol Metab*, *89*(6), 2548-2556. https://doi.org/10.1210/jc.2004-0395.

Kim, J. J., Choi, Y. M., Hong, M. A., Chae, S. J., Hwang, K., Yoon, S. H., Ku, S. Y., Suh, C. S., & Kim, S. H. (2017). FSH receptor gene p. Thr307Ala and p. Asn680Ser polymorphisms are associated with the risk of polycystic ovary syndrome. *J Assist Reprod Genet*, *34*(8), 1087-1093. https://doi.org/10.1007/s10815-017-0953-z.

Knight, P. G., & Glister, C. (2001). Potential local regulatory functions of inhibins, activins and follistatin in the ovary. *Reproduction*, *121*(4), 503-512. https://doi.org/10.1530/rep.0.1210503

Layman, L. C., Amde, S., Cohen, D. P., Jin, M., & Xie, J. (1998). The Finnish follicle-stimulating hormone receptor gene mutation is rare in North American women with 46,XX ovarian failure. *Fertil Steril*, *69*(2), 300-302. https://doi.org/10.1016/s0015-0282(97)00480-9.

Lee, H., Oh, J. Y., Sung, Y. A., Chung, H., Kim, H. L., Kim, G. S., Cho, Y. S., & Kim, J. T. (2015). Genome-wide association study identified new susceptibility loci for polycystic ovary syndrome. *Hum Reprod*, *30*(3), 723-731. https://doi.org/10.1093/humrep/deu352.

Legro, R. S. (2003). Polycystic ovary syndrome and cardiovascular disease: a premature association? *Endocr Rev*, *24*(3), 302-312. https://doi.org/10.1210/er.2003-0004.

Legro, R. S., Muhleman, D. R., Comings, D. E., Lobo, R. A., & Kovacs, B. W. (1995). A dopamine D3 receptor genotype is associated with hyperandrogenic chronic anovulation and resistant to ovulation induction with clomiphene citrate in female Hispanics. *Fertil Steril*, *63*(4), 779-784. https://doi.org/10.1016/s0015-0282(16)57481-0.

Legro, R. S., Spielman, R., Urbanek, M., Driscoll, D., Strauss, J. F., 3rd, & Dunaif, A. (1998). Phenotype and genotype in polycystic ovary syndrome. *Recent Prog Horm Res*, *53*, 217-256.

Liu, A. L., Xie, H. J., Xie, H. Y., Liu, J., Yin, J., Hu, J. S., & Peng, C. Y. (2017). Association between fat mass and obesity associated (FTO) gene rs9939609 A/T polymorphism and polycystic ovary syndrome: a systematic review and meta-analysis. *BMC Med Genet*, *18*(1), 89. https://doi.org/10.1186/s12881-017-0452-1.

Liu, X., Li, L., Chen, Z. J., Lu, Z., Shi, Y., & Zhao, Y. (2010). Genetic variants of cyclin-dependent kinase 5 regulatory subunit associated protein 1-like 1 and transcription factor 7-like 2 are not associated with polycystic ovary syndrome in Chinese women. *Gynecol Endocrinol*, *26*(2), 129-134. https://doi.org/10.3109/09513590903215490.

Lubahn, D. B., Joseph, D. R., Sullivan, P. M., Willard, H. F., French, F. S., & Wilson, E. M. (1988). Cloning of human androgen receptor complementary DNA and localization to the X chromosome. *Science*, *240*(4850), 327-330. https://doi.org/10.1126/science.3353727.

Mahmoudi, T. (2009). Genetic variation in the vitamin D receptor and polycystic ovary syndrome risk. *Fertil Steril*, *92*(4), 1381-1383. https://doi.org/10.1016/j.fertnstert.2009.05.002.

McQuillan, B. M., Beilby, J. P., Nidorf, M., Thompson, P. L., & Hung, J. (1999). Hyperhomocysteinemia but not the C677T mutation of methylenetetrahydrofolate reductase is an independent risk determinant of carotid wall thickening. The Perth Carotid Ultrasound Disease Assessment Study (CUDAS). *Circulation*, *99*(18), 2383-2388. https://doi.org/10.1161/01.cir.99.18.2383.

Menzaghi, C., Ercolino, T., Di Paola, R., Berg, A. H., Warram, J. H., Scherer, P. E., Trischitta, V., & Doria, A. (2002). A haplotype at the adiponectin locus is associated with obesity and other features of the insulin resistance syndrome. *Diabetes*, *51*(7), 2306-2312. https://doi.org/10.2337/diabetes.51.7.2306.

Mifsud, A., Ramirez, S., & Yong, E. L. (2000). Androgen receptor gene CAG trinucleotide repeats in anovulatory infertility and polycystic ovaries. *J Clin Endocrinol Metab*, *85*(9), 3484-3488. https://doi.org/10.1210/jcem.85.9.6832.

Miller, W. L. (2007). Steroidogenic acute regulatory protein (StAR), a novel mitochondrial cholesterol transporter. *Biochim Biophys Acta*, *1771*(6), 663-676. https://doi.org/10.1016/j.bbalip.2007.02.012.

Moghrabi, N., Hughes, I. A., Dunaif, A., & Andersson, S. (1998). Deleterious missense mutations and silent polymorphism in the human 17beta-hydroxysteroid dehydrogenase 3 gene (HSD17B3). *J Clin Endocrinol Metab*, *83*(8), 2855-2860. https://doi.org/10.1210/jcem.83.8.5052.

Mohanty, D., & Das, K. C. (1982). Effect of folate deficiency on the reproductive organs of female rhesus monkeys: a cytomorphological and cytokinetic study. *J Nutr*, *112*(8), 1565-1576. https://doi.org/10.1093/jn/112.8.1565.

Munir, I., Yen, H. W., Geller, D. H., Torbati, D., Bierden, R. M., Weitsman, S. R., Agarwal, S. K., & Magoffin, D. A. (2004). Insulin augmentation of 17alpha-hydroxylase activity is mediated by phosphatidyl inositol 3-kinase but not extracellular signal-regulated kinase-1/2 in human ovarian theca cells. *Endocrinology*, *145*(1), 175-183. https://doi.org/10.1210/en.2003-0329.

Nardo, L. G., Patchava, S., & Laing, I. (2008). Polycystic ovary syndrome: pathophysiology, molecular aspects and clinical implications. *Panminerva Med*, *50*(4), 267-278..

Nayak, S., Lee, P. A., & Witchel, S. F. (1998). Variants of the type II 3beta-hydroxysteroid dehydrogenase gene in children with premature pubic hair and hyperandrogenic adolescents. *Mol Genet Metab*, *64*(3), 184-192. https://doi.org/10.1006/mgme.1998.2715.

Nazouri, A. S., Khosravifar, M., Akhlaghi, A. A., Shiva, M., & Afsharian, P. (2015). No relationship between most polymorphisms of steroidogenic acute regulatory (StAR) gene with polycystic ovarian syndrome. *Int J Reprod Biomed*, *13*(12), 771-778.

Nilsson, C., Pettersson, K., Millar, R. P., Coerver, K. A., Matzuk, M. M., & Huhtaniemi, I. T. (1997). Worldwide frequency of a common genetic variant of luteinizing hormone: an international collaborative research. International Collaborative Research Group. *Fertil Steril*, *67*(6), 998-1004. https://doi.org/10.1016/s0015-0282(97)81430-6.

Ogunkolade, B. W., Boucher, B. J., Prahl, J. M., Bustin, S. A., Burrin, J. M., Noonan, K., North, B. V., Mannan, N., McDermott, M. F., DeLuca, H. F., & Hitman, G. A. (2002). Vitamin D receptor (VDR) mRNA and VDR protein levels in relation to vitamin D status, insulin secretory capacity, and VDR genotype in Bangladeshi Asians. *Diabetes*, *51*(7), 2294-2300. https://doi.org/10.2337/diabetes.51.7.2294.

Oksanen, L., Tiitinen, A., Kaprio, J., Koistinen, H. A., Karonen, S., & Kontula, K. (2000). No evidence for mutations of the leptin or leptin receptor genes in women with polycystic ovary syndrome. *Mol Hum Reprod*, *6*(10), 873-876. https://doi.org/10.1093/molehr/6.10.873.

Okuda, K., Yamada, T., Imoto, H., Komatsubara, H., & Sugimoto, O. (1994). Antigenic alteration of an anomalous human luteinizing hormone caused by two chorionic gonadotropin-type amino-acid substitutions. *Biochem Biophys Res Commun*, *200*(1), 584-590. https://doi.org/10.1006/bbrc.1994.1488.

Panidis, D., Kourtis, A., Kukuvitis, A., Farmakiotis, D., Xita, N., Georgiou, I., & Tsatsoulis, A. (2004). Association of the T45G polymorphism in exon 2 of the adiponectin gene with polycystic ovary syndrome: role of Delta4-androstenedione. *Hum Reprod, 19*(8), 1728-1733. https://doi.org/10.1093/humrep/deh336.

Papalou, O., Livadas, S., Karachalios, A., Tolia, N., Kokkoris, P., Tripolitakis, K., & Diamanti-Kandarakis, E. (2015). White blood cells levels and PCOS: direct and indirect relationship with obesity and insulin resistance, but not with hyperandogenemia. *Hormones (Athens), 14*(1), 91-100. https://doi.org/10.14310/horm.2002.1563.

Paquette, J., Giannoukakis, N., Polychronakos, C., Vafiadis, P., & Deal, C. (1998). The INS 5' variable number of tandem repeats is associated with IGF2 expression in humans. *J Biol Chem, 273*(23), 14158-14164. https://doi.org/10.1074/jbc.273.23.14158.

Peral, B., San Millán, J. L., Castello, R., Moghetti, P., & Escobar-Morreale, H. F. (2002). Comment: the methionine 196 arginine polymorphism in exon 6 of the TNF receptor 2 gene (TNFRSF1B) is associated with the polycystic ovary syndrome and hyperandrogenism. *J Clin Endocrinol Metab, 87*(8), 3977-3983. https://doi.org/10.1210/jcem.87.8.8715.

Perez Mayorga, M., Gromoll, J., Behre, H. M., Gassner, C., Nieschlag, E., & Simoni, M. (2000). Ovarian response to follicle-stimulating hormone (FSH) stimulation depends on the FSH receptor genotype. *J Clin Endocrinol Metab, 85*(9), 3365-3369. https://doi.org/10.1210/jcem.85.9.6789.

Petry, C. J., Ong, K. K., Michelmore, K. F., Artigas, S., Wingate, D. L., Balen, A. H., de Zegher, F., Ibáñez, L., & Dunger, D. B. (2005). Association of aromatase (CYP 19) gene variation with features of hyperandrogenism in two populations of young women. *Hum Reprod, 20*(7), 1837-1843. https://doi.org/10.1093/humrep/deh900.

Petry, C. J., Ong, K. K., Michelmore, K. F., Artigas, S., Wingate, D. L., Balen, A. H., de Zegher, F., Ibáñez, L., & Dunger, D. B. (2006). Associations between common variation in the aromatase gene promoter region and testosterone concentrations in two young female populations. *J Steroid Biochem Mol Biol, 98*(4-5), 199-206. https://doi.org/10.1016/j.jsbmb.2005.09.007.

Picado-Leonard, J., & Miller, W. L. (1987). Cloning and sequence of the human gene for P450c17 (steroid 17 alpha-hydroxylase/17,20 lyase): similarity with the gene for P450c21. *DNA, 6*(5), 439-448. https://doi.org/10.1089/dna.1987.6.439.

Prapas, N., Karkanaki, A., Prapas, I., Kalogiannidis, I., Katsikis, I., & Panidis, D. (2009). Genetics of polycystic ovary syndrome. *Hippokratia, 13*(4), 216-223..

Prodoehl, M. J., Hatzirodos, N., Irving-Rodgers, H. F., Zhao, Z. Z., Painter, J. N., Hickey, T. E., Gibson, M. A., Rainey, W. E., Carr, B. R., Mason, H. D., Norman, R. J., Montgomery, G. W., & Rodgers, R. J. (2009). Genetic and gene expression analyses of the polycystic ovary syndrome candidate gene fibrillin-3 and other fibrillin family members in human ovaries. *Mol Hum Reprod, 15*(12), 829-841. https://doi.org/10.1093/molehr/gap072.

Prutsch, N., Fock, V., Haslinger, P., Haider, S., Fiala, C., Pollheimer, J., & Knöfler, M. (2012). The role of interleukin-1β in human trophoblast motility. *Placenta, 33*(9), 696-703. https://doi.org/10.1016/j.placenta.2012.05.008.

Pugeat, M., Crave, J. C., Tourniaire, J., & Forest, M. G. (1996). Clinical utility of sex hormone-binding globulin measurement. *Horm Res, 45*(3-5), 148-155. https://doi.org/10.1159/000184778.

Qin, K., Ehrmann, D. A., Cox, N., Refetoff, S., & Rosenfield, R. L. (2006). Identification of a functional polymorphism of the human type 5 17beta-hydroxysteroid dehydrogenase gene associated with polycystic ovary syndrome. *J Clin Endocrinol Metab, 91*(1), 270-276. https://doi.org/10.1210/jc.2005-2012.

Rajkhowa, M., Talbot, J. A., Jones, P. W., & Clayton, R. N. (1996). Polymorphism of glycogen synthetase gene in polycystic ovary syndrome. *Clin Endocrinol (Oxf), 44*(1), 85-90. https://doi.org/10.1046/j.1365-2265.1996.658474.x.

Rajkhowa, M., Talbot, J. A., Jones, P. W., Pettersson, K., Haavisto, A. M., Huhtaniemi, I., & Clayton, R. N. (1995). Prevalence of an immunological LH beta-subunit variant in a UK population of healthy women and women with polycystic ovary syndrome. *Clin Endocrinol (Oxf), 43*(3), 297-303. https://doi.org/10.1111/j.1365-2265.1995.tb02035.x.

Ramanujam, L. N., Liao, W. X., Roy, A. C., Loganath, A., Goh, H. H., & Ng, S. C. (1999). Association of molecular variants of luteinizing hormone with menstrual disorders. *Clin Endocrinol (Oxf)*, *51*(2), 243-246. https://doi.org/10.1046/j.1365-2265.1999.00791.x.

Ranjzad, F., Mahmoudi, T., Irani Shemirani, A., Mahban, A., Nikzamir, A., Vahedi, M., Ashrafi, M., & Gourabi, H. (2012). A common variant in the adiponectin gene and polycystic ovary syndrome risk. *Mol Biol Rep*, *39*(3), 2313-2319. https://doi.org/10.1007/s11033-011-0981-1.

Rebar, R., Judd, H. L., Yen, S. S., Rakoff, J., Vandenberg, G., & Naftolin, F. (1976). Characterization of the inappropriate gonadotropin secretion in polycystic ovary syndrome. *J Clin Invest*, *57*(5), 1320-1329. https://doi.org/10.1172/jci108400.

Reis, G. V., Gontijo, N. A., Rodrigues, K. F., Alves, M. T., Ferreira, C. N., & Gomes, K. B. (2017). Vitamin D receptor polymorphisms and the polycystic ovary syndrome: A systematic review. *J Obstet Gynaecol Res*, *43*(3), 436-446. https://doi.org/10.1111/jog.13250.

Revised 2003 consensus on diagnostic criteria and long-term health risks related to polycystic ovary syndrome. (2004). *Fertil Steril*, *81*(1), 19-25. https://doi.org/10.1016/j.fertnstert.2003.10.004.

RS, L. (2009). Stein-Leventhal syndrome. *Encyclopedia britannica.*

Sáez, M. E., González-Sánchez, J. L., Ramírez-Lorca, R., Martínez-Larrad, M. T., Zabena, C., González, A., Morón, F. J., Ruiz, A., & Serrano-Ríos, M. (2008). The CAPN10 gene is associated with insulin resistance phenotypes in the Spanish population. *PLoS One*, *3*(8), e2953. https://doi.org/10.1371/journal.pone.0002953.

San Millán, J. L., Cortón, M., Villuendas, G., Sancho, J., Peral, B., & Escobar-Morreale, H. F. (2004). Association of the polycystic ovary syndrome with genomic variants related to insulin resistance, type 2 diabetes mellitus, and obesity. *J Clin Endocrinol Metab*, *89*(6), 2640-2646. https://doi.org/10.1210/jc.2003-031252.

Selby, C. (1990). Sex hormone binding globulin: origin, function and clinical significance. *Ann Clin Biochem*, *27 (Pt 6)*, 532-541. https://doi.org/10.1177/000456329002700603.

Shaikh, N., Dadachanji, R., Meherji, P., Shah, N., & Mukherjee, S. (2016). Polymorphisms and haplotypes of insulin-like factor 3 gene are associated with risk of polycystic ovary syndrome in Indian women. *Gene*, *577*(2), 180-186. https://doi.org/10.1016/j.gene.2015.11.033.

Shaikh, N., Dadachanji, R., & Mukherjee, S. (2014). Genetic markers of polycystic ovary syndrome: emphasis on insulin resistance. *International Journal of Medical Genetics*, *2014*.

Shi, Y., Guo, M., Yan, J., Sun, W., Zhang, X., Geng, L., Xu, L., & Chen, Z. (2007). Analysis of clinical characteristics in large-scale Chinese women with polycystic ovary syndrome. *Neuro Endocrinol Lett*, *28*(6), 807-810.

Shi, Y., Zhao, H., Shi, Y., Cao, Y., Yang, D., Li, Z., Zhang, B., Liang, X., Li, T., Chen, J., Shen, J., Zhao, J., You, L., Gao, X., Zhu, D., Zhao, X., Yan, Y., Qin, Y., Li, W., Yan, J., Wang, Q., Zhao, J., Geng, L., Ma, J., Zhao, Y., He, G., Zhang, A., Zou, S., Yang, A., Liu, J., Li, W., Li, B., Wan, C., Qin, Y., Shi, J., Yang, J., Jiang, H., Xu, J. E., Qi, X., Sun, Y., Zhang, Y., Hao, C., Ju, X., Zhao, D., Ren, C. E., Li, X., Zhang, W., Zhang, Y., Zhang, J., Wu, D., Zhang, C., He, L., & Chen, Z. J. (2012). Genome-wide association study identifies eight new risk loci for polycystic ovary syndrome. *Nat Genet*, *44*(9), 1020-1025. https://doi.org/10.1038/ng.2384.

Shorakae, S., Teede, H., de Courten, B., Lambert, G., Boyle, J., & Moran, L. J. (2015). The Emerging Role of Chronic Low-Grade Inflammation in the Pathophysiology of Polycystic Ovary Syndrome. *Semin Reprod Med*, *33*(4), 257-269. https://doi.org/10.1055/s-0035-1556568.

Sills, E. S., Genton, M. G., Perloe, M., Schattman, G. L., Bralley, J. A., & Tucker, M. J. (2001). Plasma homocysteine, fasting insulin, and androgen patterns among women with polycystic ovaries and infertility. *J Obstet Gynaecol Res*, *27*(3), 163-168. https://doi.org/10.1111/j.1447-0756.2001.tb01241.x.

Simoni, M., Gromoll, J., & Nieschlag, E. (1997). The follicle-stimulating hormone receptor: biochemistry, molecular biology, physiology, and pathophysiology. *Endocr Rev*, *18*(6), 739-773. https://doi.org/10.1210/edrv.18.6.0320.

Simpson, E. R., Mahendroo, M. S., Means, G. D., Kilgore, M. W., Hinshelwood, M. M., Graham-Lorence, S., Amarneh, B., Ito, Y., Fisher, C. R., Michael, M. D. (1994). Aromatase cytochrome P450, the enzyme responsible for estrogen biosynthesis. *Endocr Rev*, *15*(3), 342-355. https://doi.org/10.1210/edrv-15-3-342.

Sir-Petermann, T., Pérez-Bravo, F., Angel, B., Maliqueo, M., Calvillan, M., & Palomino, A. (2001). G972R polymorphism of IRS-1 in women with polycystic ovary syndrome. *Diabetologia, 44*(9), 1200-1201. https://doi.org/10.1007/s001250170001.

Somani, N., Harrison, S., & Bergfeld, W. F. (2008). The clinical evaluation of hirsutism. *Dermatol Ther, 21*(5), 376-391. https://doi.org/10.1111/j.1529-8019.2008.00219.x.

Sorbara, L. R., Tang, Z., Cama, A., Xia, J., Schenker, E., Kohanski, R. A., Poretsky, L., Koller, E., Taylor, S. I., & Dunaif, A. (1994). Absence of insulin receptor gene mutations in three insulin-resistant women with the polycystic ovary syndrome. *Metabolism, 43*(12), 1568-1574. https://doi.org/10.1016/0026-0495(94)90018-3.

Strachan, T., & Read, A. (1999). Instability of the human genome: mutation and DNA repair. *Human Molecular Genetics, 2*, 209-217.

Stumvoll, M., Tschritter, O., Fritsche, A., Staiger, H., Renn, W., Weisser, M., Machicao, F., & Häring, H. (2002). Association of the T-G polymorphism in adiponectin (exon 2) with obesity and insulin sensitivity: interaction with family history of type 2 diabetes. *Diabetes, 51*(1), 37-41. https://doi.org/10.2337/diabetes.51.1.37.

Tan, L., & Zhu, G. (2005). [Relationship between the microsatellite polymorphism of CYP11 alpha gene and the pathogenesis of hyperandrogenism of polycystic ovary syndrome in Chinese]. *Zhonghua Yi Xue Yi Chuan Xue Za Zhi, 22*(2), 216-218.

Tan, S., Scherag, A., Janssen, O. E., Hahn, S., Lahner, H., Dietz, T., Scherag, S., Grallert, H., Vogel, C. I., Kimmig, R., Illig, T., Mann, K., Hebebrand, J., & Hinney, A. (2010). Large effects on body mass index and insulin resistance of fat mass and obesity associated gene (FTO) variants in patients with polycystic ovary syndrome (PCOS). *BMC Med Genet, 11*, 12. https://doi.org/10.1186/1471-2350-11-12.

Tang, S. T., Wang, C. J., Tang, H. Q., Peng, W. J., Wang, Y. M., & Zhang, Q. (2012). Association of Pro12Ala polymorphism in peroxisome proliferator-activated receptor gamma with polycystic ovary syndrome: a meta-analysis. *Mol Biol Rep, 39*(10), 9649-9660. https://doi.org/10.1007/s11033-012-1830-6.

Techatraisak, K., Conway, G. S., & Rumsby, G. (1997). Frequency of a polymorphism in the regulatory region of the 17 alpha-hydroxylase-17,20-lyase (CYP17) gene in hyperandrogenic states. *Clin Endocrinol (Oxf), 46*(2), 131-134. https://doi.org/10.1046/j.1365-2265.1997.8700880.x.

Teede, H., Deeks, A., & Moran, L. (2010). Polycystic ovary syndrome: a complex condition with psychological, reproductive and metabolic manifestations that impacts on health across the lifespan. *BMC Med, 8*, 41. https://doi.org/10.1186/1741-7015-8-41.

Trimmer, E. E. (2013). Methylenetetrahydrofolate reductase: biochemical characterization and medical significance. *Curr Pharm Des, 19*(14), 2574-2593. https://doi.org/10.2174/1381612811319140008.

Tut, T. G., Ghadessy, F. J., Trifiro, M. A., Pinsky, L., & Yong, E. L. (1997). Long polyglutamine tracts in the androgen receptor are associated with reduced trans-activation, impaired sperm production, and male infertility. *J Clin Endocrinol Metab, 82*(11), 3777-3782. https://doi.org/10.1210/jcem.82.11.4385.

Urbanek, M., Du, Y., Silander, K., Collins, F. S., Steppan, C. M., Strauss, J. F., 3rd, Dunaif, A., Spielman, R. S., & Legro, R. S. (2003). Variation in resistin gene promoter not associated with polycystic ovary syndrome. *Diabetes, 52*(1), 214-217. https://doi.org/10.2337/diabetes.52.1.214.

Urbanek, M., Legro, R. S., Driscoll, D. A., Azziz, R., Ehrmann, D. A., Norman, R. J., Strauss, J. F., 3rd, Spielman, R. S., & Dunaif, A. (1999). Thirty-seven candidate genes for polycystic ovary syndrome: strongest evidence for linkage is with follistatin. *Proc Natl Acad Sci USA, 96*(15), 8573-8578. https://doi.org/10.1073/pnas.96.15.8573.

Urbanek, M., Woodroffe, A., Ewens, K. G., Diamanti-Kandarakis, E., Legro, R. S., Strauss, J. F., 3rd, Dunaif, A., & Spielman, R. S. (2005). Candidate gene region for polycystic ovary syndrome on chromosome 19p13.2. *J Clin Endocrinol Metab, 90*(12), 6623-6629. https://doi.org/10.1210/jc.2005-0622.

Urbanek, M., Wu, X., Vickery, K. R., Kao, L. C., Christenson, L. K., Schneyer, A., Legro, R. S., Driscoll, D. A., Strauss, J. F., 3rd, Dunaif, A., & Spielman, R. S. (2000). Allelic variants of the follistatin gene in polycystic ovary syndrome. *J Clin Endocrinol Metab, 85*(12), 4455-4461. https://doi.org/10.1210/jcem.85.12.7026.

Villuendas, G., San Millán, J. L., Sancho, J., & Escobar-Morreale, H. F. (2002). The -597 G-->A and -174 G-->C polymorphisms in the promoter of the IL-6 gene are associated with hyperandrogenism. *J Clin Endocrinol Metab*, *87*(3), 1134-1141. https://doi.org/10.1210/jcem.87.3.8309.

Wang, L., Xu, W., Wang, C., Tang, M., & Zhou, Y. (2017). Methylenetetrahydrofolate reductase C677T polymorphism and the risks of polycystic ovary syndrome: an updated meta-analysis of 14 studies. *Oncotarget*, *8*(35), 59509-59517. https://doi.org/10.18632/oncotarget.18472.

Wang, S., Fu, C., Wang, H., Shi, Y., Xu, X., Chen, J., Song, X., Sun, K., Wang, J., Fan, X., Wang, H., Yang, X., Huan, T., & Hui, R. (2007). Polymorphisms of the peroxisome proliferator-activated receptor-gamma coactivator-1alpha gene are associated with hypertrophic cardiomyopathy and not with hypertension hypertrophy. *Clin Chem Lab Med*, *45*(8), 962-967. https://doi.org/10.1515/cclm.2007.189.

Wang, Y., Wu, X. K., Cao, Y. X., Yi, L., Zou, Y., Qu, J. W., & Hou, L. H. (2005). [Microsatellite polymorphism of (tttta) n in the promoter of CYP11a gene in Chinese women with polycystic ovary syndrome]. *Zhonghua Yi Xue Za Zhi*, *85*(48), 3396-3400.

Waterworth, D. M., Bennett, S. T., Gharani, N., McCarthy, M. I., Hague, S., Batty, S., Conway, G. S., White, D., Todd, J. A., Franks, S., & Williamson, R. (1997). Linkage and association of insulin gene VNTR regulatory polymorphism with polycystic ovary syndrome. *Lancet*, *349*(9057), 986-990. https://doi.org/10.1016/s0140-6736(96)08368-7.

Wickenheisser, J. K., Quinn, P. G., Nelson, V. L., Legro, R. S., Strauss, J. F., 3rd, & McAllister, J. M. (2000). Differential activity of the cytochrome P450 17alpha-hydroxylase and steroidogenic acute regulatory protein gene promoters in normal and polycystic ovary syndrome theca cells. *J Clin Endocrinol Metab*, *85*(6), 2304-2311. https://doi.org/10.1210/jcem.85.6.6631.

Willer, C. J., Speliotes, E. K., Loos, R. J., Li, S., Lindgren, C. M., Heid, I. M., Berndt, S. I., Elliott, A. L., Jackson, A. U., Lamina, C., Lettre, G., Lim, N., Lyon, H. N., McCarroll, S. A., Papadakis, K., Qi, L., Randall, J. C., Roccasecca, R. M., Sanna, S., Scheet, P., Weedon, M. N., Wheeler, E., Zhao, J. H., Jacobs, L. C., Prokopenko, I., Soranzo, N., Tanaka, T., Timpson, N. J., Almgren, P., Bennett, A., Bergman, R. N., Bingham, S. A., Bonnycastle, L. L., Brown, M., Burtt, N. P., Chines, P., Coin, L., Collins, F. S., Connell, J. M., Cooper, C., Smith, G. D., Dennison, E. M., Deodhar, P., Elliott, P., Erdos, M. R., Estrada, K., Evans, D. M., Gianniny, L., Gieger, C., Gillson, C. J., Guiducci, C., Hackett, R., Hadley, D., Hall, A. S., Havulinna, A. S., Hebebrand, J., Hofman, A., Isomaa, B., Jacobs, K. B., Johnson, T., Jousilahti, P., Jovanovic, Z., Khaw, K. T., Kraft, P., Kuokkanen, M., Kuusisto, J., Laitinen, J., Lakatta, E. G., Luan, J., Luben, R. N., Mangino, M., McArdle, W. L., Meitinger, T., Mulas, A., Munroe, P. B., Narisu, N., Ness, A. R., Northstone, K., O'Rahilly, S., Purmann, C., Rees, M. G., Ridderstråle, M., Ring, S. M., Rivadeneira, F., Ruokonen, A., Sandhu, M. S., Saramies, J., Scott, L. J., Scuteri, A., Silander, K., Sims, M. A., Song, K., Stephens, J., Stevens, S., Stringham, H. M., Tung, Y. C., Valle, T. T., Van Duijn, C. M., Vimaleswaran, K. S., Vollenweider, P., Waeber, G., Wallace, C., Watanabe, R. M., Waterworth, D. M., Watkins, N., Witteman, J. C., Zeggini, E., Zhai, G., Zillikens, M. C., Altshuler, D., Caulfield, M. J., Chanock, S. J., Farooqi, I. S., Ferrucci, L., Guralnik, J. M., Hattersley, A. T., Hu, F. B., Jarvelin, M. R., Laakso, M., Mooser, V., Ong, K. K., Ouwehand, W. H., Salomaa, V., Samani, N. J., Spector, T. D., Tuomi, T., Tuomilehto, J., Uda, M., Uitterlinden, A. G., Wareham, N. J., Deloukas, P., Frayling, T. M., Groop, L. C., Hayes, R. B., Hunter, D. J., Mohlke, K. L., Peltonen, L., Schlessinger, D., Strachan, D. P., Wichmann, H. E., McCarthy, M. I., Boehnke, M., Barroso, I., Abecasis, G. R., & Hirschhorn, J. N. (2009). Six new loci associated with body mass index highlight a neuronal influence on body weight regulation. *Nat Genet*, *41*(1), 25-34. https://doi.org/10.1038/ng.287.

Willmott, M., Bartosik, D. B., & Romanoff, E. B. (1968). The effect of folic acid on superovulation in the immature rat. *J Endocrinol*, *41*(3), 439-445. https://doi.org/10.1677/joe.0.0410439.

Witchel, S. F., & Aston, C. E. (2000). The role of heterozygosity for CYP21 in the polycystic ovary syndrome. *J Pediatr Endocrinol Metab*, *13 Suppl 5*, 1315-1317.

Witchel, S. F., Lee, P. A., Suda-Hartman, M., & Hoffman, E. P. (1997). Hyperandrogenism and manifesting heterozygotes for 21-hydroxylase deficiency. *Biochem Mol Med*, *62*(2), 151-158. https://doi.org/10.1006/bmme.1997.2632.

Witchel, S. F., Lee, P. A., Suda-Hartman, M., Smith, R., & Hoffman, E. P. (1998). 17 alpha-hydroxylase/17,20-lyase dysregulation is not caused by mutations in the coding regions of CYP17. *J Pediatr Adolesc Gynecol*, *11*(3), 133-137. https://doi.org/10.1016/s1083-3188(98)70132-9.

Xie, G. B., Xu, P., Che, Y. N., Xia, Y. J., Cao, Y. X., Wang, W. J., Qiao, D., Wu, X. K., Yi, L., Gao, Q., & Wang, Y. (2013). Microsatellite polymorphism in the fibrillin 3 gene and susceptibility to PCOS: a case-control study and meta-analysis. *Reprod Biomed Online*, *26*(2), 168-174. https://doi.org/10.1016/j.rbmo.2012.10.014.

Xita, N., Georgiou, I., Chatzikyriakidou, A., Vounatsou, M., Papassotiriou, G. P., Papassotiriou, I., & Tsatsoulis, A. (2005). Effect of adiponectin gene polymorphisms on circulating adiponectin and insulin resistance indexes in women with polycystic ovary syndrome. *Clin Chem*, *51*(2), 416-423. https://doi.org/10.1373/clinchem.2004.043109.

Xita, N., Georgiou, I., & Tsatsoulis, A. (2002). The genetic basis of polycystic ovary syndrome. *Eur J Endocrinol*, *147*(6), 717-725. https://doi.org/10.1530/eje.0.1470717.

Xita, N., Tsatsoulis, A., Chatzikyriakidou, A., & Georgiou, I. (2003). Association of the (TAAAA)n repeat polymorphism in the sex hormone-binding globulin (SHBG) gene with polycystic ovary syndrome and relation to SHBG serum levels. *J Clin Endocrinol Metab*, *88*(12), 5976-5980. https://doi.org/10.1210/jc.2003-030197.

Yamada, K., Chen, Z., Rozen, R., & Matthews, R. G. (2001). Effects of common polymorphisms on the properties of recombinant human methylenetetrahydrofolate reductase. *Proc Natl Acad Sci USA*, *98*(26), 14853-14858. https://doi.org/10.1073/pnas.261469998.

Yildiz, B. O., Haznedaroğlu, I. C., Kirazli, S., & Bayraktar, M. (2002). Global fibrinolytic capacity is decreased in polycystic ovary syndrome, suggesting a prothrombotic state. *J Clin Endocrinol Metab*, *87*(8), 3871-3875. https://doi.org/10.1210/jcem.87.8.8716.

Zaki, M., Hassan, N., El-Bassyouni, H. T., Kamal, S., Basha, W., Azmy, O., & Amr, K. (2017). Association of the Pro12Ala Polymorphism with the Metabolic Parameters in Women with Polycystic Ovary Syndrome. *Open Access Maced J Med Sci*, *5*(3), 275-280. https://doi.org/10.3889/oamjms.2017.088.

Zawadzki, J. (1992). Diagnostic criteria for polycystic ovary syndrome (a rational approach). *Polycystic ovary syndrome*, 377-384.

Zhao, S., Tang, X., Shao, D., Dai, H., & Dai, S. (2003). Association study between a polymorphism of aldosterone synthetase gene and the pathogenesis of polycystic ovary syndrome. *Zhonghua Fu Chan Ke Za Zhi*, *38*(2), 94-97.

# Chapter 11

# PCOS and Genetical Inheritance: A Holistic Approach Towards the Role of Genes in the Manifestation of PCOS

**Baiza Bashir**[1]
**and Gowhar Rashid**[2,*]
[1]Department of Botany, Central University of Kashmir, Ganderbal, India
[2]Amity Medical School, Amity University Haryana, India

## Abstract

The predominant endocrinopathy among females of the prime era is polycystic ovary syndrome (PCOS). This complicated endocrine disorder primarily affects females who are of reproductive age. Genetic factors likely play a crucial part in the etiology of the condition given the naissance clustering of cases. PCOS is indeed a complex biological variable with a considerable inheritance, which may account for as much as 70% of a disorder's onset. The overlapping signs of this condition make early PCOS diagnosis difficult and confusing. Pathophysiological problems, such as insulin resistance, chronic inflammation, and hyperandrogenism, arise in PCOS women as a result of genetic variation, epigenetic modifications, and disrupted lifestyles. A specific genetic diagnostic strategy fails because numerous proteins, molecules, and signaling pathways were involved in the course of the disease at the molecular level. Four phenotypic variations of PCOS classify PCOS individuals into the vintage, ovulatory, or non-hyperandrogenic kinds. This genetic method to elucidate the pathophysiology of PCOS has recently been created. Genetic research makes it possible to pinpoint the underlying factor that led to the emergence of PCOS. Although PCOS has an autosomal dominant genetic inheritance, the most recent research has shown that the condition has several gene origins. As of yet, many genetic loci and particular genes have been shown to be connected to this illness. The paradigm for the treatment and diagnosis of PCOS, a reproductive and metabolic disorder, has evolved as a result of genome-wide heritability or associated genetic investigations.

**Keywords:** pathophysiology, genes, endocrinopathy, polymorphism, genetical inheritance, PCOS

---

* Corresponding Author's Email: gowhar9@gmail.com.

In: Polycystic Ovarian Syndrome (PCOS) and Our Biological Clock
Editors: Arpita Roy, Gowhar Rashid and Nihad Ashraf Khan
ISBN: 979-8-89113-100-2
© 2023 Nova Science Publishers, Inc.

## 1. Introduction

Females of reproductive age are susceptible to the multifactorial condition known as polycystic ovarian syndrome (PCOS). Acne, hirsutism, hyperandrogenism, oligomenorrhea, insulin resistance, amenorrhea, obesity, or infertility are all symptoms of this disorder in females. And over 40% of infertility in women is known to be related to PCOS. Furthermore, endometrial cancer is more common in PCOS-affected women (Hardiman et al., 2003). Specific genes, gene-gene interactions, and changing genes' contextual circumstances all have a role in the biological growth of PCOS. To be capable to ascertain the genetic basis of PCOS, it is crucial to recognize the main diverse gene that modifies protein function by altering both its expression and sequence (Lowe & Reddy, 2015). Cells' ability to alter their phenotypic in response to environmental changes is caused by epigenetic changes at the tissue level (Feinberg, 2007). The cellular proteome alterations in diseased tissues are described by the proteome profile (Hanash, 2003). Genetic and epigenetic factors that impact the way proteins are made affect PCOS molecular pathophysiology, which in turn influences PCOS biomarkers.

## 2. Heritability of PCOS

The most complex phenotypic traits, as well as the vast bulk of early studies on the heritability of PCOS, came to the conclusion that the condition would be most probably a dominantly inherent characteristic with low incidence and expressivity. However, more recent research has suggested that these traits are coherent with such a polygenic framework of inheritance. A chromosomal origin of PCOs ruled out by Cooper et al., also suggested that the profile of symptoms (mostly irregular menstrual cycles or hirsutism) in sisters and mothers of impacted probands probably was compatible with such an autosomal dominant form of inheritance. Extending the inclusion standards to include individuals with the polycystic ovarian structure on ultrasound led to a similar finding that the family members' pattern of characteristics was compatible with just an autosomal dominant transmission mode (Franks et al., 1997). The biochemical characteristics of the illness were found in members of the family, including male relatives, according to later research. Overall, 69% and 56% of members of the family had hyperinsulinemia or hypertriglyceridemia; 74% of female ancestors had polycystic ovaries; and 88% of male relatives had male pattern baldness (Norman et al., 1996). Legro et al., also found that sisters of PCOS probands had a higher probability of developing PCOS (22%), as well as hyperandrogenemia (24%) when they had regular menstrual periods. Twin research has been very successful in determining the heredity traits of a variety of disorders, and preliminary research with limited sample sizes came to the conclusion that polygenic or multifactorial causes of PCOS were more likely than mutations in a single gene may be accountable for the condition (Jahanfar et al., 1997); (Legro, Driscoll, Strauss, et al., 1998). In accordance with the Rotterdam criteria, 3205 females were examined in the most comprehensive twin family study, including 1332 monozygotic, 680 dizygotic twins, 474 members of dizygotic contrary sex couples, as well as 719 non-twin sisters. The association between the characteristics of PCOS of monozygotic twin pairs was substantially higher than in dizygotic of nontwin sister pairs; the relative risks of oligomenorrhea, acne, and hirsutism were 0.67 versus 0.07, 0.78 versus 0.44, and 0.86 versus 0.28, respectively. Dizygotic twin and non-twin sisters had a risk of PCOS that was 0.38 (95% CI 0.00 to 0.66) higher than that of monozygotic twin sisters, who had a risk of 0.71 (95% CI 0.43 to 0.88) overall. Inside an independent pathway model that included the 3 parameters of oligomenorrhea, hirsutism, or acne the scientists came to the conclusion that genetic diversity (79%) and specific environmental influences (21%), rather than shared environmental influences, were the main determinants of PCOS. Despite the fact that many researches, including this one, have shown that PCOS is significantly heritable, the heritability finding offers little information about the potential genes that might be at play (Vink et al., 2006).

## 3. Candidate Gene studies

The bulk of gene analysis on PCOS has employed the potential genetic strategy; this is partially because of investigator-driven theories about the etiology of PCOS, even though it is also a result of the genetic analysis technology that was available at the time the studies were conducted. In total, 241 genes with 114 SNPs that were linked to PCOS were listed in a recent database, highlighting the diversity of gene changes that have been discovered in the writings. A few interesting candidate genes within these have been found and confirmed in numerous investigations, yet it is still unknown how much these genes as a whole contribute to the pathogenesis of PCOS. Identifying gene interactions that have historically failed to hold up to scrutiny is common. The insulin receptor is the sole candidate gene whose results from GWAS investigations have been confirmed (INSR) (Jones & Goodarzi, 2016). The polymorphism mutation (D19S884) inside of the fibrillin 3 gene (FBN3) upstream of INSR was recognized by Tucci et al., as a possible cause for PCOS, however, it was unable to be determined if the susceptible loci have been within insulin genes receptor itself and within the gene region. Both investigators came to the conclusion that there had been a significant correlation with the transfer of PCOS after looking at the D19S884 marker in two bigger groups of 367 families and 453 families. These results were confirmed in a survey of Han Chinese PCOs patients; however, a smaller Spanish investigation came to the opposite conclusion, finding no connection between both the D19S884 markers and PCOS (Tucci et al., 2001); (Villuendas et al., 2003). There has been continuous research into the function of polymorphism inside the insulin response element itself given the significance of insulin resistance for the whole PCOS phenotype. Seven studies identified SNPs in INSR associated with PCOS risk, one among which was later affirmed in a significant analysis (rs2252673). Researchers also proposed a relationship between obesity-susceptibility genetics as well as PCOS in light of the strong correlation between PCOS and obesity. The rs9939609 polymorphism is associated with fat mass or obesity. An allele may be a major risk factor for PCOS sensitivity both in Asian and Caucasian subgroups, according to the results of a meta-analysis of 5 studies which included 5010 PCOS cases or 5300 controls (OR 1.43 and OR 1.33, respectively) (Liu et al., 2017) (Figure 1).

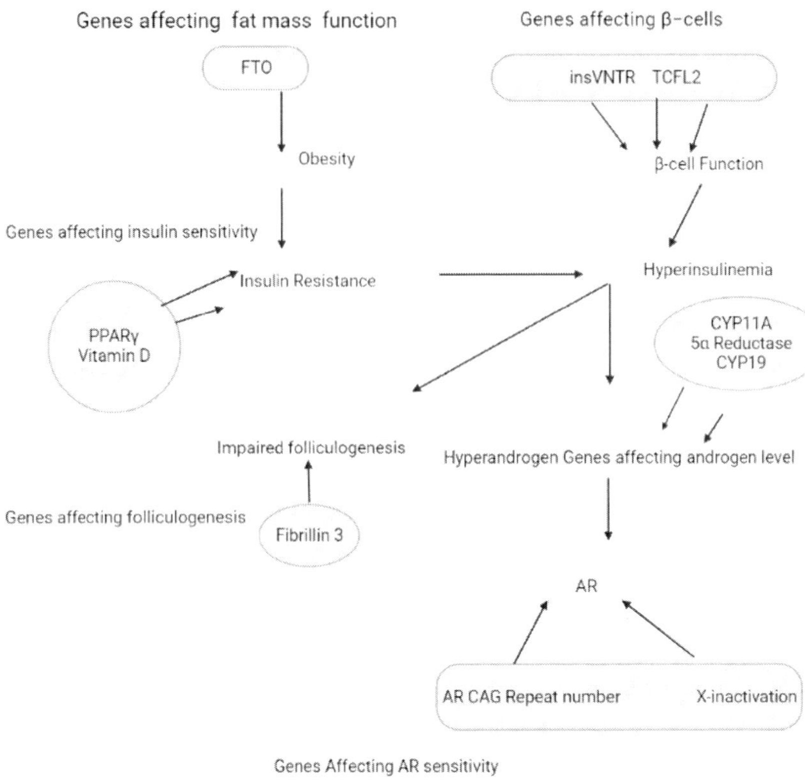


AR: Androgen receptor.

**Figure 1.** Diagram illustrating the key polycystic ovarian syndrome candidate gene studies that have been published in the literature. The major etiological pathways are represented by solid arrows, while potential gene effects are represented by dashed arrows.

Studies investigating variations in enzymes implicated inside steroidogenic pathway or susceptibility to androgen signaling has been conducted in response to genetic premises for hyperandrogenism in PCOS (Ketefian et al., 2016). Early research on the mutant androgen receptor gene repeat sequence (CAG) revealed that infertile PCOS patients had more repetitions than fertile control patients (Hickey et al., 2016). But a further meta-assessment of the function in the CAG repeats in the androgen response element came to the conclusion that the shorter repeat group was associated with androgen excess (56.25% vs. 29.14%, P0.0011) (Peng et al., 2014). In addition, SNPs in the genes of the androgen receptor signaling pathway (HSPA1A, STIP1, HSPA8, PTGES3, FKBP4, BAG1, ST13 & STUB1) were evaluated in a larger core group of 354 PCOS patients as well as 161 control individuals. A reduced odds ratio for PCOS was associated with two of these FKBP4 SNPs. A subsequent replication group only verified a single of these, rs4409904 (397 cases or 306 controls). Alternate splice variants of an androgen receptor may be linked to aberrant follicular growth and hyperandrogenemia in PCOS patients, according to a recent study (Wang et al., 2015). Studies that looked at several genes inside the steroidogenic pathway simultaneously to those involved in gonadotropin actions, fatness, energy regulation, as well as insulin action did fail to find a strong connection among variations inside the steroidogenic enzyme pathway as well as in PCOS, but they did find evidence that variations in the follistatin (a gonadotropin) gene may be (Urbanek et al., 1999).

**Table 1.** Outline of the primary polycystic ovarian syndrome candidate gene research

| S. NO | Candidacy | Study (Year) | Genes | Number of PCOs cases | References |
|---|---|---|---|---|---|
| 1 | Insulin sensitivity | (Diamanti-Kandarakis et al., 2004) | PAI-1 promoter | 162 | (Diamanti-Kandarakis et al., 2004) |
| | | (Mukherjee et al., 2007) | INSR | 180 | (Mukherjee et al., 2007) |
| | | (San-Millán & Escobar-Morreale, 2010) | PPAR-g 2 Pro 12 Ala | Meta-analysis of nine studies | (San-Millán & Escobar-Morreale, 2010) |
| | | (Mahmcudi, 2009) | FOK1 | 163 | Jay et.al.,2007 |
| 2 | Abnormal steroid production and metabolism | (Goodarzi et al., 2006) | SRD5A1, SRD5A2 (5a-reductase) | 287 | (Goodarzi et al., 2006) |
| | | (Gaasenbeek et al., 2004) | CYP11A promoter (encodes P450 11a1) | 371 | (Gaasenbeek et al., 2004) |
| 3 | Impaired folliculogenesis | (Urbanek et al., 1999) | Chromosome 19p13.2 (D19S884) | 150 families | (Urbanek et al., 1999) |
| 4 | β-cell dysfunction | (Christopoulos et al., 2008) | TCF7L2 | 183 | (Christopoulos et al., 2008) |
| | | (Barber, Bennett, Gloyn, et al., 2007) | KCNJ11 | 374 | (Barber, Bennett, Gloyn, et al., 2007) |
| | | (Powell et al., 2005) | Insulin gene VNTR | 440 | (Powell et al., 2005) |
| | | (Barber, Bennett, Groves, et al., 2007) | TCF7L2 | 369 | (Barber, Bennett, Groves, et al., 2007) |
| | | (Biyasheva et al., 2009) | TCF7L2 | 624 | (Biyasheva et al., 2009) |
| 5 | Fat mass | (Attaoua et al., 2008) | FTO | 207 | (Attaoua et al., 2008) |
| | | (Barber et al., 2008) | FTO | 463 | (Barber et al., 2008) |
| 6 | Androgen receptor and X-inactivation | (T. Hickey, 2002) | AR gene exon 1 (androgen receptor gene CAG repeat) | 122 | (T. Hickey, 2002) |
| | | (Shah et al., 2008) | AR gene exon 1 (androgen receptor gene CAG repeat) | 330 | (Shah et al., 2008) |
| | | (T. E. Hickey et al., 2006) | X-inactivation | 88 sisters of PCOS cases | (T. E. Hickey et al., 2006) |
| 7 | PCOS: polycystic ovary syndrome | VNTR Variable number of tandem repeats | FTO: Fat mass and obesity Associated | KCNJ11: potassium inwardly-rectifying channel subfamily J member 11. | |

It has been recommended that PCOS and metabolic changes are connected with an inflammatory phenotype, which may have a genetic basis in variations in the genes for inflammation cytokines such as TNF-alpha, IL-6, or IL-1 beta. A meta-analysis was performed on all articles studying polymorphisms in these genes, and 14 papers qualified for inclusion. There were a total of 802 patients and 802 controls for TNFalpha, and there was no proof that the polymorphism 308 G/A had any bearing on PCOS or obesity. 351 cases & 464 controls were found for IL-6, as well as the 174 G/C polymorphisms was examined (Table 1). Overall, no significant correlation was found; however, some evidence of relevance was found when utilizing an allelic model. The absence of a clear link between the IL-1 beta polymorphisms (511C/T) and the condition was also seen, which suggests that connections reported in earlier research utilizing sparse samples of controls and cases were eliminated by larger meta-analyses (Guo et al., 2015). Overall, the candidate gene technique is unsuitable for the research of a polygenic syndrome like PCOS, despite numerous promising findings, because it is incredibly unlikely to uncover a high-impact mutation in a specific gene when comparing just less numbers of people with or without the disorder. Furthermore, prior research has only examined population-known variants, making it unlikely that any novel variants with significant genetic impact will be found. The advent of new genomic technology has made the switch to GWAS research effective in identifying risk loci in PCOS.

## 4. Genes Associated with PCOS

Numerous genes have been investigated as potential applicants of PCOS connection. The rationale for gene finding was the pathophysiology of PCOS as it was observed. While testing of additional genes is ongoing, the majority of research has focused on a group of candidate genes.

### 4.1. Genes Associated with Sex Hormone Regulation

#### *4.1.1. FBN3*

- *Function:* A protein used for the extracellular architecture that codes for fibrillin 3.
- *Genetic studies:* A PCOS sensitivity locus was discovered by early gene mapping around a dinucleotide repeating marker on 19p13 (D19S884). Due to this locus's closeness to the insulin receptor, it is noteworthy. A further genetic investigation was conducted on 1723 people in 412 families, including 43 sisters who were impacted and 412 index cases, who are primarily of European descent. D19S884 in intron 55 of fibrillin-3, one of the 53 variations examined, provided the greatest support for a link to PCOS (p = 0.0037) (Urbanek et al., 1999).
- *Contribution to PCOS:* Although fibrillin-3 is located on chromosome 19 close to the insulin receptor gene, its precise function in PCOS is not yet established. Examination of the carrier of the A8 allele revealed elevated amounts of insulin sensitivity (17 11 U/ml A8 (+) vs. 12 4 U/ml A8 (); P = 0.008) with just an odds ratio (OR) of 1.44, independent of obesity. A8 allele carriers also had higher HOMA IR (1.94 1.1 A8(+)

vs. 1.49 0.55 A8(); P = 0.02). These metabolic alterations were not present in women with the A8 allele who did not have PCOS. Additionally, proinsulin phases as well as the proinsulin/insulin ratio were greater fasting in the siblings of PCOS patients with the A8 allele. The control of TGF familial genes, such as inhibin, activin, as well as follistatin, by fibrillins, is assumed to be the basis for fibrillin-3's involvement in PCOS (Urbanek et al., 1999). Furthermore, islet cell mass and insulin sensitivity are both increased in fibrillin-3 knockout mice (Mukherjee et al., 2007).

#### *4.1.2. SHBG*

- *Function:* A sex hormone-binding glycoprotein that the liver secretes is known as sex-hormone-binding globulin (SHBG).
- *Genetic studies:* The (TAAAA) n repeats allele inside the SHBG gene was examined by Xita et al., Comparing those with PCOS to those without, those with PCOS showed a statistically significant increase in greater frequency repeats. Lean women having PCOS or obese women having PCOS were compared, but no differences were found. Additionally, individuals with longer repeats showed lower SHBG levels (Xita et al., 2003). In contrast, Urbanek et al., extensive's investigation of 37 potential genes revealed no correlation between PCOS and SHBG levels (Urbanek et al., 1999).
- *Contribution to PCOS:* Women having PCOS commonly have low SHBG phases, and it's probable that the lengthy (TAAAA)n repeats have something to do with this. These findings need to be verified, though. Additionally, hyperinsulinemia was known to raise systemic free androgens and decrease SHBG in the liver.

#### *4.1.3. The AR Gene*

- *Function:* The gene that encodes X-linked androgen receptors.
- *Genetic studies:* N-terminal region of the androgen receptor genetic traits has polymorphic CAG trinucleotide repeats that encode a polyglutamine. In one study, 112 women having normal menstrual cycles and verified fertility were compared to 91 females with clinically diagnosed PCOS (Mifsud et al., 2000). Women who were affected and had high testosterone levels, women who had low or normal testosterone levels, and a control group had their CAG repeat length assessed. Carriage of short CAG repeats was associated statistically substantially (P = 0.004) with the anovulatory PCOS phenotype.
- *Contributions to PCOS:* One essential characteristic of PCOS is a hyperandrogenic condition. If this link is validated, it may imply that AR polymorphisms may have a role in the phenotype of PCOS despite normal testosterone levels.

#### *4.1.4. CYP21*

- *Function:* Code for the adrenal steroid 21-hydroxylase, which transforms 17-hydroxyprogesterone into 11-deoxycortisol and progesterone into deoxycorticosterone.

- *Genetic studies:* Escobar-Morreale et al., investigated the relationship between CYP21 gene alterations and 40 hirsute women. Compared to one control, eight hirsute patients were found to be heterozygote carriers of CYP21 mutations. Four of the hirsute women who were carriers revealed regular seventeen hydroxyprogesterone levels at rest and after ACTH stimulation, pointing to a PCOS-like phenotype that lacked the complete set of symptoms associated with non-classical adrenal hyperplasia (CAH). In a short study of thirty adolescent girls with hyperandrogenism (Escobar-Morreale et al., 2008), Witchel and Aston found that the commonality of CYP21 mutations was higher than that of healthy controls. They came to the conclusion that nonsense mutations displayed the non-classical CAH phenotype, whereas carriers with missense CYP21 mutations presented a PCOS phenotype (Witchel & Aston, 2000). A subsequent study included 109 women having PCOS or 95 controls, however, found no correlation (Witchel et al., 2005).
- *Contribution to PCOS:* Non-classical CAH is caused by diminished or missing action of adrenal steroid 21-hydroxylase. There is little evidence to suggest that CYP21 heterozygosity may result in elevated levels of adrenal androgen without the whole CAH syndrome. Although it is doubtful that CYP21 polymorphisms significantly contribute to PCOS, there is a chance that some CAH instances could be misdiagnosed for PCOS (Deneux et al., 2001).

### *4.1.5. Dopamine D3 Receptor*

- *Function:* The Dopamine receptor gene D3, uses inhibitory G-proteins to prevent adenylyl cyclase from being produced. GnRH & prolactin gene regulation involves D3 receptors.

  Homozygosity for a specific D3 dopamine receptor allele (the "2 allele") (Legro et al., 1995). In contrast to women who did not have homozygosity for the 2 alleles, these patients showed very erratic menstrual cycles, recurrent anovulation, and increased testosterone levels. Additionally, clomiphene doses needed to trigger ovulation in patients having homozygous 2 alleles were greater. In a later investigation, non-Hispanic Caucasian women in the Southeast of the United States were studied, but no link between PCOS and this mutation was discovered (M. Kahsar-Miller et al., 1999).
- *Contribution to PCOS:* Two key factors are at the root of dopamine's involvement in the pathophysiology of PCOS. First, excessive LH secretion is a hallmark of PCOS in women, and dopamine can be used to reduce it (Marshall & Eagleson, 1999). The second finding is that up to one-third of PCOS-afflicted women had a modest prolactinoma. In PCOS-afflicted women, a relative dopamine shortage or decreased dopamine activity may be the root of both of these issues. Before this method can be connected to a D3 receptor polymorphism as well as the impact of the 2 alleles on receptor function, however, it must first be proven (Lechin et al., 2004).

### *4.1.6. FSH-Beta*

- *Function:* Symbols that represent the follicle-stimulating hormone beta subunit.

- *Genetic studies:* The polymorphisms and mutations in exons two and three of the FSHβ gene were examined by Tong et al., in one hundred and thirty-five Chinese women having PCOS & 105 control participants(Tong et al., 2000) (Tong et.al.,2007). Although a T – C substitution which was found in exon 3, there were no missense changes found. Contrasted with the control group, PCOS patients (12.6%) had a considerably higher incidence of the CC genotype. Additionally, this gene was more frequently discovered in obese PCOS women than in PCOS-only individuals.
- *Contribution to PCOS:* Exogenous FSH administration has been shown to improve follicular development, selection, & ovulation in many PCOS patients (Franks, Mason, et al., 2000) (Franks et al., 2000). Additionally, in transgenic mice, follistatin, a regulatory protein, suppressed FSH and caused folliculogenesis to halt (Liao et al., 2000). These two elements imply that variations within the FSH gene may participate in the etiology of PCOS. These affiliation data must be verified, though.

## 4.2. Genes Associated with Insulin Resistance

### *4.2.1. CAPN10*

- *Function:* Codes the calcium-dependent cysteine protease known as Calpain-10. A type 2 diabetes whole genome scan revealed a link between insulin resistance and CAPN10 mutations (Horikawa et al., 2000).
- *Genetic studies:* Haddad et al., looked explored 4 SNPs within CAPN10 genes in one hundred and forty-six parent-child trios, 185 unconnected PCOS patients, and 525 healthy controls of European ancestry (Haddad et al., 2002). The familial-based transmissions disequilibrium test (TDT) revealed a slight correlation for one common variant, but the case-control study did not. Therefore, there is no evidence linking CAPN10 to PCOS.
- *Contributions of PCOS:* Insulin resistance have been regarded as a key component of the polycystic ovary syndrome pathophysiology. Calpain-10 is a good candidate gene for PCOS since it is related to insulin resilience. However, the findings to date do not indicate that CAPN10 has a significant impact on the etiology of PCOS.

### *4.2.2. IGF2*

- *Function:* Code to insulin-like growth factors 2, and a protein hormone that resembles insulin in terms of its molecular makeup.
- *Genetic studies:* In PCOS patients, San Millan et al., examined 15 potential genes related to insulin tolerance, obesity, as well as type 2 diabetes. The GG genotype of the IGF2 gene's ApaI variation was significantly associated with PCOS (62.9% vs. 38.1%; P = 0.018) (Millan et al., 2004).
- *Contribution of PCOS:* IGF2 expression may rise as a result of an IGF2 gene variation linked to PCOS patients. IGF2 has been shown to increase ovarian and adrenal androgen output, which may have a role in the pathophysiology of PCOs.

### *4.2.3. IRS1 and IRS2*

- *Function:* These post-receptor proteins are implicated in the signal transduction of insulin genes and encode the insulin receptor substrates 1 & 2.
- *Genetic studies:* The IRS-1 or IRS-2 gene was sequenced in Caucasian women who had PCOS and were of European descent by El Mkadem et al. The evaluation of the homeostatic model factor for insulin resilience was used to test insulin resistance. Although no mutations were observed, a relationship between insulin resistance and the IRS-1 and IRS-2 Gly1057Arg and Gly972Arg polymorphisms was found.
- *Contribution of PCOS:* Insulin resistance and PCOS go hand in hand, and insulin genetic signal transduction downstream proteins may be the culprit. Alterations in IRS1 and IRS2 expression may cause insulin resistance, a key component of polycystic ovarian syndrome pathogenesis. The implications of these variations on gene activity and/or expression, as well as the relationship between the IRS-1 as well as the IRS-2 genes and PCOs, need to be validated.

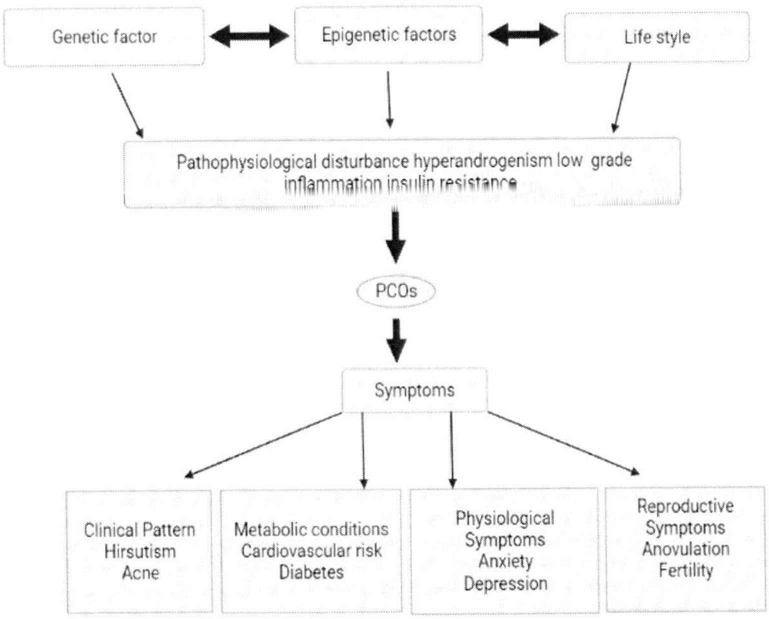


**Figure 2.** Diagram illustrating the Pathophysiological disturbance and symptoms.

Unrelated to obesity, insulin signaling deficiency is a significant clinical indication from PCOs (insulin resilience). The pathogenies of PCOS also involve the glyco-oxidative pathway and the modified insulin gene expression pathway (Cortón et al., 2007); (Dunaif, 1997). Low insulin activity as a result of high oxidative stress leads to hyperandrogenism (Figure 2).

## 5. Genes with Specific Functions in PCOS Pathophysiology

### 5.1. Gene Involved in the Production of Adrenal and Ovarian Steroids

Numerous genes have been connected to PCOS hyperandrogenism through assessment and identification methods. The gene CYP19, which may be found on the 15q21.2 chromosome, is in charge of the aromatase p450 activities needed for the production of estrogen. Low aromatase activity is seen in PCOS patients who are lean and fat (Takayama, 2004). The conversion of progesterone to 17-hydroxyprogesterone as well as the pregnenolone to the 17-hydroxypregnenolone is catalyzed by the enzyme P450c17, which is encoded by CYP17. It was discovered that PCOS is linked to a mutation in the promoter area and CYP17 overexpression in theca cells (Wickenheisser et al., 2000). An enzyme that converts 17-hydroxyprogesterone to 11-deoxycortisol as part of the production of steroid hormones is encoded by the CYP21 gene. Ineffective steroid anabolism caused by the enzyme's inactivity further contributes to PCOS (Witchel & Aston, 2000). CYP11a encodes the enzyme that is involved in the phase that limits how quickly cholesterol is converted to progesterone. Due to polymorphism and variation in CYP11a, numerous investigations by scientists have discovered a link between the two conditions (Franks, Gilling-Smith, et al., 2000) (Wang et al., 2015).

### 5.2. Insulin Action and Secretion-Related Genes

Humans have a gene called CAPN10 that codes for the protein called calpain-10. The family of cysteine proteases known as Calpains is calcium-dependent. A significant subunit is encoded by this gene. Because it lacks the calcium-binding domain that is similar to calmodulin and instead contains a divergent C-terminal domain, calpain-10 (CAPN10) is an unusual calpain (Zhang et al., 2014). This gene is situated in the NIDDM1 area and is linked to type 2 and non-insulin-dependent diabetic mellitus (NIDDM). For this gene, several different transcript versions have been reported. Moreover, CAPN10 is a gene that codes for proteins. Type 1 diabetes 2 or PCOS are illnesses linked to CAPN10. The integrin system and ERK signaling are two of its related pathways. Cytoskeletal complexation and nutrient cysteine-type endopeptidase activity are two copies of ontology (GO) annotations associated with this gene. CAPN3 is a significant paralog of this gene (Sáez et al., 2008). Patients with PCOS experience abnormal insulin levels. The CAPN10 mutation has been linked to PCOS in earlier research. The first type 2 diabetes risk gene to be discovered was the CAPN10 gene. The CAPN10 gene contains several single nucleotide polymorphisms as well. The polymorphisms of UCSNP-19 and UCSNP-63 have both been linked to PCOS. UCSNP-45, UCSNP-63, or UCSNP-19 genotypes are risk factors for PCOS, according to a second study on Asian women. The link between the CAPN10 polymorphism and the metabolic characteristic of PCOS has been studied using a variety of case-control or meta-assessment studies in various research groups (Shen et al., 2013).

## 5.3. Genes Affecting the Effect of Steroid Hormones

### *5.3.1. Gene for the Androgen Receptor*

The androgen receptor gene, which has eleven exons or codes for a 90kb tri-domain protein, is situated on the q arm of chromosomal X. Chromosome X mutant or cellular structural disruptions are both known causes of PCOS in people. Numerous investigations have demonstrated that elevated androgen levels cause irregular menstruation, anovulation, and the development of ovarian microcysts. Additionally, experimental investigations suggested that androgen exposure during fetal development contributes to the adult onset of PCOS. Genetic variation in an exon 1 for the AR gene with a CAG repeat determines androgen activity as well as the prevalence of PCOs (Schüring et al., 2012). According to numerous studies, the androgen genetic trait may contribute to the growth of PCOS in the Chinese or Caucasian population by increasing the frequency of the short AR CAG repeat. This polymorphism is also connected to higher androgen sensitivity and upregulated androgen receptors. Studies from Slovenia, India, Croatia, and Korea, however, could not discover any links between PCOS and CAG repeat length. According to a study comparing PCOS families, the XCI (X chromosome inactivity pattern) is significantly linked to the pathophysiology of the condition. Sisters with different XCI profiles have more varied PCOS symptoms than sisters with the same XCI profile (T. Hickey, 2002). Additionally, the preovulatory follicular development gene BMP15 (Xp11.2), which is linked to the XCI pattern, can be affected. BMP15 expression is correlated with elevated FSH transcription and secretion but not with LH expression. According to another study, there is no correlation among the length of AG CAG allele, hirsutism, XCI patterns, and AR CAG BM levels to the DHEAS hormone. According to Chaudhary et al., the XCI pattern may directly affect the phases of the hormones LH and FSH, which affect the levels of the genes that are necessary for follicular growth (gonadotropins and other genes) (Chaudhary et al., 2021).

### *5.3.2. Gene for Sex Hormone-Binding Globulin*

On chromosome 17p13-p12, there is a gene called the sexual hormone-binding globulin (SHBG), which produces a protein with 373 amino acids. In the body, sex hormone levels are controlled by androgen (testosterone and estrogen) interacting with SHBG protein. The manufacture of SHBG via hepatocytes is regulated by metabolic variables like testosterone and insulin (Plymate et al., 1988). Females with PCOS have decreased levels of SHBG, which is a result of hyperinsulinemia's inhibition of SHBG production. Single nucleotide variation in SHBG has been related to PCOS in a number of studies on the subject (Chen et al., 2019).

## 5.4. Gonadotropin-Related Gene

### *5.4.1. Hormone and Receptor for Lutein*

Androgen overload and ovulatory in PCOS are caused by the luteinizing hormone's altered amount and disrupted functions. A follicular-stimulating hormone is inhibited by extra luteinizing hormone adversely, which further reduces estrogen production by androgen transfer and increases the concentration of androgen in the ovaries. A study on PCOS women found follicle-stimulating receptor point mutation B sub-unit at (Trp8Arg and IIg15Thr), even though this mutation was also found in 15% of non-PCOs woman populations (Nilsson et al., 1997).

### *5.4.2. Receptor for Follicular Stimulating Hormone*

Hormonal instability in PCOS women is brought on by a change in the receptor gene that causes the structural distortion of an encoded protein. A G-protein-associated receptor is produced by this gene, which is located within the p arm of chromosome 2 or contains 14 exons. This receptor is necessary for the development of the gonadal organ. There was a high-frequency variation in this gene in a study of women from North Iraq (Baban et al., 2017).

## 5.5. Additional Genes

### *5.5.1. PCOS1*

The gene, commonly referred to as PCOS1, is located on chromosome 19p13.2. Several researchers have examined this gene to determine the link. The first instance of this gene being found in two sisters was in 1971; additionally, this study was repeated in 2005. The study used a sizable sampling of 367 PCOS families (Urbanek et al., 1999) (Table 2).

**Table 2.** Different Genes Are Involved in the PCOS Pathogenesis

| S.NO | Different gene categories involved in PCOS | Genes under categories |
|---|---|---|
| 1 | Gene Involved in the Production of Adrenal and Ovarian Steroids. | CYP17<br>CYP19<br>CYP21<br>CYP11a<br>CYP21 |
| 2 | Insulin Action and Secretion-Related Genes | CAPN10<br>INS<br>INS<br>IRS-1<br>IRS-2 |
| 3 | Genes Affecting the Effect of Steroid Hormones | SHBR<br>AR |
| 4 | Gonadotropin-related gene | LH<br>FSHR<br>AMH |
| 5 | Other Genes | PCO<br>FTO<br>SRD5A<br>SRD5B |

According to the study, D19S884, a dinucleotide-repeats found within an intron of the FBN3 (Fibrillin 3) gene 105 bp'3 to the exon 55, may be responsible again for transcription of the neighboring gene as well as for INSR because the findings of an earlier study by the same scientific team were replicated. Additionally, it was determined that D19S884 may have a role in the post-translational conversion of FBN3 into mRNA (Table 2) (Urbanek et al., 1999).

### *5.5.2. SRD5A and SRD5B*

A study was conducted in 1999 to assess the activities of SRD5A among PCOS women, and it was shown to be high. Additionally, SRD5B's cytogenetic position is 2p23.1. Further research revealed that PCOS patients with the SRD5A variant have hirsutism, but those with the SRD5B variant experience PCOS protection (Goodarzi et al., 2006).

#### *5.5.3. Fat Mass Obesity (FTO)*

This chromosome 16 gene, linked to obesity or type 2 diabetes, produces the alpha-ketoglutarate enzyme (q arm). In Pakistan, PCOS women were linked to the single nucleotide polymorphism rs9939609. Compared to the general people, PCOS women were said to have a significantly higher level of this polymorphism (Rizwan et al., n.d.).

## 6. Family Studies

Based on the clustering of instances in families, it appears that PCOS has a genetic component. The greatest genetically inherited trait in familial cases appears to be hyperandrogenemia. There are a number of problems that have impeded the genetic analysis of PCOS. Large pedigrees for linkage study are hard to come by because PCOS is linked to infertility. Furthermore, due to which use of several diagnostic criteria as well as the heterogeneity of PCOS, family studies cannot be easily compared. Furthermore, a distinct PCOS male phenotype has not yet been discovered (Fauser et al., 2004).

Despite these obstacles, most investigations point to a dominantly transmitted characteristic with modest penetrance & variable confirmed. This route of inheritance might be in line with the diverse clinical manifestations of PCOS. However, it is impossible to rule out polygenic, genetic heterogeneity, or multifactorial inheritance. The familial research is summarised in Table 3.

Cooper et al., evaluated 18 people with Stein-Leventhal syndrome in the first systematic genetic investigation (Cooper et al., 1968). Sisters of cases experienced oligomenorrhea, hirsutism, & enlarged ovaries far more frequently than sisters of controls. Additionally, male relatives were more likely to exhibit hirsutism or "pelosity."

Givens and colleagues at the University of Tennessee in Memphis conducted studies in the 1970s that suggested PCOS might be inherited dominantly via the X chromosome. The presence of hirsutism and the polycystic or bilaterally large ovaries served as diagnostic criteria. Givens et al., identified 2 families in the first report that had several members impacted throughout more than two generations. Acanthosis nigricans, insulin sensitivity, and hypertension were common in 1 kindred, and affect females had infarction in the fifth decade. The majority of subjects were African Americans (Givens et al., 1971). The maturational stoppage of spermatogenesis was seen in some males in a third kindred. Wilroy et colleagues calculated that, after excluding index cases, 47% of the affected females children were female. 89% of daughters in a male's progeny with an increased Luteinizing hormone stimulating hormone (FSH) ratios were affected. It is compatible with X-linked dominant inheritance that nearly all affected males' daughters also had health issues (Cohen et al., 1975).

Ferriman and Purdie evaluated a control cohort of 179 women in the UK together with 381 patients who had hirsutism and/or oligomenorrhea. The most inherited traits were found in hirsute women with larger ovaries. 38 1st relatives had hirsutism, Thirty had oligomenorrhea, and 19 had infertility out of 188 patients having hirsutism as well as enlarged ovaries. There were 73, 15, and 10 first-degree relatives of 96 patients having hirsutism but normal-sized ovary who exhibited the aforementioned features, respectively. Numbers 7, 8, & 8 were found in 179 controls. Male family members of hirsute women had a considerably higher rate of baldness (FERRIMAN & PURDIE, 1979).

Additional evidence supporting the heritability of PCOS, specifically autosomal dominant inheritance, was supplied by later British investigations. Hague et al. employed ultrasonography criteria and either LH hypersecretion or hyperandrogenemia to estimate the prevalence of PCOS in afflicted persons' relatives. PCOS was discovered in 24 of 36 (67%) mothers and 45 of 52 (87%) sisters of probands. Doubts concerning the specificity of the diagnostic criteria were raised because the regularity of impacted relatives was significantly higher than 50% indicated either for autosomal dominant or Cross dominant inheritance. Such a skewed segregation ratio would need the use of non-Mendelian mechanisms. More likely, the diagnosis was falsely positive due to overly sensitive criteria (HAGUE et al., 1988).

The regularity of afflicted relatives in PCOs was closer to 50% predicted with autosomal dominant inheritance in later British investigations. Carey et al. did genetic research. Ten probands' first-degree relatives were investigated. 58 of the 62 informants were subjected to ultrasonography screening. 51% of the 58 first-degree women relatives were impacted (Carey et al., 1993).

Lunde et al. conducted family investigations in Norway. Only 6–15% of first-degree relatives were impacted, according to Lunde et al., who used hirsutism as well oligomenorrhea as inclusion criteria. According to Norman et al., 23, there were significantly more impacted relatives in 15 probands. By ultrasonography, 13 of 15 (87%) of the sisters had high testosterone (T), 10 of 15 (66%) had hyperinsulinemia, and 11 of 15 (73%) have polycystic ovaries (Lunde et al., 1989); (Norman et al., 1996).

Legro et al., in the US (Pennsylvania) evaluated 80 probands who were diagnosed with oligomenorrhea (6 menses/year) due to increased testosterone; non-classical 21-hydroxylase deficit was excluded. They discovered that 36 of the 80 (45%) sisters were affected by hyperandrogenemia (Legro, Driscoll, Strauss Iii, et al., 1998).

Govind et al., studied 10 control women and 29 probands. The diagnostic criteria included polycystic ovary on ultrasound, together either with or without the clinical and biochemical signs of PCOs; 61% of female 1$^{st}$ relatives were affected, while 22% of male first-degree relatives had male-pattern baldness that started early (before age 30). When compared to the control family, the prevalence was substantially higher. A total of 71 PCOS proband siblings were examined; 39 (55%) of them had the condition, which is congruent with inherited dominant inheritance (Govind et al., 1999).

**Table 3.** Summary of studies assessing the frequency of PCOS in female relatives.

| Author | Diagnostic criteria | Frequency of Specific traits assessed | Affected sisters (%) | Affected mothers (%) | Overall affected first-degree female relatives (%) |
|---|---|---|---|---|---|
| (Givens et al., 1971) | Oligomenorrhea, hirsutism, and polycystic ovaries (exam and surgery) | Oligomenorrhea | | | 16/67 (24%) |
| | | Hirsutism | | | 28/54 (52%) |
| (FERRIMAN & PURDIE, 1979) | Hirsutism and/or oligomenorrhea (60% with polycystic ovaries by air Contrast gynecography) | Hirsutism | 30/337 (9%) | 32/284 (5%) | |
| | | Oligomenorrhea | 32/337 (9%) | 24\284 (8%) | |
| (Lunde et al., 1989) | Menstrual dysfunction, hyperandrogenism, obesity, infertility, and polycystic ovaries (transabdominal ultrasound) | Hirsutism | 8\129(6%) | 17\132(13%) | |
| | | Oligomenorrhea | 19/129 (15%) | 16\132 (12%) | |
| (Cooper et al., 1968) | Oligomenorrhea, hirsutism, polycystic ovaries (culdoscopy, gynecography, or wedge resection) | Oligomenorrhea | 9\19(47%) | 4\13(31%) | |
| | | Hirsutism | 14\24 (58%) | 4\13 (31%) | |
| | | Elevated 24-hour urinary 17-ketosteroids | 12/19 (63%) | 2/7 (29%) | |
| | | Enlarged ovaries | 10\19 (53%) | 0\7 (0%0 | |
| (HAGUE et al., 1988) | Menstrual irregularities, hirsutism, infertility, obesity and multicystic ovaries (wedge resection) | Hirsutism | | | 28/107 (26% |
| | | Oligomenorrhea | | | 19/107 (18%) |
| (Norman et al., 1996) | Elevated androgens, decreased SHBG, polycystic ovaries (ultrasound) | Polycystic ovaries (ultrasound) | 11/15 (73%) | 1/1 (100%) | |
| | | Increased testosterone or androstenedione | 13/15 (87%) | 1\5(20%) | |
| | | Hyperinsulinemia | 10/15 (66%) | 5\5(100%) | |
| (Govind et al., 1999) | Polycystic ovaries (ultrasound) | Polycystic ovaries | 35/53 (66%) | 15/29 (52%) | 50/82 (61%) |
| (M. Kahsar-Miller et al., 1999) | Oligomenorrhea and either\hirsutism or <brelevated testosterone | Polycystic ovaries | 35/53 (66%) | 15/29 (52%) | 50\82(61%) |
| | | PCOS as defined | 16\50(32%) | 19\78(24%) | |
| (Legro, Driscoll, Strauss, et al., 1998) | Elevated testosterone and oligomenorrhea | Hyperadrogenemia | 36/80 (45%) | | |
| (Carey et al., 1994) | Polycystic ovaries by transabdominal ultrasound | Polycystic ovaries (ultrasound) | | | 37/50 (74%) |
| | | Elevated testosterone | | | 16/50 (32%) |

In families of 93 cohorts of PCOS, Kahsar-Miller and colleagues looked examined the frequency of oligomenorrhea either hirsutism or high testosterone of all Ist female relatives. First-degree relatives were shown to have a considerably greater risk of PCOS than the general population, indicating a hereditary component to the condition (M. D. Kahsar-Miller et al., 2001).

Conway et al. demonstrated that the level of relatedness between a PCOS group was 4 times higher than overall average relatedness as one of a large random selection of a similar database, which was used to assess the degree of heredity in PCOS and seek a founder effect (Conway et al., 2014).

## 7. Genetic Identification Application

Precision medicine, often known as genetic disease detection, is a clinical or preventive technique. Variations in diabetes mellitus type 2 disease, single nucleotide variants myocardial infarction in coronary heart disease, and associations between diseases or phenotypic comorbidities have all been discussed using genetic-risk scores in various research. This idea has already been applied to GWAS of Chinese women to identify genetic loci among PCOS women, as well as core group studies have been reported with English women. Recently, several genetic loci that could be used for disease diagnosis, prognosis, and treatment have been found (Brower et al., 2015).

## Conclusion

Pathophysiologically speaking, PCOS is a complex disease. As a diverse condition with multiple endocrinologic anomalies in the release of hormones, receptor activation, and post-receptor action, PCOS can be seen as the last common pathway. It is obvious that the combination of various susceptibility factors and environmental variables results in this complex disease. Over the last ten years, numerous loci & genes have produced evidence suggesting a link with PCOS, and there is now strong epidemiologic evidence to corroborate this. The intricacy of mammalian female reproduction endocrinology is ultimately what predisposes one to the risk of poor functioning across numerous pathways, so it is likely that multiple genes will contribute to an individual's susceptibility to PCOS. A number of pathways have obvious signals, but further functional research is required to fully understand their roles in pathogenesis. This is true even while genetic studies have proven the roles of major pathways like resistance to insulin and secretion of gonadotropin and receptor function.

## References

Attaoua, R., Ait El Mkadem, S., Radian, S., Fica, S., Hanzu, F., Albu, A., Gheorghiu, M., Coculescu, M., & Grigorescu, F. (2008). FTO gene associates to metabolic syndrome in women with polycystic ovary syndrome. *Biochemical and Biophysical Research Communications*, *373*(2), 230–234. https://doi.org/10.1016/J.BBRC.2008.06.039.

Baban, A. Sh. Sh., Korsheed, S. H., & Hayawi, A. Y. (2017). The FSHR Polymorphisms Association With Polycystic Ovary Syndrome in Women of Erbil, Kurdistan in North of Iraq. *Ibn AL-Haitham Journal For Pure and Applied Sciences*, 257–272. https://doi.org/10.30526/2017.IHSCICONF.1799.

Barber, T. M., Bennett, A. J., Gloyn, A. L., Groves, C. J., Sovio, U., Ruokonen, A., Martikainen, H., Pouta, A., Taponen, S., Weedon, M. N., Hartikainen, A. L., Wass, J. A. H., Järvelin, M. R., Zeggini, E., Franks, S., & McCarthy, M. I. (2007). Relationship between E23K (an established type II diabetes-susceptibility variant within KCNJ11), polycystic ovary syndrome and androgen levels. *European Journal of Human Genetics : EJHG*, *15*(6), 679–684. https://doi.org/10.1038/SJ.EJHG.5201802.

Barber, T. M., Bennett, A. J., Groves, C. J., Sovio, U., Ruokonen, A., Martikainen, H., Pouta, A., Hartikainen, A. L., Elliott, P., Lindgren, C. M., Freathy, R. M., Koch, K., Ouwehand, W. H., Karpe, F., Conway, G. S., Wass, J. A. H., Järvelin, M. R., Franks, S., & McCarthy, M. I. (2008). Association of variants in the fat mass and obesity associated (FTO) gene with polycystic ovary syndrome. *Diabetologia*, *51*(7), 1153–1158. https://doi.org/10.1007/S00125-008-1028-6.

Barber, T. M., Bennett, A. J., Groves, C. J., Sovio, U., Ruokonen, A., Martikainen, H., Pouta, A., Hartikainen, A. L., Elliott, P., Wass, J. A. H., Järvelin, M. R., Zeggini, E., Franks, S., & McCarthy, M. I. (2007). Disparate genetic influences on polycystic ovary syndrome (PCOS) and type 2 diabetes revealed by a lack of association between common variants within the TCF7L2 gene and PCOS. *Diabetologia*, *50*(11), 2318–2322. https://doi.org/10.1007/S00125-007-0804-Z.

Biyasheva, A., Legro, R. S., Dunaif, A., & Urbanek, M. (2009). Evidence for association between polycystic ovary syndrome (PCOS) and TCF7L2 and glucose intolerance in women with PCOS and TCF7L2. *The Journal of Clinical Endocrinology and Metabolism*, *94*(7), 2617–2625. https://doi.org/10.1210/JC.2008-1664.

Brower, M. A., Jones, M. R., Rotter, J. I., Krauss, R. M., Legro, R. S., Azziz, R., & Goodarzi, M. O. (2015). Further investigation in europeans of susceptibility variants for polycystic ovary syndrome discovered in genome-wide association studies of Chinese individuals. *The Journal of Clinical Endocrinology and Metabolism*, *100*(1), E182–E186. https://doi.org/10.1210/JC.2014-2689.

Carey, A. H., Chan, K. L., Short, F., White, D., Williamson, R., & Franks, S. (1993). Evidence for a single gene effect causing polycystic ovaries and male pattern baldness. *Clinical Endocrinology*, *38*(6), 653–658. https://doi.org/10.1111/J.1365-2265.1993.TB02150.X.

Carey, A. H., Waterworth, D., Patel, K., White, D., Little, J., Novelli, P., Franks, S., & Williamson, R. (1994). Polycystic ovaries and premature male pattern baldness are associated with one allele of the steroid metabolism gene CYP17. *Human Molecular Genetics*, *3*(10), 1873–1876. https://doi.org/10.1093/HMG/3.10.1873.

Chaudhary, H., Patel, J., Jain, N. K., & Joshi, R. (2021). The role of polymorphism in various potential genes on polycystic ovary syndrome susceptibility and pathogenesis. *Journal of Ovarian Research*, *14*(1). https://doi.org/10.1186/S13048-021-00879-W.

Chen, B., Xu, P., Wang, J., & Zhang, C. (2019). The role of MiRNA in polycystic ovary syndrome (PCOS). *Gene*, *706*, 91–96. https://doi.org/10.1016/J.GENE.2019.04.082.

Christopoulos, P., Mastorakos, G., Gazouli, M., Panidis, D., Deligeoroglou, E., Katsikis, I., Papadias, K., Diamandi-Kandarakis, E., & Creatsas, G. (2008). Genetic variants in TCF7L2 and KCNJ11 genes in a Greek population with polycystic ovary syndrome. *Gynecological Endocrinology: The Official Journal of the International Society of Gynecological Endocrinology*, *24*(9), 486–490. https://doi.org/10.1080/09513590802196379.

Cohen, P. N., Givens, J. R., Wiser, W. L., Wilroy, R. S., Summitt, R. L., Coleman, S. A., & Andersen, R. N. (1975). Polycystic Ovarian Disease, Maturation Arrest of Spermiogenesis, and Klinefelter's Syndrome in Siblings of a Family with Familial Hirsutism. *Fertility and Sterility*, *26*(12), 1228–1238. https://doi.org/10.1016/S0015-0282(16)41539-6.

Conway, G., Dewailly, D., Diamanti-Kandarakis, E., Escobar-Morreale, H. F., Franks, S., Gambineri, A., Kelestimur, F., Macut, D., Micic, D., Pasquali, R., Pfeifer, M., Pignatelli, D., Pugeat, M., & Yildiz, B. O. (2014). The polycystic ovary syndrome: a position statement from the European Society of Endocrinology. *European Journal of Endocrinology*, *171*(4), P1–P29. https://doi.org/10.1530/EJE-14-0253.

Cooper, H. E., Spellacy, W. N., Prem, K. A., & Cohen, W. D. (1968). Hereditary factors in the Stein-Leventhal syndrome. *American Journal of Obstetrics and Gynecology, 100*(3), 371–387. https://doi.org/10.1016/S0002-9378(15)33704-2.

Cortón, M., Botella-Carretero, J. I., Benguría, A., Villuendas, G., Zaballos, A., San Millán, J. L., Escobar-Morreale, H. F., & Peral, B. (2007). Differential gene expression profile in omental adipose tissue in women with polycystic ovary syndrome. *The Journal of Clinical Endocrinology and Metabolism, 92*(1), 328–337. https://doi.org/10.1210/JC.2006-1665.

Deneux, C., Tardy, V., Anne, D., Mornet, E., Billaud, L., Charron, D., Morel, Y., & Kuttenn, F. (2001). Phenotype-genotype correlation in 56 women with nonclassical congenital adrenal hyperplasia due to 21-hydroxylase deficiency. *The Journal of Clinical Endocrinology and Metabolism, 86*(1), 207–213. https://doi.org/10.1210/JCEM.86.1.7131.

Diamanti-Kandarakis, E., Palioniko, G., Alexandraki, K., Bergiele, A., Koutsouba, T., & Bartzis, M. (2004). The prevalence of 4G5G polymorphism of plasminogen activator inhibitor-1 (PAI-1) gene in polycystic ovarian syndrome and its association with plasma PAI-1 levels. *European Journal of Endocrinology, 150*(6), 793–798. https://doi.org/10.1530/EJE.0.1500793.

Dunaif, A. (1997). Insulin resistance and the polycystic ovary syndrome: mechanism and implications for pathogenesis. *Endocrine Reviews, 18*(6), 774–800. https://doi.org/10.1210/EDRV.18.6.0318.

Escobar-Morreale, H. F., Sanchón, R., & San Millán, J. L. (2008). A prospective study of the prevalence of nonclassical congenital adrenal hyperplasia among women presenting with hyperandrogenic symptoms and signs. *The Journal of Clinical Endocrinology and Metabolism, 93*(2), 527–533. https://doi.org/10.1210/JC.2007-2053.

Fauser, B. C. J. M., Tarlatzis, Fauser, Chang, Aziz, Legro, Dewailly, Franks, Balen, Bouchard, Dahlgren, Devoto, Diamanti, Dunaif, Filicori, Homburg, Ibanez, Laven, Magoffin, … Lobo. (2004). Revised 2003 consensus on diagnostic criteria and long-term health risks related to polycystic ovary syndrome (PCOS). *Human Reproduction (Oxford, England), 19*(1), 41–47. https://doi.org/10.1093/HUMREP/DEH098.

Feinberg, A. P. (2007). Phenotypic plasticity and the epigenetics of human disease. *Nature, 447*(7143), 433–440. https://doi.org/10.1038/NATURE05919.

FERRIMAN, D., & PURDIE, A. W. (1979). The inheritance of polycystic ovarian disease and a possible relationship to premature balding. *Clinical Endocrinology, 11*(3), 291–300. https://doi.org/10.1111/J.1365-2265.1979.TB03077.X.

Franks, S., Gharani, N., Waterworth, D., Batty, S., White, D., Williamson, R., & McCarthy, M. (1997). The genetic basis of polycystic ovary syndrome. *Human Reproduction (Oxford, England), 12*(12), 2641–2648. https://doi.org/10.1093/HUMREP/12.12.2641.

Franks, S., Gilling-Smith, C., Gharani, N., & McCarthy, M. (2000). Pathogenesis of polycystic ovary syndrome: evidence for a genetically determined disorder of ovarian androgen production. *Human Fertility (Cambridge, England), 3*(2), 77–79. https://doi.org/10.1080/1464727002000198731.

Franks, S., Mason, H., & Willis, D. (2000). Follicular dynamics in the polycystic ovary syndrome. *Molecular and Cellular Endocrinology, 163*(1–2), 49–52. https://doi.org/10.1016/S0303-7207(99)00239-7.

Gaasenbeek, M., Powell, B. L., Sovio, U., Haddad, L., Gharani, N., Bennett, A., Groves, C. J., Rush, K., Goh, M. J., Conway, G. S., Ruokonen, A., Martikainen, H., Pouta, A., Taponen, S., Hartikainen, A. L., Halford, S., Järvelin, M. R., Franks, S., & McCarthy, M. I. (2004). Large-scale analysis of the relationship between CYP11A promoter variation, polycystic ovarian syndrome, and serum testosterone. *The Journal of Clinical Endocrinology and Metabolism, 89*(5), 2408–2413. https://doi.org/10.1210/JC.2003-031640.

Givens, J. R., Wiser, W. L., Coleman, S. A., Wilroy, R. S., Andersen, R. N., & Fish, S. A. (1971). Familial ovarian hyperthecosis: A study of two families. *American Journal of Obstetrics and Gynecology, 110*(7), 959–972. https://doi.org/10.1016/0002-9378(71)90550-3.

Goodarzi, M. O., Shah, N. A., Antoine, H. J., Pall, M., Guo, X., & Azziz, R. (2006). Variants in the 5alpha-reductase type 1 and type 2 genes are associated with polycystic ovary syndrome and the severity of hirsutism in affected women. *The Journal of Clinical Endocrinology and Metabolism, 91*(10), 4085–4091. https://doi.org/10.1210/JC.2006-0227.

Govind, A., Obhrai, M. S., & Clayton, R. N. (1999). Polycystic Ovaries Are Inherited as an Autosomal Dominant Trait: Analysis of 29 Polycystic Ovary Syndrome and 10 Control Families. *The Journal of Clinical Endocrinology & Metabolism*, *84*(1), 38–43. https://doi.org/10.1210/JCEM.84.1.5382.

Guo, R., Zheng, Y., Yang, J., & Zheng, N. (2015). Association of TNF-alpha, IL-6 and IL-1beta gene polymorphisms with polycystic ovary syndrome: a meta-analysis. *BMC Genetics*, *16*(1). https://doi.org/10.1186/S12863-015-0165-4.

Haddad, L., Evans, J. C., Gharani, N., Robertson, C., Rush, K., Wiltshire, S., Frayling, T. M., Wilkin, T. J., Demaine, A., Millward, A., Hattersley, A. T., Conway, G., Cox, N. J., Bell, G. I., Franks, S., & Mccarthy, M. I. (2002). Oxford OX3 7BN, United Kingdom; Plymouth Postgraduate Medical School. *J Clin Endocrinol Metab*, *87*, 2606–2610. https://academic.oup.com/jcem/article/87/6/2606/2846940.

Hague, W. M., Adams, J., Reeders, S. T., Peto, T. E. A., & Jacobs, H. S. (1988). Familial Polycystic Ovaries: A Genetic Disease? *Clinical Endocrinology*, *29*(6), 593–605. https://doi.org/10.1111/J.1365-2265.1988.TB03707.X.

Hanash, S. (2003). Disease proteomics. *Nature*, *422*(6928), 226–232. https://doi.org/10.1038/NATURE01514.

Hardiman, P., Pillay, O. S., & Atiomo, W. (2003). Polycystic ovary syndrome and endometrial carcinoma. *Lancet*, *361*(9371), 1810–1812. https://doi.org/10.1016/S0140-6736(03)13409-5.

Hickey, T. (2002). The Androgen Receptor CAG Repeat Polymorphism and X-Chromosome Inactivation in Australian Caucasian Women with Infertility Related to Polycystic Ovary Syndrome. *Journal of Clinical Endocrinology & Metabolism*, *87*(1), 161–165. https://doi.org/10.1210/JC.87.1.161.

Hickey, T. E., Legro, R. S., & Norman, R. J. (2006). Epigenetic modification of the X chromosome influences susceptibility to polycystic ovary syndrome. *The Journal of Clinical Endocrinology and Metabolism*, *91*(7), 2789–2791. https://doi.org/10.1210/JC.2006-0069.

Horikawa, Y., Oda, N., Cox, N. J., Li, X., Orho-Melander, M., Hara, M., Hinokio, Y., Lindner, T. H., Mashima, H., Schwarz, P. E. H., del Bosque-Plata, L., Horikawa, Y., Oda, Y., Yoshiuchi, I., Colilla, S., Polonsky, K. S., Wei, S., Concannon, P., Iwasaki, N., Schulze, J., Baier, L. J., Bogardus, C., Groop, L., Boerwinkle, E., Harris, C. L., Bell, G. I. (2000). Genetic variation in the gene encoding calpain 10 is associated with type 2 diabetes mellitus. *Nature Genetics*, *26*(2), 163–175. https://doi.org/10.1038/79876.

Jahanfar, S., Eden, J. A., Nguyen, T., Wang, X. L., & Wilcken, D. E. L. (1997). A twin study of polycystic ovary syndrome and lipids. *Gynecological Endocrinology*, *11*(2), 111–117. https://doi.org/10.3109/09513599709152521.

Jones, M. R., & Goodarzi, M. O. (2016). Genetic determinants of polycystic ovary syndrome: progress and future directions. *Fertility and Sterility*, *106*(1), 25–32. https://doi.org/10.1016/J.FERTNSTERT.2016.04.040.

Kahsar-Miller, M., Boots, L. R., & Azziz, R. (1999). Dopamine D3 receptor polymorphism is not associated with the polycystic ovary syndrome. *Fertility and Sterility*, *71*(3), 436–438. https://doi.org/10.1016/S0015-0282(98)00485-3.

Kahsar-Miller, M. D., Nixon, C., Boots, L. R., Go, R. C., & Azziz, R. (2001). Prevalence of polycystic ovary syndrome (PCOS) in first-degree relatives of patients with PCOS. *Fertility and Sterility*, *75*(1), 53–58. https://doi.org/10.1016/S0015-0282(00)01662-9.

Ketefian, A., Jones, M. R., Krauss, R. M., Chen, Y. D. I., Legro, R. S., Azziz, R., & Goodarzi, M. O. (2016). Association study of androgen signaling pathway genes in polycystic ovary syndrome. *Fertility and Sterility*, *105*(2), 467-473.e4. https://doi.org/10.1016/J.FERTNSTERT.2015.09.043.

Lechin, F., van der Dijs, B., & Spritzer, P. M. (2004). Neuroendocrine profiling in PCOS [3] (multiple letters). *Fertility and Sterility*, *82*(3), 765–766. https://doi.org/10.1016/j.fertnstert.2004.06.008.

Legro, R. S., Driscoll, D., Strauss Iii, J. F., Fox, J., & Dunaif, A. (1998). Evidence for a genetic basis for hyperandrogenemia in polycystic ovary syndrome. *Medical Sciences*, *95*, 14956–14960. www.pnas.org.

Legro, R. S., Driscoll, D., Strauss, J. F., Fox, J., & Dunaif, A. (1998). Evidence for a genetic basis for hyperandrogenemia in polycystic ovary syndrome. *Proceedings of the National Academy of Sciences of the United States of America*, *95*(25), 14956–14960. https://doi.org/10.1073/PNAS.95.25.14956.

Legro, R. S., Muhleman, D. R., Comings, D. E., Lobo, R. A., & Kovacs, B. W. (1995). A dopamine D3 receptor genotype is associated with hyperandrogenic chronic anovulation and resistant to ovulation induction with clomiphene citrate in female Hispanics. *Fertility and Sterility*, *63*(4), 779–784. https://doi.org/10.1016/S0015-0282(16)57481-0.

Liao, W. X., Roy, A. C., & Ng, S. C. (2000). Preliminary investigation of follistatin gene mutations in women with polycystic ovary syndrome. *Molecular Human Reproduction*, *6*(7), 587–590. https://doi.org/10.1093/MOLEHR/6.7.587.

Liu, A. L., Xie, H. J., Xie, H. Y., Liu, J., Yin, J., Hu, J. S., & Peng, C. Y. (2017). Association between fat mass and obesity associated (FTO) gene rs9939609 A/T polymorphism and polycystic ovary syndrome: a systematic review and meta-analysis. *BMC Medical Genetics*, *18*(1). https://doi.org/10.1186/S12881-017-0452-1.

Lowe, W. L., & Reddy, T. E. (2015). Genomic approaches for understanding the genetics of complex disease. *Genome Research*, *25*(10), 1432–1441. https://doi.org/10.1101/GR.190603.115.

Lunde, O., Magnus, P., Sandvik, L., & Høglo, S. (1989). Familial Clustering in the Polycystic Ovarian Syndrome. *Gynecologic and Obstetric Investigation*, *28*(1), 23–30. https://doi.org/10.1159/000293493.

Mahmoudi, T. (2009). Genetic variation in the vitamin D receptor and polycystic ovary syndrome risk. *Fertility and Sterility*, *92*(4), 1381–1383. https://doi.org/10.1016/J.FERTNSTERT.2009.05.002.

Marshall, J. C., & Eagleson, C. A. (1999). Neuroendocrine aspects of polycystic ovary syndrome. *Endocrinology and Metabolism Clinics of North America*, *28*(2), 295–324. https://doi.org/10.1016/S0889-8529(05)70071-2.

Mifsud, A., Ramirez, S., & Yong, E. L. (2000). Androgen receptor gene CAG trinucleotide repeats in anovulatory infertility and polycystic ovaries. *The Journal of Clinical Endocrinology and Metabolism*, *85*(9), 3484–3488. https://doi.org/10.1210/JCEM.85.9.6832.

Mukherjee, A., Sidis, Y., Mahan, A., Raher, M. J., Xia, Y., Rosen, E. D., Bloch, K. D., Thomas, M. K., & Schneyer, A. L. (2007). FSTL3 deletion reveals roles for TGF-beta family ligands in glucose and fat homeostasis in adults. *Proceedings of the National Academy of Sciences of the United States of America*, *104*(4), 1348–1353. https://doi.org/10.1073/PNAS.0607966104.

Nilsson, C., Matzuk, M. M., Pettersson, K., Huhtaniemi, I. T., Millar, R. P., Coerver, K. A., Savontaus, M. L., Punab, M., Pisarek, H., Kula, K., Pettersson, T. M., van Santbrink, E. J. B., Fauser, B. C. J. M., Clayton, R. N., Beck-Peccoz, P., Fujieda, K., Aribarg, A., & Wang, C. N. (1997). Worldwide frequency of a common genetic variant of luteinizing hormone: An international collaborative research. *Fertility and Sterility*, *67*(6), 998–1004. https://doi.org/10.1016/S0015-0282(97)81430-6.

Norman, R. J., Masters, S., & Hague, W. (1996). Hyperinsulinemia is common in family members of women with polycystic ovary syndrome. *Fertility and Sterility*, *66*(6), 942–947. https://doi.org/10.1016/S0015-0282(16)58687-7.

Peng, C. Y., Xie, H. J., Guo, Z. F., Nie, Y. L., Chen, J., Zhou, J. M., & Yin, J. (2014). The association between androgen receptor gene CAG polymorphism and polycystic ovary syndrome: a case-control study and meta-analysis. *Journal of Assisted Reproduction and Genetics*, *31*(9), 1211–1219. https://doi.org/10.1007/S10815-014-0286-0.

Powell, B. L., Haddad, L., Bennett, A., Gharani, N., Sovio, U., Groves, C. J., Rush, K., Goh, M. J., Conway, G. S., Ruokonen, A., Martikainen, H., Pouta, A., Taponen, S., Hartikainen, A. L., Halford, S., Zeggini, E., Järvelin, M. R., Franks, S., & McCarthy, M. I. (2005). Analysis of multiple data sets reveals no association between the insulin gene variable number tandem repeat element and polycystic ovary syndrome or related traits. *The Journal of Clinical Endocrinology and Metabolism*, *90*(5), 2988–2993. https://doi.org/10.1210/JC.2004-2485.

Rizwan, S., Ghazanvi, S., Rasheed, N., Ullah, M. I. 2018, undefined. (n.d.). Association of FTO Common RS9939609 Polymor-phism with Obesity and Polycystic Ovarian Syndrome in Pakistani Women. *Article.Scholarena.Co*. Retrieved February 19, 2023, from http://article.scholarena.co/Association-of-FTO-Common-RS9939609-Polymorphism-with-Obesity-and-Polycystic-Ovarian-Syndrome-in-Pakistani-Women.pdf.

Sáez, M. E., González-Sánchez, J. L., Ramírez-Lorca, R., Martínez-Larrad, M. T., Zabena, C., González, A., Morón, F. J., Ruiz, A., & Serrano-Ríos, M. (2008). The CAPN10 gene is associated with insulin resistance phenotypes in the Spanish population. *PloS One*, *3*(8). https://doi.org/10.1371/JOURNAL.PONE.0002953.

San-Millán, J. L., & Escobar-Morreale, H. F. (2010). The role of genetic variation in peroxisome proliferator-activated receptors in the polycystic ovary syndrome (PCOS): an original case-control study followed by systematic review and meta-analysis of existing evidence. *Clinical Endocrinology*, *72*(3), 383–392. https://doi.org/10.1111/J.1365-2265.2009.03679.X.

Schüring, A. N., Welp, A., Gromoll, J., Zitzmann, M., Sonntag, B., Nieschlag, E., Greb, R. R., & Kiesel, L. (2012). Role of the CAG repeat polymorphism of the androgen receptor gene in polycystic ovary syndrome (PCOS). *Experimental and Clinical Endocrinology & Diabetes: Official Journal, German Society of Endocrinology [and] German Diabetes Association*, *120*(2), 73–79. https://doi.org/10.1055/S-0031-1291343.

Shah, N. A., Antoine, H. J., Pall, M., Taylor, K. D., Azziz, R., & Goodarzi, M. O. (2008). Association of androgen receptor CAG repeat polymorphism and polycystic ovary syndrome. *The Journal of Clinical Endocrinology and Metabolism*, *93*(5), 1939–1945. https://doi.org/10.1210/JC.2008-0038.

Shen, W., Li, T., Hu, Y., Liu, H., & Song, M. (2013). Calpain-10 genetic polymorphisms and polycystic ovary syndrome risk: a meta-analysis and meta-regression. *Gene*, *531*(2), 426–434. https://doi.org/10.1016/J.GENE.2013.08.072.

Takayama, H. (2004). Chemistry and pharmacology of analgesic indole alkaloids from the rubiaceous plant, Mitragyna speciosa. *Chemical & Pharmaceutical Bulletin*, *52*(8), 916–928. https://doi.org/10.1248/CPB.52.916.

Tong, Y., Liao, W. X., Roy, A. C., & Ng, S. C. (2000). Association of AccI polymorphism in the follicle-stimulating hormone beta gene with polycystic ovary syndrome. *Fertility and Sterility*, *74*(6), 1233–1236. https://doi.org/10.1016/S0015-0282(00)01616-2.

Tucci, S., Futterweit, W., Concepcion, E. S., Greenberg, D. A., Villanueva, R., Davies, T. F., & Tomer, Y. (2001). Evidence for association of polycystic ovary syndrome in caucasian women with a marker at the insulin receptor gene locus. *The Journal. of Clinical Endocrinology and Metabolism*, *86*(1), 446–449. https://doi.org/10.1210/JCEM.86.1.7274.

Urbanek, M., Legro, R. S., Driscoll, D. A., Azziz, R., Ehrmann, D. A., Norman, R. J., Strauss, J. F., Spielman, R. S., & Dunaif, A. (1999). Thirty-seven candidate genes for polycystic ovary syndrome: strongest evidence for linkage is with follistatin. *Proceedings of the National Academy of Sciences of the United States of America*, *96*(15), 8573–8578. https://doi.org/10.1073/PNAS.96.15.8573.

Villuendas, G., Escobar-Morreale, H. F., Tosi, F., Sancho, J., Moghetti, P., & San Millán, J. L. (2003). Association between the D19S884 marker at the insulin receptor gene locus and polycystic ovary syndrome [2]. *Fertility and Sterility*, *79*(1), 219–220. https://doi.org/10.1016/S0015-0282(02)04570-3.

Vink, J. M., Sadrzadeh, S., Lambalk, C. B., & Boomsma, D. I. (2006). Heritability of polycystic ovary syndrome in a Dutch twin-family study. *The Journal of Clinical Endocrinology and Metabolism*, *91*(6), 2100–2104. https://doi.org/10.1210/JC.2005-1494.

Wang, F., Pan, J., Liu, Y., Meng, Q., Lv, P., Qu, F., Ding, G. L., Klausen, C., Leung, P. C. K., Chan, H. C., Yao, W., Zhou, C. Y., Shi, B., Zhang, J., Sheng, J., & Huang, H. (2015). Alternative splicing of the androgen receptor in polycystic ovary syndrome. *Proceedings of the National Academy of Sciences of the United States of America*, *112*(15), 4743–4748. https://doi.org/10.1073/PNAS.1418216112.

Wickenheisser, J. K., Quinn, P. G., Nelson, V. L., Legro, R. S., Strauss, J. F., & McAllister., J. M. (2000). Differential activity of the cytochrome P450 17alpha-hydroxylase and steroidogenic acute regulatory protein gene promoters in normal and polycystic ovary syndrome theca cells. *The Journal of Clinical Endocrinology and Metabolism*, *85*(6), 2304–2311. https://doi.org/10.1210/JCEM.85.6.6631.

Witchel, S. F., & Aston, C. E. (2000). The role of heterozygosity for CYP21 in the polycystic ovary syndrome. *Journal of Pediatric Endocrinology & Metabolism: JPEM*, *13 Suppl 5*(SUPPL. 5), 1315–1317. https://europepmc.org/article/med/11117678.

Witchel, S. F., Kahsar-Miller, M., Aston, C. E., White, C., & Azziz, R. (2005). Prevalence of CYP21 mutations and IRS1 variant among women with polycystic ovary syndrome and adrenal androgen excess. *Fertility and Sterility*, *83*(2), 371–375. https://doi.org/10.1016/J.FERTNSTERT.2004.10.027.

Zhang, D., Cong, J., Shen, H., Wu, Q., & Wu, X. (2014). Genome-wide identification of aberrantly methylated promoters in ovarian tissue of prenatally androgenized rats. *Fertility and Sterility*, *102*(5), 1458–1467. https://doi.org/10.1016/J.FERTNSTERT.2014.07.1203.

Chapter 12

# Several Diagnostic Tools and Tests for the Analysis of PCOS and Their Current Advancements

**Haleema Ahmad**[1,*]
**Mohd Salik Usmani**[2]
**Humaira Maryam**[1]
**Labiba Shahnawaz**[1]
**and Aiman Fatima**[1]
[1]Department of Biochemistry, Faculty of Life Science, Aligarh Muslim University, Aligarh, India
[2]Jawaharlal Nehru Medical College, Faculty of Medicine, Aligarh Muslim University, Aligarh, India

## Abstract

Polycystic ovarian syndrome (PCOS), which affects women of reproductive age, is the most common and widespread endocrine disorder. Infertility, insulin resistance, obesity, and cardiovascular disorders are just a few of the health concerns brought on by this syndrome. PCOS is a polygenic, multifactorial, autoimmune, inflammatory, and dysregulated steroid state condition that mostly manifests as a result of poor lifestyle choices. There is no defined test that can accurately identify polycystic ovary syndrome (PCOS). PCOS in afflicted females may now be identified due to the development of biochemical testing, ultrasound imaging, and laparoscopy. Analysing ultrasound pictures, which provide vital information such as the number, size, and position of follicles might help overcome the significant difficulty of studying these types of disorders in females. Hyperandrogenism and persistent anovulation are the illness's defining symptoms; the amount of androgen is crucial for the diagnosis of PCOS, which is made when there is no known pituitary or adrenal pathology. Laparoscopic techniques are also applied for its detection. However, there aren't many reliable, objective tests that can definitively identify and comprehend PCOS. There is a combination of diagnostic and screening tests to identify PCOS in females. This chapter describes the understanding and explanation of different tools and techniques used in the detection of PCOS and its advancement with time.

**Keywords**: laparoscopy, ultrasonography, androgen, ovarian health, PCOS, insulin

* Corresponding Author's Email: sheikhzaaraahmad@gmail.com.

In: Polycystic Ovarian Syndrome (PCOS) and Our Biological Clock
Editors: Arpita Roy, Gowhar Rashid and Nihad Ashraf Khan
ISBN: 979-8-89113-100-2
© 2023 Nova Science Publishers, Inc.

## 1. Introduction

In 1935, Stein and Leventhal described a rare gynecological illness, that would eventually be known as PCOS. At the time, none of them could have envisioned the level of interest and debate that would follow. PCOS was first identified in seven women, who at best might be characterized as having hirsutism, obesity, amenorrhea, and enlarged bilateral polycystic ovaries as a result of the disease ("Amenorrhea associated with bilateral polycystic ovaries," 1935). Since then, so much has changed in our knowledge of PCOS that none of the initially noted symptoms—not even the presence of several microscopic ovarian "cysts," after which the disease was named—are now thought to be a persistent finding in the condition (Dunaif & Thomas, 2001). Despite being one of the most prevalent endocrine diseases affecting women, PCOS's diagnosis, treatment, and long-term health consequences are still up for debate. Anovulation and androgen excess has always been seen as PCOS's defining characteristics. Although both symptoms continue to be the most common in PCOS patients, none is currently thought to be a strict need for the disease (Azziz et al., 2004). The phenotypic range of PCOS has significantly expanded after polycystic ovaries as detected by ultrasonography was included as a diagnostic diagnosis. One of the most prevalent endocrine illnesses affecting women is PCOS. Using biochemical and/or clinical data, epidemiological studies have produced prevalence estimates in women of reproductive age ranging from 6.5% to 8% (Asuncion et al., 2000; Diamanti-Kandarakis et al., 1999; Knochenhauer et al., 1998), and ultrasound-based investigations have suggested a prevalence of 20% or higher. Regardless of BMI or central adiposity, Diamanti-Kandarakis et al., found that the hyperandrogenic and anovulatory phenotypes of PCOS were the most insulin resistant in the largest research to evaluate the phenotypic range of the condition (Diamanti-Kandarakis & Panidis, 2007). In order to diagnose and assess a sizable research population, several doctors and ultrasonographers collaborated in order to clarify distinctions among PCOS phenotypes. Each research subject was only included if at least two doctors concurred that they could clearly see symptoms and indicators of PCOS. From a sizable group of non-hirsute, consistently menstruation women with confirmed ovulatory cycles, cut-off levels for biochemical hyperandrogenism were painstakingly determined. Finally, each transvaginal ultrasound recording was analyzed by a separate ultrasonographer. Although these researchers made excellent efforts, it is likely that the lack of precision and dependability that is evident in the evaluation of PCOS traits would hinder future efforts to validate these findings for various populations (Barth, Yasmin, & Balen, 2007; Fraser & Kovacs, 2004).

However, it is a complicated multigenetic condition in which insulin resistance, hyperinsulinism, dysregulation of steroidogenesis, and abnormal gonadotropin release all play a part. In addition to the usual physical exam findings of acne, hirsutism, obesity, and acanthosis nigricans, the diagnosis is supported by laboratory evidence of hyperandrogenism, including elevated free testosterone, androstenedione, and dehydroepiandrosterone sulfate (DHEAS), decreased sex hormone-binding globulin (SHBG), and increased luteinizing hormone (LH). After a time of normal menstruation, chronic anovulation and irregular menses may start; on ultrasonography, the polycystic ovaries may or may not be seen.; the excess androgen may manifest as hirsutism, acne, and male-pattern hair loss in variable degrees. There is strong evidence that PCOS is a chronic condition, with early symptoms appearing before puberty and occasionally manifesting as premature adrenarche (PA) (Ibanez, Potau, Francois, & de Zegher,

1998; Ibanez et al., 1993). Regardless of their current weight, girls who are born small for gestational age (SGA) are more likely to develop PA and, as a result, PCOS (Ibanez et al., 1998). The diagnosis of PCOS may take longer due to the varied nature of the symptoms, which might change over time. Furthermore, environmental variables including weight increase may have an impact on the disease's metabolic component and development. The classic PCOS patient is therefore usually overweight and has the related metabolic issues of obesity and insulin resistance, in addition to the aforementioned signs and symptoms. PCOS affects 4% to 12% of women of reproductive age. Many clinicians find it difficult to identify this common disease due to a lack of well-defined diagnostic criteria (Sheehan, 2004). It is essential to accurately diagnose the disease phenotypes in order to give PCOS patients individualized treatment opportunities. However, the diagnostic standards for the various phenotypes are primarily based on symptoms, physical examinations, and laboratory findings (Ni et al., 2020). The three most important diagnostic methods include analysis of biochemical/metabolic markers, sonography, and laparoscopy.

Hyperandrogenism, which presents clinically as hirsutism, acne, and alopecia, is the defining characteristic of PCOS. Hyperandrogenism is a result of both the adrenals and the ovaries producing too much androgen. (Ashraf, Nabi, Rasool, Rashid, & Amin, 2019). The discovery of decreased or increased levels of a single hormone is not the basis for the diagnosis of hyperandrogenism. Many different hormone levels are analyzed in order to suggest the occurrence of hyperandrogenism. It is also believed that compensatory hyperinsulinemia causes hyperandrogenism in PCOS patients because many of them appear to have insulin resistance. Blood progesterone, thyroid, and prolactin levels are also analyzed for anovulation (la Marca et al., 2000). Lipid profile is also assessed along with other hormones like Anti Mullerian hormone. An internal transvaginal ultrasound (a form of sonography) is used for the analysis of the womb and ovaries and is considered the most common method for diagnosing PCOS. The laparoscopic analysis assesses fallopian tubes and looks for associated endometriosis.

## 2. Tools and Techniques Used for the Detection of PCOS

### 2.1. Biochemical/ Serum Analysis

FSH, LH, Insulin, and circulating male hormones may all be measured using blood testing. The quantity of free testosterone, which is not attached to the protein that transports it around in the bloodstream, is more significant than other circulating male hormones, such as testosterone. In PCOS, a male hormone precursor is frequently elevated. Dehydroepiandrosterone sulfate (DHEAS), one of the most often increased male hormones in PCOS, is known as this. Male hormone blood levels are not as essential as the signs of excess male hormones. The ratio of the FSH and LH levels in the blood will be reversed in a sizable portion of PCOS patients. FSH levels are often a little higher than LH levels. The role of different hormones in PCOS is summarized (Table 1).

***Hyperandrogenism***

A biochemical test for hyperandrogenism is typically performed on serum samples to measure TT (total testosterone), sex hormone binding globulin (SHBG), dehydroepiandrosterone sulfate

(DHEAS), 17-hydroxyprogesterone (17-OHP), androstenedione (A), and free testosterone, as well as to calculate the free androgen index (FAI = (TT/SHBG)100). Serum levels of all these androgens are frequently elevated in PCOS patients compared to healthy women. The ovaries are primarily responsible for hyperandrogenism, with the adrenal glands and fatty tissue also playing significant roles (Diamanti-Kandarakis & Dunaif, 2012).

**Table 1.** Table showing the effect of PCOS on androgen levels in serum

| S. No. | ANDROGEN | NORMAL LEVEL | LEVEL IN PCOS |
|---|---|---|---|
| 1. | Testosterone | 15 to 70 ng/dL | ≤ 150 ng/dL (≤ 5.2 nmol/L) |
| 2. | DHEA (Age dependent) | 395 to 17 (μg/dL) or 0.46 to 10.66 (μmol/L) | Slightly elevated |
| 3. | Free testosterone | 35 - 155 pg/mL, or 3.50 - 15.50 ng/dL | ≤ 200 pg/dL (≤ 20 ng/dL) |
| 4. | SHBG | 24.6 - 122 nmol/L | Slightly decreased |
| 5. | Androstenedione | 0.7 to 3.1 ng/mL | Elevated levels |
| 6. | 17-hydroxyprogesterone (Age dependent) | 200 (ng/dL) to 600 ng/dL | Elevated levels |

***Hyperinsulinemia***

Another significant factor in PCOS patients is hyperinsulinemia, which is made more severe by the build-up of visceral fat brought on by hyperandrogenism. The production of adrenal androgen is increased as a result of hyperinsulinemia's stimulation of the adrenal axis of hypothalamic-pituitary- both centrally and peripherally (Diamanti-Kandarakis et al., 1999; Diamanti-Kandarakis & Panidis, 2007). In women with PCOS, DHEA-S levels are related to insulin resistance. The hepatic production of SHBG is reduced by testosterone and insulin, which raises free testosterone levels. In return, testosterone lessens the sensitivity of oestradiol and progesterone's effects on the hypothalamus and pituitary's feedback mechanisms (Chan et al., 2005).

Several women with PCOS also have impaired metabolism of glucose, which is another cause for worry along with ovulation, the function of the menstrual cycle, hirsutism, and acne. While it is simple to identify diabetes mellitus and reduced glucose tolerance, the identification and importance of insulin resistance as a precursor condition are unappreciated. Women with PCOS are at risk for coronary artery disease, metabolic syndrome, and insulin resistance can be the earliest significant indication of metabolic illness. Insulin resistance IR and dyslipidemia are linked to teenage obesity (Bougle, Zunquin, Sesboue, & Sabatier, 2010). Adolescent obesity and PCOS-related ovulatory dysfunction are frequently correlated (Kasa-Vubu, Jain, & Welch, 2010). Long-standing suspicions of a genetic basis for PCOS exist (Deligeoroglou, Kouskouti, & Christopoulos, 2009), and findings correlate genetic polymorphisms with obesity and metabolic abnormalities in PCOS (Tan et al., 2010). Some support the regular administration of oral glucose tolerance tests to all PCOS women (la Marca et al., 2000). Diagnosis of glucose metabolism may be more crucial in young women since dyslipidemia often precedes problems in glucose metabolism in teenagers (Fulghesu et al., 2010). Diabetes Miletus is identified by fasting plasma glucose (taken after 8 hours of fasting) value of approximately 126 mg/dL, another glucose value (taken after 2 hours) of 200 mg/dL following a glucose tolerance test which is oral, the value of approximately 200 mg/dL, along with the presence of symptoms of diabetes verified by either of the following tests. Another indicator of DM is hemoglobin AIC > 6.5% (Gillett, 2009). A 2h threshold of 140–200 mg/dL on the oral glucose tolerance test serves as the definition of impaired glucose tolerance. Unexpectedly, 15% of obese teenagers are affected by abnormal and altered glucose tolerance (Ghergherechi & Tabrizi, 2010; Tan et al., 2010). 10% of PCOS women develop diabetes, and up to 70% of them are insulin-resistant (Ovalle & Azziz, 2002). In just three years, the rate of conversion to impaired glucose metabolism in PCOS women with originally normal glucose metabolism can reach 25% (Pesant & Baillargeon, 2011). Even more concerning, teenagers with PCOS frequently have insulin abnormalities (Bhattacharya & Ghosh, 2010).

When insulin cannot effectively facilitate the impacts of its actions on the metabolism of glucose, it builds up in the bloodstream and causes insulin resistance. The following techniques are used to assess insulin sensitivity, classified according to their levels of accuracy: fasting glucose, homeostasis model assessment (HOMA), oral glucose tolerance test (OGTT), frequently sampled intravenous glucose tolerance test (FSIVGTT), and euglycemic hyperinsulinemic clamp (De Leo et al., 2016).

### *Anovulation*

Anovulation is the most important cause of irregular menstruation in women suffering from PCOS. Women diagnosed with PCOS but claim to have regular menstrual cycles can suffer from ovulatory dysfunction (Lujan, Chizen, & Pierson, 2008). Different hormones like progesterone, thyroid, and prolactin are analyzed for anovulation. The release of an egg stimulates the production of progesterone in a normal cycle. This hormone is responsible for a woman's body's ability to maintain regular periods. During an anovulatory cycle, if there is a lack of progesterone then it may result in heavy bleeding and the woman can mistakenly take this bleeding for her period (Sanchez et al., 2016). Prolactin levels that are too elevated, can lead to the abnormal production of other hormones like estrogen and progesterone. This can cause drastic changes sometimes even leading to the alteration of ovulation (Crosignani, Bianchedi, Riccaboni, & Vegetti, 1999). TSH blood levels can be easily used to identify hypothyroidism which is of two types (Andersen, Pedersen, Bruun, & Laurberg, 2002). Subclinical hypothyroidism is indicated by a slight elevation in levels of TSH and normal levels of T3 and T4, whereas clinical hypothyroidism is indicated by elevated TSH levels along with decreased levels of T3 and T4 (Raber, Gessl, Nowotny, & Vierhapper, 2003). More people have subclinical hypothyroidism. It may directly cause anovulation or raise prolactin indirectly (Raber et al., 2003).

### *Lipid Profile for PCOS*

The lipoprotein profile in obese PCOS patients is characterized by increased plasma triglycerides along with HDL-C (decreased lipoprotein cholesterol) concentrations, similar to those in type 2 diabetes patients. In PCOS, LDL-C (low-density lipoprotein cholesterol) levels are most often only slightly increased.

### *Anti-Mullerian HORMONE*

The anti-Müllerian hormone is produced by the pre-antral and small antral follicles within the ovary (AMH) of granulosa cells. Due to a larger number of antral follicles and an increased production per antral follicle, it is significantly higher in women with PCOS. It is believed to play an inhibitory role in the development of follicles and may be crucial in the etiology of anovulation in polycystic ovary syndrome. Assessment of serum AMH levels has been suggested as a diagnostic method because it is extremely helpful in identifying PCOS (Bhide & Homburg, 2016).

## 2.2. Sonography

Medical ultrasonography or sonography is a technique that employs ultrasound waves to generate images of internal tissues and organs such as the abdomen, liver, gall bladder, pancreas, blood vessels, etc., which otherwise were not visible using older techniques such as X-ray imaging. X-ray imaging employs electromagnetic radiation to generate images of body parts that absorb some of the X-rays and transmit the rest, such as bones. Ultrasonography uses high-frequency ultrasound waves that are emitted into the body and the echoes produced are processed to generate an image using the ultrasound machine (Figure 1). The ultrasound machine is safer to use compared to X-rays which pose a threat of radiation to the exposed individuals. Ultrasound is a preferred choice for imaging the brain, heart, uterus, and fetus (Edler & Lindstrom, 2004). Ultrasound is a technique that was adopted from sound navigation and ranging (SONAR) technology used by the military to spot submarines during the first world war (Edler & Lindstrom, 2004).

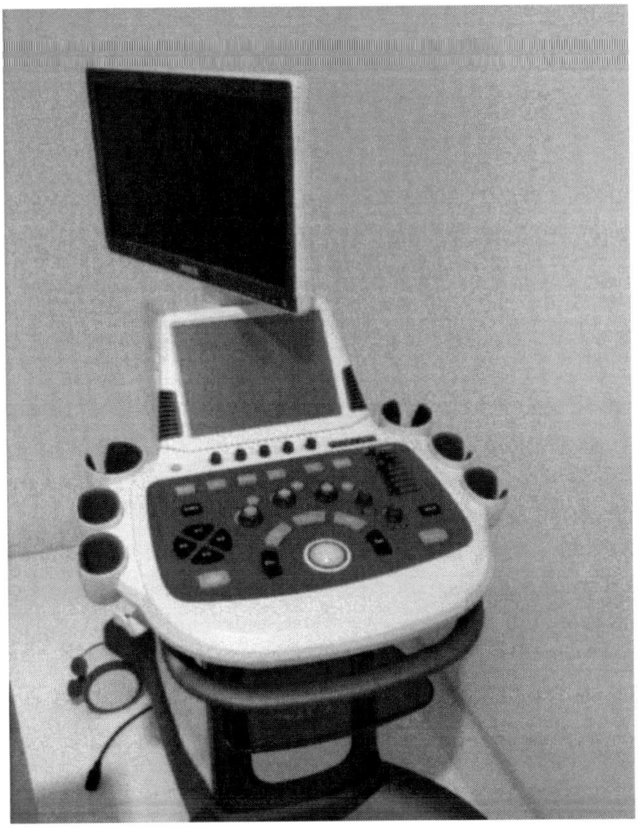

**Figure 1.** Ultrasound sonography machine, source: Pixabay License.

***The Basic Working of Ultrasound Technology***

Ultrasound machines depend on the physical properties of the ultrasound waves for accurately producing images of the body parts. These physical properties include reflection, refraction, and attenuation. Sound waves are mechanical waves that create particle displacement and pressure changes as they travel from one point to the other. Sound waves, unlike electromagnetic radiation, generate an echo as they interact with the different organs and tissues. The echoes produced are captured by the machine and are recorded as echo strength, echo direction, and time of arrival of echoes from the tissues. The production and detection of echoes is the basic principle upon which ultrasound machines rely for diagnostic purposes (Aldrich, 2007).

The sound waves are defined by the frequency at which they are emitted. The frequency ranges from 2- 10 MHz for clinical purposes. The propagation speed of the sound waves with which they can travel through a medium, for example, the soft tissues, is dependent on the physical properties of the medium, namely the density of the tissues and how stiff they are. Acoustic impedance is a property of the medium, which is defined as the product of the propagation speed of the soundwave and the density of the medium through which it travels. When the acoustic impedance of two mediums is different, they will produce an echo when soundwaves interact with it at the boundary, however, if the acoustic impedance is the same for two mediums no echo will be produced. This property is important for correctly diagnosing various ailments using ultrasound imaging. The bones and organs filled with air produce very large echoes and any organs or tissues behind these areas of the body cannot be imaged, and hence must be avoided for correctly visualizing the tissues behind these parts of the body (Aldrich, 2007; Shriki, 2014). The ultrasound beam comes from a transducer. This ultrasound transducer is a device that converts electrical signals to mechanical energy sound using piezoelectric materials. Ultrasound is pulsed through the body using a probe and the sound waves which echo back are detected by the same probe and are recorded by the computer where the information is converted into an image (Shriki, 2014).

Ultrasound has been used to detect small ovarian follicles, observe developing fetuses, and the uterine lining, and investigate general ovarian health. It is useful for diagnosing polycystic ovarian syndrome (PCOS). According to the Rotterdam criteria, 12 or more small ovarian follicles must be observed in the suspected ovary for diagnosis. An ovarian volume of 10 ml is also used as a diagnostic criterion for PCOS (Bozkurt et al., 2021; Teede et al., 2018). When the ovaries of patients with PCOS are scanned, frequently transvaginal, certain abnormalities are observed. The tiny growing follicles often rest just below the ovary's surface; they do not penetrate the ovary's interior. These follicles, which on ultrasound can resemble block holes, are typically 6 to 10 mm in diameter and form a ring around the ovarian surface. The ovary has a completely white center that is visible. Because it resembles a string of black pearls around a white neck, this sign is also known as the "pearl string" sign. On an ultrasound examination, polycystic ovaries may also seem to be larger than normal.

## 2.3. Laparoscopy

Laparoscopy also known as keyhole surgery is a surgical procedure used to access the organs, particularly of the abdominal region of the body for medical diagnosis and treatment. The term is derived from the Greek words 'laparo' meaning the flank or abdominal wall, and 'skopein' meaning to examine. Laparoscopy is the examination of the abdominal cavity using an endoscope or a laparoscope. A laparoscope is a thin tube-like tool that has a light source and a camera at the end used for seeing the inside of the abdomen and associated organs without having to cut open the abdomen by surgery (Figure 2). Laparoscopy is minimally invasive and requires only a small opening compared to regular surgical procedures to perform the treatment (Shabanzadeh & Sorensen, 2012). The chances of infection post-surgery are low, and the recovery period and the duration of the hospital stay are shorter making it a preferred procedure used by doctors to treat disorders of the hepatobiliary system, the abdominal organs, malignancies, ovarian and uterine conditions, etc. (Philipose & Sinha, 1994; Soper, Brunt, & Kerbl, 1994).

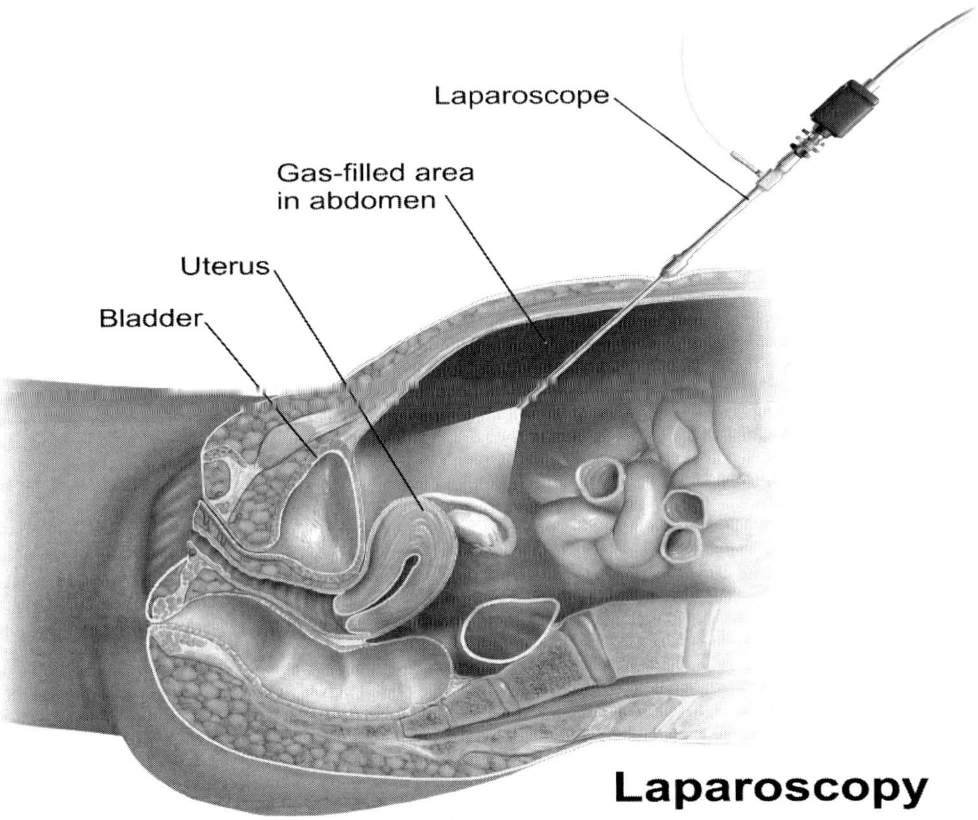


Source: Blausen.com staff (2014). "Medical Gallery of Blausen Medical 2014."

**Figure 2.** Laparoscopy in PCOS.

Laparoscopy has been used in gynecology for many years to diagnose and treat problems related to infertility in women. Diagnostic laparoscopy is used to diagnose conditions causing infertility problems like polycystic ovarian syndrome. However, a pelvic laparoscopy is done for diagnostic purposes only if other diagnostic tests like sonography and hormonal tests are unable to clarify the symptoms. A laparoscopy is frequently performed on PCOS patients, especially on those who are having problems becoming pregnant. A surgery known as a laparoscopy involves giving the patient a brief general anesthesia, making a tiny incision in the umbilicus, and inserting a telescope to see the pelvic contents, including the uterus, tubes, and ovaries. PCOS ovaries seem something like ping-pong balls during laparoscopy. The ovary's white capsule is thicker, and it frequently has a highly spherical shape. The condition of the fallopian tubes will also be evaluated, and any endometriosis that may be present will be checked for, during the laparoscopy.

Polycystic ovaries appear smooth glossy and tightly stretched on the surface with characteristic vascular patterns or loops present when observed with a laparoscope. They appear like ping-pong balls and subcapsular cysts are present on the ovaries. Small transparent or yellowish cysts are observed in the ovarian sections. These observations confirm whether a patient has polycystic ovarian syndrome or not, along with the other diagnostic tests (De Leo et al., 2016).

## 3. Current Advancements in Tools and Techniques

The current advancement in Biochemical/ Serum Analysis is based on the Microparticle Enzyme Immunoassay (MEIA) technology and Chemiluminescent Immunoassay (CLIA) technology. The ratio of luteinizing hormone (LH)/FSH has been used to assist in the diagnosis of polycystic ovary disease. Steroid hormone tests using mass spectrometry are physicochemical analytical methods that identify the analyte by figuring out the usual mass-to-charge ratios of the relevant molecule or its characteristic fragments. Mass spectrometry enables better specificity compared to conventional isotopic and non-isotopic immunoassay methods. Targeted steroid hormone analysis of several analytes from a single sample is made possible by liquid chromatography coupled with tandem mass spectrometry (LC-MS/MS) (Kulle, Riepe, Melchior, Hiort, & Holterhus, 2010; T. Søeborg et al., 2013; Tue Søeborg et al., 2014; Wudy & Choi, 2016). Using both targeted and nontargeted methods, simultaneous measurement of steroid hormones and metabolites is possible with gas chromatography and mass spectrometry (GC- MS) (Wudy & Choi, 2016).

With the significant advancements in ultrasonic imaging technology, images are now much crisper and more distinct. Increased processing rates have been made possible by real-time computer imaging, which results in better photos. For the past few years, volumetric ultrasound technology has been developed. Compared to conventional sonograms, the images created by these cutting-edge ultrasounds offer more depth and complexity. They can also be used, among other things, to look for cancer and assess cardiac function. This type of ultrasound is so-called because it may provide images that more accurately mimic how organs and systems actually look while also having more visual volume than a flat appearance. In some cases, these ultrasounds can greatly simplify the diagnosis. Natural orifice transluminal endoscopic surgery (NOTES), a new advancement in laparoscopic surgery, uses natural orifices to get access to the peritoneal cavity without making any incisions or cutting through the anterior abdominal wall. Using tools in one bodily cavity, often the peritoneal cavity, this treatment is carried out utilizing currently available endoscopic procedures (Atallah, Martin-Perez, Keller, Burke, & Hunter, 2015). Via a natural entrance, such as the mouth, anus, vagina, or urethra, or occasionally through incisions to construct internal orifices, the cavity is accessed with an endoscope (Ahmed & Paraskeva, 2011). Hybrid NOTES procedures, typically used in combination with laparoscopic tools, combine a NOTES approach with direct transcutaneous access to the cavity (Ahmed & Paraskeva, 2011). The transesophageal, transgastric, trans colonic, and transvaginal methods have all been used to enter the peritoneal cavity.

## Conclusion

Polycystic ovarian syndrome is a complicated illness that necessitates the use of several therapeutic and diagnostic approaches, depending on the reason a patient seeks therapy. A personalized diagnosis and treatment strategy should be developed for females who exhibit PCOS symptoms. It's important to pay attention to the history, physical exam, and laboratory findings to spot females who are PCOS-prone. Hyper androgenicity and irregular menstrual cycles are two of the primary clinical signs of PCOS. Most PCOS sufferers exhibit indications of metabolic dysregulation, including insulin resistance, which is not only unrelated to but exacerbated by obesity. Despite differences in symptoms brought on by a person's lifestyle and stage of life, PCOS seems to afflict people all over the world at a comparable rate. As a result, it needs to be properly identified and treated. Practitioners must determine a woman's risk for factors that led her to seek PCOS diagnosis and treatment, also regardless of BMI, serum evaluations and biochemical analysis should likely be performed on all PCOS patients. Surgical treatments like laparoscopy and hysteroscopy are used to identify and treat gynecological conditions like PCOS, endometriosis uterine fibroids, ovarian cysts or tumors, etc. Both of these are less intrusive forms of surgery than the more traditional ones. Many doctors find it difficult to diagnose polycystic ovarian syndrome (PCOS), a prevalent condition, because there is no known test to specifically diagnose it and because there are no established diagnostic criteria. Nevertheless, symptoms, physical examinations, and test results are the key components of the diagnostic criteria for the various phenotypes. With the advancement in science and technology, more reliable and cost-efficient methods shall develop. With the advent of artificial intelligence PCOS diagnosis and detection might see a new horizon over time.

## References


Ahmed, I., & Paraskeva, P. (2011). A clinical review of single-incision laparoscopic surgery. *The Surgeon, 9*(6), 341-351. doi:https://doi.org/10.1016/j.surge.2011.06.003.

Aldrich, J. E. (2007). Basic physics of ultrasound imaging. *Crit. Care Med., 35*(5 Suppl), S131-137. doi:10.1097/01.CCM.0000260624.99430.22.

Amenorrhea associated with bilateral polycystic ovaries. (1935). *American Journal of Obstetrics and Gynecology, 29*(2), 181-191. doi:https://doi.org/10.1016/S0002-9378(15)30642-6.

Andersen, S., Pedersen, K. M., Bruun, N. H., & Laurberg, P. (2002). Narrow individual variations in serum T(4) and T(3) in normal subjects: a clue to the understanding of subclinical thyroid disease. *J. Clin. Endocrinol. Metab., 87*(3), 1068-1072. doi:10.1210/jcem.87.3.8165.

Ashraf, S., Nabi, M., Rasool, S. U. A., Rashid, F., & Amin, S. (2019). Hyperandrogenism in polycystic ovarian syndrome and role of CYP gene variants: a review. *Egyptian Journal of Medical Human Genetics, 20*(1), 25. doi:10.1186/s43042-019-0031-4.

Asuncion, M., Calvo, R. M., San Millan, J. L., Sancho, J., Avila, S., & Escobar-Morreale, H. F. (2000). A prospective study of the prevalence of the polycystic ovary syndrome in unselected Caucasian women from Spain. *J. Clin. Endocrinol. Metab., 85*(7), 2434-2438. doi:10.1210/jcem.85.7.6682.

Atallah, S., Martin-Perez, B., Keller, D., Burke, J., & Hunter, L. (2015). Natural-orifice transluminal endoscopic surgery. *British Journal of Surgery, 102*(2), e73-e92. doi:10.1002/bjs.9710.

Azziz, R., Woods, K. S., Reyna, R., Key, T. J., Knochenhauer, E. S., & Yildiz, B. O. (2004). The prevalence and features of the polycystic ovary syndrome in an unselected population. *J. Clin. Endocrinol. Metab., 89*(6), 2745-2749. doi:10.1210/jc.2003-032046.

Barth, J. H., Yasmin, E., & Balen, A. H. (2007). The diagnosis of polycystic ovary syndrome: the criteria are insufficiently robust for clinical research. *Clin. Endocrinol. (Oxf), 67*(6), 811-815. doi:10.1111/j.1365-2265.2007.02932.x.

Bhattacharya, S. M., & Ghosh, M. (2010). Insulin resistance and adolescent girls with polycystic ovary syndrome. *J. Pediatr. Adolesc. Gynecol., 23*(3), 158-161. doi:10.1016/j.jpag.2009.10.004.

Bhide, P., & Homburg, R. (2016). Anti-Mullerian hormone and polycystic ovary syndrome. *Best Pract. Res. Clin. Obstet. Gynaecol., 37*, 38-45. doi:10.1016/j.bpobgyn.2016.03.004.

Bougle, D., Zunquin, G., Sesboue, B., & Sabatier, J. P. (2010). Relationships of cardiorespiratory fitness with metabolic risk factors, inflammation, and liver transaminases in overweight youths. *Int. J. Pediatr., 2010*, 580897. doi:10.1155/2010/580897.

Bozkurt, M., Kara Bozkurt, D., Kurban, D., Takmaz, T., Sevket, O., & Ozcan, P. (2021). 2-D and 3-D ultrasonographic characteristics of the ovary in women with PCOS and multifollicular ovaries. *J. Obstet. Gynaecol., 41*(6), 920-926. doi:10.1080/01443615.2020.1803244.

Chan, O., Inouye, K., Akirav, E., Park, E., Riddell, M. C., Vranic, M., & Matthews, S. G. (2005). Insulin alone increases hypothalamo-pituitary-adrenal activity, and diabetes lowers peak stress responses. *Endocrinology, 146*(3), 1382-1390. doi:10.1210/en.2004-0607.

Crosignani, P. G., Bianchedi, D., Riccaboni, A., & Vegetti, W. (1999). Management of anovulatory infertility. *Hum. Reprod., 14 Suppl 1*, 108-119. doi:10.1093/humrep/14.suppl_1.108.

De Leo, V., Musacchio, M. C., Cappelli, V., Massaro, M. G., Morgante, G., & Petraglia, F. (2016). Genetic, hormonal and metabolic aspects of PCOS: an update. *Reprod. Biol. Endocrinol., 14*(1), 38. doi:10.1186/s12958-016-0173-x.

Deligeoroglou, E., Kouskouti, C., & Christopoulos, P. (2009). The role of genes in the polycystic ovary syndrome: predisposition and mechanisms. *Gynecol. Endocrinol., 25*(9), 603-609. doi:10.1080/09513590903015619.

Diamanti-Kandarakis, E., & Dunaif, A. (2012). Insulin resistance and the polycystic ovary syndrome revisited: an update on mechanisms and implications. *Endocr. Rev, 33*(6), 981-1030. doi:10.1210/er.2011-1034.

Diamanti-Kandarakis, E., Kouli, C. R., Bergiele, A. T., Filandra, F. A., Tsianateli, T. C., Spina, G. G., Zapanti, E. D., & Bartzis, M. I. (1999). A survey of the polycystic ovary syndrome in the Greek island of Lesbos: hormonal and metabolic profile. *J. Clin. Endocrinol. Metab., 84*(11), 4006-4011. doi:10.1210/jcem.84.11.6148.

Diamanti-Kandarakis, E., & Panidis, D. (2007). Unravelling the phenotypic map of polycystic ovary syndrome (PCOS): a prospective study of 634 women with PCOS. *Clin. Endocrinol. (Oxf), 67*(5), 735-742. doi:10.1111/j.1365-2265.2007.02954.x.

Dunaif, A., & Thomas, A. (2001). Current concepts in the polycystic ovary syndrome. *Annu. Rev. Med., 52*, 401-419. doi:10.1146/annurev.med.52.1.401.

Edler, I., & Lindstrom, K. (2004). The history of echocardiography. *Ultrasound. Med. Biol., 30*(12), 1565-1644. doi:10.1016/S0301-5629(99)00056-3.

Fraser, I. S., & Kovacs, G. (2004). Current recommendations for the diagnostic evaluation and follow-up of patients presenting with symptomatic polycystic ovary syndrome. *Best Pract. Res. Clin. Obstet. Gynaecol., 18*(5), 813-823. doi:10.1016/j.bpobgyn.2004.06.009.

Fulghesu, A., Magnini, R., Portoghese, E., Angioni, S., Minerba, L., & Melis, G. B. (2010). Obesity-related lipid profile and altered insulin incretion in adolescents with polycystic ovary syndrome. *J. Adolesc. Health, 46*(5), 474-481. doi:10.1016/j.jadohealth.2009.10.008.

Ghergherechi, R., & Tabrizi, A. (2010). Prevalence of impaired glucose tolerance and insulin resistance among obese children and adolescents. *Ther. Clin. Risk Manag., 6*, 345-349. doi:10.2147/tcrm.s12033.

Gillett, M. J. (2009). International Expert Committee report on the role of the A1c assay in the diagnosis of diabetes: Diabetes Care 2009; 32(7): 1327-1334. *Clin. Biochem. Rev., 30*(4), 197-200. Retrieved from https://www.ncbi.nlm.nih.gov/pubmed/20011212.

Ibanez, L., Potau, N., Francois, I., & de Zegher, F. (1998). Precocious pubarche, hyperinsulinism, and ovarian hyperandrogenism in girls: relation to reduced fetal growth. *J. Clin. Endocrinol. Metab., 83*(10), 3558-3562. doi:10.1210/jcem.83.10.5205.

Ibanez, L., Potau, N., Virdis, R., Zampolli, M., Terzi, C., Gussinye, M., Carrascosa, A., & Vicens-Calvet, E. (1993). Postpubertal outcome in girls diagnosed of premature pubarche during childhood: increased frequency of functional ovarian hyperandrogenism. *J. Clin. Endocrinol. Metab., 76*(6), 1599-1603. doi:10.1210/jcem.76.6.8501168.

Kasa-Vubu, J. Z., Jain, V., & Welch, K. (2010). Impact of fatness, insulin, and gynecological age on luteinizing hormone secretory dynamics in adolescent females. *Fertil. Steril., 94*(1), 221-229. doi:10.1016/j.fertnstert.2009.02.072.

Knochenhauer, E. S., Key, T. J., Kahsar-Miller, M., Waggoner, W., Boots, L. R., & Azziz, R. (1998). Prevalence of the polycystic ovary syndrome in unselected black and white women of the southeastern United States: a prospective study. *J. Clin. Endocrinol. Metab., 83*(9), 3078-3082. doi:10.1210/jcem.83.9.5090.

Kulle, A. E., Riepe, F. G., Melchior, D., Hiort, O., & Holterhus, P. M. (2010). A Novel Ultrapressure Liquid Chromatography Tandem Mass Spectrometry Method for the Simultaneous Determination of Androstenedione, Testosterone, and Dihydrotestosterone in Pediatric Blood Samples: Age- and Sex-Specific Reference Data. *The Journal of Clinical Endocrinology & Metabolism, 95*(5), 2399-2409. doi:10.1210/jc.2009-1670.

La Marca, A., Egbe, T. O., Morgante, G., Paglia, T., Cianci, A., & De Leo, V. (2000). Metformin treatment reduces ovarian cytochrome P-450c17alpha response to human chorionic gonadotrophin in women with insulin resistance-related polycystic ovary syndrome. *Hum. Reprod., 15*(1), 21-23. doi:10.1093/humrep/15.1.21.

Lujan, M. E., Chizen, D. R., & Pierson, R. A. (2008). Diagnostic criteria for polycystic ovary syndrome: pitfalls and controversies. *J. Obstet. Gynaecol. Can., 30*(8), 671-679. doi:10.1016/S1701-2163(16)32915-2.

Ni, C. M., Huang, W. L., Jiang, Y. M., Xu, J., Duan, R., Zhu, Y. L., Zhu, X.-P., Fan, X.-M., Luo, G.-A., Wang, Y.-M., Li, Y.-Y., He, Q., & Xu, L. (2020). Improving the accuracy and efficacy of diagnosing polycystic ovary syndrome by integrating metabolomics with clinical characteristics: study protocol for a randomized controlled trial. *Trials, 21*(1), 169. doi:10.1186/s13063-020-4060-6.

Ovalle, F., & Azziz, R. (2002). Insulin resistance, polycystic ovary syndrome, and type 2 diabetes mellitus. *Fertil. Steril., 77*(6), 1095-1105. doi:10.1016/s0015-0282(02)03111-4.

Pesant, M. H., & Baillargeon, J. P. (2011). Clinically useful predictors of conversion to abnormal glucose tolerance in women with polycystic ovary syndrome. *Fertil. Steril., 95*(1), 210-215. doi:10.1016/j.fertnstert.2010.06.036.

Philipose, K. J., & Sinha, B. (1994). Laparoscopic Surgery. *Med. J. Armed. Forces India, 50*(2), 137-143. doi:10.1016/S0377-1237(17)31019-5.

Raber, W., Gessl, A., Nowotny, P., & Vierhapper, H. (2003). Hyperprolactinaemia in hypothyroidism: clinical significance and impact of TSH normalization. *Clin. Endocrinol. (Oxf), 58*(2), 185-191. doi:10.1046/j.1365-2265.2003.01694.x.

Sanchez, E. G., Giviziez, C. R., Sanchez, H. M., Agostinho, P. L., Barros, P. S., & Approbato, M. S. (2016). Low progesterone levels and ovulation by ultrasound assessment in infertile patients. *JBRA Assist. Reprod., 20*(1), 13-16. doi:10.5935/1518-0557.20160004.

Shabanzadeh, D. M., & Sorensen, L. T. (2012). Laparoscopic surgery compared with open surgery decreases surgical site infection in obese patients: a systematic review and meta-analysis. *Ann. Surg., 256*(6), 934-945. doi:10.1097/SLA.0b013e318269a46b.

Sheehan, M. T. (2004). Polycystic ovarian syndrome: diagnosis and management. *Clin. Med. Res., 2*(1), 13-27. doi:10.3121/cmr.2.1.13.

Shriki, J. (2014). Ultrasound physics. *Crit. Care Clin., 30*(1), 1-24, v. doi:10.1016/j.ccc.2013.08.004.

Søeborg, T., Frederiksen, H., Fruekilde, P., Johannsen, T. H., Juul, A., & Andersson, A. M. (2013). Serum concentrations of DHEA, DHEAS, 17α-hydroxyprogesterone, Δ4-androstenedione and testosterone in children determined by TurboFlow-LC–MS/MS. *Clinica Chimica Acta, 419*, 95-101. doi:https://doi.org/10.1016/j.cca.2013.01.019.

Søeborg, T., Frederiksen, H., Mouritsen, A., Johannsen, T. H., Main, K. M., Jørgensen, N., Petersen, J. H., Andersson, A.-M., & Juul, A. (2014). Sex, age, pubertal development and use of oral contraceptives in relation to serum concentrations of DHEA, DHEAS, 17α-hydroxyprogesterone, Δ4-androstenedione, testosterone and their ratios in children, adolescents and young adults. *Clinica Chimica Acta, 437*, 6-13. doi:https://doi.org/10.1016/j.cca.2014.06.018.

Soper, N. J., Brunt, L. M., & Kerbl, K. (1994). Laparoscopic general surgery. *N. Engl. J. Med., 330*(6), 409-419. doi:10.1056/NEJM199402103300608.

Tan, S., Scherag, A., Janssen, O. E., Hahn, S., Lahner, H., Dietz, T., Scherag, S., Grallert, H., Vogel, C. I. G., Kimmig, R., Illig, T., Mann, K., Hebebrand, J., Hinney, A. (2010). Large effects on body mass index and insulin resistance of fat mass and obesity associated gene (FTO) variants in patients with polycystic ovary syndrome (PCOS). *BMC Med. Genet., 11*, 12. doi:10.1186/1471-2350-11-12.

Teede, H. J., Misso, M. L., Costello, M. F., Dokras, A., Laven, J., Moran, L., Piltonen, T., Norman, R. J., International, P. N. (2018). Recommendations from the international evidence-based guideline for the assessment and management of polycystic ovary syndrome. *Hum. Reprod., 33*(9), 1602-1618. doi:10.1093/humrep/dey256.

Wudy, S. A., & Choi, M. H. (2016). Steroid LC–MS has come of age. *The Journal of Steroid Biochemistry and Molecular Biology, 162*, 1-3. doi:https://doi.org/10.1016/j.jsbmb.2016.05.010.

# Chapter 13

# A Holistic Approach Towards Several Biomarkers for the Early Detection of PCOS

**Deepali Siwan***
Department of Pharmacology, Delhi PharmaceuticalSciences Research University (DPSRU), New Delhi, India

## Abstract

Furthermost prevalent endocrinal illness in females with a vast range of clinical manifestations is polycystic ovarian syndrome (PCOS). This condition causes many health problems, including infertility, insulin resistance, obesity, and cardiovascular concerns. PCOS is an autoimmune, polygenic, systemic, immunological, dysregulated steroid status, an inflammatory condition primarily resulting from poor lifestyle choices. Numerous predisposing factors, including genetic and epigenetic abnormalities, might contribute to the changes that PCOS-affected women experience. Environmental variables have a less significant impact in terms of worsening insulin resistance. A molecular genetic code might be used to identify PCOS, protein, and enzyme markers. The genetic markers linked to PCOS do not help enable real-time detection; instead, they could only be used to validate PCOS in people now displaying the characteristic symptoms. Indicators of proteins and enzymes were commonly used to monitor the individual condition and predict the onset of PCOS problems. Insulin resistance and the emergence of PCOS have been revealed to have a strong relationship with adipose tissue proteins. The examination of several parameters is therefore necessary for the PCOS diagnosis. To better understand the intricate metabolic processes in patients with PCOS, we concentrated on identifying several distinct metabolites in women with the condition via a holistic approach. This comprehensive analysis using a variety of biomarkers may make it easier to develop improved PCOS management strategies.

**Keywords:** ovarian disease, biochemical evaluation, biomarkers, PCOS, fertility, reproductive health

---

* Corresponding Author's Email: deepalisiwan6@gmail.com.

In: Polycystic Ovarian Syndrome (PCOS) and Our Biological Clock
Editors: Arpita Roy, Gowhar Rashid and Nihad Ashraf Khan
ISBN: 979-8-89113-100-2
© 2023 Nova Science Publishers, Inc.

## 1. Introduction

The co-occurrence of hirsutism, hyperandrogenism, and ovulatory disruption defines the complex illness known as PCOS (polycystic ovary syndrome). Between 6% and 20% of premenopausal women have PCOS (using the most recent, broadest definitions) (Asuncio´n et al., 2000). This condition possesses a phenotypic range of 2-5, maybe the predominant physiological simultaneously physiological disease in many women of childbearing (Azziz et al., 2004). Consequently, the worldwide and local healthcare authorities, particularly the pharmaceutical business, have not shown the same interest in PCOS as the scientific community. Stein and Leventhal (Yildiz et al., 2012) first described PCOS as a combination of amenorrhea, continuous anovulation, impotence, excess weight, and enlarged cystic ovaries in 1935. Hirsutism, which refers to the development of terminal hair with a typical pattern in females, was also included in their initial diagnosis. However, "E28.2 polycystic ovarian syndrome," commonly known as sclerotic ovaries disease or Stein-Leventhal syndrome, was not even included in the 10th edition of the International Classification of Diseases until 1990. Furthermore, the majority of prescription drugs used to treat the symptoms of PCOS, such as oral contraceptives, antiandrogens, insulin stimulators, and aromatase inhibitors, are being used off-label as neither the Food and Drug Administration nor the European Medicines Agency has consistently approved a drug created solely for the treatment of PCOS (RADOSH, 2009). The existing registration of clinical trials is an example of the pharmaceutical industry's lack of interest in PCOS. Whereas 28 profitable experiments on PCOS were certified at ClinicalTrials.gov now, after August 2017, 4,632 studies addressed diabetes mellitus, even though both conditions have comparable global prevalence ([illegible] et al., [illegible]). As a result, from the standpoint of pharmaceutical therapy, PCOS may now be regarded as an orphan condition that adversely affects women who are sexually active most frequently.

The lack of understanding of PCOS among clients, doctors, and even researchers and its long-term effects on patients and their family's health has restricted the distribution of assets for advancement and research into this study area. This is the most plausible reason for medical experts' lack of enthusiasm in addition to the pharmaceutical sector (Dokras et al., 2017). The insufficiency of PCOS's name, its diverse character, the perennially contentious problem of its definition, and the numerous unanswered questions regarding its origin and pathophysiology are possible causes of this misconception.

Our review discusses the most recent developments and presents gaps in scientific understanding of PCOS to outline concise, straightforward guidelines for accurate diagnosis and long-term therapeutic care. While most of these suggestions are based on and by the most recent evidence-based clinical recommendations for the treatment of PCOS, there are a few instances where they are based solely on my personal experience or a small number of studies, in which case, as a result of scientific proof is made clear.

## 2. Aetiology and Pathophysiology

It is believed that a mix of inherited, genomic, and prenatal ecological variables influence the complicated pathogenesis of PCOS. The two least prevalent and essential indications of the condition, hyperandrogenism, and hyperinsulinemia, are present between 75 and 95 percent, including all women with PCOS (Figure 1). The major genetically inherited phenotypic characteristic in afflicted women and the principal reason for hyperandrogenism is ovarian androgen hypersecretion (Legro et al., 1998). By boosting androgen production in theca cells, elevated concentrations of luteinizing hormone (LH) arise in reaction to increased gonadotropin-releasing hormone (GnRH) release and, likely furthermore, the lack of negative feedback from progesterone, worsen ovarian hyperandrogenism (Escobar-Morreale, 2018). In patients with PCOS, theca cell intrinsic malfunction also leads to high ovarian levels of testosterone (Gilling-Smith et al., 1997). Furthermore, theca cell hyperandrogenism, connected to PCOS-positive women's higher quantity of ovarian antral follicles, further enhances the amount of tiny antral follicles and gonadotropin-independent preantral follicles (Nisenblat and Norman 2009; Webber et al., 2003) motes primary follicular recruitment. Preantral follicles exhibit the highest levels of androgen receptor (AR) expression, indicating that androgens' direct effects are felt at these initial stages of folliculogenesis (Lenie & Smitz, 2009). In addition, the comparatively lower amounts of follicle-stimulating hormone (FSH) compared to LH levels impede both follicular maturation and expansion (Taylor et al., 1997).

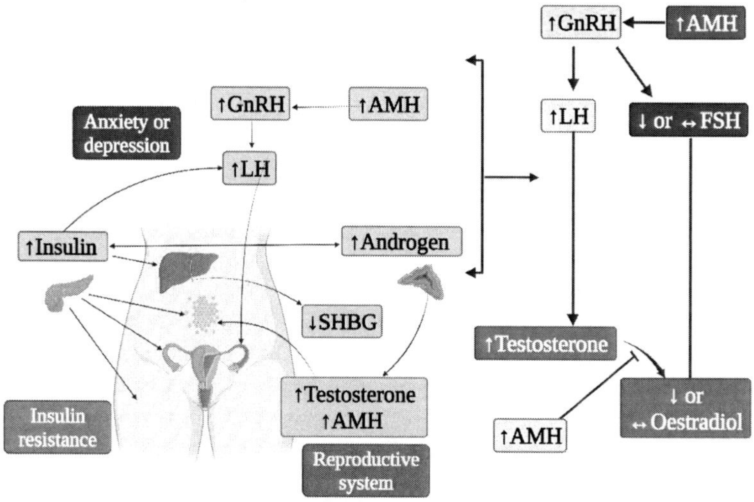


**Figure 1.** PCOS is connected to psychological disorders, including anxiety and depression and metabolic and reproductive problems. Gonadotropin stimulation is necessary for ovarian steroidogenesis. Among PCOS patients, the gonadotropin-releasing hormone (GnRH) pulse generators resist the harmful. The adverse effects of ovarian steroids, which the androgen-receptor blocker flutamide may reverse be reversed by the androgen-receptor blocker flutamide, are most likely caused by androgen excess. A major factor in the hyperandrogenaemia experienced by women with PCOS is the hypersecretion of luteinizing hormone (LH), brought on by the increased GnRH pulse frequency. This condition, characterized by hypersecretion of LH, is a sign of PCOS. drives theca cell hyperandrogenism. In addition to being obese, women with PCOS also have hyperinsulinemia, which increases the synthesis of testosterone in the theca cells, exacerbates LH hypersecretion, and decreases the formation of sex hormone-binding globulin (SHBG) in the liver, all of which contribute to hyperandrogenaemia. Reduced follicle-stimulating hormone (FSH) release prevents follicles from becoming more extensive and mature. Since there are so many preantral and tiny antral follicles, women with PCOS also produce too much anti-Müllerian hormone (AMH). AMH prevents the aromatase gene CYP19A1 from being expressed, which prevents androgens from converting to estrogens and contributes to higher androgen levels. Increased GnRH neuron activity and LH production regulated by GnRH are directly stimulated by elevated AMH levels, which may further promote ovarian hyperandrogenism. Obesity increases the incidence of PCOS in women, worsens the syndrome's symptoms overall, and also results in PCOS. ↓, decreased; ↑, increased; ↔, unchanged.

Insulin sensitivity, which leads to hyperinsulinemia, lowers the production of sex hormone-binding proteins in the liver globulin (SHBG) and the production of androgens development via ovarian theca cells. These outcomes work in concert. when combined with LH's stimulatory effects and elevated testosterone levels in the blood and free form (Baillargeon & Carpentier, 2007). Furthermore, hyperinsulinemia increases LH receptors, inhibiting the development of follicles and theca cells, which worsens androgen-dependent male sexual dysfunction anovulation (Barbierit et al., 1986; Barbieri, Smith, and Ryan 1988). Further mechanistic research is needed (Thong et al., 2020) since it is still unclear whether congenital adrenal hyperplasia or impaired insulin is the leading cause of PCOS. What is known is that PCOS medications that target dual androgen production and insulin sensitivity help women with reproductive and metabolic symptoms. This finding illustrates how crucial it is to pinpoint the primary causes of PCOS to create fresh therapy approaches that are mechanism-based Figure 1.

## 3. Variables That Raise the Risk of Developing PCOS

According to the incidence rate, a common endocrine disorder is PCOS which impacts 4%–8% of all under-women who can procreate, per the NIH/NICHD guidelines (Azziz et al., 2004; Michelmore et al., 1999; Knochenhauer et al., 1998; Asunción et al., 2000). The occurrence of PCOS has subsequently been revealed to vary depending upon this clinical guideline, according to different studies (see Table 1) (March et al., 2010). According to this research, the prevalence estimates determined using Rotterdam standards were primarily approximately two to three times greater than those found utilizing NIH/NICHD recommendations. The family background of PCOS is a potential risk factor. PCOS is thought to be an inherited genetic illness based on the grouping of instances in families (Franks et al., 1997; Legro et al., 1998). A high PCOS prevalence or its characteristics among close family members indicate hereditary factors (Amato and Simpson 2004; Crosignani and Nicolosi 2001). Additionally, monozygotic twins have been found to have higher concordance than dizygotic twins. The method of inheritance still needs to be clarified. The variety of PCOS phenotypes, the challenge of phenotyping men, postmenopausal women, and adolescent girls, and the challenge of gathering sufficient sample sizes to provide adequate statistical power are all issues that hamper the growth in this field, though (Goodarzi et al., 2011). The locus sites found in Han Chinese people's genome-wide association analyses were on chromosomes 2p16.3, 2p21, and 9q33.3 (Amato & Simpson, 2004). In particular, the chromosome 2p21 THADA and genome 9p33.3 DENND1A susceptibility loci chromosome 2p21 THADA and genome 9p33.3 DENND1A susceptibility loci, in particular, showed replicated in European populations. Sharing the same susceptibility genes shows that PCOS is a long-standing condition that predates human migration out of Africa (Hart et al., 2004). Several disorders are connected to a higher prevalence of PCOS. A healthy personality has been found to reduce body weight, abdominal fat, and testosterone, improve insulin sensitivity, and reduce hirsutism in women with PCOS. A history of weight gain frequently precedes the emergence of the clinical manifestations of PCOS (Sirmans & Pate, 2013) and a history of weight gain often precedes hirsutism (Lim et al., 2019). 28.3% of obese women referred for weight reduction help had PCOS (Álvarez-Blasco et al., 2006). The PCOS prevalence did not differ substantially in an unselected sample depending on the obesity class (Herzog, 2006; Yildiz et al., 2008). Underweight, average weight, overweight, mildly, moderately, and severely obese women had PCOS prevalence rates of 8.2%, 9.8%, 9.9%, 5.2%, 12.4%, and 11.5%, respectively. The scientists concluded to the conclusion that obesity may somewhat raise the risk of PCOS. In women with epilepsy, there has been a documented rise in the prevalence of reproductive problems, including PCOS (Herzog, 2006). Using NIH diagnostic criteria, Bilo et al. (Bilo et al., 2001) identified PCOS in 13 of 50 women (26%) experiencing seizures. Observations about epilepsy, independently of antiepileptic medications, increased the incidence of PCOS and are supported by the fact that among the 16 individuals with epilepsy who were not taking medication at the time of performance, five (31%) had PCOS. When given to women with epilepsy, the antiepileptic medication valproic acid, often epilepsy treatment and bipolar disorder, including migraines, is linked to symptoms of polycystic ovary syndrome. These characteristics include irregular menstrual cycles, polycystic ovarian morphology, and increased serum testosterone (Betts et al., 2003; Isojarvi et al., 1993). Fasting serum glucose, body mass index, and testosterone levels were reduced in epileptic women who were given lamotrigine instead of valproic acid. Hence, the confounding effects of medication must be considered in research that examines the link between epilepsy, bipolar disorder, and PCOS. Type 1, 2, and gestational diabetes have all been associated with increased PCOS prevalence. Escobar-Morre-Ale et al., examined 85 White women with type 1 diabetes mellitus for PCOS using the NIH/NICHD criteria. PCOS was discovered in 16 of these women (18.8%). After that, 42 women with type 1 diabetes and 38 controls with similar age and BMI were screened for PCOS using the ESHRE/ASRM criteria (Codner et al., 2006). PCO occurs in 82% of women with type 2 diabetes, making them frequent (Codner et al., 2006). There are 26.7% additional patients having type 2 diabetes who also have PCOS, based on NIH/NICHD standards (Peppard et al., 2001). Six of the 94 women (6.4%) without gestational diabetes and 15 of the 94 women (16%) having gestational had a confirmed diagnosis of PCOS ($P = 0.03$) (Kashanian et al., 2008). Several variables have been linked to a higher risk of PCOS in children (Rosenfield, 2007). Low birth weight, congenital virilization, and increased birth weight in girls born to obese moms are all prenatal risk factors. Risk factors that emerge later in infancy include early pubarche, abnormal progress puberty, obesity syndromes, hyperpigmentation nigricans, and metabolic syndrome. Many of these risk factors and chronically irregular menstrual periods in adolescents should raise suspicions of PCOS (Nicandri & Hoeger, 2012).

**Table 1.** Representation of the incidence of polycystic ovarian syndrome (PCOS) based on various clinical criteria

| S. No. | Country (Females) | NIH/NICHD standard | ESHRE/ASRM standard | High androgen and PCOS societal standards | Reference |
|---|---|---|---|---|---|
| 1. | 392 (Turkish) | 6.1% | 19.9% | 15.3% | (March et al., 2010) |
| 2. | 929 (Iranian) | 7.1% | 14.6% | 11.7% | (Franks et al., 1997) |
| 3. | 820 (Iranian) | 7% | 15.2% | 7.92% | (March et al., 2010) |
| 4. | 728 (Australian) | 8.7% | 17.8% | 12.0% | (Yildiz et al., 2012) |

Abbreviation: NIH/NICHD: National Institutes of Health/National Institute of Child Health and Human Disease; ESHRE/ASRM: European Society for Human Reproduction and Embryology/American Society for Reproductive Medicine.

## 4. Molecular-Based Method to Detect PCOS

Across laboratories and countries, PCOS is defined and diagnosed differently. While the European diagnostic standards need the ovaries to seem abnormal, the North American. The numerous biochemical signs of hyperandrogenism or hyperandrogenaemia are used as diagnostic criteria. Enzymes, peptides, and genetic markers may be used to provide a biochemical diagnosis. The numerous PCOS diagnostic indicators, along with their benefits and drawbacks, are covered in this section. Studies have revealed a significant genetic link between PCOS development and an autosomal dominant inheritance pattern. A woman typically has a 30–50% probability of developing PCOS if her relatives have the condition. According to twin studies, monozygotic identical twins had a double high risk of getting Dizygotic twin daughters with PCOS had a double as high-risk of getting PCOS as dizygotic twins, according to twin studies. Researchers have discovered over 100 susceptibility genes linked to PCOS (Stepto et al., 2013). Numerous research suggests that it could have ontogenetic traits. Even though heredity demonstrates a close family bond, different family members may exhibit different phenotypic traits (Panda et al., 2016). According to Shaikh, Dadachanji, and Mukherjee (2014), environmental variables and other anomalies are also involved in the formation of PCOS and contribute to it added to its hereditary component. Additionally, PCOS is significantly related to many different conditions, such as hyperinsulinemia and hyperandrogenemia, indicating that it is a heterogenic syndrome. As a result, understanding the molecular underpinnings of various disorders is necessary to inquire into the genetic origin of PCOS (Shaikh et al., 2014). Several genes that control the production of androgen and insulin have been linked to PCOS. Insulin resistance, defined as the host cells' failure to react to insulin production, is one of the most significant associated disorders. A quick examination of insulin action reveals that it participates in a multistep process that activates INSR and IGF-1 receptors, among other cellular receptors (Urbanek et al., 1999). The INSR is a significant insulin receptor composed of two alpha and two beta components in a tetrameric configuration. Insulin primarily stimulates the INSR, which activates tyrosine kinases, activating a long, intricate signaling cascade. Research conducted by (Shaikh et al., 2014) on the genes associated with 37 PCOS candidates revealed that both muscle fibers and adipose tissues had post-signaling defects of INSR. D19S884, located on chromosome 19 P13.2.13, is one of the markers that has shown a substantial connection with INSR deficiency and is related to PCOS. IRS is a different chemical linked to the activation of INSR. INSR can interface components of insulin sensitivity such as PI3K, Fyn, and Crk, thanks to the phosphorylation of IRS. Dunaif, Wu, Lee, and Diamanti-Kandarakis (Dunaif et al., 2001) show defective skeletal muscle IRS molecules in PCOS candidates (Shaikh, Dadachanji, and Mukherjee 2014; Diamanti-Kandarakis et al., 2009; Gharani et al., 1997). PPARγ, ENPP1, and Calpain-10 are additional insulin signaling molecules linked to PCOS. Polymorphism is a problem with these markers. The abovementioned study found that these indicators did not appear in all PCOS patients. It is still being determined precisely what function they play in the etiology of PCOS. As previously stated, several additional conditions are linked to PCOS, and numerous studies have described how these other disorders may influence PCOS's pathogenesis. Although PCOS manifests a range of symptoms, the fundamental feature is aberrant hormonal release, or an excessive number of male hormones, which causes problems with periodic bleeding with the development of cysts on the ovaries. To comprehend the genetic underpinnings of PCOS, it is crucial to look at the irregularities in steroidogenesis at the atomic threshold. The aberrant rise of circulating androgen, one of the diagnostic signs of PCOS, is caused by an overabundance ovaries' theca cells, which are responsible for generating androstenedione and testosterone. This is brought on by the steroidogenic enzymes' improved transcription and mRNA stability.

Historically, hyperandrogenism and CYP17 have been linked. It records the P450c17α enzyme, the preventive step in producing androgens. Individuals with high testosterone and PCOS had high P450c17α activity, possibly related to the enormous androgen production. On chromosome 10q24.3, CYP17 resides. However, other investigations did not support the link between the mutation of CYP17 and PCOS manifestation. This gene's precise function has yet to be established. Another gene, CYP11A, is regarded as a potential applicant for PCOS and hyperandrogenism. The CYP11A gene produces the enzyme needed to break the cholesterol terminal branch and prepare it for translation into androgen, the first stage of androgenesis. Repeats of (tttta) in the CYP11A promoter (528 bp) in this gene characterize a polymorphism. In 20 pedigrees with the condition, this genotype had a high correlation with PCOS [(Eisenberg et al., 2017). Although these genes were associated with PCOS, several were unreliable for making an early diagnosis. This is caused by the lack of a population-wide standard expression pattern and the existence of additional genes that affect how hyperandrogenism manifests. Serum miRNA-20b and miRNA-429 can be used to test for anovulatory women, according to a new analysis by Eisenberg et al., (Sørensen et al., 2014). In the study, there were 18 PCOS-positive women, 15 menopausal women who regularly ovulated, and 7 women that regularly ovulated. RT-PCR was used as the detecting technique. According to the findings, PCOS and anovulatory women had greater concentrations of miRNA20b & miRNA-429 than women who were ovulating naturally (Sørensen et al., 2014). MiRNA impacts how follicular cells are produced and how follicular growth is controlled. It demonstrates varying concentrations throughout the luteal cycles. By attaching to the 3' in the 3' untranslated mRNA, miRNA can regulate the expression of specific genes. Rendering the target mRNA is unstable; this prevents translation. The precise function of miRNA in PCOS isn't yet known. However, follicular fluids and patients' serum have substantially increased specific miRNA. A study used the expression of rat models to understand miRNA's role in PCOS. DHT was employed in the study to simulate human hyperandrogenic levels. Compared with the control, wherein 17 miRNA showed depression, the study of something like the ovaries in such animals revealed a hyper increase of 72 miRNA. Another study clarified miRNAs' role in controlling death and differentiation in ovarian cells, possibly related to aberrant miRNAs in PCOS (Panda et al., 2016). According to Zao et al., (2017), there may be a connection between the methylation of the o-PPARGC1A regulators in leukocytes and PCOS patients' mitochondria. According to the cross-sectional study, PCOS patients had higher levels of methylated PPARGC1A promoter than healthy controls. Additionally, it shows that PCOS sufferers have less mitochondrial DNA than healthy women. According to the study, there may be a connection between these indicators and patients with PCOS metabolic problems. The study offers epigenetics as one reason for the increased methylation PPARGC1A promoter in leukocytes. Inevitably, hypermethylation of the PPARGC1A promoters results from androgen enhancement of the patient's genome's epigenetic alteration. The mitochondrial DNA and the PPARGC1A promoters in leukocytes contribute significantly to human physiological processes, such as regulating cholesterol control and blood pressure management. The ratio of the PPARGC1A activator in leukocytes to mitochondrial DNA can be employed to identify metabolic risks in PCOS.

Recent research has suggested potential PCOS indicators that might be utilized as conclusive markers with both assessment and screening in the future. Among the indicators, D19S884 demonstrated high PCOS specificity. The microsatellite is inside the fibrillin gene's intron (Diamanti-Kandarakis et al., 2009). Although the fibrillin gene regulates TGF-B, its precise function in PCOS is unknown. TCF7L2, another crucial gene, is used in treating type 2 diabetes. The IRSN mutation has also demonstrated a significant association with PCOS. MiRNA has proven to be helpful for screening purposes in detecting anovulation patients. However, it can only indicate that the patient's ovulation cycle is defective (Gilling-Smith et al., 1994). As was established, PCOS is a complicated disease linked to many illnesses, many of which have hereditary roots, including anomalies in the insulin receptors. Due to various circumstances, including variance, external conditions, and changes in the causative agents in PCOS, evaluating these genetic markers' efficacy may, in many instances, be unsuccessful. Many research sought to relate individual genes in patients' genomes to PCOS, while others attempted to use association studies to show an accurate screening device for illness. While some research seemed effective in identifying a relevant marker, others revealed that this marker lacks specificity and plays no meaningful function in testing. This is tied to the test's varying clarity and responsiveness settings. Besides illustration, following corrective testing, the POMC gene rs12473543, previously believed to be associated with PCOS, failed to provide any meaningful value. Historical theories linking specific genes, such as follistatin and lamin, to PCOS have not provided a conclusive diagnosis. Even though most of these genes were detected in high frequency among PCOS patients, none are definitive for diagnosing PCOS. While some of them are recognized to have a part in the illness, others remain to have an unclear function. Finding a valuable genetic trait for PCOS is extremely difficult due to the non-specificity and symptoms that PCOS shares with other endocrinal diseases. The regular operation of the organism can be impacted by changes in enzyme function, whether caused by restriction or lack of activity. As a result, polycystic ovarian syndrome Is one of the symptoms that might result from an enzyme modification in the ovaries (PCOS). As mentioned previously, compared to normal theca, theca cells of polycystic ovaries produce more androstenedione and progesterone in vitro (Stone & Hechter, 1955). This shows that the progesterone biosynthesis level or higher is where the suspected steroidogenesis problem occurs. Initially limiting the rate of the beginning of the sex mechanism for steroid production is the transformation of sterol to pregnenolone, which is catalyzed by the cholesterol side-chain cleaving enzyme cytochrome P450scc (Mason et al., 1994). High expression of this enzyme may boost androgen synthesis, according to the theory. Aromatase (cytochrome P450arom), a secondary steroidogenic enzyme, catalyzes the transformation of C19 steroids (androgens) into C18 estrogens. Granulosa cells with anovulation polycystic ovaries have a markedly higher rate of estradiol synthesis than those from normal ovaries when exposed to FSH in vitro. This demonstrates that PCOS has an abnormal control of this enzyme. On the other hand, two other investigations have shown instances where aromatase insufficiency was linked to hyperandrogenemia (Ito et al., 1993). These results also imply that a change in the control of this enzyme may bring on PCOS. P450scc and P450arom enzymes were the subjects of research to look at their potential role in PCOS/MPB. The long reach of chromosome 15 contains the genes for P450scc (CYP11a) & P450arom (CYP19), both found at locations 15q24 and 15q21.1, respectively (Kruglyak et al., 1996). PCOS/MPB pedigrees underwent either statistical or non-parametric linkage studies because of the uncertainty surrounding the segregation hypothesis for PCOS. The CYP11a promoter region underwent mutation screening as well. To conduct an interaction study on Europid women with PCOS, a case-control study collection of sequentially detected CYP11a intragenic biomarkers was used. The GENEHUNTER program performed parametric or non-parametric linkage analysis for each probable locus (Artimani et al., 2016; Mooser et al., 1995). The studies used the placement moreover, the chromosomal sequence of the microsatellite elements. The CYP19 gene was excluded since there was no proof of excessive gene exchange across the entire region. The CYP11a locus non-parametric data demonstrated excess allele sharing. According to the findings from these data, the CYP11a (ac)n/D15S169 locus may be connected to almost 60% of the pedigrees. The CYP11a protein expression received mutation screening since any harmful changes in CYP11a are anticipated to result in upregulation. Multiple cAMP-regulated elements that increase baseline transcriptional activity and elements that suppress expression are likely to present in this area. Evaluation by genotyping was utilized to analyze 1.85kb of sequence in 10 afflicted and abandoned by eight lineage members using 25 PCR amplification. No variations to the authored sequence were found in any individual, except variations in the number of tandem repeats of the two single-nucleotide polymorphisms present in this region—a dinucleotide (ac)n repeat and a large number of members (tttta) n repeat—at positions 1376 and 528 from the ATG start of translation site, respectively. The CYP11a (tttta)n markers of those participating in the case-control study were analyzed. Our data analysis found four alleles—216, 226, 236, and 241—with reported frequencies of 0.59, 0.28, 0.04, and 0.09, respectively. To prevent repeating allele comparisons for uncommon alleles, individuals were split into two groups depending on their genotype: those with at least one copy of the common, four-repeat unit alleles (216+) and those without the 216 alleles (designated 216-). The entire data set revealed a correlation between this mutation and serum testosterone levels. When the genotype distributions of the whole data set's blood testosterone levels were examined, the proportion of people with 216-genotypes in each quartile was 0.44, 0.23, 0.18, and 0.13 (from highest to lowest). Only women with PCOS showed the link between the CYP11a genotype and testosterone in the subgroup analysis. There was no discernible distinction between the control participants or the PCO groups between the average testosterone levels of 216- and 216+ people. However, the tiny sample sizes in these groups increased the risk of mistakes. The genotype distributions for CYP11a were then compared between subject groups. Between PCOS women and a combined standard control/PCO group, the whole data set—including those for which testosterone levels were unavailable—was examined. A substantial change in the genotype distribution between these groups was found. This was because blood testosterone production and CYP11a genotype correlate only in the PCOS group did blood testosterone production, and CYP11a genotype correlates. According to the data, it is possible that the aromatase gene (CYP19) is not a significant risk factor for PCOS/MPB. On the other hand, the linkage information for the side chain cleavage gene CYP11a suggests that this gene plays a role in the etiology of PCOS. The association findings indicate that allelic variants of CYP11a play a part in developing gynecomastia, which is connected to PCOS. The fact that this gene is associated with hirsutism but not with the ovulatory state suggests that CYP11a plays a significant role in the emergence of hirsutism in PCOS. Elevated serum concentrations and CYP11a alleles (tttta) markers have been significantly correlated. Allelic variations of this percentage enzyme may impact the androgen content synthesis. However, this link can only be proven in the PCOS subgroup. Small sample numbers may be to blame for the inability to show the connection between PCOS (polycystic ovary sufferers with no symptoms; quiet) and regular groups. As an alternative, this locus may modify possible that this locus modifies the evolution of ovarian alterations by combining with other hereditary and environmental variables, affecting, in turn affecting, how PCOS manifests clinically. The protein expression of CYP11a contains CYP11a (tttta)n, and sequencing examination of the nearby areas has not turned up any additional mutations that are expected to have significant pathogenic implications. The suspected mutation, however, may be found elsewhere, so only 1.85 kb of the DNA was examined. In recent years, several gene-connected VNTRs (variable number tandem repeats) were linked to the regulation of genes, including the VNTR for the insulin gene (Mooser et al., 1995; Zhang et al., 2015). Also, a direct link has been established between the alleles of a (tttta)n repeated polymorphism in the 5′ flanking region of the apolipoprotein(a) gene and plasma concentrations of Lp (a) (Zhang et al., 2015). Expression studies have revealed that constructs with eight copies of the apolipoprotein(a) (tttta) sequence exhibit a 5-fold higher transcriptional activity than those with nine copies (Zhang et al., 2015). The (tttta) repetitive polymorphism in CYP11a has not yet been given a regulatory role. Thus, more research into the agent region of this gene is necessary to understand how it affects the control of such a gene. Allelic variations of the CYP11a gene influence the cause of hyperandrogenism. This, in turn, could be enough to result in ovarian morphological changes or work in concert with additional biological factors to change how PCOS manifests phenotypically. The expression of genes differs from individual to individual. The sent differently in PCO persons and PCOS patients, as is proven by the fact that it is insufficient to utilize genetic indications or enzymes for a conclusive verdict of PCOS. Individuals with PCOS are presently tested for a wide range of protein markers. However, most of these are employed for prognosis, monitoring, and stopping additional consequences like cardiovascular disease. Elevated intestinal permeability may be related to PCOS etiology. Increased gut permeability is connected to chronic fatigue condition, overweight, and irritable bowel disorder and promotes the growth of the illness. Zonulin, a physiologic mediator in the zonula corresponding to the vibrio cholera zonula, reversibly regulates gut permeability. This non-invasive marker detects enhanced intestinal immunity and gut permeability in the small intestine. Its significance in detecting metabolic disorders has recently come to light (Polak et al., 2017). Anthropometry measurements were acquired from the control and the experimental groups. The serum zonulin concentration was determined by ELISA (sensitivity 0.01ng/ml) to validate the connection between high serum zonulin stages and the emergence of PCOS. Serum zonulin levels are strongly linked to diabetes, and dyslipidemia, besides the severity of menstruation problems. It has been established that elevated protein concentrations are associated with PCOS. Some research linked the importance of stomach sensitivity to PCOS and discovered indicated individuals with PCOS had higher levels of zonulin than those without the condition. It is hypothesized that changes in gut permeability compromise the intestinal barrier, make it easier for infectious agents to enter the body, and increase gamma interferon production. Although several studies have shown the use of serum zonulin as a biomarker in detecting PCOS, the molecular relationship between zonulin and PCOS development still needs to be understood. This imitation can be enhanced by measuring cytokines such as tumor necrosis factor, interleukin-6, and b-1 interleukin (Lau & Muniandy, 2011). One of the locations where the adipocytokine adiponectin, which matures adipocytes make, is secreted is the visceral adipose tissue. Serum adiponectin levels in obese people are known to decrease, which causes them to become more insulin resistant and develop polycystic ovarian syndrome (Artimani et al., 2016). Type 2 diabetes has been linked to the marker adiponectin and insulin resistance. Blood adiponectin in urinary samples was measured using an ELISA technique in a cross-sectional observational study to gauge the extent of underlying insulin resistance in PCOS patients (Badawy and Elnashar 2011). It is known that there is a correlation between the level of serum adiponectin and the degree of insulin sensitivity in PCOS women. Increasing insulin sensitivity and Obesity are inversely linked to lower adiponectin amounts in PCOS patients. As was already established, "polycystic ovarian syndrome" refers to a group of metabolic disorders. The two most notable include hyperinsulinemia and insulin sensitivity. The study mentioned above also showed that diabetes mellitus type 2 in people with PCOS is caused mostly by low blood insulin levels. Adiponectin, since it improves insulin sensitivity and impairs beta cell activity. Additionally, it showed that obese PCOS individuals had lower blood adiponectin levels than those of average weight. Although the pathogenesis of PCOS remains, interesting material has been found that low levels of adiponectin, increased levels of androgens, and anomalies in metabolism all contribute to the disease's development. The serum amount of adiponectin is regarded as a reliable biomarker for PCOS and the severity of insulin sensitivity. Additionally, it helps clinicians forecast and prognosticate future consequences, such as systemic morbidity.

## 5. Different Options for the Treatment and Management of PCOS

### 5.1. Therapy of Diseases Induced by Androgens

Eczema, scalp psoriasis, and alopecia are the three androgen-related PCOS symptoms of PCOS that are most often reported. Each patient's symptoms differ; some individuals only have one or two symptoms, while others have all three. In most cases, premenopausal women use oral contraceptive pills (OCPs) as their first pharmacologic treatment for hirsutism (Al Wattar et al., 2021). Because pharmacologic therapies do not provide them with the desired results they want, women frequently prefer mechanical hair removal methods like laser hair removal (Shah et al., 2018). The hair growth cycle to hair growth cycle often requires at least 6 months of therapy to notice a reaction. Antiandrogens could be included when there is no progress after six months of medication. Management of acne with OCPs and antiandrogens has proved successful. Isotretinoin may help approximately people with severe acne (Badawy and Elnashar 2011; Dokras et al., 2017). OCPs & androgen blockers are utilized in treating alopecia despite the paucity of available data (Dokras et al., 2017).

For individuals who do not want to get pregnant, hormonal contraception contraceptives (CHC) OCPs are an excellent therapy choice. They are frequently used as the initial course of treatment for hirsutism and eczema brought on by PCOS. CHCs encourage counterproductive LH production, which reduces the ovaries' ability to synthesize androgens. CHCs lower androgens in numerous ways that CHCs lower androgens include: 1) increasing the liver's development of sex hormone-binding globulin, which lowers percolating levels of free androgen; 2) lowering the production of adrenal androgen; and 3) suppressing central testosterone conversion to dihydrotestosterone and adhesion of dihydrotestosterone to specific proteins. Different progestins have different levels of androgenic activity. Less androgenic progestins, including norethindrone, desogestrel, and norgestimate, are frequently found in recent OCPs (Dokras et al., 2017). Drospirenone is a spironolactone analog, a more recent progestin with anti-mineralocorticoid action and androgen receptor antagonist properties. Patients taking spironolactone should be checked for potassium status and treated cautiously if they are at a higher risk of hyperkalemia (Dokras et al., 2017; Badawy and Elnashar 2011). Dienogest is a further modern progestin with antiandrogenic characteristics (Badawy and Elnashar 2011). The effectiveness of various low-dosage CHCs may vary, although no concrete proof exists. Although there are dangers connected with CHCs, for most PCOS patients, the advantages exceed the disadvantages (Badawy and Elnashar 2011). Aldosterone antagonist spironolactone functions primarily as an anti-androgen by antagonistically interacting with the androgen receptor. Additionally, it competes with specific proteins in hair follicles, inhibits the steroidogenesis of the adrenal and ovarian glands, and directly inhibits 5-reductase activity (Padilla et al., 2018). One to two split dosages of 25–200 mg daily are utilized. Spironolactone is frequently used with OCPs to treat PCOS-related symptoms since it can be used alone; it might lead to irregular menstruation and run the feminization of a male embryo or fetus susceptibility unless the individual falls pregnant (Rajashekar et al., 2022) (Bates & Propst, 2012). By increasing insulin sensitivity, thiazolidinediones and metformin lower insulin levels, lowering testosterone levels in the blood (Bates & Propst, 2012). Furthermore, these Medications have a part in treating since they are more likely to occur in PCOS women with insulin sensitivity, leading to myocardial infarctions and metabolic conditions (Goudarzi et al., 2014). On the afflicted areas of the forehead and chin, it should be applied twice each, at least eight hours apart (Bates & Propst, 2012).

## 5.2. Therapy for Diseases Associated with Menstruation

Along with patients' complaints of irregular menstruation, PCOS related, frequently chronic anovulation might raise a patient's risk of uterine fibroids and cancer. Endometrial proliferation can be reduced using periodic progesterone or a low-dosage CHC combining estrogen and progestin (Padilla et al., 2018). The primary suggested therapy for dysmenorrhea associated with PCOS and increased menstrual regularity is low-dosage CHCs (Bates & Propst, 2012). Besides many other metabolic advantages, weight loss can raise circulating testosterone levels in PCOS patients (Padilla et al., 2018). With a 5% reduction in starting weight, weight loss advantages can be seen (Amker et al., 2004). Acupuncture is a complementary therapy that is becoming more and more popular. Acupuncture's main benefits are diminished hyperandrogenism and enhanced menstrual regularity (Bates & Propst, 2012; Pasquali et al., 2003).

It is recommended that management for overweight or obese PCOS individuals begin with losing weight. Obesity, anovulation (Frøen et al., 2001), and reproductive loss (Gjønnaess, 1994) are related. Additionally, obesity is linked to a decreased response to reproductive therapies such as laparoscopic ovarian surgery, gonadotropins, and clomiphene citrate (Homburg, 2003). According to observational studies, 5% to 10% weight loss can boost ovulation and the likelihood of pregnancy (Escobar-Morreale et al., 2005). An increase in cycle consistency, an increase in ovulation, and an increase in spontaneous conception have all been linked to bariatric surgery (Eid et al., 2005).

The medication of this first choice for PCOS-afflicted women to induce ovulation is clomiphene citrate (Balen, 2013). A somewhat selective estrogen receptor modulator is clomiphene citrate. A shift in the gonadotropin-releasing hormone (GnRH) pulse frequency induced by its anti-estrogenic action in the hypothalamus causes an increase in the construction of follicle-stimulating (FSH) from the pituitary gland. The cumulative live birth rate for therapy up to six cycles varies from 50% to 60%, whereas the conception rate with clomiphene is between 70% and 85% every cycle (Costello et al., 2012). The primary clomiphene citrate medication is 50 mg daily for 5 days after a natural and progestin-induced discontinuation hemorrhage. If no ovulation occurs, the dosage is raised by 50 mg every cycle, up to a daily maximum of 150 mg. Six ovulatory cycles are often the number of rotations at most (Wiweko & Susanto, 2017). The patient is deemed clomiphene refractory if ovulation can be achieved at 150 mg/day dosages. Using clomiphene results in the inability to become pregnant after six ovulatory cycles (Morin-Papunen et al., 2012). Biguanide metformin is frequently used as an antihyperglycemic medication. It has been thoroughly examined in cases of infertility linked to PCOS. Inside its 2008 consensus conference, the ESHRE/ASRM concluded that metformin is less effective than clomiphene at starting eggs, and there is no advantage to supplementing metformin with clomiphene (Casper & Mitwally, 2011; Wiweko & Susanto, 2017). Compared to placebo or no therapy, metformin boosted the number of ovulation and clinical pregnancy but not the rate of live births in a randomized controlled trial meta-analysis (Kjøtrød et al., 2011). However, metformin boosted compares healthy fertility rate to placebo in an ample multicentre, randomized, double-blind, placebo-controlled research (41.9% versus 28.8%, P = 0.014), with the most considerable advantageous impact shown in obese women (Casper & Mitwally, 2011; Pritts, 2010). These findings align with other research that looked at the effects of administration with metformin for three months before fertility treatment sperm injection (IVF/ICSI) (Pritts, 2010). These findings imply that metformin, when given three months before and contemporaneous with conventional infertility therapies, may significantly enhance a significant role in strengthening live birth rates, even if its effect in ovulation induction in PCOS has been restricted. The synthesis of androstenedione, estradiol, and estrone via testosterone is prevented by aromatase inhibitors, as is the synthesis of these hormones from testosterone. This decrease in estrogenic activity releases the hypothalamus from unfavorable scrutiny, resulting in a rise in the secretion of FSH (Misso et al., 2012). Letrozole, the far more popular ovarian-stimulating aromatase antagonist, is given in dosages ranging from 2.5 to 7.5 mg daily for five days beginning on the third day of the menstrual cycle (Dokras et al., 2011). The lack of oestrogenic effects on the endometrium, a shorter half-life than clomiphene, and a rate greater of mono follicular ovulation are all alleged benefits of letrozole (Misso et al., 2012). Letrozole medication was linked to a greater ovulation rate per individual, according to a recent comprehensive review and conceptual of randomized controlled trials comparing letrozole with clomiphene. Letrozole did not raise the rate of live births per person, ovulation per cycle, or pregnancy (Kar, 2012). Since that review, letrozole use has been linked to a markedly increased pregnancy ratc (21.56% in the ovulation induction group compared to 7.84% in the clomiphene collective, P = 0.015) but an equivalent ovulation incidence (73.08% in the letrozole group compared 60.78% inside the clomiphene group, P = 0.39) in (Legro et al., 2012) treatment-nave infertile women with PCOS (Perales-Puchalt & Legro, 2013). The Birth with Polycystic Ovary Syndrome II trial compared the rates of children born for clomiphene and letrozole in 750 infertile PCOS patients (Christin-Maitre & Hugues, 2003; Wiweko & Susanto, 2017). The trial's findings will clarify how letrozole induces ovulation in PCOS patients. The ESHRE/ASRM classifies laparoscopic ovarian drilling (LOD) and gonadotropin stimulation of ovulation as second-line treatments for ovulation induction (Wiweko & Susanto, 2017). Gonadotropin is the preferred therapy for women who don't want surgery because it's less intrusive. LOD is chosen when a patient has additional surgical reasons or cannot keep up with the multiple follow-up appointments necessary with gonadotropin treatment (Goudarzi et al.,

2014). The growth of a single follicle leading to a singleton live birth is the objective of FSH injection for ovulation induction. Multiple pregnancies and polycystic ovary syndrome (OHSS) are risks connected with ovulation induction. A low-dose step-up regimen is advised since women having PCOS are extremely sensitive to the outcomes of FSH (Homburg et al., 2012). Once follicular growth is visible, the initial dose of 37.5-50 IU of FSH daily is increased to 25-37.5 IU every 7-14 days. Sequential ultrasound and plasma oestradiol levels are used to aid in the titration of the FSH dose and determine whether human chorionic gonadotropin should be administered to begin ovulation (Amker et al., 2004; Gjonnaess, 1984). Cycle cancellation is suggested if more than two follicles measure more than 16 mm or if one counts more than 16 mm upwards of two follicles measured and over 16 mm or if only one counts more than 16 mm, cycle cancellation is suggested. Cycle cancellation is advised when two other follicles measure more than 14 mm, when more than two follicles measure more than 16 mm, or when one measures more than 16 mm and two other follicles measure more than 14 mm (Saha et al., 2013). In recent research, the effectiveness of clomiphene vs the low-dose step-up FSH strategy for the first three cycles of infertility therapy in anovulatory women with PCOS was compared. According to protocol analysis, the low-dose step-up of the pregnancy rate increased due to FSH medication. overall (52.1% compared to 41.2%, P = 0.021) throughout the first phase (30% against 14.6%, P = 0.003) and in total living birth rates (47.4% versus 36.9%, P = 0.031) (Amker et al., 2004; Sirmans & Pate, 2013, 2014). Contrarily, gonadotropin therapy is more expensive and inconvenient than clomiphene therapy. LOD entails drilling between four and ten holes in the ovary's stroma and surface using a laser or electrocautery. It is prescribed to treat infertility in PCOS clomiphene-resistant patients (Saha et al., 2013). In 92% of women, a single therapy establishes ovulatory menstrual periods, and in 58% of women, it causes conception (Sirmans & Pate, 2013, 2014). Physique mass index of $35 grams, blood testosterone levels of $4.5 nmol/L, unbound androgen index of 15, and extent of infertility of 3 years are indicators of a poor response with LOD. At baseline, serum LH values of $10 IU/L are substantially related to a higher chance of pregnancy (Heijnen et al., 2006; Hughes et al., 2007). Regarding ovulation or pregnancy, LOD and clomiphene did not differ when used as first-line therapy (Heijnen et al., 2006). According to a Cochrane analysis, LOD is comparable to live birth. Three to six rounds of gonadotropins can result in conception rates without putting the patient in danger of multiple pregnancies or OHSS (Heijnen et al., 2006). A recent thorough analysis and meta-analysis showed that LOD with or without pharmaceutical ovulation outline treatment was compared to pharmacologic ovulation induction among women with clomiphene-resistant PCOS. There were no distinctions between the groups according to ovarian frequency or live fertility rate. However, the LOD group did not have any cases of OHSS, and LOD was linked to a decreased rate of pregnancy complications (OR 0.21, 95% CI 0.08-0.58, P = 0.002). In vitro fertilization (IVF) has been recommended as a third-line medication for treating infertility by the 2008 Thessaloniki, resulting low PCOS agreement working group. When using traditional IVF, women with PCOS experience pregnancy, miscarriage, and live birth rates comparable to those without the condition (Heijnen et al., 2006). Women observed more cycle cancellations with PCOS. In addition, PCOS-afflicted women recovered more oocytes with a lower fertilization rate each cycle.

## Conclusion

The most common endocrine condition of the mechanism of fertilization in women, PCOS, is complicated and impacted by ecological, physiological, and metabolic factors. It may result in temporary health problems. morbid conditions, including diabetes and heart disease. Hirsutism, sudden weight gain, hormonal irregularities, oligo/anovulation, premature ovarian failure, metabolic abnormalities, hyperandrogenaemia, and elevated testosterone levels are typically seen in PCOS patients. Despite the lack of a clear pathophysiology for the disorder, the primary defects are thought to be caused by insulin sensitivity, luteinizing hormone, and follicle-stimulating hormone levels, which lead to excessive androgen and testosterone production. Elevated doses of LH compared to FSH also cause oligomenorrhea or oligo-ovulation and difficulties conceiving. After the existence of androgenemia, androgenic, and an/oligoovulation, PCOS is diagnosed in individuals by ruling out all other potential endocrinopathies. While some locations rely on the look of the ovaries for diagnosis, other methods include the use of numerous gene, protein, and enzyme markers. 43 genes have been extracted and have been linked to PCOS. These genetic markers are those involved in controlling insulin action and androgen production. These genetic markers, however, can only confirm PCOS in people who have already shown the telltale symptoms, making them ineffective for early detection. For prediction and patient monitoring, protein and enzyme indicators are frequently employed to stop the progression of PCOS problems, including CVD. As a result of its ability to control menstruation and improve the likelihood of conceiving in both androgen receptor and non-androgenic types of PCOS, metformin is currently administered to individuals with the condition. According to a recent method, testosterone levels are significantly reduced after taking myoinositol, gymnemic acid, and L-methyl folate, especially in individuals who are fat or overweight. PCOS patients are encouraged to maintain a healthy lifestyle to avoid the onset of obesity, diabetes, cardiovascular disease, and other morbidities due to reduced metabolism.

## References

Al Wattar, B. H., Fisher, M., Bevington, L., Talaulikar, V., Davies, M., Conway, G., & Yasmin, E. (2021). Clinical Practice Guidelines on the Diagnosis and Management of Polycystic Ovary Syndrome: A Systematic Review and Quality Assessment Study. *The Journal of Clinical Endocrinology and Metabolism*, *106*(8), 2436–2446. https://doi.org/10.1210/CLINEM/DGAB232.

Álvarez-Blasco, F., Botella-Carretero, J. I., San Millán, J. L., & Escobar-Morreale, H. F. (2006). Prevalence and characteristics of the polycystic ovary syndrome in overweight and obese women. *Archives of Internal Medicine*, *166*(19), 2081–2086. https://doi.org/10.1001/ARCHINTE.166.19.2081.

Amato, P., & Simpson, J. L. (2004). The genetics of polycystic ovary syndrome. *Best Practice and Research: Clinical Obstetrics and Gynaecology*, *18*(5 SPEC. ISS.), 707–718. https://doi.org/10.1016/j.bpobgyn.2004.05.002.

Amker, S. A. K., Li, T. C., & Ledger, W. L. (2004). Ovulation induction using laparoscopic ovarian drilling in women with polycystic ovarian syndrome: predictors of success. *Human Reproduction (Oxford, England)*, *19*(8), 1719–1724. https://doi.org/10.1093/HUMREP/DEH343.

Artimani, T., Saidijam, M., Aflatoonian, R., Ashrafi, M., Amiri, I., Yavangi, M., Soleimani Asl, S., Shabab, N., Karimi, J., & Mehdizadeh, M. (2016). Downregulation of adiponectin system in granulosa cells and low levels of HMW adiponectin in PCOS. *Journal of Assisted Reproduction and Genetics*, *33*(1), 101–110. https://doi.org/10.1007/S10815-015-0620-1.

Asunción, M., Calvo, R. M., San Millán, J. L., Sancho, J., Avila, S., & Escobar-Morreale, H. F. (2000). A prospective study of the prevalence of the polycystic ovary syndrome in unselected Caucasian women from Spain. *The Journal of Clinical Endocrinology and Metabolism*, *85*(7), 2434–2438. https://doi.org/10.1210/JCEM.85.7.6682.

Azziz, R., Woods, K. S., Reyna, R., Key, T. J., Knochenhauer, E. S., & Yildiz, B. O. (2004a). The prevalence and features of the polycystic ovary syndrome in an unselected population. *The Journal of Clinical Endocrinology and Metabolism*, *89*(6), 2745–2749. https://doi.org/10.1210/JC.2003-032046.

Azziz, R., Woods, K. S., Reyna, R., Key, T. J., Knochenhauer, E. S., & Yildiz, B. O. (2004b). The prevalence and features of the polycystic ovary syndrome in an unselected population. *The Journal of Clinical Endocrinology and Metabolism*, *89*(6), 2745–2749. https://doi.org/10.1210/JC.2003-032046.

Badawy, A., & Elnashar, A. (2011a). Treatment options for polycystic ovary syndrome. *International Journal of Women's Health*, *3*(1), 25–35. https://doi.org/10.2147/IJWH.S11304.

Badawy, A., & Elnashar, A. (2011b). Treatment options for polycystic ovary syndrome. *International Journal of Women's Health*, *3*(1), 25–35. https://doi.org/10.2147/IJWH.S11304.

Baillargeon, J. P., & Carpentier, A. (2007). Role of insulin in the hyperandrogenemia of lean women with polycystic ovary syndrome and normal insulin sensitivity. *Fertility and Sterility*, *88*(4), 886–893. https://doi.org/10.1016/J.FERTNSTERT.2006.12.055.

Balen, A. H. (2013). Ovulation induction in the management of anovulatory polycystic ovary syndrome. *Molecular and Cellular Endocrinology*, *373*(1–2), 77–82. https://doi.org/10.1016/J.MCE.2012.10.008.

Barbieri, R. L., Smith, S., & Ryan, K. J. (1988). The role of hyperinsulinemia in the pathogenesis of ovarian hyperandrogenism. *Fertility and Sterility*, *50*(2), 197–212. https://doi.org/10.1016/S0015-0282(16)60060-2.

Bates, G. W., & Propst, A. M. (2012). Polycystic Ovarian Syndrome Management Options. *Obstetrics and Gynecology Clinics of North America*, *39*(4), 495–506. https://doi.org/10.1016/J.OGC.2012.10.001.

Betts, T., Yarrow, H., Dutton, N., Greenhill, L., & Rolfe, T. (2003). A study of anticonvulsant medication on ovarian function in a group of women with epilepsy who have only ever taken one anticonvulsant compared with a group of women without epilepsy. *Seizure*, *12*(6), 323–329. https://doi.org/10.1016/S1059-1311(03)00065-7.

Bilo, L., Meo, R., Valentino, R., Di Carlo, C., Striano, S., & Nappi, C. (2001). Characterization of reproductive endocrine disorders in women with epilepsy. *The Journal of Clinical Endocrinology and Metabolism*, *86*(7), 2950–2956. https://doi.org/10.1210/JCEM.86.7.7633.

Casper, R. F., & Mitwally, M. F. M. (2011). Use of the aromatase inhibitor letrozole for ovulation induction in women with polycystic ovarian syndrome. *Clinical Obstetrics and Gynecology*, *54*(4), 685–695. https://doi.org/10.1097/GRF.0B013E3182353D0F.

Christin-Maitre, S., & Hugues, J. N. (2003). A comparative randomized multicentric study comparing the step-up versus step-down protocol in polycystic ovary syndrome. *Human Reproduction (Oxford, England)*, *18*(8), 1626–1631. https://doi.org/10.1093/HUMREP/DEG336.

Codner, E., Soto, N., Lopez, P., Trejo, L., Ávila, A., Eyzaguirre, F. C., Íniguez, G., & Cassorla, F. (2006). Diagnostic criteria for polycystic ovary syndrome and ovarian morphology in women with type 1 diabetes mellitus. *The Journal of Clinical Endocrinology and Metabolism*, *91*(6), 2250–2256. https://doi.org/10.1210/JC.2006-0108.

Costello, M. F., Misso, M. L., Wong, J., Hart, R., Rombauts, L., Melder, A., Norman, R. J., & Teede, H. J. (2012). The treatment of infertility in polycystic ovary syndrome: a brief update. *The Australian & New Zealand Journal of Obstetrics & Gynaecology*, *52*(4), 400–403. https://doi.org/10.1111/J.1479-828X.2012.01448.X.

Crosignani, P. G., & Nicolosi, A. E. (2001). Polycystic ovarian disease: heritability and heterogeneity. *Human Reproduction Update*, *7*(1), 3–7. https://doi.org/10.1093/HUMUPD/7.1.3.

Diamanti-Kandarakis, E., Bourguignon, J. P., Giudice, L. C., Hauser, R., Prins, G. S., Soto, A. M., Zoeller, R. T., & Gore, A. C. (2009). Endocrine-disrupting chemicals: an Endocrine Society scientific statement. *Endocrine Reviews*, *30*(4), 293–342. https://doi.org/10.1210/ER.2009-0002.

Dokras, A., Clifton, S., Futterweit, W., & Wild, R. (2011). Increased risk for abnormal depression scores in women with polycystic ovary syndrome: a systematic review and meta-analysis. *Obstetrics and Gynecology*, *117*(1), 145–152. https://doi.org/10.1097/AOG.0B013E318202B0A4.

Dokras, A., Saini, S., Gibson-Helm, M., Schulkin, J., Cooney, L., & Teede, H. (2017). Gaps in knowledge among physicians regarding diagnostic criteria and management of polycystic ovary syndrome. *Fertility and Sterility*, *107*(6), 1380-1386.e1. https://doi.org/10.1016/J.FERTNSTERT.2017.04.011.

Dunaif, A., Wu, X., Lee, A., & Diamanti-Kandarakis, E. (2001). Defects in insulin receptor signaling in vivo in the polycystic ovary syndrome (PCOS). *American Journal of Physiology. Endocrinology and Metabolism*, *281*(2). https://doi.org/10.1152/AJPENDO.2001.281.2.E392.

Eid, G. M., Cottam, D. R., Velcu, L. M., Mattar, S. G., Korytkowski, M. T., Gosman, G., Hindi, P., & Schauer, P. R. (2005). Effective treatment of polycystic ovarian syndrome with Roux-en-Y gastric bypass. *Surgery for Obesity and Related Diseases: Official Journal of the American Society for Bariatric Surgery*, *1*(2), 77–80. https://doi.org/10.1016/J.SOARD.2005.02.008.

Eisenberg, I., Nahmias, N., Novoselsky Persky, M., Greenfield, C., Goldman-Wohl, D., Hurwitz, A., Haimov-Kochman, R., Yagel, S., & Imbar, T. (2017). Elevated circulating micro-ribonucleic acid (miRNA)-200b and miRNA-429 levels in anovulatory women. *Fertility and Sterility*, *107*(1), 269–275. https://doi.org/10.1016/J.FERTNSTERT.2016.10.003.

Escobar-Morreale, H. F. (2018). Polycystic ovary syndrome: definition, aetiology, diagnosis and treatment. *Nature Reviews. Endocrinology*, *14*(5), 270–284. https://doi.org/10.1038/NRENDO.2018.24.

Escobar-Morreale, H. F., Botella-Carretero, J. I., Álvarez-Blasco, F., Sancho, J., & San Millán, J. L. (2005). The polycystic ovary syndrome associated with morbid obesity may resolve after weight loss induced by bariatric surgery. *The Journal of Clinical Endocrinology and Metabolism*, *90*(12), 6364–6369. https://doi.org/10.1210/JC.2005-1490.

Franks, S., Gharani, N., Waterworth, D., Batty, S., White, D., Williamson, R., & McCarthy, M. (1997). The genetic basis of polycystic ovary syndrome. *Human Reproduction (Oxford, England)*, *12*(12), 2641–2648. https://doi.org/10.1093/HUMREP/12.12.2641.

Frøen, J. F., Arnestad, M., Frey, K., Vege, Å., Saugstad, O. D., & Stray-Pedersen, B. (2001). Risk factors for sudden intrauterine unexplained death: Epidemiologic characteristics of singleton cases in Oslo, Norway, 1986-1995. *American Journal of Obstetrics and Gynecology*, *184*(4), 694–702. https://doi.org/10.1067/mob.2001.110697.

Gharani, N., Waterworth, D. M., Batty, S., White, D., Gilling-Smith, C., Conway, G. S., McCarthy, M., Franks, S., & Williamson, R. (1997). Association of the steroid synthesis gene CYP11a with polycystic ovary syndrome and hyperandrogenism. *Human Molecular Genetics*, *6*(3), 397–402. https://doi.org/10.1093/HMG/6.3.397.

Gilling-Smith, C., Story, H., Rogers, V., & Franks, S. (1997). Evidence for a primary abnormality of thecal cell steroidogenesis in the polycystic ovary syndrome. *Clinical Endocrinology*, *47*(1), 93–99. https://doi.org/10.1046/J.1365-2265.1997.2321049.X.

Gilling-Smith, C., Willis, D. S., Beard, R. W., & Franks, S. (1994). Hypersecretion of androstenedione by isolated thecal cells from polycystic ovaries. *The Journal of Clinical Endocrinology and Metabolism*, *79*(4), 1158–1165. https://doi.org/10.1210/JCEM.79.4.7962289.

Gjonnaess, H. (1984). Polycystic ovarian syndrome treated by ovarian electrocautery through the laparoscope. *Fertility and Sterility*, *41*(1), 20–25. https://doi.org/10.1016/S0015-0282(16)47534-5.

Gjønnaess, H. (1994). Ovarian electrocautery in the treatment of women with polycystic ovary syndrome (PCOS). Factors affecting the results. *Acta Obstetricia et Gynecologica Scandinavica*, *73*(5), 407–412. https://doi.org/10.3109/00016349409006253.

Goodarzi, M. O., Dumesic, D. A., Chazenbalk, G., & Azziz, R. (2011). Polycystic ovary syndrome: etiology, pathogenesis and diagnosis. *Nature Reviews. Endocrinology*, *7*(4), 219–231. https://doi.org/10.1038/NRENDO.2010.217.

Goudarzi, Z. M., Fallahzadeh, H., Aflatoonian, A., & Mirzaei, M. (2014). Laparoscopic ovarian electrocautery versus gonadotropin therapy in infertile women with clomiphene citrate-resistant polycystic ovary syndrome: A systematic review and meta-analysis. *Iranian Journal of Reproductive Medicine*, *12*(8), 531. /pmc/articles/PMC4233311/.

Hart, R., Hickey, M., & Franks, S. (2004). Definitions, prevalence and symptoms of polycystic ovaries and polycystic ovary syndrome. *Best Practice and Research: Clinical Obstetrics and Gynaecology*, *18*(5 SPEC. ISS.), 671–683. https://doi.org/10.1016/j.bpobgyn.2004.05.001.

Heijnen, E. M. E. W., Eijkemans, M. J. C., Hughes, E. G., Laven, J. S. E., Macklon, N. S., & Fauser, B. C. J. M. (2006). A meta-analysis of outcomes of conventional IVF in women with polycystic ovary syndrome. *Human Reproduction Update*, *12*(1), 13–21. https://doi.org/10.1093/HUMUPD/DMI036.

Herzog, A. G. (2006). Menstrual disorders in women with epilepsy. *Neurology*, *66*(6 Suppl 3). https://doi.org/10.1212/WNL.66.66_SUPPL_3.S23.

Homburg, R. (2003). The management of infertility associated with polycystic ovary syndrome. *Reproductive Biology and Endocrinology : RB&E*, *1*. https://doi.org/10.1186/1477-7827-1-109.

Homburg, R., Hendriks, M. L., König, T. E., Anderson, R. A., Balen, A. H., Brincat, M., Child, T., Davies, M., D'Hooghe, T., Martinez, A., Rajkhowa, M., Rueda-Saenz, R., Hompes, P., & Lambalk, C. B. (2012). Clomifene citrate or low-dose FSH for the first-line treatment of infertile women with anovulation associated with polycystic ovary syndrome: a prospective randomized multinational study. *Human Reproduction (Oxford, England)*, *27*(2), 468–473. https://doi.org/10.1093/HUMREP/DER401.

Hughes, E., Brown, J., Collins, J. J., Farquhar, C., Fedorkow, D. M., & Vandekerckhove, P. (2007). Ovulation suppression for endometriosis. *The Cochrane Database of Systematic Reviews*, *2007*(3), CD000155. https://doi.org/10.1002/14651858.CD000155.PUB2.

Isojarvi, J., Laatikainen, T. J., Pakarinen, A. J., Juntunen, K., & Myllyla, V. V. (1993). Polycystic ovaries and hyperandrogenism in women taking valproate for epilepsy. *The New England Journal of Medicine*, *329*(19), 1383–1388. https://doi.org/10.1056/NEJM199311043291904.

Ito, Y., Fisher, C. R., Conte, F. A., Grumbach, M. M., & Simpson, E. R. (1993). Molecular basis of aromatase deficiency in an adult female with sexual infantilism and polycystic ovaries. *Proceedings of the National Academy of Sciences of the United States of America*, *90*(24), 11673–11677. https://doi.org/10.1073/PNAS.90.24.11673.

Kar, S. (2012). Clomiphene citrate or letrozole as first-line ovulation induction drug in infertile PCOS women: A prospective randomized trial. *Journal of Human Reproductive Sciences*, *5*(3), 262–265. https://doi.org/10.4103/0974-1208.106338.

Kashanian, M., Fazy, Z., & Pirak, A. (2008). Evaluation of the relationship between gestational diabetes and a history of polycystic ovarian syndrome. *Diabetes Research and Clinical Practice*, *80*(2), 289–292. https://doi.org/10.1016/J.DIABRES.2007.12.022.

Kjøtrød, S. B., Carlsen, S. M., Rasmussen, P. E., Holst-Larsen, T., Mellembakken, J., Thurin-Kjellberg, A., Haapaniemikouru, K., Morin-Papunen, L., Humaidan, P., Sunde, A., & Von Düring, V. (2011). Use of metformin before and during assisted reproductive technology in non-obese young infertile women with polycystic ovary syndrome: a prospective, randomized, double-blind, multi-centre study. *Human Reproduction (Oxford, England)*, *26*(8), 2045–2053. https://doi.org/10.1093/HUMREP/DER154.

Knochenhauer, E. S., Key, T. J., Kahsar-Miller, M., Waggoner, W., Boots, L. R., & Azziz, R. (1998). Prevalence of the polycystic ovary syndrome in unselected black and white women of the southeastern United States: a prospective study. *The Journal of Clinical Endocrinology and Metabolism*, *83*(9), 3078–3082. https://doi.org/10.1210/JCEM.83.9.5090.

Kruglyak, L., Daly, M. J., Reeve-Daly, M. P., & Lander, E. S. (1996). Parametric and nonparametric linkage analysis: a unified multipoint approach. *American Journal of Human Genetics*, *58*(6), 1347–1363. https://www.ncbi.nlm.nih.gov/pmc/articles/pmid/8651312/?tool=EBI.

Lau, C. H., & Muniandy, S. (2011). Novel adiponectin-resistin (AR) and insulin resistance (IRAR) indexes are useful integrated diagnostic biomarkers for insulin resistance, type 2 diabetes and metabolic syndrome: a case control study. *Cardiovascular Diabetology*, *10*. https://doi.org/10.1186/1475-2840-10-8.

Legro, R. S., Driscoll, D., Strauss, J. F., Fox, J., & Dunaif, A. (1998a). Evidence for a genetic basis for hyperandrogenemia in polycystic ovary syndrome. *Proceedings of the National Academy of Sciences of the United States of America*, *95*(25), 14956–14960. https://doi.org/10.1073/PNAS.95.25.14956.

Legro, R. S., Driscoll, D., Strauss, J. F., Fox, J., & Dunaif, A. (1998b). Evidence for a genetic basis for hyperandrogenemia in polycystic ovary syndrome. *Proceedings of the National Academy of Sciences of the United States of America*, *95*(25), 14956. https://doi.org/10.1073/PNAS.95.25.14956.

Legro, R. S., Kunselman, A. R., Brzyski, R. G., Casson, P. R., Diamond, M. P., Schlaff, W. D., Christman, G. M., Coutifaris, C., Taylor, H. S., Eisenberg, E., Santoro, N., & Zhang, H. (2012). The Pregnancy in Polycystic Ovary Syndrome II (PPCOS II) trial: rationale and design of a double-blind randomized trial of clomiphene citrate and letrozole for the treatment of infertility in women with polycystic ovary syndrome. *Contemporary Clinical Trials*, *33*(3), 470–481. https://doi.org/10.1016/J.CCT.2011.12.005.

Lenie, S., & Smitz, J. (2009). Functional AR signaling is evident in an in vitro mouse follicle culture bioassay that encompasses most stages of folliculogenesis. *Biology of Reproduction*, *80*(4), 685–695. https://doi.org/10.1095/BIOLREPROD.107.067280.

Lim, S. S., Hutchison, S. K., Van Ryswyk, E., Norman, R. J., Teede, H. J., & Moran, L. J. (2019). Lifestyle changes in women with polycystic ovary syndrome. *The Cochrane Database of Systematic Reviews*, *3*(3). https://doi.org/10.1002/14651858.CD007506.PUB4.

March, W. A., Moore, V. M., Willson, K. J., Phillips, D. I. W., Norman, R. J., & Davies, M. J. (2010). The prevalence of polycystic ovary syndrome in a community sample assessed under contrasting diagnostic criteria. *Human Reproduction (Oxford, England)*, *25*(2), 544–551. https://doi.org/10.1093/HUMREP/DEP399.

Mason, H. D., Willis, D. S., Beard, R. W., Winston, R. M. L., Margara, R., & Franks, S. (1994). Estradiol production by granulosa cells of normal and polycystic ovaries: relationship to menstrual cycle history and concentrations of gonadotropins and sex steroids in follicular fluid. *The Journal of Clinical Endocrinology and Metabolism*, *79*(5), 1355–1360. https://doi.org/10.1210/JCEM.79.5.7962330.

Michelmore, K. F., Balen, A. H., Dunger, D. B., & Vessey, M. P. (1999). Polycystic ovaries and associated clinical and biochemical features in young women. *Clinical Endocrinology*, *51*(6), 779–786. https://doi.org/10.1046/J.1365-2265.1999.00886.X.

Misso, M. L., Wong, J. L. A., Teede, H. J., Hart, R., Rombauts, L., Melder, A. M., Norman, R. J., & Costello, M. F. (2012). Aromatase inhibitors for PCOS: a systematic review and meta-analysis. *Human Reproduction Update*, *18*(3), 301–312. https://doi.org/10.1093/HUMUPD/DMS003.

Mooser, V., Mancini, F. P., Bopp, S., Pethö-schramm, A., Guerra, R., Boerwinkle, E., Müller, H. J., & Hobbs, H. H. (1995). Sequence polymorphisms in the apo(a) gene associated with specific levels of Lp(a) in plasma. *Human Molecular Genetics*, *4*(2), 173–181. https://doi.org/10.1093/HMG/4.2.173.

Morin-Papunen, L., Rantala, A. S., Unkila-Kallio, L., Tiitinen, A., Hippeläinen, M., Perheentupa, A., Tinkanen, H., Bloigu, R., Puukka, K., Ruokonen, A., & Tapanainen, J. S. (2012). Metformin improves pregnancy and live-birth rates in women with polycystic ovary syndrome (PCOS): a multicenter, double-blind, placebo-controlled randomized trial. *The Journal of Clinical Endocrinology and Metabolism*, *97*(5), 1492–1500. https://doi.org/10.1210/JC.2011-3061.

Nicandri, K. F., & Hoeger, K. (2012). Diagnosis and treatment of polycystic ovarian syndrome in adolescents. *Current Opinion in Endocrinology, Diabetes, and Obesity*, *19*(6), 497–504. https://doi.org/10.1097/MED.0B013E32835A1A03.

Nisenblat, V., & Norman, R. J. (2009). Androgens and polycystic ovary syndrome. *Current Opinion in Endocrinology, Diabetes, and Obesity*, *16*(3), 224–231. https://doi.org/10.1097/MED.0B013E32832AFD4D.

Padilla, O., Arya, S., Noble, L. S., & Plavsic, S. K. (2018). Saline infusion sonography: Tips and tricks for improved visualization of the uterine cavity. *Donald School Journal of Ultrasound in Obstetrics and Gynecology*, *12*(1), 32–51. https://doi.org/10.5005/JP-JOURNALS-10009-1550.

Panda, P. K., Rane, R., Ravichandran, R., Singh, S., & Panchal, H. (2016). Genetics of PCOS: A systematic bioinformatics approach to unveil the proteins responsible for PCOS. *Genomics Data*, *8*, 52–60. https://doi.org/10.1016/J.GDATA.2016.03.008.

Pasquali, R., Pelusi, C., Genghini, S., Cacciari, M., & Gambineri, A. (2003). Obesity and reproductive disorders in women. *Human Reproduction Update*, *9*(4), 359–372. https://doi.org/10.1093/HUMUPD/DMG024.

Peppard, H. R., Marfori, J., Iuorno, M. J., & Nestler, J. E. (2001). Prevalence of polycystic ovary syndrome among premenopausal women with type 2 diabetes. *Diabetes Care*, *24*(6), 1050–1052. https://doi.org/10.2337/DIACARE.24.6.1050.

Perales-Puchalt, A., & Legro, R. S. (2013). Ovulation induction in women with polycystic ovary syndrome. *Steroids*, *78*(8), 767–772. https://doi.org/10.1016/J.STEROIDS.2013.05.005.

Polak, K., Czyzyk, A., Simoncini, T., & Meczekalski, B. (2017). New markers of insulin resistance in polycystic ovary syndrome. *Journal of Endocrinological Investigation*, *40*(1). https://doi.org/10.1007/S40618-016-0523-8.

Pritts, E. A. (2010). Letrozole for ovulation induction and controlled ovarian hyperstimulation. *Current Opinion in Obstetrics & Gynecology*, *22*(4), 289–294. https://doi.org/10.1097/GCO.0B013E32833BEEBF.

RADOSH, L. (2009). Drug Treatments for Polycystic Ovary Syndrome. *American Family Physician*, *79*(8), 671–676. https://www.aafp.org/pubs/afp/issues/2009/0415/p671.html.

Rajashekar, S., Ravindran, S. G., Kakarla, M., Gambo, M. A., Salama, M. Y., Ismail, N. H., Tavalla, P., Uppal, P., Mohammed, S. A., & Hamid, P. (2022). Spironolactone Versus Oral Contraceptive Pills in the Treatment of Adolescent Polycystic Ovarian Syndrome: A Systematic Review. *Cureus*, *14*(5). https://doi.org/10.7759/CUREUS.25340.

Rosenfield, R. L. (2007). Clinical review: Identifying children at risk for polycystic ovary syndrome. *The Journal of Clinical Endocrinology and Metabolism*, *92*(3), 787–796. https://doi.org/10.1210/JC.2006-2012.

Saha, L., Kaur, S., & Saha, P. (2013). N-acetyl cysteine in clomiphene citrate resistant polycystic ovary syndrome: A review of reported outcomes. *Journal of Pharmacology & Pharmacotherapeutics*, *4*(3), 187. https://doi.org/10.4103/0976-500X.114597.

Shah, D., Patil, M., & Group, O. behalf of the N. P. W. (2018). Consensus Statement on the Use of Oral Contraceptive Pills in Polycystic Ovarian Syndrome Women in India. *Journal of Human Reproductive Sciences*, *11*(2), 96. https://doi.org/10.4103/JHRS.JHRS_72_18.

Shaikh, N., Dadachanji, R., & Mukherjee, S. (2014). Genetic Markers of Polycystic Ovary Syndrome: Emphasis on Insulin Resistance. *International Journal of Medical Genetics*, *2014*, 1–10. https://doi.org/10.1155/2014/478972.

Sirmans, S. M., & Pate, K. A. (2013). Epidemiology, diagnosis, and management of polycystic ovary syndrome. *Clinical Epidemiology*, *6*(1), 1–13. https://doi.org/10.2147/CLEP.S37559.

Sirmans, S. M., & Pate, K. A. (2014). Epidemiology, diagnosis, and management of polycystic ovary syndrome. *Clinical Epidemiology*, *6*(1), 1. https://doi.org/10.2147/CLEP.S37559.

Sørensen, A. E., Wissing, M. L., Salö, S., Englund, A. L. M., & Dalgaard, L. T. (2014). MicroRNAs Related to Polycystic Ovary Syndrome (PCOS). *Genes*, *5*(3), 684–708. https://doi.org/10.3390/GENES5030684.

Soriguer, F., Goday, A., Bosch-Comas, A., Bordiú, E., Calle-Pascual, A., Carmena, R., Casamitjana, R., Castaño, L., Castell, C., Catalá, M., Delgado, E., Franch, J., Gaztambide, S., Girbés, J., Gomis, R., Gutiérrez, G., López-Alba, A., Martínez-Larrad, M. T., Menéndez, E., … Vendrell, J. (2011). Prevalence of diabetes mellitus and impaired glucose regulation in Spain: the Di@bet.es Study. *Diabetologia*, *55*(1), 88–93. https://doi.org/10.1007/S00125-011-2336-9.

Stepto, N. K., Cassar, S., Joham, A. E., Hutchison, S. K., Harrison, C. L., Goldstein, R. F., & Teede, H. J. (2013). Women with polycystic ovary syndrome have intrinsic insulin resistance on euglycaemic-hyperinsulaemic clamp. *Human Reproduction (Oxford, England)*, *28*(3), 777–784. https://doi.org/10.1093/HUMREP/DES463.

Stone, D., & Hechter, O. (1955). Studies on ACTH action in perfused bovine adrenals: aspects of progesterone as an intermediary in corticosteroidogenesis. *Archives of Biochemistry and Biophysics*, *54*(1), 121–128. https://doi.org/10.1016/0003-9861(55)90014-X.

Taylor, A. E., McCourt, B., Martin, K. A., Anderson, E. J., Adams, J. M., Schoenfeld, D., & Hall, J. E. (1997). Determinants of abnormal gonadotropin secretion in clinically defined women with polycystic ovary syndrome. *The Journal of Clinical Endocrinology and Metabolism*, *82*(7), 2248–2256. https://doi.org/10.1210/JCEM.82.7.4105.

Thong, E. P., Codner, E., Laven, J. S. E., & Teede, H. (2020). Diabetes: a metabolic and reproductive disorder in women. *The Lancet. Diabetes & Endocrinology*, *8*(2), 134–149. https://doi.org/10.1016/S2213-8587(19)30345-6.

Urbanek, M., Legro, R. S., Driscoll, D. A., Azziz, R., Ehrmann, D. A., Norman, R. J., Strauss, J. F., Spielman, R. S., & Dunaif, A. (1999). Thirty-seven candidate genes for polycystic ovary syndrome: strongest evidence for linkage is with follistatin. *Proceedings of the National Academy of Sciences of the United States of America*, *96*(15), 8573–8578. https://doi.org/10.1073/PNAS.96.15.8573.

Webber, L. J., Stubbs, S., Stark, J., Trew, G. H., Margara, R., Hardy, K., & Franks, S. (2003). Formation and early development of follicles in the polycystic ovary. *Lancet*, *362*(9389), 1017–1021. https://doi.org/10.1016/S0140-6736(03)14410-8.

Wiweko, B., & Susanto, C. (2017). The Effect of Metformin and Cinnamon on Serum Anti-Mullerian Hormone in Women Having PCOS: A Double-Blind, Randomized, Controlled Trial. *Journal of Human Reproductive Sciences*, *10*(1), 31–36. https://doi.org/10.4103/JHRS.JHRS_90_16.

Yildiz, B. O., Bozdag, G., Yapici, Z., Esinler, I., & Yarali, H. (2012). Prevalence, phenotype and cardiometabolic risk of polycystic ovary syndrome under different diagnostic criteria. *Human Reproduction (Oxford, England)*, *27*(10), 3067–3073. https://doi.org/10.1093/HUMREP/DES232.

Yildiz, B. O., Knochenhauer, E. S., & Azziz, R. (2008). Impact of obesity on the risk for polycystic ovary syndrome. *The Journal of Clinical Endocrinology and Metabolism*, *93*(1), 162–168. https://doi.org/10.1210/JC.2007-1834.

Zhang, D., Zhang, L., Yue, F., Zheng, Y., & Russell, R. (2015). Serum zonulin is elevated in women with polycystic ovary syndrome and correlates with insulin resistance and severity of anovulation. *European Journal of Endocrinology*, *172*(1), 29–36. https://doi.org/10.1530/EJE-14-0589.

# Chapter 14

# Case Studies: A Collection of Mild to Severe Cases of PCOS Patients: A Major Cause of Infertility

**Nikhil Maheshwari***
Department of Biochemistry, Faculty of Life Sciences, Aligarh Muslim University, Aligarh

## Abstract

Polycystic ovary syndrome (PCOS) was earlier called the Stein-Leventhal syndrome and was defined as common endocrine and metabolic disorder. Females of the reproductive (18-40 years) age are more prone to PCOS and are advised to regularly monitor diabetes, cardiovascular risk factors, and blood cholesterol. PCOS is a heterogenic, inheritable multifactorial syndrome that is categorized in phenotypes A, B, C & D on the bases of its clinical description. The cause of PCOS is not well illustrated but genetic and environmental factors play a pivotal role. In PCOS tiny cysts develop in the ovaries during reproductive age. It can be diagnosed by increased levels of testosterone and luteinizing hormone (LH) in the blood, amenorrhea or oligomenorrhea, and infertility. Ultrasonography identified the slightly enlarged ovaries with the appearance of many small follicles (cysts) in PCOS patients. PCOS at early stages shows the increased susceptibility of type-2 diabetes mellitus (T2DM) in gestation, hypercholesterolemia, hypertension, apnoea, and obesity. Prolonged PCOS leads to severe health risks like an increased rate of heart stroke and long-term insulin resistance in later life. It also causes hepatic steatosis, depression, pre-eclampsia, irregular menstrual cycle, hirsutism, baldness, endometrial carcinoma, and mainly infertility. The prevention and cure of PCOS are based on the type, prevalence, severity, and symptoms. The risk of PCOS is reduced or can be prevented by adopting a healthful lifestyle based on a balanced diet, routine physical activity exercise, and avoiding nicotine consumption. Laparoscopic ovarian drilling (LOD), oophorectomy, and assisted reproductive technology (ART) are also suggested in severe PCOS cases.

**Keywords:** PCOS, prevalence, phenotypes, symptoms, treatment, case studies

* Corresponding Author's Email: nikhil.5795@gmail.com.

In: Polycystic Ovarian Syndrome (PCOS) and Our Biological Clock
Editors: Arpita Roy, Gowhar Rashid and Nihad Ashraf Khan
ISBN: 979-8-89113-100-2
© 2023 Nova Science Publishers, Inc.

# 1. Introduction

Polycystic ovarian syndrome (PCOS) is a hormonal abnormality adversely affecting the female of reproductive age. Indeed the 4-21% prevalence of PCOS has been reported by following the Rotterdam criteria of diagnosis (Delcour et al. 2019) in females. In PCOS numerous fluid-filled cysts develop in the ovaries which contain immature follicles. The early symptoms of PCOS include irregular menstruation, hyperandrogenism, and polycystic ovaries. Being a complex disorder PCOS not only involves the reproductive system but also is linked to obesity, dyslipidemia, hypertension, type-2 diabetes mellitus (T2DM), and metabolic syndrome. The root cause of the occurrence of PCOS is still unknown but various pathophysiological factors are involved. The association of PCOS with female infertility is well documented. Severe cases of PCOS also lead to pathologies like endometrial carcinoma, hepatic steatosis, malignant ovaries, and cardiovascular diseases. Because PCOS is a multifactorial disorder where individual genes, gene-environment interaction, and gene-gene interactions are also involved (Khan et al. 2019). Prevention and cure of PCOS is difficult but adopting a healthy lifestyle along with proper medication can minimize the risk of the syndrome.

## 1.1. General Literature

Stein and Leventhal reported 7 instances of PCOS for the first time with symptoms like oversized polycystic ovaries, infertility, and amenorrhea (Stein and Leventhal 1935). Laquer and Butenandt identified the hormone testosterone followed by androgens assay (Laquer and Butenandt 1935). Later it was reported that androgens are produced by not only the adrenal gland but also the ovaries. Findings further show the association of hyperandrogenism with PCOS in women (Ginsburg and Havard 1975).

PCOS causes anovulatory infertility in women and affects a significant population across the globe. Kovanci and Buster reported a 5-10% prevalence of PCOS around the world (Kovanci and Buster 2015). Etiological studies show that it mainly affects reproductive-aged women (8-13%). PCOS is a polygenic, multifactorial, and complex disease so because of overlapping symptoms its diagnosis is often difficult. Although progress has been done in its diagnosis and management, the molecular mechanisms and signaling pathways involved are yet to be analyzed (Khan et al. 2019).

PCOS is associated with 40% of infertility cases and causes ovulatory dysfunction and hyperandrogenism in females (Krysiak et al. 2006)

## 1.2. Inheritance of PCOS

Degenerative ovaries were seen in a case study in 1844. Studies were continued and various cellular mechanisms, biochemical changes, genetic determinants, and environmental risk factors involved in PCOS were decoded. Cooper and Colleagues later reported the genetic aspect of PCOS for the first time in 1968 (Cooper et al. 1968). Factual data shows that in 1972 sterile woman was diagnosed with tiny shiny ovaries.

Carey et al. monitored the body mass index (BMI), degree of hirsutism, gonadotropins, prolactin, and testosterone level in the serum of all the members of a family (Carey et al. 1993). They noted irregular menstrual, reproductive history, obesity, glucose, insulin level, and baldness. Results of the study showed that first-degree female members of PCOS patients are 51% more prone to being affected. They postulate that alleles of the same gene cause androgenetic alopecia in PCOS which disturbs the production and function of androgens. The ontogenetic drift in both sexes governs the stages of androgenetic baldness. The varying nature of other genes could be an elucidation of the somewhat variable phenotype. The onset of early baldness was linked to observable traits of individuals (accurate phenotype) for definite male carriers. PCOS penetrates each family at more than a 90% rate by autosomal dominant inheritance.

Jahanfar et al. examine the genetic factors in PCOS in 19 monozygotic and 15 dizygotic female twins using the classic twin model (Jahanfar et al. 1995). The BMI, level of fasting insulin, and androstanediol glucuronide were influenced by genetic factors. They postulate that PCOS is induced by one autosomal defective gene or polygenic factor and may be an X-linked syndrome. The pathogenesis of PCOS perhaps involves intrauterine and extrauterine environmental factors.

Jahanfar et al. studied the effect of genetic and androgenic factors and PCOS on the circulating lipid fractions in a subset of 19 identical and 15 fraternal female twin pairs. The discordant twins suffering from PCOS show equivalent levels of lipids to their conjoined twins. They postulate that genetic factors significantly regulate the level of circulating lipoprotein (High-Density Lipoprotein-Cholesterol, apolipoprotein-B, and total cholesterol) (Jahanfar et al. 1997).

Vink et al. analyzed the hereditary of PCOS in 1332 genetically identical twins and 1873 fraternal twins/singleton sisters of twins (they share 50% common genes of their segregating genes). Inheritable factors depend on the familial aggregation of genes in PCOS cases. Results of this study confirm the involvement of familial factors in PCOS and show, twice the resemblance of monozygotic twin sisters for PCOS to fraternal twins and other sisters with a polychoric correlation of 0.71 and 0.38, respectively. A univariate examination reveals the strong influence of inheritable traits on the variance in PCOS patients. A trivariate-genetic study based on hirsutism, acne, and oligomenorrhea confirmed the involvement of genetic factors in familial components in PCOS (Vink et al. 2005).

### 1.3. Incidence and Prevalence

In 1990, NIH (National Institutes of Health) proposed the diagnostic criteria for PCOS, and the prevalence of PCOS is determined from the number of criteria followed. The prevalence of PCOS determined in divergent populations is shown in Table 1.

**Table 1.** The data shows the prevalence of PCOS in various populations around the world

| S. No. | Year | Race/Country/ Other sources | Gender | Prevalence of PCOS (%) | References |
|---|---|---|---|---|---|
| 1. | 1998 | Caucasian and black races | Female | 4.0% | Knochenhauer et al. 1998 |
| 2. | 1999 | Oxford University | Female | 6.8% | Michelmore et al. 1999 |
| 3. | 2000 | Greek, Spanish, and Caucasian | Female | 6.8% | Asunción et al. 2000 |
| 4. | 2010 | Karachi, Pakistan | Infertile female | 40% | Baqai et al. 2010 |
| 5. | 2011 | Indian | The female of reproductive age | 9.13% | Nidhi et al. 2011 |
| 6. | 2013 | Chinese | The female of reproductive age | 5.6% | Li et al. 2013 |
| 7. | 2015 | South Asian, Pakistan | Female | 50% | Akram and Roohi, 2015 |
| 8. | 2017 | White and black populations | 400 females (18-45 years) | 6.6% (white 8%, black 4%) | Chan et al. 2017 |
| 9. | 2020 | Chinese | Females of 20-24 years | 15% | Yang et al. 2022 |

## 1.4. Phenotypes of PCOS and its Clinical Description

There are four categories of PCOS based on phenotype A, B, C, and D. Metabolic dysfunction in all four phenotypes can be diagnosed by ultrasonography and predicted by common symptoms like obesity, hyperandrogenic oligo-anovulation, degree of menstrual irregularities, and ovaries with multiple cysts (Ehrmann et al. 2006; Brower et al. 2013). NIH criteria recognized phenotypes A and B only, the AES-PCOS accepted the phenotypes A, B, and C, whereas the Rotterdam consensus declared all four categories of phenotypes.

### *1.4.1. Phenotype-A and B*

Phenotype-A is the most identified PCOS (44-65%) followed by B (8-33%), both phenotypes are termed classic PCOS (Khan et al. 2019). Women suffering from phenotypes A and B can be characterized by menstrual dysfunction, increased insulin secretion and resistance, and risk for metabolic syndrome. They also show specific symptoms like hepatic steatosis, atherogenic dyslipidemia, and elevated level of anti-mullerian hormone (Goverde et al. 2009; Sahmay et al. 2013; Lizneva et al. 2016).

### *1.4.2. Phenotype-C (Ovulatory PCOS)*

Phenotype-C ovulatory PCOS can be distinguished from classic and non-hyperandrogenic PCOS in patients by elevated serum insulin, androgens, hirsutism, and atherogenic lipids. Metabolic disorders are commonly seen in ovulatory PCOS in comparison to other phenotypes. Phenotype-C is identified in 3-29% of cases of PCOS (Guastella et al. 2010).

### *1.4.3. Phenotype-D (Non-hyperandrogenic PCOS)*

Phenotype-D is reported in 0-23% of cases of PCOS (Jamil et al. 2016). Non-hyperandrogenic PCOS is identified by enhanced levels of sex hormone-binding globulin, decreased T3 and T4 levels, and LH/FSH ratio when compared to healthy controls. Normally women show normal androgen, intermittent irregularities in mensuration, and the lowest metabolic disorder in phenotype-D PCOS (Khan et al. 2019).

Since PCOS is a multifactorial syndrome, not all the investigations agree with the phenotypic classification of PCOS. Intrinsic activation of theca cell steroidogenesis enhances the level of androgens causing subcellular damage in theca cells in PCOS patients. Intrinsic stimulation affects granulosa cells by enhancing the level of anti-mullerian hormone in the serum of PCOS patients when compared to healthy women (Pellatt et al. 2007; Azziz et al. 2009; Villarroel et al. 2011). Several studies documented the defective apoptotic pathways in maturing follicles which increase the numbers of pre-small antral follicles in PCOS women (Webber et al. 2003; Das et al. 2008). The defective insulin signaling and gene expression pathways due to intrinsic abrasion, have also been reported in women with PCOS (Dunaif 1997; Corton et al. 2007). Glyco-oxidative stress and oxidative stress-mediated insulin resistance leading to hypergonadism have been linked with the underlying pathology of PCOS in women (Gonzalez et al. 2006; Victor et al. 2009).

## 1.5. Genetics and Mutations Involved in PCOS

Since PCOS is a heterogenic complex disease, the genetics within families and between families varies but it is linked to a common pathway. The related gene within a family has not been identified and the hereditary of various genes remain different in PCOS patients from the same family. Genome screening and linkage analysis come up with negative results in such families (Abbott et al. 2002). Genetic testing for PCOS proves to be impractical and is limited to finding the known risk of the disease. Case-control studies of PCOS conducted on a large population and genome-wide association studies (GWAS) would be helpful to decode the genetic association (Urbanek et al. 1999).

Till now no study has reported the true penetration of causative gene/mutation conducted in multiple families. Genes or mutations documented in familial aggregation exhibit a low penetrance linked to other covariant, environmental, and hormonal factors to cause PCOS (Table 2).

# 2. Mild and Severe Cases of PCOS

PCOS is a physiological disorder that negatively affects various systems like metabolic, endocrine, reproductive, and psychological in the body. To delineate the pathophysiology of PCOS, the symptoms, diagnosis, and possible treatment are discussed below.

### 2.1. Symptoms

In PCOS patients symptoms differ from mild to severe. Women with mild PCOS show unwanted hair, low energy, mood swings, and insomnia, and it is unpredictable when it becomes abnormal or severe. Women suffering from severe PCOS may experience infertility, irregular menstruation, obesity, acne, T2DM, and hyperandrogenism. The key symptoms of long-term PCOS condition are given in Figure 1. In certain cases, pathophysiological conditions like non-alcoholic steatohepatitis, endometrial cancer, and miscarriage or premature birth are also observed in severe PCOS cases.

### 2.2. Diagnosis

PCOS symptoms can be identified by the Rotterdam criteria which are based on the symptoms like increased androgen level, irregular menstruation, and polycystic ovaries (Ajmal et al. 2019). Various criteria set by agencies or scientists for PCOS diagnosis are depicted in Table 3 (Diamanti-Kandarakis and Legro 2006).

**Table 2.** The direct and indirect role and association of various genes with PCOS

| S. No. | Gene | Cytogenic location and function | Involvement of gene | Inference | References |
|---|---|---|---|---|---|
| 1. | CYP11a | Encodes an enzyme to covert cholesterol to progesterone | Ovarian and adrenal steroidogenesis | Polymorphs and variation as associated factors with PCOS | Gharani et al. 1997<br>Diamanti-Kandarakis et al. 2000<br>Wang et al. 2006 |
| | | | | Unable to replicate the results | Gaasenbeek et al. 2004 |
| 2. | CYP21 | Encodes an enzyme to covert 17-hydroxyprogesterone to 11-deoxycortisol | Ovarian and adrenal steroidogenesis | Ineffective anabolism of steroidogenesis leading to PCOS | Witchel and Aston 2000 |
| | | | | Association of heterozygous CYP21 to PCOS with hyperandrogenemia | |
| | | | | No direct association of CYP21 variation with PCOS | Witchel et al. 2005 |
| 3. | CYP17 | Encodes an enzyme to covert progesterone and pregnenolone into 17-hydroxyprogesterone and 17-hydroxypregnenolone | Ovarian and adrenal steroidogenesis | Increased level of androgens in PCOS patients | Rosenfield et al. 1990 |
| | | | | Increased expression in theca cells | Wickenheisser et al. 2000 |
| | | | | Polymorph in the promoter region which is linked with PCOS | Carey et al. 1994 |
| 4. | CYP19A1 | 15q21.2, encodes an enzyme aromatase p450 required for estrogen synthesis. | Ovarian and adrenal steroidogenesis | Decreased activity of aromatase in PCOS patients | Bulun et al. 2004 |
| 5. | Androgen Receptor Gene (AR) | Xq12 on the 'q' arm of the X-chromosome, consists of 11 axons and encodes a tri-domain protein of 92 kb | Steroid hormone | GWAS find a novel variation in the gene to be the cause of PCOS | Urbanek et al. 2007 |
| 6. | Sex Hormone-Binding Globulin (SHBG) Gene | 17p13-p12, synthesized 373 amino acid proteins in the liver which regulates sex hormone levels. Its synthesis is regulated by insulin and androgens. | Steroid hormone | Low SHBG level in PCOS patients, inhibitory control of hyperinsulinemia on SHBG synthesis | Nestler et al. 1991 |
| | | | | SNP in the SHBG gene was linked with PCOS | Chen et al. 2010 |
| 7. | Luteinizing Hormone (LH) Receptor Gene | Regulate and synthesize LH | Gonadotropin | Enhanced level of LH suppresses FSH level by negative feedback | Nardo et al. 2008 |
| | | | | The polymorphic β-subunit gene of LH is linked to PCOS | Roy et al. 1996 |
| | | | | A point mutation is reported in a β-subunit gene (Trp8Arg and Ilg15Thr) as well as in 15% of the normal population | Furui et al. 1994 |
| 8. | AMH | Cytogenetic location 13.3 on the long arm of chromosome 19, encodes a protein involved in infertility | Gonadotropin | Variation in the AMH is linked to PCOS | Cate et al. 1986 |
| | | | | GWAS and whole exome sequencing find several variants of the AMH gene linked to PCOS | Gorsic et al. 2017 |

| S. No. | Gene | Cytogenic location and function | Involvement of gene | Inference | References |
|---|---|---|---|---|---|
| 9. | FSHR | 2p16.3 on the 'p' arm of chromosome 2, having 14 exons, encodes G-coupled receptor protein needed for the development of gonads | Gonadotropin | Increased expression of the gene in PCOS patients | Baban et al. 2018 |
| 10. | Insulin gene (INS) | INS regulates the androgen production in theca cells. The transcriptional rate of the INS sandwich gene and IGF-II is governed by polymorphic VNTR | Action and secretion of insulin | Enhanced insulin level provokes phosphoinositide 3-kinase/protein kinase B pathway in PCOS theca cells to increase androgen synthesis | Baillargeon et al. 2007 |
| | | | | Polymorphic VNTR is linked to PCOS | Waterworth et al. 1997 |
| 11. | INSR | Encodes turmeric protein (2α2β) | Action and secretion of insulin | D19S884 part of chromosome region 19p13.2 (contains INSR gene) was associated with PCOS | Urbanek et al. 2005 |
| 12. | IRS proteins | The binding of insulin to its receptor autophosphorylates them, then tyrosine kinase activity of INSR phosphorylates IRS-1 and IRS-2, further used in downstream steps | Action and secretion of insulin | Increased expression of Arg972 IRS-1 in PCOS patients | Sir-Petermann et al. 2001 |
| | | | | Higher expression of Gly972Arg in IRS-1 in PCOS patients | Dilek et al. 2005 |
| 13. | Calpain10 gene | Located on the long arm of 'q' of chromosome 2 having 12 exons, encodes the heterodimeric calcium-dependent cysteine protease. Calpain10 is linked to T2DM | Action and secretion of insulin | Affects the secretion and metabolism of insulin, so considered a candidate gene causing PCOS | Ajmal et al. 2019 |
| 14. | FTO gene | 16q12.2 on the 'q' arm of chromosome 16 and encodes the enzyme α-ketoglutarate, show an association between T2DM and obesity | Fat mass obesity | SNP rs9939609 was significantly increased in PCOS-affected women | Rizwan et al. 2018 |
| 15. | PCOS1 | 19p13.2 region on chromosome 19, also known as the PCO gene | Fat mass obesity | Found to be associated with PCOS in several cases | Urbanek et al. 2005 |
| 16. | SRD5A2 and SRD5A1 | 2p23.1 on chromosome | Fat mass obesity | SRD5A2 is involved in protection against PCOS while the SRD5A1 variant is linked to hirsutism and PCOS | Goodarzi et al. 2006 |

(AMH, anti-Müllerian hormone; Arg, arginine; CYP, cytochrome P450; FSHR, follicle stimulating hormone receptor; FTO, fat mass and obesity-associated; Gly, glycine; GWAS, genome-wide association studies; IGF, insulin like growth factor; INS, insulin; INSR, insulin receptor; IRS, insulin receptor substrate; LH, luteinizing hormone; PCOS, polycystic ovarian syndrome; SHBG, sex hormone binding globulin; SNP, single nucleotide polymorphisms; SRD5A1 and SRD5A2, steroid 5 alpha reductase 1 and 2; T2DM, type 2 diabetes mellitus; VNTR, variable number of tandem repeats)

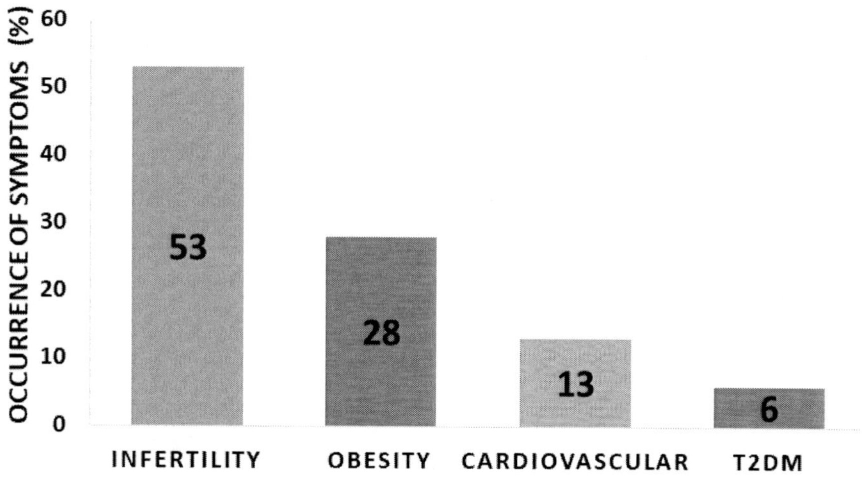


**Figure 1.** Occurrence of signs and symptoms of PCOS in women.

**Table 3.** Diagnostic measures for PCOS

| S. No. | Year | Agencies/criteria | Criteria |
|---|---|---|---|
| 1. | 1990 | NIH | Prolonged anovulation, increased androgens level |
| 2. | 2003 | Rotterdam | irregular ovulation and infertility, Polycystic ovaries, Hyperandrogenism |
| 3. | 2006, 2009 | AE-PCOS society | Hyperandrogenism, ovarian dysfunction, polycystic ovaries |
| 4. | 2012 | NIH | Hyperandrogenism, oligo-anovulation, antral follicular count≥12, ovarian volume ≥10 $cm^3$ |
| 5. | 2018 | ESHRE | Hyperandrogenism, oligo-anovulation, antral follicular count≥20 only with endovaginal ultrasound transducers (8MHz), ovarian volume ≥10 $cm^3$ |

(AE, Androgen Excess; ESHRE, European Society of Human Reproduction and Embryology; NIH, National Health Institute; PCOS, Polycystic ovary syndrome)

In order to effectively treat PCOS, the proper diagnosis of types of PCOS is mandatory. The four types of PCOS are given below in Table 4.

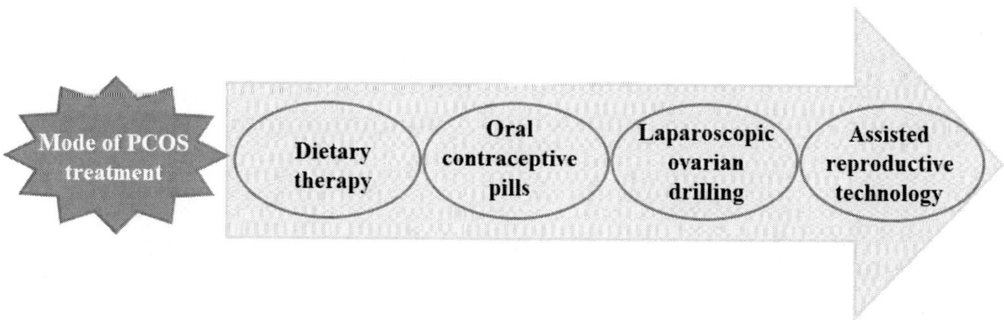


**Figure 2.** Possible mode of PCOS treatment.

**Table 4.** The types, prevalence, and symptoms of PCOS

| S. No. | Type of PCOS | Prevalence/severity/ causative agents | Symptoms | Diagnostic measures | Precaution/ treatment |
|---|---|---|---|---|---|
| 1. | Insulin resistance PCOS | 70%, most common, smoking, pollution, excessive intake of sugars, and trans | hyperinsulinemia, obesity, fatigue, brain fog, hyperandrogenism, hirsutism, acne, alopecia | HbA1c, blood sugar level, fasting insulin | Regular exercise, quit sugar and trans fat, Micro-macronutrients supplementation |
| 2. | Pill-induced PCOS | 2%, the second most common PCOS, occurs 3-6 months after oral intake of contraceptives like Ginet, Yasmin, Yaz | No insulin resistance | High blood LH level | Micro-macronutrients Herbs like chaste trees and peonies, Good sleep and reduce stress level |
| 3. | Adrenal PCOS | 10%, | No hyperandrogenism | High DHEA-S level, | Manage stress, good sleep, Avoid caffeine, micronutrients, and herbal supplementation |
| 4. | Inflammatory PCOS | chronic inflammation stimulates the ovaries to secrete excess testosterone, leading to anovulation | headaches, joints pain, fatigue, eczema, and bowel issues like IBS | Normal fasting glucose and insulin, abnormal CBC and Vit-D C-reactive protein ≥ 5 | Improve gut health, avoid food triggers, and natural anti-inflammatories Magnesium supplementation |
| Always first consult a practitioner for effective prescription and dosages | | | | | |

(CBC, complete blood count; DHEA-S, dehydroepiandrosterone sulfate; HbA1c, hemoglobin A1c; IBS, irritable bowel syndrome; LH, luteinizing hormone; PCOS, polycystic ovarian syndrome; Vit, vitamin)

Sometimes PCOS can be misdiagnosed as hypothalamic amenorrhoea due to overlapping symptoms like excess hair growth, mild acne, and the appearance of a polycystic ovary. It can be distinguished from the higher LH: FSH ratio in PCOS (3:1) while the much lower LH: FSH ratio in hypothalamic amenorrhoea.

## 3. A Future Perspective on the Treatment

Currently, PCOS is incurable and the possible therapeutic options are given in Figure 2. Almost 30% of PCOS patients are diagnosed with obesity and dietary therapies can recover PCOS symptoms like irregular mensuration, annulations, and insulin resistance (Gu et al. 2022). In the long term, dietary therapy remains ineffective, therefore bariatric surgery can be done for promising results (Crave et al. 1995).

Oral contraceptive pills (OCPs) can regulate endocrine deformity, hirsutism, and acne and are safer than other remedies due to less risk of endometrial carcinoma. OCPs increases the level of SHBG and decreases FSH and LH level resulting in decreased ovarian androgens and free testosterone. OCPs treatment has several adverse effects including, depression, cardiac risks, impaired glycolytic pathways, insulin resistance, hyperglycemia, and diabetes mellitus (Rimm et al. 1992). During infertility treatment, Clomid, FSH, LH and sometimes Letrozole are prescribed by doctors.

Laparoscopic ovarian drilling (LOD) is used when both Clomid medications for ovulation and wedge resection surgery fail. LOD increases the SHBG level and improves insulin resistance and production of ovarian androgens, and the rate of miscarriages with a success rate of 84%. LOD treatment can be assessed by the level of antimullerian hormone in the serum of women. Cyst aspiration techniques can remove fluids from non-cancerous cysts which can improve the fertility of women. Oophorectomy is a surgical process to prevent PCOS, endometriosis, and ovarian cancer by removing one or both ovaries.

In assisted reproductive technology (ART) external gonadotropin stimulus is given to ovulate multiple follicles in ovaries, but this stimulus leads to ovarian hyperstimulation syndrome (OHSS) in PCOS patients (Tummon et al. 2005). Interventional procedures like IVF, IVM fertilization, and laparoscopic drilling also go with several secondary diseases (Melo et al. 2015). During these procedures, intake of Spironolactone or Eflornithine medicines to prevent hair growth can lead to birth defects.

## 4. Case Studies

### 4.1. Case Study 1: (Sachdeva et al. 2019)

*A clinical trial based on the clomiphene-induced changes in the hormonal and metabolic profile of different PCOS phenotypes*- This study was conducted on 164 women suffering from PCOS-derived infertility in an Infertility Clinic, PGIMER, Chandigarh, India.

#### *4.1.1. Recommendation and Treatment*

According to the NIH (National Institute of Health) guidelines, patients were grouped into four phenotypes and given an increasing dose of clomiphene (50-150 mg/day) in three cycles. Each phenotype was screened for hormonal and metabolic profile, clinical history, and ultrasonography.

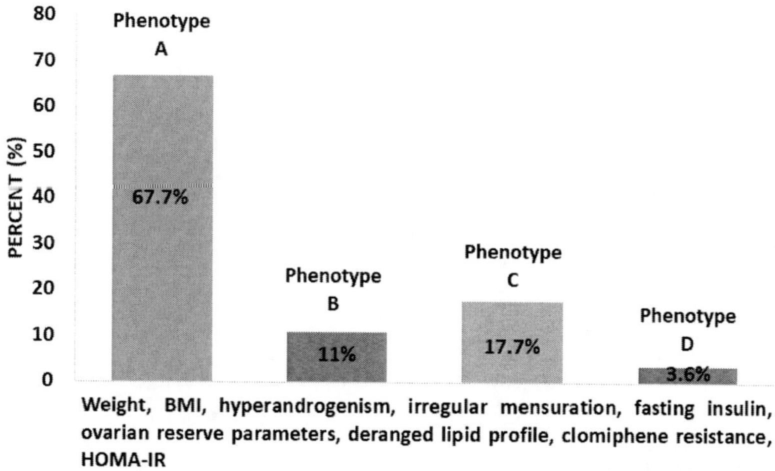


(BMI, body mass index, HOMA-IR, homeostatic model assessment of insulin resistance)

**Figure 3.** Prevalence of phenotype A, B, C, and D to various pathological conditions in response to clomiphene treatment.

The levels of LH-FSH ratio and Vitamin D were not altered significantly, no notable changes were seen in the waist-hip ratio, waist circumference, blood sugar, and hypertension among various PCOS phenotypes. Full-blown phenotype-A is the most severe PCOS and shows a higher risk of cardiovascular diseases and adverse metabolic outcomes. However, phenotype-D is considered the least severe PCOS. This phenotypic categorization of PCOS patients will be helpful in forecasting the PCOS patients about the severity of the syndrome and PCOS-derived infertility (Figure 3).

## 4.2. Case Study 2: (NHS 2018; NICE, 2018, 2020)

*A woman with PCOS who is trying to conceive:* Sheila (35 years) is seeking advice on naturopathy to sustain her pregnancy. She has stopped consuming contraceptives that were prescribed to her a year ago to control the PCOS symptoms. However, she started gaining weight again, and now gained even more weight due to her anxiety. Sheila was asked to visit a fertility clinic, but her appointment has been delayed by 4 months. She is not on any medication now. She has no addiction but smokes sometimes.

### *4.2.1. Advice and Recommendations*

Sheila's concern should be carefully listened to and advised to lose weight to increase her fertility. Explain to her that for successful reproductive procedures body mass index should be ranged between 19 -30 (NICE 2017). She should be advised to follow routine exercise and a healthy diet plan to decrease her weight and smoking cessation services.

Sheila should be referred to consult her general practitioner in need so that she can monitor her glucose tolerance test to screen for T2DM and anxiety (NICE 2018). Advise her to take 400 μg of folic acid daily or another multivitamin supplement to prepare her body for pre-conception, and other pre-pregnancy caution like ensuring her all the vaccinations to date (NHS 2018).

## 4.3. Case Study 3: (Vaniqa 2017; Tucker 2019; NHS 2019)

*A woman with PCOS who wants information on how to manage symptoms*- Johanna, 25 years old girl asked the pharmacist how to manage unwanted facial hair and acne. Johanna confirms that she is suffering from PCOS and consuming combined oral contraceptives for the last three months. She told that her mensural cycle is now more regular and less painful but the facial hairs and acne are still there. She confirmed that she has no genealogy of cardiovascular disorder and she joined a gymnasium to maintain her fitness.

### *4.3.1. Advice and Recommendations*

After 3 months of medication, Johanna got relief in her symptoms, so she does not need to visit a dermatologist or general practitioner. She should follow the same treatment for at least six months to get maximum relief. Thus, she should be assured that it may take another 3 months before the full effect of the treatment is achieved. Johanna should be asked to continue with her running club and consume a nutritious balanced diet.

She was suggested benzoyl peroxide (5%) as facial gel or as facewash (10%) to apply on her acne. To get better results, she should use it on her face by applying a cleanser and sunscreen moisturizer instead of using it on individual lesions. Johanna should be advised that complete treatment will take at least 6 weeks and assessed thereafter (Tucker 2019). She should be asked to use non-comedogenic makeup if it is available.

Even after following a 6 months treatment, the acne and facial hair persist, Johana should be asked to consult her general practitioner for a prescription for topical cream for facial hirsutism or topical retinoids/antibiotics for acne. Moreover, she should be advised to do hair removal by laser or other advanced techniques because facial hirsutism cream has common side effects like acne (Vaniqa 2017; NHS 2019).

### 4.4. Case Study 4: (Warren and Arslanian, 2006)

*A suspected case of PCOS in the teenager-* A patient and her 12-year-old daughter, Nadia visit the pharmacy. She was suffering from long and painful mensural periods and mild pimples.

#### *4.4.1. Advice and Recommendations*

Nadia should be asked to record the regularity and duration of her periods and the intensity of the pain. If she feels exhausted then this could be a sign of anemia. Describe to her that mild acne usually occurs during puberty due to hormonal changes, but leading a healthy lifestyle is more important. She was advised to keep her body hydrated, consume nutritious-healthy food, do routine exercise, and avoid picking spots to sustain good skincare.

Prescribe Nadia to take paracetamol 500 mg and 200-400 mg ibuprofen up to four times a day to control the pain during her periods, as recommended in the SmPC, However, if the symptoms persist, she should consult the general practitioners for further advice.

Diagnosis of PCOS in adolescents should be based on genealogy, excluding the other causes of Cushing's syndrome and proper laboratory testing. The lack of controlled clinical trials complicates the pharmacological treatment of PCOS in such patients. Therapeutic options include lifestyle interventions, oral contraceptives, and insulin sensitizers. Long-term follow-up is also needed to assess the effectiveness of these approaches in modifying the natural history of the reproductive and metabolic outcomes, without causing undue harm.

## 5. Conclusion

PCOS is a widespread endocrine and metabolic syndrome in females of reproductive age. Since incidences of PCOS are increasing day by day, it is linked to hypertension, obesity, visceral adiposity, T2DM, metabolic disorders, hyperandrogenism, male pattern baldness, polycystic ovaries, female infertility, and coronary heart diseases. Severe PCOS leads to endometrial carcinoma, ovarian malignancies, steatohepatitis, miscarriage, and premature birth. Apart from environmental factors, several candidate genes are also linked to the etiology of PCOS. Genetic defects alter the metabolic pathways leading to ovarian dysfunction and PCOS progression. Adopting a healthy lifestyle is the first line of PCOS management which includes a healthy diet, regular exercise, maintaining healthy sleep and mood, and weight loss. OCPs, LOD and

ART can also manage PCOS conditions with various side effects in patients. Keeping in mind all these pathologies, a core team of a gynecologist, physicians, endocrinologists, and obstetricians will help PCOS patients.

## References


Abbott, D. H., Dumesic, D. A., and Franks, S. (2002). Developmental origin of polycystic ovary syndrome- A hypothesis. *J Endocrinol.*, 174, 1-5. doi:10.1677/joe.0.1740001.

Ajmal, N., Khan, S. Z., and Shaikh, R. (2019). X polycystic ovary syndrome (PCOS) and genetic predisposition: a review article. *Eur J Obstet Gynecol Reprod Biol X.*, 3, 100060. doi:10.1016/j.eurox.2019.100060.

Ajmal, N., Khan, S. Z., and Shaikh, R. (2019). Polycystic ovary syndrome (PCOS) and genetic predisposition: A review article.

Akram, M., and Roohi, N. (2015). Endocrine correlates of polycystic ovary syndrome in Pakistani women. *J Coll Physicians Surg Pakistan.*, 25, 22–26.

Asunción, M., Calvo, R. M., N JL, S. M., Sancho, J., Avila, S., and Escobar-Morreale, H. F. (2000). A prospective study of the prevalence of the polycystic ovary syndrome in unselected Caucasian women from Spain. *J Clin Endocrinol Metab.*, 85, 2434–2438.

Azziz, R., Carmina, E., Dewailly, D., Diamanti-Kandarakis, E., Escobar-Morreale, H. F., Futterweit, W., Janssen, O. E., Legro, R. S., Norman, R. J., Taylor, A. E., and Witchel, S. F. (2009). The androgen excess and PCOS Society criteria for the polycystic ovary syndrome: the complete task force report. *Fertil Steril.*, 91, 456–488. doi:10.1016/j.fertnstert.2008.06.035.

Baban, A. S. S., Korsheed, S. H., and Al Hayawi, A. Y. (2018). The FSHR polymorphisms association with polycystic ovary syndrome in women of Erbil, Kurdistan in North of Iraq. *Ibn AL- Haitham J Pure Appl Sci.*, 262, doi:10.30526/2017.IHSCICONF.1799

Baillargeon, J. P., and Carpentier, A. (2007). Role of insulin in the hyperandrogenemia of lean women with polycystic ovary syndrome and normal insulin sensitivity. *Fertil Steril.*, 88,886–893. doi:10.1016/j.fertnstert.2006.12.055

Baqai, Z., Khanam, M., and Parveen, S. (2010). Prevalence of PCOS in infertile patients. *Med Chanel.*, 16, 255–260.

Brower, M., Brennan, K., Pall, M., and Azziz, R. (2013). The severity of menstrual dysfunction as a predictor of insulin resistance in PCOS. *J Clin Endocrinol Metab.*, 98,1967-1971. doi:10.1210/jc.2013-2815.

Bulun, S. E., Takayama, K., Suzuki, T., Sasano, H., Yilmaz, B., and Sebastian, S. (2004). Organization of the human aromatase p450 (CYP19) gene. *Seminars in Reproductive Medicine*, 22(1), 5–9. doi:10.1055/s-2004-823022

Butenandt, A., and Hanisch, G. (1935). Testosterone. The transformation of dehydroandrosterone into androstenediol and testosterone; a method for producing testosterone from cholesterin. *Hoppe-Seyler's Z Physiol Chem.*, 237, 89-98.

Carey, A. H., Chan, K. L., Short, F., White, D., Williamson, R., and Franks, S. (1993). Evidence for a single gene effect causing polycystic ovaries and male pattern baldness. *Clin Endocrinol (Oxf).*, 38(6), 653-8. doi: 10.1111/j.1365-2265.1993.tb02150.x. PMID: 8334753.

Carey, A. H., Waterworth, D., Patel, K., White, D., Little, J., Novelli, P., Franks, S., Williamson, R. (1994). Polycystic ovaries and premature male pattern baldness are associated with one allele of the steroid metabolism gene CYP17. *Hum Mol Genet.*, 3, 1873-1876. doi:10.1093/hmg/3.10.1873

Cate, R. L., Mattaliano, R. J., Hession, C., Tizard, R., Farber, N. M., Cheung, A., Ninfa, E. G., Frey, A. Z., Gash, D. J., and Chow, E. P. (1986). Isolation of the bovine and human genes for müllerian inhibiting substance and expression of the human gene in animal cells. *Cell.*, 45, 685–698. doi:10.1016/0092-8674(86)90783-X

Chan, J. L., Kar, S., Vanky, E., Morin-Papunen, L., Piltonen, T., Puurunen, J., Tapanainen, J. S., Maciel, G. A. R., Hayashida, S. A. Y., Soares, J. M. Jr., Baracat, E. C., Mellembakken, J. R., and Dokras, A. (2017). Racial and ethnic differences in the prevalence of metabolic syndrome and its components of metabolic syndrome in women with polycystic ovary syndrome: a regional cross-sectional study. *Am J Obstet Gynecol.*, 217, 189.e1–189.e8. doi:10.1016/j.ajog.2017.04.007.

Chen, C., Smothers, J., Lange, A., Nestler, J. E., Strauss Iii, J. F., Wickham Iii, E. P. (2010). Sex hormone-binding globulin genetic variation: associations with type 2 diabetes mellitus and polycystic ovary syndrome. *Minerva Endocrinol.*, 35(4), 271–280.

Chen, C., Smothers, J., Lange, A., Nestler, J. E., Strauss Iii, J. F., and Wickham Iii, E. P. (2010). Sex hormone-binding globulin genetic variation: associations with type 2 diabetes mellitus and polycystic ovary syndrome. *Minerva Endocrinol.*, 35(4), 271–280.

Cooper, H. E., Spellacy, W. N., Prem, K. A., and Cohen, W. D. (1968). Hereditary factors in the Stein-Leventhal syndrome. *Am J Obstet Gynecol.*, 100, 371-387. doi:10.1016/S0002-9378(15)33704-2.

Cortón, M., Botella-Carretero, J. I., Benguría, A., Villuendas, G., Zaballos, A., San, and Millan, J. L., Escobar-Morreale, H. F., and Peral, B. (2007). Differential gene expression profile in omental adipose tissue in women with polycystic ovary syndrome. *J Clin Endocrinol Metab.*, 92, 328–337. doi:10.1210/jc.2006-1665.

Crave, J. C., Fimbel, S., Lejeune, H., Cugnardey, N., Déchaud, H., and Pugeat, M. (1995). Effects of diet and metformin administration on sex hormone-binding globulin, androgens, and insulin in hirsute and obese women. *J Clin Endocrinol Metab.*, 80, 2057–2062.

Das, M., Djahanbakhch, O., Hacihanefioglu, B., Saridogan, E., Ikram, M., Ghali, L., Raveendran, M., and Storey, A. (2008). Granulosa cell survival and proliferation are altered in polycystic ovary syndrome. *J Clin Endocrinol Metab.*, 93, 881–887. doi:10.1210/jc.2007-1650.

Delcour, C., Robin, G., Young, J., and Dewailly, D. (2019). PCOS and Hyperprolactinemia: what do we know in 2019? *Clin Med Insights Reprod Health.*, 13, 1179558119871921. doi: 10.1177/1179558119871921.

Diamanti-Kandarakis, E., Bartzis, M. I., Bergiele, A. T., Tsianateli, T. C., and Kouli, C. R., (2000). Microsatellite polymorphism (tttta)(n) at −528 base pairs of gene CYP11α influences hyperandrogenemia in patients with polycystic ovary syndrome. *Fertil Steril.*, 73, 735–741.doi:10.1016/S0015-0282(99)00628-7.

Diamanti-Kandarakis, E. K. H., and Legro, R. S. (2006). The role of genes and environment in the etiology of PCOS. *Endocrine*, 30, 19–26.

Dilek, S., Ertunc, D., Tok, E. C., Erdal, E. M., and Aktas, A. (2005). Association of Gly972Arg variant of insulin receptor substrate-1 with metabolic features in women with polycystic ovary syndrome. *Fertil Steril.*, 84, 407–412. doi:10.1016/j.fertnstert.2005.01.133.

Dunaif, A. (1997). Insulin resistance and the polycystic ovary syndrome: mechanism and implications for pathogenesis. *Endocr Rev.*, 7, 345–349.

Ehrmann, D. A., Liljenquist, D. R., Kasza, K., Azziz, R., Legro, R. S., and Ghazzi, M. N., and PCOS/Troglitazone Study Group. (2006). Prevalence and predictors of the metabolic syndrome in women with polycystic ovary syndrome. *J Clin Endocrinol Metab.*, 91, 48–53. doi:10.1210/jc.2005-1329.

Furui, K., Suganuma, N., Tsukahara, S. I., Asada, Y., Kikkawa, F., Tanaka, M., Ozawa, T., and Tomoda, Y. (1994). Identification of two point mutations in the gene coding luteinizing hormone (LH) β-subunit, associated with immunologically anomalous LH variants. *J Clin Endocrinol Metab.*, 78, 107–113.

Gaasenbeek, M., Powell, B. L., Sovio, U., Haddad, L., Gharani, N., Bennett, A., Groves, C. J., Rush, K., Goh, M. J., Conway, G. S., Ruokonen, A., Martikainen, H., Pouta, A., Taponen, S., Hartikainen, A. L., Halford, S., Järvelin, M. R., Franks, S., and McCarthy, M. I. (2004). Large-scale analysis of the relationship between CYP11A promoter variation, polycystic ovarian syndrome, and serum testosterone. *J Clin Endocrinol Metab.*, 89, 2408–2413. doi:10.1210/jc.2003-031640.

Gharani, N., Waterworth, D. M., Batty, S., White, D., Gilling-Smith, C., Conway, G. S., McCarthy, M., Franks, S., and Williamson, R. (1997). Association of the steroid synthesis gene CYP11a with polycystic ovary syndrome and hyperandrogenism. *Hum Mol Genet.*, 6, 397-402. doi:10.1093/hmg/6.3.397.

Ginsburg, J., and Havard, C. W. (1976). Polycystic ovary syndrome. *Br Med J.*, 2(6038), 737-740.

González, F., Rote, N. S., Minium, J., and Kirwan, J. P. (2006). Reactive oxygen species-induced oxidative stress in the development of insulin resistance and hyperandrogenism in polycystic ovary syndrome. *J Clin Endocrinol Metab.*, 91, 336–340. doi:10.1210/jc.2005-1696.

Goodarzi, M. O., Shah, N. A., Antoine, H. J., Pall, M., Guo, X., and Azziz, R. (2006). Variants in the 5α-reductase type 1 and type 2 genes are associated with polycystic ovary syndrome and the severity of hirsutism in affected women. *J Clin Endocrinol Metab.*, 91, 4085–4091. doi:10.1210/jc.2006-0227.

Gorsic, L. K., Kosova, G., Werstein, B., Sisk, R., Legro, R. S., Hayes, M. G., Teixeira, J. M., Dunaif, A., and Urbanek, M. (2017). Pathogenic anti-Müllerian hormone variants in polycystic ovary syndrome. *J Clin Endocrinol Metab.*, 102, 2862–2872. doi:10.1210/jc.2017-00612.

Goverde, A. J., Van, Koert, A. J. B., Eijkemans, M. J., Knauff, E. A., Westerveld, H. E., Fauser, B. C., and Broekmans, F. J. (2009). Indicators for metabolic disturbances in anovulatory women with polycystic ovary syndrome diagnosed according to the Rotterdam consensus criteria. *Hum Reprod.*, 24, 710–717.

Gu, Y., Zhou, G., Zhou, F., Wu, Q., Ma, C., Zhang, Y., Ding, J., and Hua, K. (2022). Life Modifications and PCOS: Old Story But New Tales. *Front. Endocrinol.*, 13, 808898. doi: 10.3389/fendo.2022.808898.

Guastella, E., Longo, R. A., and Carmina, E. (2010). Clinical and endocrine characteristics of the main polycystic ovary syndrome phenotypes. *Fertil Steril.*, 94, 2197–2201. doi:10.1016/j.fertnstert.2010.02.014.

Jahanfar, S., Eden, J. A., Nguyen, T., Wang, X. L., and Wilcken, D. E. (1997). A twin study of polycystic ovary syndrome and lipids. *Gynecol Endocrinol.*, 11(2), 111-7. doi: 10.3109/09513599709152521. PMID: 9174852.

Jahanfar, S., Eden, J. A., Warren, P., Seppälä, M., and Nguyen, T. V. (1995). A twin study of polycystic ovary syndrome. *Fertil Steril.*, 63(3), 478-86. PMID: 7531655.

Jamil, A. S., Alalaf, S. K., Al-Tawil, N. G., and Al-Shawaf, T. (2016). Comparison of clinical and hormonal characteristics among four phenotypes of polycystic ovary syndrome based on the Rotterdam criteria. *Arch Gynecol Obstet.*, 293, 447–456. doi:10.1007/s00404-015-3889-5.

Khan, M. J., Ullah, A., and Basit, S. (2019). Genetic Basis of Polycystic Ovary Syndrome (PCOS): Current Perspectives. *Appl Clin Genet.*, 12, 249-260. doi: 10.2147/TACG.S200341.

Knochenhauer, E. S., Key, T. J., Kahsar-Miller, M., Waggoner, W., Boots, L. R., and Azziz, R. (1998). Prevalence of the polycystic ovary syndrome in unselected black and white women of the Southeastern United States: a prospective study. *J Clin Endocrinol Metab.*, 83, 3078–3082.

Kovanci, E., and Buster, J. E. (2015). Polycystic ovary syndrome. *Clin Gynecol.*, 2015. Second Edition.

Krysiak, R., Okopie, B., Gdula-Dymek, A., and Herman, Z. S. (2006). Update on the management of polycystic ovary syndrome. *Pharmacol Rep.*, 58, 614.

Li, R., Zhang, Q., Yang, D., Li, S., Lu, S., Wu, X., Wei, Z., Song, X., Wang, X., Fu, S., Lin, J., Zhu, Y., Jiang, Y., Feng, HL., and Qiao, J. (2013). Prevalence of polycystic ovary syndrome in women in China: a large community-based study. *Hum Reprod.*, 28, 2562–2569.

Lizneva, D., Suturina, L., Walker, W., Brakta, S., Gavrilova-Jordan, L., and Azziz, R. (2016). Criteria, prevalence, and phenotypes of polycystic ovary syndrome. *Fertil Steril.*, 106, 6–15. doi:10.1016/j.fertnstert.2016.05.003.

Melo, A. S., Ferriani, R. A., and Navarro, P. A. (2015). Treatment of infertility in women with polycystic ovary syndrome: approach to clinical practice. *Clinics.*, 70, 765–769. doi:10.6061/clinics.

Michelmore, K. F., Balen, A. H., Dunger, D. B., and Vessey, M. P. (1999). Polycystic ovaries and associated clinical and biochemical features in young women. *Clin Endocrinol (Oxf).*, 51, 779–786. doi:10.1046/j.1365-2265.1999.00886.x.

Nardo, L. G., Patchava, S., and Laing, I. (2008). Polycystic ovary syndrome: pathophysiology, molecular aspects and clinical implications. *Panminerva Med.*, 50, 267–278.

National Institute for Health and Care Excellence. (2017). Fertility problems: assessment and treatment. Clinical guideline [CG156]. Available at: https://www.nice.org.uk/guidance/cg156 (accessed March 2020).

National Institute for Health and Care Excellence. (2019). Polycystic ovary syndrome. Clinical Knowledge Summary. 2018. Available at: https://cks.nice.org.uk/polycystic-ovary-syndrome (accessed March 2020).

Nestler, J. E., Powers, L. P., Matt, D. W., Steingold, K. A., Plymate, S. R., Rittmaster, R. S., Clore, J. N., and Blackard, W. G. (1991). A direct effect of hyperinsulinemia on serum sex hormone-binding globulin levels in obese women with the polycystic ovary syndrome. *J Clin Endocrinol Metab.*, 72, 83–89. doi:10.1210/jcem-72-1-83.

NHS. (2018). Trying to get pregnant. Available at: https://www.nhs.uk/conditions/pregnancy-and-baby/getting-pregnant/ (accessed March 2020).

NHS. (2019). Polycystic ovary syndrome. Available at: https://www.nhs.uk/conditions/polycystic-ovary-syndrome-pcos/ (accessed March 2020).

Nidhi, R., Padmalatha, V., Nagarathna, R., and Amritanshu, R. (2011). Prevalence of polycystic ovarian syndrome in Indian adolescents. *J Pediatr Adolesc Gynecol.*, 24, 223–227. doi:10.1016/j.jpag.2011.03.002.

Pellatt, L., Hanna, L., Brincat, M., Galea, R., Brain, H., Whitehead, S., and Mason, H. (2007). Granulosa cell production of anti-Müllerian hormone is increased in polycystic ovaries. *J Clin Endocrinol Metab.*, 92, 240–245. doi:10.1210/jc.2006-1582.

Rebecca, L. (2013). A Case Study of Polycystic Ovarian Syndrome" (2013). Honors Theses. 85. https://encompass.eku.edu/honors_theses/85.

Rimm, E. B., Manson, J. E., Stampfer, M. J., Colditz, G. A., Willett, W. C., Rosner, B., Hennekens, C. H., and Speizer, F. E. (1992). Oral contraceptive use and the risk of Type 2 (non-insulin-dependent) diabetes mellitus in a large prospective study of women. *Diabetologia.*, 35, 967–972. doi:10.1007/BF00401427.

Rizwan, S., Ghazanvi, S., Rasheed, N., and Mi, U. (2018). Association of FTO common RS9939609 polymorphism with obesity and association of FTO common RS9939609 polymorphism with obesity and polycystic ovarian syndrome in Pakistani women. *J Med Res Biol Stud*, 1, 2018.

Rosenfield, R. L., Barnes, R. B., Cara, J. F., and Lucky, A. W. (1990). Dysregulation of cytochrome P450c17α as the cause of polycystic ovarian syndrome. *Fertil Steril.*, 53, 785–791. doi:10.1016/S0015-0282(16)53510-9.

Roy, A. C., Liao, W. X., Chen, Y., Arulkumaran, S., and Ratnam, S. S. (1996). Identification of seven novel mutations in LH?-Subunit gene by SSCP. *Mol Cell Biochem.*, 165(2), 151–153. doi:10.1007/BF00229477.

Sachdeva, G., Gainder, S., Suri, V., Sachdeva, N., and Chopra, S. (2019). Comparison of the different PCOS phenotypes based on clinical metabolic, and hormonal profile, and their response to clomiphene. *Indian J Endocr Metab.*, 23, 326-31.

Sahmay, S., Atakul, N., Oncul, M., Tuten, A., Aydogan, B., and Seyisoglu, H. (2013). Serum anti-mullerian hormone levels in the main phenotypes of polycystic ovary syndrome. *Eur J Obstet Gynecol Reprod Biol.*, 170, 157-161. doi:10.1016/j.ejogrb.2013.05.019.

Sir-Petermann, T., Pérez-Bravo, F., Angel, B., Maliqueo, M., Calvillan, M., and Palomino, A. (2001). G972R polymorphism of IRS-1 in women with polycystic ovary syndrome [3]. *Diabetologia.*, 44, 1200–1201.

Stein, I. F., and Leventhal, M. L. (1935). Amenorrhea associated with bilateral polycystic ovaries. *Am J Obstet Gynecol.*, 29, 181-191.

Tucker, R. (2019). Case-based learning; acne vulgaris. *Pharm J.*, 302(7926), 359–363. doi: 10.1211/PJ.2019.20206226.

Tummon, I., Gavrilova-Jordan, L., Allemand, M. C., and Session, D. (2005). Polycystic ovaries and ovarian hyperstimulation syndrome: a systematic review. *Acta Obstet Gynecol Scand.*, 84, 611–616.

Urbanek, M., Legro, R. S., Driscoll, D. A., Azziz, R., Ehrmann, D. A., Norman, R. J., Strauss, J. F., 3rd. Spielman, R. S., and Dunaif, A. (1999). Thirty-seven candidate genes for polycystic ovary syndrome: strongest evidence for linkage is with follistatin. *Proc Natl Acad Sci U S A.*, 96, 8573–8578 doi:10.1073/pnas.96.15.8573.

Urbanek, M., Woodroffe, A., Ewens, K. G., Diamanti-Kandarakis, E., Legro, R. S., Strauss, J. F., 3rd. Dunaif, A., and Spielman, R. S. (2005). Candidate gene region for polycystic ovary syndrome on chromosome 19p13.2. *J Clin Endocrinol Metab.*, 90(12), 6623–6629. doi:10.1210/jc.2005-0622.

Urbanek, M. (2007). The genetics of the polycystic ovary syndrome. *Nature Clin Pract Endocrinol Metab.*, 3,103–111.doi:10.1038/ncpendmet0400.

Vaniqa, A. (2017). Electronic medicines compendium. Available at: https://www.medicines.org.uk/emc (accessed March 2020).

Victor, V. M., Rocha, M., Bañuls, C., Sanchez-Serrano, M., Sola, E., Gomez, M., and Hernandez-Mijares, A. (2009). Mitochondrial complex I impairment in leukocytes from polycystic ovary syndrome patients with insulin resistance. *J Clin Endocrinol Metab.*, 94, 3505–3512. doi:10.1210/jc.2009-0466.

Villarroel, C., Merino, P. M., López, P., Eyzaguirre, F. C., Van, Velzen, A., Iñiguez, G., and Codner, E. (2011). Polycystic ovarian morphology in adolescents with regular menstrual cycles is associated with elevated anti-Mllerian hormone. *Hum Reprod.*, 26, 2861–2868. doi:10.1093/humrep/der223.

Vink, J. M., Sadrzadeh, S., Lambalk, C. B., and Boomsma, D. I. (2006). Heritability of polycystic ovary syndrome in a Dutch twin-family study. *J Clin Endocrinol Metab.*, 91(6), 2100-4. doi: 10.1210/jc.2005-1494. Epub 2005 Oct 11. PMID: 16219714.

Wang, Y., Wu, X. K., Cao, Y., Yi, L., and Chen, J. (2006). A microsatellite polymorphism (tttta)n in the promoter of the CYP11a gene in Chinese women with polycystic ovary syndrome. *Fertil Steril.*, 86, 223–226.

Warren-Ulanch, J., and Arslanian, S. (2006). Treatment of PCOS in adolescence. *Best Pract Res Clin Endocrinol Metab.*, 20(2), 311–330. doi: 10.1016/j.beem.2006.02.002.

Waterworth, D. M., Bennett, S. T., Gharani, N., McCarthy, M. I., Hague, S., Batty, S., Conway, G. S., White, D., Todd, J. A., Franks, S., and Williamson, R. (1997). Linkage and association of insulin gene VNTR regulatory polymorphism with polycystic ovary syndrome. *Lancet.*, 349, 986–990. doi:10.1016/S0140-6736(96)08368-7.

Webber, L. J., Stubbs, S., Stark, J., Trew, G. H., Margara, R., Hardy, K., and Franks, S. (2003). Formation and early development of follicles in the polycystic ovary. *Lancet.*, 362, 1017–1021. doi:10.1016/S0140-6736(03)14410-8.

Wickenheisser, J. K., Quinn, P. G., Nelson, V. L., Legro, R. S., Strauss, J. F., and Mcallister, J. M. (2000). Differential activity of the cytochrome P450 17α-hydroxylase and steroidogenic acute regulatory protein gene promoters in normal and polycystic ovary syndrome theca cells. *J Clin Endocrinol Metab.*, 85, 2304–2311.

Wickham, E. P., Ewens, K. G., Legro, R. S., Dunaif, A., Nestler, J. E., and Strauss, J. F. (2011). Polymorphisms in the SHBG gene influence serum SHBG levels in women with polycystic ovary syndrome. *J Clin Endocrinol Metab.*, 96, 719-727. doi:10.1210/jc.2010-1842.

Witchel, S. F., and Aston, C. E. (2000). The role of heterozygosity for CYP21 in the polycystic ovary syndrome. *J Pediatr Endocrinol Metab.*, 13, 1315–1317

Witchel, S. F., Kahsar-Miller, M., Aston, C. E., White, C., and Azziz, R. (2005). Prevalence of CYP21 mutations and IRS1 variant among women with polycystic ovary syndrome and adrenal androgen excess. *Fertil Steril.*, 83, 371–375. doi:10.1016/j.fertnstert.2004.10.027.

Yang, R., Qin, Li, Q., and Zhou, Z. (2022). Changes in the prevalence of polycystic ovary syndrome in China over the past decade. *The Lancet Regional Health- Western Pacific*, 25, 100494. https://doi.org/10.1016/j.lanwpc.2022.100494.

## Chapter 15

# Epigenetic Markers in the Pathogenesis of Polycystic Ovary Syndrome

**Syed Douhath Yousuf**[1]
**Saliha Rizvi**[2]
**Gowhar Rashid**[3]
**and Mohammad Ashraf Ganie**[4,*]

[1]Department of Clinical Biochemistry, Sher-i-Kashmir Institute of Medical Sciences, SKIMS, Soura, Srinagar, Jammu and Kashmir, India
[2]Department of Biotechnology, Era University, Lucknow, India
[3]Department of Amity Medical School, Amity University Haryana, India
[4]Department of Endocrinology, Sher-i-Kashmir Institute of Medical Sciences, SKIMS, Soura, Srinagar, Jammu and Kashmir, India

## Abstract

Epigenetic modifications have been recently found to be implicated in polycystic ovary syndrome (PCOS) pathogenesis. Numerous studies revealed that women with PCOS have altered DNA methylation and miRNA profiles, which may be brought on by environmental factors like nutrition and/or obesity. Because of the heterogeneity in the phenotype expression between people and family lineages, emphasis has been focused on genetic and epigenetic modifications in an attempt to explain these variations. Therefore, accurate investigation of the genetic and epigenetic mechanisms is fundamental to understanding this condition, which may help to improve the molecular profiling for specific PCOS phenotypes and thus lead to accuracy of diagnosis and individualized future treatment options. The objective of this chapter is to give updated information to the readers on the epigenetic changes studied so far in patients with PCOS.

**Keywords:** DNA methylation, epigenetic markers, genetics, GWAS, miRNAs, polycystic ovary syndrome, SNP

* Corresponding Author's Email: ashraf.endo@gmail.com.

In: Polycystic Ovarian Syndrome (PCOS) and Our Biological Clock
Editors: Arpita Roy, Gowhar Rashid and Nihad Ashraf Khan
ISBN: 979-8-89113-100-2
© 2023 Nova Science Publishers, Inc.

## 1. Introduction

Polycystic ovary syndrome (PCOS) is one of the most prevalent endocrine diseases, impacting approximately 5-20% of adult women of childbearing age ("Revised 2003 consensus on diagnostic criteria and long-term health risks related to polycystic ovary syndrome (PCOS)," 2004). It is a heterogeneous and complex condition with multiple factors like non-functional ovaries, high androgen levels, and polycystic ovaries all of which can contribute to an infertile state in women (Eiras et al., 2022). Apart from its reproductive repercussions, PCOS is linked with several other complications like metabolic disorders, insulin resistance (IR), high BMI, type 2 diabetes (T2D), and cardiovascular complications.

The pathogenesis of PCOS is influenced by both genetic and environmental variables (Vázquez-Martínez et al., 2019). IR and maternal hyperandrogenism can be passed down to children, and obesity brought on by an imbalance between caloric consumption and energy exertion can raise androgen production and have an impact on how severe IR is, both of which can add to the development of PCOS (Merkin et al., 2016). To date, attempts to understand the genetic foundation of PCOS have concentrated on candidate genes selected from rational paths such as steroid synthesis or insulin signaling. Despite several good findings, no genes are universally recognized as essential in PCOS pathogenesis, owing to a dearth of replication of positive results. Recent studies have focused on the epigenetic process of PCOS as environmental and hormonal changes have a direct impact on clinical symptoms and the onset of PCOS. Ambient factors affecting epigenetic modifications, like intrauterine hormonal and metabolic shifts affecting the growth of embryos and adulthood lifestyle, are examples of environmental epigenetic modifications which in a variety of clinical symptoms, may all contribute to PCOS development.

In this chapter, we attempted to understand the different factors affecting the mechanism of regulation of epigenetics in PCOS, highlighting DNA methylation, transcriptome, and miRNA profiles in PCOS patients. It encompasses the central role of DNA methylation as an epigenetic modification affecting the phenotype of disease trait PCOS women that also accounts for future epigenetic inheritance of disease genotype. Apart from this histone alterations also provide for strong paternal germline intergenerational inheritance. The chapter also discusses the role of small non-coding RNAs and how the heritability of metabolic characteristics may potentially be influenced by alterations in the levels of these non-coding RNAs in adipose tissue, skeletal muscle, ovarian tissue, and cumulus granulosa cells. MicroRNA (miRNA) plays a role in steroid synthesis, cell death, and cell growth of ovarian cells and have been linked to PCOS in numerous genome-wide investigations (Mu et al., 2021; Sirotkin et al., 2010). The methylation levels of different genes reported in PCOS disrupt several biochemical networks and physiological functions which could be analyzed with ease in peripheral blood, serum, and plasma. Furthermore, the information provided in the chapter could help in identifying novel methods for future research resulting in proper and accurate diagnosis and a more personalized and efficient future therapy. These possible epigenetic indicators of PCOS might also prove to be beneficial for the management of related comorbidities.

## 2. Epigenetics

The etiology and pathophysiology of this disease may be influenced by environmental and epigenetic factors that affect gene expression at transcription and post-transcriptional levels. Silent features of genes controlling PCOS functional features include epigenetic regulation of expression, DNA methylation/histone modification, enhancer-binding, binding of the transcription factor, promoter function, and gene expression profile. Significant epigenetic and transcriptome differences have been found in the blood, serum, adipose tissue, oocytes, follicular fluid, and skeletal muscle of women with PCOS, which may contribute to the pathogenesis. These modifications imply that alteration in the expression of genes that determine tissue function, as well as the emergence of PCOS and associated comorbidities, are likely to be influenced by tissue-specific DNA methylation patterns. PCOS and its accompanying complications like ineffectiveness to insulin, high androgen levels, persistent anovulation, high BMI, and other endocrine/metabolic abnormalities are linked to a disturbance in the expression of miRNA and non-coding RNAs, in addition to altered DNA methylation. Further research into DNA/histone methylation and miRNA patterns could increase diagnosis accuracy and lead to new therapeutic options in the future. To treat related comorbidities and improve the quality of life for PCOS women, this chapter aims to present updated information on the linked non-coding RNAs (ncRNAs) and miRNAs as possible epigenetic markers of PCOS.

Early studies of embryonic development (Maass et al., 2014; Mu et al., 2021; Slack, 2002) and cellular phenotypic maintenance during mitosis (Nanney, 1958) were the primary topics of epigenetics research before shifting to the role of methylation of DNA and its implication in the regulation of transcription of specific genes and differentiation of cells (Holliday & Pugh, 1975; Nanney, 1958). Epigenetics is now commonly used to describe a variety of biological elements and functions involved in gene expression, and chromatin structure, including DNA modification, nuclear architecture, and ncRNAs (Bird, 2007; Cavalli & Heard, 2019; Goldberg et al., 2007) (Figure 1).

Notably, epigenetic changes in daughter cells after mitotic or meiotic division are not only heritable but also reversible. As a result, epigenetic mechanisms may serve as a link between early-life exposures and later phenotypic diversity and may play a role in disease transmission as well as therapeutic interventions.

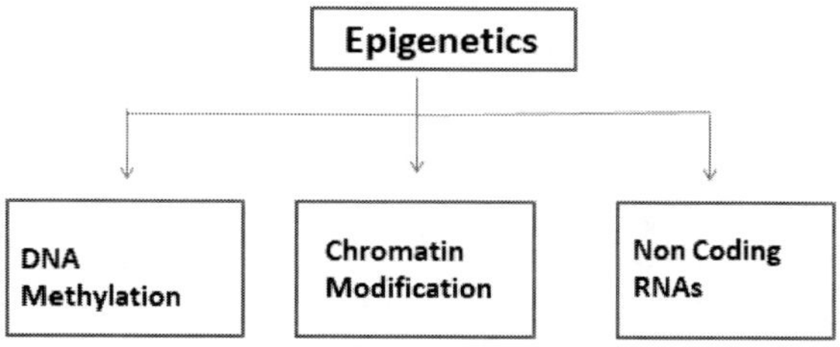


**Figure 1**. Major Epigenetic Processes.

## 2.1. DNA Methylation

One of the most extensively researched epigenetic processes is DNA methylation, which is essential for the regulation of gene expression in health and illness. The methylation of DNA at gene bodies, CpG islands (containing coding and non-coding sequences in a transcriptome), imprinting regulatory loci, and jumping genes. It is linked with slower transcription levels and genomic imprinting.

The maintenance, formation along with erasure of DNA methylation have all been studied extensively. DNA (cytosine-5) methyltransferase 1 (DNMT1) and the E3 ubiquitin-protein ligase UHRF (Bostick et al., 2007; Sharif et al., 2007; Song et al., 2011), attach to hemimethylated CpG dinucleotides selectively at replication forks while keeping the methylation pattern precise during DNA replication. UHRF1 then recruits DNMT1, which then releases its self-suppression and methylates the newly synthesized DNA strand (Bourc'his et al., 2001; Okano et al., 1999). DNMT3A and DNMT3B are the two primary de novo DNA methylation enzymes in mammals (Barau et al., 2016; Kriaucionis & Heintz, 2009). DNMT3L is a germline-specific gene that is required in maternal genomic imprinting. This gene has no catalytic action, but its association with DNMT3A and DNMT3B provides the methyltransferase function (Tahiliani et al., 2009). De novo methylation activity is also present in DNMT3C (Ito et al., 2011).

DNA methylation, in essence, ensures genetic stability. The methylcytosine dioxygenases namely TET1, TET2, and TET3, on other hand, demethylate DNA by oxidizing methylcytosine. 5- methylcytosine is gradually transformed to 5 formyl cytosine, 5-hydroxymethylcytosine, and 5- carboxyl cytosine in this process (Greenberg & Bourc'his, 2019; Tang et al., 2015; L. Wang et al., 2014). Two crucial rounds of global DNA methylation erasure that remove acquired epimutations take place during early embryogenesis and germline development. This erasure, however, is insufficient, as around 20% of DNA methylation loci (6–8% of CpGs) retain methylation in every cycle (Skvortsova et al., 2018). Therefore, more than 116,000 genomic sites stay hypermethylated in human primordial germ cells even after global demethylation(Steger & Balhorn, 2018). DNA sequences around transposable elements and imprinting regulatory regions are largely resistant to demethylation. Some single-copy DNA sequences, on the other hand, remain unmethylated and may play a role in epigenetic inheritance (Hammoud et al., 2009).

## 2.2. Chromatin Modifications

Most nucleosomes in animals are substituted by protamines to help with the compaction of the paternal DNA during spermatogenesis (Steger & Balhorn, 2018). Some locations may still have modifications in nucleosomes and histones, which will epigenetically affect embryonic development and possibly transfer regulatory states, particularly those that contain important developmental genes and miRNA clusters (Hammoud et al., 2009). Mammalian eggs transmit to embryonic cells both activating (H3K4me3) and inhibitory (H3K27me3) histone alterations, which may have an impact on how embryonic development is controlled. Maternal imprinting in rodent embryos is significantly influenced by transcriptional suppression mediated by H3K27me3, which is distinct from DNA methylation (Inoue et al., 2017). Across numerous mitotic and meiotic cell cycles, intrinsic heterochromatin (defined by the H3K9me3 change) can be epigenetically transmitted in cis in rodents and yeast (Dahl et al., 2016). Histone alterations also provide for strong paternal germline intergenerational inheritance (Brykczynska et al., 2010; Erkek et al., 2013; Peters et al., 2001).

### 2.3. Small Noncoding RNAs

Numerous RNAs that are non-coding, such as miRNAs, siRNAs, tsRNAs and piRNAs serve in different species as heritable controllers of genomic elements and play a role in both embryonic development and the transfer of acquired traits (Duempelmann et al., 2020). Various short RNAs, for example, control transcriptional or post-transcriptional processes within or outside chromatin, triggering shifts in gene expression that last a long time in reaction to environmental cues (Zhang et al., 2019). Also, extrinsic signals that cause phenotypic alterations affect the number and sequence of these small RNAs in germline cells. Apart from DNA, ncRNAs found in mammalian sperm are reportedly found to act as a reservoir of male heritable traits (Zhang et al., 2019). Studies have demonstrated a causative link between changed metabolic and behavioural traits in the progeny and sperm RNAs from male rodents subjected to a variety of environmental stressors, such as social stress or an unhealthy diet. The transmission of traits to children is also linked to the loss of small RNA sequences in parents (Gapp et al., 2014). Thus, the heritability of metabolic characteristics may potentially be influenced by RNA alterations (Zhang et al., 2021).

## 3. Epigenetic Changes in PCOS Women

### 3.1. Epigenetic Changes in PCOS Women's Adipose Tissue

Women with PCOS exhibit abnormal morphology in their adipose tissue, including larger fat cells, high-fat mass, and slowed adiponectin synthesis (Jonkhout et al., 2017). There were 440 locations with different CpG methylation identified in a study that looked at the universal DNA methylation patterns in subcutaneous adipose tissue of PCOS women and matched controls, of which 33 were linked to 30 diversely expressed genes (Kokosar et al., 2016).

The 600 kb stretch surrounding these uniquely expressed and methylated genes is discovered to be correlated with pathway regulation of adipogenesis, inflammation, sex hormone metabolism, energy metabolism, and regulation of glucose using at the transcriptional level.

Another study looked at the methylation of DNA at genes associated with PCOS and examined single-nucleotide polymorphisms (SNPs) in subcutaneous adipose tissue in PCOS cases and controls to see if there were any PCOS-specific changes (Mannerås-Holm et al., 2011). The researchers found diverse patterns of DNA methylation at genes responsible for measurable phenotypes, as well as reduced methylation at the *LHCGR* gene and greater methylation at the INSR gene in PCOS, demonstrating the significance of local genetic variation in gene regulation (Dahlman et al., 2015).

Loss of weight or medical treatments like low-frequency electrical stimulation can reverse DNA methylation patterns in subcutaneous adipose tissue, demonstrating flexibility (Jones et al., 2015). Due to the ease of access, human investigations have concentrated on subcutaneous fat, while primates subjected to mother androgens during gestation have been the only species in which visceral adipose tissue has been studied. Only a few of the overall reported genes are uniquely transcribed in subcutaneous adipose tissue and displayed a different DNA methylation pattern in omental adipose tissue (Dahlman et al., 2015; Kokosar et al., 2018).

It was discovered that regions with varying levels of methylation overlay with variably synthesized genes for cell metabolism and cAMP signaling and were abundant in transcription factor binding motifs (Carbone et al., 2019). Furthermore, 97 miRNAs have been related to changed glucose and lipid metabolism, dysfunction of the reproductive system, and distinct expression in women with and without PCOS (Xu et al., 2010). The overexpressed *miR-93* was discovered to be highly associated with PCOS.It causes IR by suppressing the *GLUT4* gene. Experiments in women with PCOS demonstrated that *miR-93* expression is adverse to the expression of *MCM7* (Chen et al., 2013) (Table 1).

### 3.2. Epigenetic Alterations in Skeletal Muscle of PCOS Women

Skeletal muscle absorbs the vast bulk of the blood's supply of glucose. IR is related to abnormalities in insulin signalling in skeletal muscle in women with PCOS, which is a T2D risk factor. To present, a single study looked into the methylation level of DNA in skeletal muscle, in PCOS women. Even though the researchers discovered 85 differently expressed transcripts, after statistical adjustment for multiple comparisons, only two CpG sites had variable methylation (Nilsson et al., 2018).

The minimal number of relationships found could be due to the study's short sample size, 30% of differently expressed genes were linked with methylation of DNA at CpG islands proximal to skeletal muscle genes, indicating that methylation of DNA couldn't impact these genes' expression (Benrick et al., 2020). Alterations induced by electrical stimulation in gene expression and DNA methylation in skeletal muscle. *miR-485-3p* was found to be increased in skeletal muscles where it suppresses *PGC-1* and causes PCOS women to become insulin resistant (Skov et al., 2007) (Table 1).

### 3.3. Epigenetic Alterations in Ovarian Tissue and Cumulus Granulosa Cells of PCOS Women

The arrest of follicular maturation causes oligoovulation or anovulation, which is one of the most common symptoms of PCOS. Due to the scarcity and difficulty of obtaining ovarian tissue of PCOS subjects, only limited data on DNA methylation profiles in human ovarian tissue have been reported with controversial findings. Hypermethylated genomic regions were detected at CpG loci coasts and high CpG promoters in PCOS, but lesser DNA methylation levels were observed within genes. In women with PCOS, however, CpG islands and CpG island coasts were hypomethylated, according to another study. Furthermore, the two investigations assessed DNA methylation using distinct methods: focused assays or whole genome sequencing (X. X. Wang et al., 2014; Yu et al., 2015). Nonetheless, the findings of this research imply that genes implicated in glucose metabolism, hormone activity, inflammation, and insulin signaling cascade are methylated differently in PCOS as compared to control subjects. Importantly, genome wide association studies (GWAS) have linked polymorphisms in *CYP19A1* to PCOS, and higher levels of methylation in *CYP19A1* promoter coincide with altered androgen levels seen in PCOS subjects (Yu et al., 2013). Changes in DNA methylation, on the other hand, contribute mildly to the altered gene expression seen in ovarian tissue from PCOS women, as has been reported in other tissues (Yu et al., 2013).

Several investigations of DNA methylation in ovarian granulosa cells, which play a key role in folliculogenesis and steroidogenesis, have been done. Comparatively speaking to other cell categories, cumulus granulosa cells were easily accessible since they may typically be pulled off from the oocytes undergoing in vitro maturation while in vitro fertilization and are in metaphase II (MII). Hypomethylation at the promoters of *YAP1, LHCGR*, NCOR1, and HDAC3 has been linked to ovarian disease, apart from granulosa cell proliferation, increase in expression of LH receptor, and disturbed hormonal signaling (Qu et al., 2012; P. Wang et al., 2014).

The low levels of methylation at CpG loci at 5′ UTR of transposon namely, *LINE1* identified in granulosa cells, is an indicator of the cumulative hypomethylation of DNA. *CYP19A1 and PPARG* promoter regions, on the other hand, are hypermethylated, indicating that androgen metabolism is suppressed (Xu et al., 2016). The genome-wide studies on DNA methylation in granulosa cells, of obese PCOS cases, showed 5,202 and 6,936 (compared to healthy control women) unique methylation profiles at CpG loci on comparing with non-obese PCOS cases and healthy controls respectively. Women with PCOS were found to have double the number of variably methylated CpG loci as compared to healthy non-obese controls (Sagvekar et al., 2019).

This finding implies that obesity has an impact on granulosa cell epigenetic programming, which might relate to PCOS pathogenesis. A study that employed next generation sequencing technique, discovered reduced methylation in 977 CpG loci encoding 2,063 genes and hypermethylation at 2,509 CpG sites within 1,777 transcripts. The ovarian form, function, and hormonal regulation are all linked to these differential methylation genes (Sagvekar et al., 2019).

In granulosa cells, miRNAs influence both folliculogenesis and steroid production. The loss of Dicer1 activity in granulosa cells in rodents causes sterility and a variety of other abnormalities, such as the quick activation of primordial follicles that ultimately degenerate (Imbar & Eisenberg, 2014). In women with PCOS, *miR-15a* and *miR-182* levels (that regulate steroidogenesis, proliferation, and cell death) are significantly reduced in granulocytes, whereas the expression of *miR-93 and miR-21* is significantly enhanced (Nagaraja et al., 2008; Naji et al., 2017).

The growth factors belonging to the transforming growth factor (TGF) family had been linked to granulosa cell development and differentiation. The expression of miR-24 (which lowers oestradiol secretion by inhibiting TGF signaling) is higher in PCOS subjects. Furthermore, the miR-27a-3p expression has been linked to hormonal dysregulation and granulosa cell death, suggesting that it may play a role in the pathogenesis of PCOS (Table 1). Despite this accumulating body of findings, the effect of epigenetic modifications in PCOS etiology is yet unknown (Lei et al., 2010; Naji et al., 2018). More research should be undertaken to understand the genetic pathways to examine the phenotypic effects of epigenetic modifications in different tissues, both common and distinct. The pathophysiology of PCOS may also be connected to crosstalk between these pathways.

**Table 1.** Differentially methylated genes and miRNA expression reported in tissues from patients with PCOS

| S No. | Tissues | DNA Methylation | Upregulated miRNA | Downregulated miRNA |
|---|---|---|---|---|
| 1. | Adipose tissue | Decreased methylation of DNA in *the LHCGR* gene. Higher methylation of DNA in INSR gene (Dahlman et al., 2015) | *miR-93 (Chen et al., 2013)* | -- |
| 2. | Skeletal muscles | 85 genes showed altered expressions and altered methylation of two CpG loci (Nilsson et al., 2018). Accounting for 30% of altered gene expression due to methylation on CpG loci (Benrick et al., 2020). | *miR-485-3p (Skov et al., 2007)* | -- |
| 3. | Ovarian tissue and cumulus granulosa cells | Increase in DNA methylation at *CYP19A1* promoter (Yu et al., 2013).<br>Hypomethylation at promoters of *LHCGR, YAP1, HDAC3 and NCOR1 (Qu et al., 2012; P. Wang et al., 2014)*<br>Decreased methylation levels at CpG loci at 5′ UTR in *LINE (Xu et al., 2016).*<br>Increase in the frequency of methylation at *CYP19A1 and PPARG* promoters (Xu et al., 2016). | *miR-93*<br>*miR-21*<br>*miR-24*<br>*miR-27a-3p*<br>(Lei et al., 2010; Nagaraja et al., 2008; Naji et al., 2017; Naji et al., 2018) | *miR-15a*<br>*miR-182*<br>(Nagaraja et al., 2008; Naji et al., 2017) |
| 4. | Peripheral blood, serum, and plasma | The promoters of *FST* (which encodes follistatin), *LMNA* (which encodes Lamin A/C), and *PPARGC1A* (peroxisome proliferator-activated receptor gamma coactivator-1) have all seen an increase in DNA methylation<br>(Li et al., 2017; Sang et al., 2014). | *miR-19a*<br>*miR-16*<br>*miR-30c*<br>*miR-24*<br>*miR-146a*<br>*miR-106b*<br>*miR-222*<br>*miR-106 (Ding et al., 2015; Hosseini et al., 2017; Long et al., 2014)* | miR-320 (Ding et al., 2015; Hosseini et al., 2017; Long et al., 2014) |

## 3.4. Epigenetic Alterations in Peripheral Blood, Serum, and Plasma of PCOS Women

Along with genome-wide methylation studies on DNA carried out in PCOS women, research targeting the analysis of methylation levels of different genes has been reported. The promoters of *FST* (follistatin), *LMNA* (Lamin A/C), and *PPARGC1A* (peroxisome proliferator-activated receptor gamma coactivator-1) have observed a heightened methylation level. In PCOS cases, lower amounts of this epigenetic marker are located in the promoters of the *LHCGR* gene (encodes the LH receptor) and the *EPHX1* gene (encodes epoxide hydrolase 1) compared to controls (Li et al., 2017; Sang et al., 2014). PCOS disrupts several biochemical networks and physiological functions like follicular formation, which were linked to changes in DNA methylation. Infertility, steroidogenesis, glucose metabolism, and insulin signaling are some of the topics that have been studied (Eldar-Geva et al., 2001; Hai et al., 2015; Vandenbeek et al., 2018).

MiRNAs are long-lasting, resistant to ribozyme action, and easily detectable in serum. As a result, miRNAs might serve as non-invasive biomarkers for PCOS. According to several studies, levels of these small RNAs are reportedly different in PCOS cases as compared to controls (Munker & Calin, 2011; Murri et al., 2013). Long et al. used miRNA arrays and reported a heightened expression of *miR-24, miR-16, miR-30c, miR-19a, miR-146a, miR-320, miR-222, miR-186, and miR-106b* in PCOS women's serum, whereas *miR-320* was found to be downregulated. The *miR-146a, miR-30c, and miR-222* showed a statistically significant increase in PCOS cases (Long et al., 2014).

Out of the different miRNA reported *miR-146a, miR-222, and miR-30c* was recommended to be viable biomarker for PCOS based on sensitivity and specificity study. The *rs2910164 and rs2858060* polymorphisms in *miR-146a and miR-222* are strongly related to a higher incidence of PCOS. Apart from the *rs2910164* polymorphism in *miR-146a* polymorphism was also found to be significantly associated with PCOS risk in another study (Ding et al., 2015; Hosseini et al., 2017) (Table 1).

## Conclusion

It is difficult to comprehend the processes underpinning the pathophysiology of PCOS and its effects on female reproduction because it is a heterogeneous, multifactorial, and complicated disease. The variety of clinical symptoms seen in PCOS points to a pathophysiology that involves several different variables in combination. PCOS develops throughout life due to a combination of genetic susceptibility (candidate genes), a significant environmental impact brought on by lifestyle modifications, obesity, and hormonal and metabolic disruptors. The chapter intended to give a summary of recent studies on PCOS, DNA methylation, and other epigenetic issues. Developmental PCOS or its related clinical abnormalities after delivery may be brought on by environmental-driven epigenetic alterations brought on due to an unfavorable environment (increased secretion of androgens) in the uterus during the development of the embryo in primitive stages. Clinical manifestations of PCOS and its effect on overall body hemostasis, however, have a high degree of flexibility and can change or even go away throughout a lifetime. Through epigenetic changes in gene expression, changes in lifestyle, such as increased physical exercise and a healthy diet, have a direct impact on metabolic diseases and enhance fertility in PCOS patients. The discovery of potential molecular markers and epigenetic alterations linked to the various PCOS phenotypes, including IR, hyperandrogenism, chronic anovulation, obesity, and other related alterations, may help guide treatment and enhance fertility in affected patients.

## Future Perspective

Individualized medicine combined with targeted therapy appears to be a viable treatment option for this illness. Molecular profiling could help identify which populations in a community should be evaluated and treated with eradication therapy before permanent effects like infertility, T2D, and CVD occur. The ultimate goal of studying the molecular basis of any disease is to develop individualized treatments. However, more investigation is further needed to clarify the part played by epigenetic alterations in the etiology of PCOS.

## References


Barau, J., Teissandier, A., Zamudio, N., Roy, S., Nalesso, V., Hérault, Y., Guillou, F., & Bourc'his, D. (2016). The DNA methyltransferase DNMT3C protects male germ cells from transposon activity. *Science*, *354*(6314), 909-912. https://doi.org/10.1126/science.aah5143.

Benrick, A., Pillon, N. J., Nilsson, E., Lindgren, E., Krook, A., Ling, C., & Stener-Victorin, E. (2020). Electroacupuncture Mimics Exercise-Induced Changes in Skeletal Muscle Gene Expression in Women With Polycystic Ovary Syndrome. *J Clin Endocrinol Metab*, *105*(6), 2027-2041. https://doi.org/10.1210/clinem/dgaa165.

Bird, A. (2007). Perceptions of epigenetics. *Nature*, *447*(7143), 396-398. https://doi.org/10.1038/nature05913.

Bostick, M., Kim, J. K., Estève, P. O., Clark, A., Pradhan, S., & Jacobsen, S. E. (2007). UHRF1 plays a role in maintaining DNA methylation in mammalian cells. *Science*, *317*(5845), 1760-1764. https://doi.org/10.1126/science.1147939.

Bourc'his, D., Xu, G. L., Lin, C. S., Bollman, B., & Bestor, T. H. (2001). Dnmt3L and the establishment of maternal genomic imprints. *Science*, *294*(5551), 2536-2539. https://doi.org/10.1126/science.1065848.

Brykczynska, U., Hisano, M., Erkek, S., Ramos, L., Oakeley, E. J., Roloff, T. C., Beisel, C., Schübeler, D., Stadler, M. B., & Peters, A. H. (2010). Repressive and active histone methylation mark distinct promoters in human and mouse spermatozoa. *Nat Struct Mol Biol*, *17*(6), 679-687. https://doi.org/10.1038/nsmb.1821.

Carbone, L., Davis, B. A., Fei, S. S., White, A., Nevonen, K. A., Takahashi, D., Vinson, A., True, C., Roberts, C. T., Jr., & Varlamov, O. (2019). Synergistic Effects of Hyperandrogenemia and Obesogenic Western-style Diet on Transcription and DNA Methylation in Visceral Adipose Tissue of Nonhuman Primates. *Sci Rep*, *9*(1), 19232. https://doi.org/10.1038/s41598-019-55291-8.

Cavalli, G., & Heard, E. (2019). Advances in epigenetics link genetics to the environment and disease. *Nature*, *571*(7766), 489-499. https://doi.org/10.1038/s41586-019-1411-0.

Chen, Y. H., Heneidi, S., Lee, J. M., Layman, L. C., Stepp, D. W., Gamboa, G. M., Chen, B. S., Chazenbalk, G., & Azziz, R. (2013). miRNA-93 inhibits GLUT4 and is overexpressed in adipose tissue of polycystic ovary syndrome patients and women with insulin resistance. *Diabetes*, *62*(7), 2278-2286. https://doi.org/10.2337/db12-0963.

Dahl, J. A., Jung, I., Aanes, H., Greggains, G. D., Manaf, A., Lerdrup, M., Li, G., Kuan, S., Li, B., Lee, A. Y., Preissl, S., Jermstad, I., Haugen, M. H., Suganthan, R., Bjørås, M., Hansen, K., Dalen, K. T., Fedorcsak, P., Ren, B., & Klungland, A. (2016). Broad histone H3K4me3 domains in mouse oocytes modulate maternal-to-zygotic transition. *Nature*, *537*(7621), 548-552. https://doi.org/10.1038/nature19360.

Dahlman, I., Sinha, I., Gao, H., Brodin, D., Thorell, A., Rydén, M., Andersson, D. P., Henriksson, J., Perfilyev, A., Ling, C., Dahlman-Wright, K., & Arner, P. (2015). The fat cell epigenetic signature in post-obese women is characterized by global hypomethylation and differential DNA methylation of adipogenesis genes. *Int J Obes (Lond)*, *39*(6), 910-919. https://doi.org/10.1038/ijo.2015.31.

Ding, C. F., Chen, W. Q., Zhu, Y. T., Bo, Y. L., Hu, H. M., & Zheng, R. H. (2015). Circulating microRNAs in patients with polycystic ovary syndrome. *Hum Fertil (Camb)*, *18*(1), 22-29. https://doi.org/10.3109/14647273.2014.956811.

Duempelmann, L., Skribbe, M., & Bühler, M. (2020). Small RNAs in the Transgenerational Inheritance of Epigenetic Information. *Trends Genet*, *36*(3), 203-214. https://doi.org/10.1016/j.tig.2019.12.001.

Eiras, M. C., Pinheiro, D. P., Romcy, K. A. M., Ferriani, R. A., Reis, R. M. D., & Furtado, C. L. M. (2022). Polycystic Ovary Syndrome: the Epigenetics Behind the Disease. *Reprod Sci*, *29*(3), 680-694. https://doi.org/10.1007/s43032-021-00516-3.

Eldar-Geva, T., Spitz, I. M., Groome, N. P., Margalioth, E. J., & Homburg, R. (2001). Follistatin and activin A serum concentrations in obese and non-obese patients with polycystic ovary syndrome. *Hum Reprod*, *16*(12), 2552-2556. https://doi.org/10.1093/humrep/16.12.2552.

Erkek, S., Hisano, M., Liang, C. Y., Gill, M., Murr, R., Dieker, J., Schübeler, D., van der Vlag, J., Stadler, M. B., & Peters, A. H. (2013). Molecular determinants of nucleosome retention at CpG-rich sequences in mouse spermatozoa. *Nat Struct Mol Biol*, *20*(7), 868-875. https://doi.org/10.1038/nsmb.2599.

Gapp, K., Jawaid, A., Sarkies, P., Bohacek, J., Pelczar, P., Prados, J., Farinelli, L., Miska, E., & Mansuy, I. M. (2014). Implication of sperm RNAs in transgenerational inheritance of the effects of early trauma in mice. *Nat Neurosci*, *17*(5), 667-669. https://doi.org/10.1038/nn.3695.

Goldberg, A. D., Allis, C. D., & Bernstein, E. (2007). Epigenetics: a landscape takes shape. *Cell*, *128*(4), 635-638. https://doi.org/10.1016/j.cell.2007.02.006.

Greenberg, M. V. C., & Bourc'his, D. (2019). The diverse roles of DNA methylation in mammalian development and disease. *Nat Rev Mol Cell Biol*, *20*(10), 590-607. https://doi.org/10.1038/s41580-019-0159-6.

Hai, L., McGee, S. R., Rabideau, A. C., Paquet, M., & Narayan, P. (2015). Infertility in Female Mice with a Gain-of-Function Mutation in the Luteinizing Hormone Receptor Is Due to Irregular Estrous Cyclicity, Anovulation, Hormonal Alterations, and Polycystic Ovaries. *Biol Reprod*, *93*(1), 16. https://doi.org/10.1095/biolreprod.115.129072.

Hammoud, S. S., Nix, D. A., Zhang, H., Purwar, J., Carrell, D. T., & Cairns, B. R. (2009). Distinctive chromatin in human sperm packages genes for embryo development. *Nature*, *460*(7254), 473-478. https://doi.org/10.1038/nature08162.

Holliday, R., & Pugh, J. E. (1975). DNA modification mechanisms and gene activity during development. *Science*, *187*(4173), 226-232.

Hosseini, A. H., Kohan, L., Aledavood, A., & Rostami, S. (2017). Association of miR-146a rs2910164 and miR-222 rs2858060 polymorphisms with the risk of polycystic ovary syndrome in Iranian women: A case-control study. *Taiwan J Obstet Gynecol*, *56*(5), 652-656. https://doi.org/10.1016/j.tjog.2017.08.014.

Imbar, T., & Eisenberg, I. (2014). Regulatory role of microRNAs in ovarian function. *Fertil Steril*, *101*(6), 1524-1530. https://doi.org/10.1016/j.fertnstert.2014.04.024.

Inoue, A., Jiang, L., Lu, F., Suzuki, T., & Zhang, Y. (2017). Maternal H3K27me3 controls DNA methylation-independent imprinting. *Nature*, *547*(7664), 419-424. https://doi.org/10.1038/nature23262.

Ito, S., Shen, L., Dai, Q., Wu, S. C., Collins, L. B., Swenberg, J. A., He, C., & Zhang, Y. (2011). Tet proteins can convert 5-methylcytosine to 5-formylcytosine and 5-carboxylcytosine. *Science*, *333*(6047), 1300-1303. https://doi.org/10.1126/science.1210597.

Jones, M. R., Brower, M. A., Xu, N., Cui, J., Mengesha, E., Chen, Y. D., Taylor, K. D., Azziz, R., & Goodarzi, M. O. (2015). Systems Genetics Reveals the Functional Context of PCOS Loci and Identifies Genetic and Molecular Mechanisms of Disease Heterogeneity. *PLoS Genet*, *11*(8), e1005455. https://doi.org/10.1371/journal.pgen.1005455.

Jonkhout, N., Tran, J., Smith, M. A., Schonrock, N., Mattick, J. S., & Novoa, E. M. (2017). The RNA modification landscape in human disease. *Rna*, *23*(12), 1754-1769. https://doi.org/10.1261/rna.063503.117.

Kokosar, M., Benrick, A., Perfilyev, A., Fornes, R., Nilsson, E., Maliqueo, M., Behre, C. J., Sazonova, A., Ohlsson, C., Ling, C., & Stener-Victorin, E. (2016). Epigenetic and Transcriptional Alterations in Human Adipose Tissue of Polycystic Ovary Syndrome. *Sci Rep*, *6*, 22883. https://doi.org/10.1038/srep22883.

Kokosar, M., Benrick, A., Perfilyev, A., Nilsson, E., Källman, T., Ohlsson, C., Ling, C., & Stener-Victorin, E. (2018). A Single Bout of Electroacupuncture Remodels Epigenetic and Transcriptional Changes in Adipose Tissue in Polycystic Ovary Syndrome. *Sci Rep*, *8*(1), 1878. https://doi.org/10.1038/s41598-017-17919-5.

Kriaucionis, S., & Heintz, N. (2009). The nuclear DNA base 5-hydroxymethylcytosine is present in Purkinje neurons and the brain. *Science*, *324*(5929), 929-930. https://doi.org/10.1126/science.1169786.

Lei, L., Jin, S., Gonzalez, G., Behringer, R. R., & Woodruff, T. K. (2010). The regulatory role of Dicer in folliculogenesis in mice. *Mol Cell Endocrinol*, *315*(1-2), 63-73. https://doi.org/10.1016/j.mce.2009.09.021.

Li, S., Zhu, D., Duan, H., Ren, A., Glintborg, D., Andersen, M., Skov, V., Thomassen, M., Kruse, T., & Tan, Q. (2017). Differential DNA methylation patterns of polycystic ovarian syndrome in whole blood of Chinese women. *Oncotarget*, *8*(13), 20656-20666. https://doi.org/10.18632/oncotarget.9327.

Long, W., Zhao, C., Ji, C., Ding, H., Cui, Y., Guo, X., Shen, R., & Liu, J. (2014). Characterization of serum microRNAs profile of PCOS and identification of novel non-invasive biomarkers. *Cell Physiol Biochem*, *33*(5), 1304-1315. https://doi.org/10.1159/000358698.

Maass, P. G., Luft, F. C., & Bähring, S. (2014). Long non-coding RNA in health and disease. *J Mol Med (Berl)*, *92*(4), 337-346. https://doi.org/10.1007/s00109-014-1131-8.

Mannerås-Holm, L., Leonhardt, H., Kullberg, J., Jennische, E., Odén, A., Holm, G., Hellström, M., Lönn, L., Olivecrona, G., Stener-Victorin, E., & Lönn, M. (2011). Adipose tissue has aberrant morphology and function in PCOS: enlarged adipocytes and low serum adiponectin, but not circulating sex steroids, are strongly associated with insulin resistance. *J Clin Endocrinol Metab*, *96*(2), E304-311. https://doi.org/10.1210/jc.2010-1290.

Merkin, S. S., Phy, J. L., Sites, C. K., & Yang, D. (2016). Environmental determinants of polycystic ovary syndrome. *Fertil Steril*, *106*(1), 16-24. https://doi.org/10.1016/j.fertnstert.2016.05.011.

Mu, L., Sun, X., Tu, M., & Zhang, D. (2021). Non-coding RNAs in polycystic ovary syndrome: a systematic review and meta-analysis. *Reprod Biol Endocrinol*, *19*(1), 10. https://doi.org/10.1186/s12958-020-00687-9.

Munker, R., & Calin, G. A. (2011). MicroRNA profiling in cancer. *Clin Sci (Lond)*, *121*(4), 141-158. https://doi.org/10.1042/cs20110005.

Murri, M., Insenser, M., Fernández-Durán, E., San-Millán, J. L., & Escobar-Morreale, H. F. (2013). Effects of polycystic ovary syndrome (PCOS), sex hormones, and obesity on circulating miRNA-21, miRNA-27b, miRNA-103, and miRNA-155 expression. *J Clin Endocrinol Metab*, *98*(11), E1835-1844. https://doi.org/10.1210/jc.2013-2218.

Nagaraja, A. K., Andreu-Vieyra, C., Franco, H. L., Ma, L., Chen, R., Han, D. Y., Zhu, H., Agno, J. E., Gunaratne, P. H., DeMayo, F. J., & Matzuk, M. M. (2008). Deletion of Dicer in somatic cells of the female reproductive tract causes sterility. *Mol Endocrinol*, *22*(10), 2336-2352. https://doi.org/10.1210/me.2008-0142.

Naji, M., Aleyasin, A., Nekoonam, S., Arefian, E., Mahdian, R., & Amidi, F. (2017). Differential Expression of miR-93 and miR-21 in Granulosa Cells and Follicular Fluid of Polycystic Ovary Syndrome Associating with Different Phenotypes. *Sci Rep*, *7*(1), 14671. https://doi.org/10.1038/s41598-017-13250-1.

Naji, M., Nekoonam, S., Aleyasin, A., Arefian, E., Mahdian, R., Azizi, E., Shabani Nashtaei, M., & Amidi, F. (2018). Expression of miR-15a, miR-145, and miR-182 in granulosa lutein cells, follicular fluid, and serum of women with polycystic ovary syndrome (PCOS). *Arch Gynecol Obstet*, *297*(1), 221-231. https://doi.org/10.1007/s00404-017-4570-y.

Nanney, D. L. (1958). EPIGENETIC CONTROL SYSTEMS. *Proc Natl Acad Sci USA*, *44*(7), 712-717. https://doi.org/10.1073/pnas.44.7.712.

Nilsson, E., Benrick, A., Kokosar, M., Krook, A., Lindgren, E., Källman, T., Martis, M. M., Højlund, K., Ling, C., & Stener-Victorin, E. (2018). Transcriptional and Epigenetic Changes Influencing Skeletal Muscle Metabolism in Women With Polycystic Ovary Syndrome. *J Clin Endocrinol Metab*, *103*(12), 4465-4477. https://doi.org/10.1210/jc.2018-00935.

Okano, M., Bell, D. W., Haber, D. A., & Li, E. (1999). DNA methyltransferases Dnmt3a and Dnmt3b are essential for de novo methylation and mammalian development. *Cell*, *99*(3), 247-257. https://doi.org/10.1016/s0092-8674(00)81656-6.

Peters, A. H., O'Carroll, D., Scherthan, H., Mechtler, K., Sauer, S., Schöfer, C., Weipoltshammer, K., Pagani, M., Lachner, M., Kohlmaier, A., Opravil, S., Doyle, M., Sibilia, M., & Jenuwein, T. (2001). Loss of the Suv39h histone methyltransferases impairs mammalian heterochromatin and genome stability. *Cell*, *107*(3), 323-337. https://doi.org/10.1016/s0092-8674(01)00542-6.

Qu, F., Wang, F. F., Yin, R., Ding, G. L., El-Prince, M., Gao, Q., Shi, B. W., Pan, H. H., Huang, Y. T., Jin, M., Leung, P. C., Sheng, J. Z., & Huang, H. F. (2012). A molecular mechanism underlying ovarian dysfunction of polycystic ovary syndrome: hyperandrogenism induces epigenetic alterations in the granulosa cells. *J Mol Med (Berl)*, *90*(8), 911-923. https://doi.org/10.1007/s00109-012-0881-4.

Revised 2003 consensus on diagnostic criteria and long-term health risks related to polycystic ovary syndrome (PCOS). (2004). *Hum Reprod*, *19*(1), 41-47. https://doi.org/10.1093/humrep/deh098.

Sagvekar, P., Kumar, P., Mangoli, V., Desai, S., & Mukherjee, S. (2019). DNA methylome profiling of granulosa cells reveals altered methylation in genes regulating vital ovarian functions in polycystic ovary syndrome. *Clin Epigenetics*, *11*(1), 61. https://doi.org/10.1186/s13148-019-0657-6.

Sang, Q., Li, X., Wang, H., Wang, H., Zhang, S., Feng, R., Xu, Y., Li, Q., Zhao, X., Xing, Q., Jin, L., He, L., & Wang, L. (2014). Quantitative methylation level of the EPHX1 promoter in peripheral blood DNA is associated with polycystic ovary syndrome. *PLoS One*, *9*(2), e88013. https://doi.org/10.1371/journal.pone.0088013.

Sharif, J., Muto, M., Takebayashi, S., Suetake, I., Iwamatsu, A., Endo, T. A., Shinga, J., Mizutani-Koseki, Y., Toyoda, T., Okamura, K., Tajima, S., Mitsuya, K., Okano, M., & Koseki, H. (2007). The SRA protein Np95 mediates epigenetic inheritance by recruiting Dnmt1 to methylated DNA. *Nature*, *450*(7171), 908-912. https://doi.org/10.1038/nature06397 .

Sirotkin, A. V., Lauková, M., Ovcharenko, D., Brenaut, P., & Mlyncek, M. (2010). Identification of microRNAs controlling human ovarian cell proliferation and apoptosis. *J Cell Physiol*, *223*(1), 49-56. https://doi.org/10.1002/jcp.21999.

Skov, V., Glintborg, D., Knudsen, S., Jensen, T., Kruse, T. A., Tan, Q., Brusgaard, K., Beck-Nielsen, H., & Højlund, K. (2007). Reduced expression of nuclear-encoded genes involved in mitochondrial oxidative metabolism in skeletal muscle of insulin-resistant women with polycystic ovary syndrome. *Diabetes*, *56*(9), 2349-2355. https://doi.org/10.2337/db07-0275.

Skvortsova, K., Iovino, N., & Bogdanović, O. (2018). Functions and mechanisms of epigenetic inheritance in animals. *Nat Rev Mol Cell Biol*, *19*(12), 774-790. https://doi.org/10.1038/s41580-018-0074-2.

Slack, J. M. (2002). Conrad Hal Waddington: the last Renaissance biologist? *Nat Rev Genet*, *3*(11), 889-895. https://doi.org/10.1038/nrg933.

Song, J., Rechkoblit, O., Bestor, T. H., & Patel, D. J. (2011). Structure of DNMT1-DNA complex reveals a role for autoinhibition in maintenance DNA methylation. *Science*, *331*(6020), 1036-1040. https://doi.org/10.1126/science.1195380.

Steger, K., & Balhorn, R. (2018). Sperm nuclear protamines: A checkpoint to control sperm chromatin quality. *Anat Histol Embryol*, *47*(4), 273-279. https://doi.org/10.1111/ahe.12361.

Tahiliani, M., Koh, K. P., Shen, Y., Pastor, W. A., Bandukwala, H., Brudno, Y., Agarwal, S., Iyer, L. M., Liu, D. R., Aravind, L., & Rao, A. (2009). Conversion of 5-methylcytosine to 5-hydroxymethylcytosine in mammalian DNA by MLL partner TET1. *Science*, *324*(5929), 930-935. https://doi.org/10.1126/science.1170116.

Tang, W. W., Dietmann, S., Irie, N., Leitch, H. G., Floros, V. I., Bradshaw, C. R., Hackett, J. A., Chinnery, P. F., & Surani, M. A. (2015). A Unique Gene Regulatory Network Resets the Human Germline Epigenome for Development. *Cell*, *161*(6), 1453-1467. https://doi.org/10.1016/j.cell.2015.04.053.

Vandenbeek, R., Khan, N. P., & Estall, J. L. (2018). Linking Metabolic Disease With the PGC-1α Gly482Ser Polymorphism. *Endocrinology*, *159*(2), 853-865. https://doi.org/10.1210/en.2017-00872.

Vázquez-Martínez, E. R., Gómez-Viais, Y. I., García-Gómez, E., Reyes-Mayoral, C., Reyes-Muñoz, E., Camacho-Arroyo, I., & Cerbón, M. (2019). DNA methylation in the pathogenesis of polycystic ovary syndrome. *Reproduction*, *158*(1), R27-r40. https://doi.org/10.1530/rep-18-0449.

Wang, L., Zhang, J., Duan, J., Gao, X., Zhu, W., Lu, X., Yang, L., Zhang, J., Li, G., Ci, W., Li, W., Zhou, Q., Aluru, N., Tang, F., He, C., Huang, X., & Liu, J. (2014). Programming and inheritance of parental DNA methylomes in mammals. *Cell*, *157*(4), 979-991. https://doi.org/10.1016/j.cell.2014.04.017.

Wang, P., Zhao, H., Li, T., Zhang, W., Wu, K., Li, M., Bian, Y., Liu, H., Ning, Y., Li, G., & Chen, Z. J. (2014). Hypomethylation of the LH/choriogonadotropin receptor promoter region is a potential mechanism underlying susceptibility to polycystic ovary syndrome. *Endocrinology*, *155*(4), 1445-1452. https://doi.org/10.1210/en.2013-1764.

Wang, X. X., Wei, J. Z., Jiao, J., Jiang, S. Y., Yu, D. H., & Li, D. (2014). Genome-wide DNA methylation and gene expression patterns provide insight into polycystic ovary syndrome development. *Oncotarget*, *5*(16), 6603-6610. https://doi.org/10.18632/oncotarget.2224.

Xu, J., Bao, X., Peng, Z., Wang, L., Du, L., Niu, W., & Sun, Y. (2016). Comprehensive analysis of genome-wide DNA methylation across human polycystic ovary syndrome ovary granulosa cell. *Oncotarget*, *7*(19), 27899-27909. https://doi.org/10.18632/oncotarget.8544.

Xu, N., Azziz, R., & Goodarzi, M. O. (2010). Epigenetics in polycystic ovary syndrome: a pilot study of global DNA methylation. *Fertil Steril*, *94*(2), 781-783.e781. https://doi.org/10.1016/j.fertnstert.2009.10.020.

Yu, Y. Y., Sun, C. X., Liu, Y. K., Li, Y., Wang, L., & Zhang, W. (2013). Promoter methylation of CYP19A1 gene in Chinese polycystic ovary syndrome patients. *Gynecol Obstet Invest*, *76*(4), 209-213. https://doi.org/10.1159/000355314.

Yu, Y. Y., Sun, C. X., Liu, Y. K., Li, Y., Wang, L., & Zhang, W. (2015). Genome-wide screen of ovary-specific DNA methylation in polycystic ovary syndrome. *Fertil Steril*, *104*(1), 145-153.e146. https://doi.org/10.1016/j.fertnstert.2015.04.005.

Zhang, Y., Ren, L., Sun, X., Zhang, Z., Liu, J., Xin, Y., Yu, J., Jia, Y., Sheng, J., Hu, G. F., Zhao, R., & He, B. (2021). Angiogenin mediates paternal inflammation-induced metabolic disorders in offspring through sperm tsRNAs. *Nat Commun*, *12*(1), 6673. https://doi.org/10.1038/s41467-021-26909-1.

Zhang, Y., Shi, J., Rassoulzadegan, M., Tuorto, F., & Chen, Q. (2019). Sperm RNA code programmes the metabolic health of offspring. *Nat Rev Endocrinol*, *15*(8), 489-498. https://doi.org/10.1038/s41574-019-0226-2.

## Chapter 16

# A Conclusion and Novel Approach Towards PCOS: A Lifestyle Disorder and Several Measures to Mitigate or Eliminate Its Effects

**Ananya Chakraborty***

Department of Biotechnology, Adamas University, Kolkata, India

## Abstract

PCOS influences the quality of life and can exacerbate worry and stress levels due to painful signs and the diagnosis process. A healthy lifestyle is important to manage PCOS including modification in regular exercise, a balanced diet, and achieving and managing a healthy weight. Energy homeostasis anomalies may also be present in PCOS women. The substrate oxidation or carbohydrate-to-fat oxidation ratio is related to the respiratory leverage ratio or respiratory quotient (RQ). RQ is reportedly elevated in PCOS-affected women. The ability to switch from lipid oxidation in fasting circumstances to lipid access in non-fasting conditions, also known as metabolic flexibility, is assessed by contrasting RQ during the fasting phase with an insulin-rich state. Many healthy foods and diets can help to control PCOS. A healthy diet includes plenty of vegetables and fruits, lean protein, whole grains, low-fat dairy products, and less consumption of processed foods and sugars. Limiting saturated fat, cholesterol, and sodium can also help to control PCOS. Importantly, children and adolescents who engage in moderate to vigorous physical activity every day for at least 60 minutes have improved physical and mental health. Due to this issue, not all PCOS teenagers may have lower LH levels after LSM according to our findings.

**Keywords**: respiratory quotient, diet management, physical and mental health, healthy lifestyle, artificial intelligence, exercise

## 1. Introduction

Excess stress can wreak havoc on health in any situation, but it is especially harmful when they have polycystic ovary syndrome (PCOS). Yoga is beneficial for so many different aspects of a

* Corresponding Author's Email: ananya6899@gmail.com.

In: Polycystic Ovarian Syndrome (PCOS) and Our Biological Clock
Editors: Arpita Roy, Gowhar Rashid and Nihad Ashraf Khan
ISBN: 979-8-89113-100-2
© 2023 Nova Science Publishers, Inc.

person's life, including emotional stability and physical health. Yoga can help to improve our emotional stability and mood by helping to reduce stress and anxiety. Additionally, yoga can help to improve our physical health by helping to improve flexibility and balance. In general, a diet rich in fibre, low in sugar, and low in calories are likely to be beneficial. The disorder known as polycystic ovarian syndrome is linked to a higher risk of obesity, type 2 diabetes, and heart disease. To manage these risks, it is important to maintain a healthy weight and to make sure that our diet includes enough fibre, fruits, vegetables, and whole grains.

Lifestyle diseases, which share risk factors with prolonged exposure to three modifiable lifestyle behaviours: poor eating, smoking, and inactivity, can cause chronic diseases like heart disease, diabetes, stroke, obesity, and metabolic syndrome. Smoking, which can result in lung cancer, heart disease, type II diabetes, obesity, and stroke, as well as insufficient physical exercise, poor diet, drinking, and substance misuse issues affects PCOS indirectly. Overall, these all come under the section of a healthy lifestyle and omitting some of these can lead to a change in internal operations which might cause PCOS. People who battle with a lifestyle disorder can believe that to feel "normal," they must adhere to a specific set of rules. This can be very challenging because following these guidelines frequently requires making significant adjustments to how one lives. The respiratory quotient (RQ) is a measure of how efficiently a person breathes. Persons with a high RQ usually breathe more air than those with a low RQ which is common in PCOS women.

Many medications are prescribed to treat PCOS. These medications can improve the symptoms of PCOS, such as acne, excess hair growth, and difficulty losing weight. Some of the most used medications to treat PCOS include birth control pills, testosterone therapy, and spironolactone. Birth control pills are one of the most used medications to treat PCOS. Birth control pills function by blocking the release of eggs from the ovaries.

Medical science is constantly evolving, and many novel approaches are being developed that could improve patient care. Gene therapy is a new approach to treating diseases that uses genetic instructions to modify or delete disease-causing genes. This technology has been used to treat conditions such as cancer and is being developed as a treatment for other diseases, including Alzheimer's and Parkinson's. PCOS is a highly complex and heterogeneous disorder. Although variations between and within families, the genetic cause of PCOS is linked to a common mechanism. PCOS is a common condition that reflects a harmful impact on women of reproductive age. About one in ten women develop the condition, and it can lead to several health problems, including obesity, infertility, and chronic pain. There is no definitive test for PCOS, and diagnosis can be difficult. However, there are various ways to detect PCOS in women. Some of the most common methods include blood tests, hormone tests, and ultrasound tests. One of the most common methods for detecting PCOS is a blood test. This test measures levels of certain hormones, including testosterone, insulin, and glucose. In this chapter, there will be the critical justification of different innovative approaches that can solve complications of PCOS.

## 2. Different Aspects of PCOS

### 2.1. Importance of a Balanced and Nutritious Diet on PCOS

PCOS affects the quality of life and can exacerbate worry and depression caused by symptoms. A healthy lifestyle includes a balanced diet, regular exercise, and achieving weight maintenance (Alshammari et al., 2020). Regular exercise can be extremely helpful in the treatment of PCOS. It helps fight against obesity by burning calories and boosting muscle mass, which reduces insulin resistance. Up to 15% of women of reproductive age have PCOS, a prevalent condition that affects the ovaries. Prior research is suggested that PCOS may be linked to psychiatric and mood issues (Barrea et al., 2023). In addition to affecting the quality of life, PCOS can make anxiety and sadness worse due to symptoms. A balanced diet, obtaining and maintaining a healthy weight, and frequent exercise are all components of a healthy lifestyle. Anomalies in energy homeostasis may also exist in PCOS women.

PCOS can increase a patient's risk of Type 2 diabetes and heart disease. Even though PCOS is currently incurable, lifestyle and dietary adjustments, such as better food, more exercise, cosmetic procedures, and medication, may help with the symptoms. Making a few little modifications to their lifestyle can help them treat PCOS naturally. To lower inflammation and assist regulate insulin levels, an optimal PCOS diet might forego alcohol and tobacco in addition to sugar, animal fats, processed meals, and dairy items. According to research, having PCOS symptoms such as excessive hair loss, weight changes, acne, and fertility issues can have a detrimental impact on self-confidence, mood, and body image. The ovaries are thus stimulated to create additional hormones, including testosterone, because of the high insulin levels. In turn, this causes problems like weight gain, irregular menstruation periods, and hair growth.

## 2.2. Challenges of the Respiratory System due to PCOS

The respiratory leverage ratio or respiratory quotient is connected to the substrate oxidation or carbohydrate-to-fat oxidation ratio (RQ). According to reports, women with PCOS had higher RQ levels. By comparing RQ during the hungry phase with an insulin-rich state, metabolic flexibility, sometimes referred to as the ability to switch from lipid oxidation to lipid access, is evaluated (Brutocao et al., 2018). Diets and meals rich in nutrients with reducing saturated fat, cholesterol, and salt can help manage PCOS. A balanced diet includes plenty of fruits and vegetables, lean protein, whole grains, low-fat dairy products, and less processed food and sugar. Importantly, the physical and mental health of kids and teenagers who exercise every day for at least 60 minutes is better when they conduct moderate to strenuous physical activity. Different data suggest that not all PCOS teenagers have reduced LH levels following LSM because of a lack of physical activity. It should be kept in mind that during adolescence, height is not stable, which may affect BMI estimates.

## 2.3. Effects of Hormones on PCOS

PCOS is a condition that is defined by an increase in the levels of testosterone and a decrease in the levels of progesterone. This can lead to several problems, including an increased risk of developing other conditions, such as high blood pressure, diabetes, and obesity. One of the main problems associated with PCOS is a mismatch between the levels of the hormone testosterone and progesterone (Chang & Coffler, 2007). This can lead to an increase in the levels of testosterone and a decrease in the levels of progesterone, which cause problems with the rhythm of the body's natural clock. PCOS is a common hormonal disorder that can lead to a host of health problems, including osteoporosis. PCOS is characterized by an imbalance of testosterone and oestrogen, which can cause increased levels of the male sex hormone in women and an excess of the female sex hormone in the body. This can lead to an increase in the size and number of the ovaries, as well as an increase in the production of male hormones. Women with PCOS are often obese because they have difficulty regulating their weight. Their insulin levels are high, and this makes it difficult for them to burn calories. They also have trouble getting rid of fat. In addition, PCOS can lead to other problems, such as irregular periods and infertility. If left untreated, PCOS can lead to obesity and other health problems, such as cancer, heart disease, and Type II diabetes.

Insulin resistance, a disorder in which the body has difficulty using insulin, is also linked to PCOS. A primary risk factor for type 2 diabetes, which is characterized by high blood sugar levels, is insulin resistance. PCOS is a complex condition that is often difficult to diagnose. Symptoms may vary from woman to woman and may go unrecognized for years.

There is a strong correlation between PCOS and an elevated level of androgens in women. Androgens are a group of hormones that are responsible for the development of male characteristics in women, such as increased muscle mass and aggression. The increase in androgens can lead to the development of PCOS, a condition that is characterized by an irregular menstrual cycle, excess hair growth, and difficulty with fertility. Androgens also play a role in the development of obesity, insulin resistance, and heart disease, all of which are common problems in women with PCOS. There is increasing evidence that PCOS, or polycystic ovary syndrome, is a condition that can be caused by an increased level of androgens. Androgens are hormones that are responsible for the development of male reproductive organs, such as the testicles. PCOS is a condition that is characterized by excessive production of androgens. Although the precise cause of PCOS is unknown, several reasons could apply. Genetic predisposition, obesity, androgen receptor mutations, androgen receptor activator medications, and environmental variables are some of the factors that may lead to the development of PCOS.

## 2.4. Effect of Polymorphism on PCOS

Polymorphism is a term used to describe a person's genetic makeup that produces different results in different situations. When it comes to PCOS, polymorphism has been shown to play a role in the development of the disorder. PCOS is a health condition that affects women of reproductive age. The disorder is characterized by irregular periods, excess hair growth, and difficulty getting pregnant. PCOS is a complex condition that is caused by a variety of factors, including genetics. Studies have shown that PCOS is associated with polymorphism in the genes that control the menstrual cycle. Complex illnesses with unidentified aetiology, such as PCOS, may be attributed to genetic polymorphisms linked to individual differences and variations. Iranian women with PCOS have been found to carry several prominent genetic markers with established biological activities. Genetic variations in the population are caused by mutations in the human genome. Even though many of these are thought to be "normal" variations, many of them cause human disease and are often kept in the population by a delicate balance between selection and mutation. The genetic variation in exon 1 of the AR gene, which contains CAG repeats, suggests a connection between the incidence of PCOS and AR activity. One of the main treatments for PCOS is anti-musician hormone therapy (AMH). AMH is a hormone that helps to regulate the level of testosterone in the body. AMH levels are usually low in women with PCOS. This is because the ovaries in these women do not produce enough AMH. AMH therapy can help to regulate testosterone levels and improve the symptoms of PCOS.

## 2.5. PCOS as a Genetic Disorder

The autosomal dominant pattern of inheritance in PCOS families, which may be brought on by the same gene, is congruent with how PCO and PMPB are inherited. Families of women without PCOS did not experience this genetic influence. Another gene implicated in the development and progression of PCOS is Cytochrome P450, Family 21, subfamily A member 2. It has 10 exons and is located on chromosome 6p21.33. A heterozygous mutation in CYP21A2 may be involved in the aetiology of PCOS. There have been discussions on genes like Cytochrome family p450, CAPN10, Insulin gene, FTO, AR, and FSHR. The gene for androgen receptor (AR).

PCOS is a condition that is extremely complex and heterogeneous. The genetic basis of PCOS is connected to a common mechanism despite variations across and within families. Due to complexity and variety, a genetic material or nuclear factor in a single family has not been described. The autosomal dominant pattern of inheritance in PCOS families, which may be brought on by the same gene, is congruent with how PCO and PMPB are inherited. Families of women without PCOS did not experience this genetic influence. Up to 70% of women with PCOS go on to have daughters who also have the condition, but the genetic variation does not fully account for the high incidence within families; according to some genome-wide linkage maps of PCOS susceptibility, genetics only accounts for 10% of the condition's heritability.

PCOS is a condition that affects a woman's reproductive system. It is a common condition, affecting up to one in five women. A combination of genetics and lifestyle causes PCOS (Couillaud et al., 2019). There is no one cause of PCOS, but it is often linked to obesity, insulin resistance, and diabetes. These three factors can interfere with a woman's reproductive system, leading to PCOS. One of the main symptoms of PCOS is irregular or absent menstrual cycles. This can make it difficult for a woman to conceive. Other common symptoms of PCOS include heavy periods, acne, and hair growth on the face and chest.

Clinic-based research is shown that women with PCOS are more likely than comparison groups of women without the condition to experience sleep disruptions and abnormalities, such as obstructive sleep apnoea and excessive daytime sleepiness. It is also known that unhealthy habits leading to obesity, hyperinsulinemia, insulin resistance, and hyperandrogenism are risk factors for the development of PCOS in women. A crucial component of controlling PCOS is changing their diet. Insulin is a hormone the body uses to control high blood sugar levels, and people with PCOS typically have greater levels of this hormone. The body may stop paying attention to the hormone if insulin levels are consistently high. Blood sugar levels could consequently continue to be excessive.

## 3. Novel Approches

Many novel approaches are being developed to treat PCOS, and many of these are still in the early stages of development. Studies have shown that treating PCOS with drugs that target the insulin-signalling pathway can be very effective in treating the condition. These drugs include things like metformin and thiazolidinediones, which work by decreasing the amount of insulin that is produced by the pancreas. Many women with PCOS also have problems with their ovaries, which can lead to development. There is no one-size-fits-all answer to this question, as the effects of PCOS on a person's overall health and well-being will vary depending on the extent and severity of the condition. However, some tips on how to mitigate or eliminate the effects of PCOS on a person's life include the following:

- Regularly monitoring blood sugar levels and adjusting lifestyle and diet accordingly;
- Taking prescribed medications as prescribed by a doctor to treat the condition;
- Reducing stress levels;
- Ensuring a healthy weight; and
- Maintaining a healthy balance of exercise and rest.

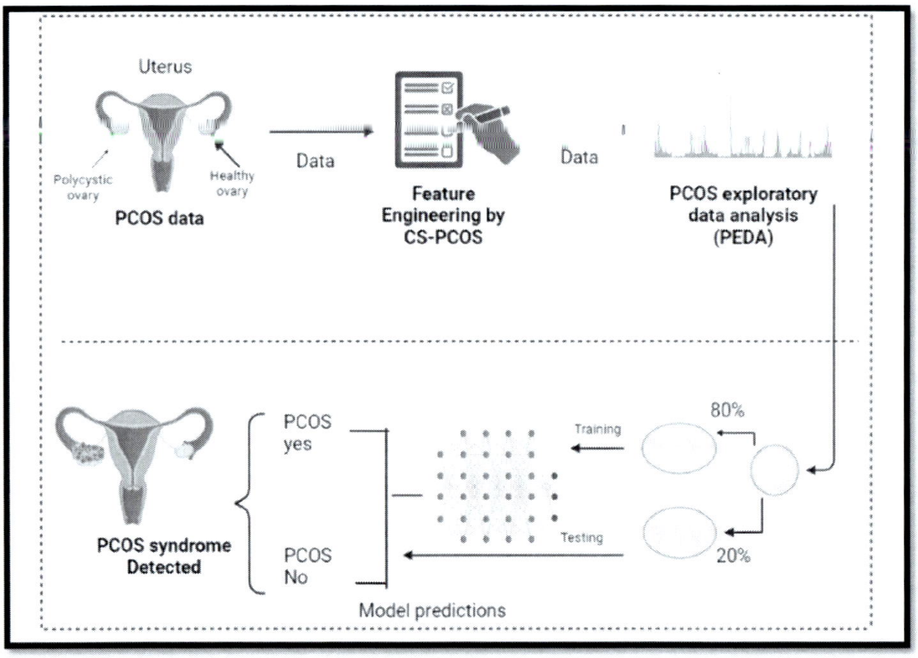


**Figure 1.** PCOS detection process. This figure shows the detailed process through which data will be analysed and the AI-dependent process that ensures the presence of PCOS. Initially, it shows PCOS data collection from patients and is transferred to an automated system for detailed analysis. Furthermore, testing and training are used for confirming the PCOS.

For PCOS patients who are trying to get pregnant, clomiphene may be the first medication suggested. The monthly production of an egg from the ovaries is encouraged by clomiphene (ovulation). Metformin may be suggested as a backup medication if clomiphene is unable to promote ovulation. PCOS's clinical symptoms are made worse by obesity. Problems with reproduction such as irregular menstrual cycles, decreased fertility, a drop in ovulation frequency, polycystic ovaries on ultrasound, and excessive levels of male hormones are among these clinical features like testosterone (Denny et al., 2019). Acne and undesirable hair growth on the face or body can both be caused by raised hormone levels. *Figure 1 illustrates* a flow diagram of data collection and exploratory analysis through (PEDA). Finally, through training machine learning and AI- dependent analysis predicts the presence of PCOS. Additionally, PCOS is linked to metabolic characteristics, abnormal cholesterol levels, including elevated insulin levels or insulin resistance, and risk factors for heart disease and diabetes (Guan et al., 2020). Because of its symptoms or because it has been identified as a chronic disease, PCOS can aggravate anxiety and depression and harm the quality of life. PCOS cannot be cured, but its symptoms can be managed.

### 3.1. Novel Approach of CS-PCOS Method in PCOS

The chi squared PCOS (CSPCOS) mechanism is a unique feature selection method that is suggested. Comparatively, the 10 hyper-parametrized machine learning algorithms are used. The Gaussian naive Bayes (GNB) surpassed machine learning models and innovative studies when using the innovative CS-PCOS technique (Nasim et al., 2022). Chi-squared PCOS method is a widely used statistical method for analysing data. This method is used to determine the association between two variables. The CS-PCOS method is used to choose the dataset features with the highest relevance values before creating machine learning models. The suggested model by the authors outperformed machine learning methods and previously proposed state-of-the-art studies by employing the CS-PCOS strategy (Guerain, 2020). The most notable indicators with a significant impact on PCOS prediction include prolactin (PRL), thyroid stimulating hormone (TSH), relative risk (RR-breaths), blood pressure (systolic and diastolic), and pregnancy.

### 3.2. Significant Dietary Change for PCOS Treatment

Additionally, it was discovered that people with PCOS consumed more low- and free-fat milk. According to the findings of previous studies, low-fat milk, and PCOS have a beneficial link. Dairy products with little fat may raise levels of insulin-like growth factor I. They need to make sure to include plenty of vegetables, fruits, and whole grains in their meals, as these foods are high in fibre and nutrients that are beneficial for PCOS. Additionally, bananas have a mild GI, making it safe for people with PCOS to consume them in moderation. Overindulgence, however, could cause spikes or rises in blood glucose levels. According to studies, a balanced diet can help manage and prevent polycystic ovarian syndrome (PCOS). It is a terrific approach to receive the vital vitamins, minerals, and fibre required to lessen and prevent chronic disease to consume dried fruits including dates, black raisins, apricots, and Anjeer. Red grapes, blackberries, papaya, blueberries, cherries, and melon are just a few examples of coloured fruits that are high in antioxidants and fibre while being low in glycaemic index, making them beneficial for PCOS sufferers. They also state their desires for sweets. Bananas are a wonderful source of potassium, fibre, and vitamins. They do, however, have a moderate GI, which can cause blood sugar levels to rise. Therefore, if you have PCOS, it is better to ingest bananas in moderation. PCOS sufferers can feed curd but should be careful with their quantity sizes. Curd can provide the patient's body with the required nutrients and has a considerably lower carbohydrate level than other dairy products.

### 3.3. Reduction of Stress to Improve Health Condition in PCOS Patients

Moreover, there is a lot of debate surrounding the effects of reducing stress levels in PCOS. Some people believe that it can improve symptoms while others feel that it can aggravate them. It is important to discuss the effects of stress levels in PCOS with doctors if they are experiencing them. The most common symptom of PCOS is ovulation problems. Stress can worsen ovulation problems by increasing the number of stress hormones in the patient's body. These hormones can interfere with the body's natural ovulation process. When ovulation problems occur, it is more difficult to get pregnant. Stress can increase levels of the stress hormone cortisol, which can lead to an increased risk of developing PCOS. Cortisol can also damage the cells in the reproductive system, leading to infertility. Coping with stress can be difficult for people with PCOS. Many people with PCOS experience heightened levels of stress due to the condition.

Stress is known to be brought on by PCOS itself, especially when it comes to the condition's visible signs like excessive body and facial hair. Anxiety and sadness might result from this tension. Women with PCOS who are younger are more likely to be affected. Furthermore, compared to lean patients, participants with PCOS who were overweight had greater amylase activity. The subjects with PCOS had significantly higher pulse rates, BMIs, adiposity, and waist-hip ratios (WHRs) than the controls. Between BMI or WHR, as appropriate, and -amylase activity among PCOS patients, a substantial association could be inferred. These findings point to a significant relationship between the subsequently proved changes in the body composition characteristics of PCOS patients. Salivary amylase (SAA) and corticosteroids have been identified as sensitive biomarkers for alterations brought on by stress in the body and as being crucial for maintaining metabolic homeostasis. These signify the sympathetic-adrenal medullary (SAM) and hypothalamic-pituitary-adrenal (HPA) axes being activated, respectively.

### 3.4. AI-Based PCOS Prediction for Better Treatment

There is currently no accurate diagnostic test for PCOS, which affects up to one-third of all women of reproductive age. However, several diagnostic methods are being developed that are based on artificial intelligence (AI). One such method is called the PCOS Detection AI Suite. This is a tool that uses a variety of AI algorithms to detect the presence of PCOS. The tool is based on several different factors, including the levels of circulating hormones, the size and shape of the ovaries, and the levels of inflammation in the abdomen.

The inclusion of AI-based analysis can support the medical system for the early identification and prediction of PCOS using ideal and basic but effective clinical and metabolic criteria that serve as an early marker for this condition. Understand the early prediction process will likely be subjective. There is no right or wrong way to predict PCOS, and each woman will develop her approach over time. AI may be able to diagnose PCOS by learning features in self-correcting elements. Various research projects to identify and diagnose PCOS use AI techniques such as neural networks, Convolution Neural Networks (CNN), logistic regression, Bayesian Classifiers, support vector machines, k-nearest neighbours, and others.

### 3.5. Observation of PCOS through the Menstrual Cycle

Although the development of PCOS throughout the early adolescent years is not fully understood, it appears to entail aberrant hypothalamic-pituitary-ovarian-adrenal axis activity and morphologic ovarian abnormalities. Early detection and prompt inhibition of excessive ovarian androgen production are essential for reducing the clinical symptoms of PCOS in young teenage girls. However, many women with PCOS start to experience problems with their menstrual cycles and fertility around age 25 or 26 and should seek treatment if these issues become severe or persistent. In general, women with PCOS should visit their doctor for an evaluation if they have any of the following symptoms irregular menstrual cycles often shorter than usual, heavier periods, or both, and poor fertility. Observation of PCOS through the menstrual cycle is a very important step in the diagnosis of PCOS. A woman with PCOS may have irregular periods, which can vary in length, severity, and frequency. They may also have an increased number of acne breakouts, and difficulty getting pregnant. To diagnose PCOS, a doctor will ask about menstrual cycles and other symptoms. A patient will also perform a physical examination and may order tests, such as a blood test to measure levels of insulin and other hormones.

### 3.6. Significance of Ultrasound in PCOS

Studying these conditions in women is a significant challenge that can be overcome by analysing ultrasound scans, which contain crucial information including the number, size, and location of follicles (Gupta et al., 2022). However, there are currently no reliable objective tests that can diagnose and comprehend PCOS with full certainty. This encourages us to consider developing a way to identify PCOS early and stop subsequent difficulties. The implementation of an automatic PCOS diagnosis tool would decrease the amount of time required physically trace follicles and evaluate the geometric properties of each follicle. As reflected in Figure 2, geometric transformation, segmentation, and feature extraction are important factors for the detection of PCOS. The use of a K-Nearest Neighbours Algorithm (KNN) classifier to classify the ultrasonic picture based on several extractions of features criteria. To accurately identify the disease, pre-processing, segmenting, and deleting irrelevant data are used. This study suggests the most effective way to identify a patient to spare doctors' time. Up to 97% accuracy was achieved using the entire approach as described. The implementation of automatic PCOS early detection is complete (Guerain, 2020). By providing information on the number of follicles found, texture, and geometric parameters like area, perimeter, smoothness, compactness, and accuracy, the system delivers a complete diagnosis of an ultrasound image. The system offers KNN algorithm comparison results. The project's future scope can be used to reduce the processing time required by the KNN method.

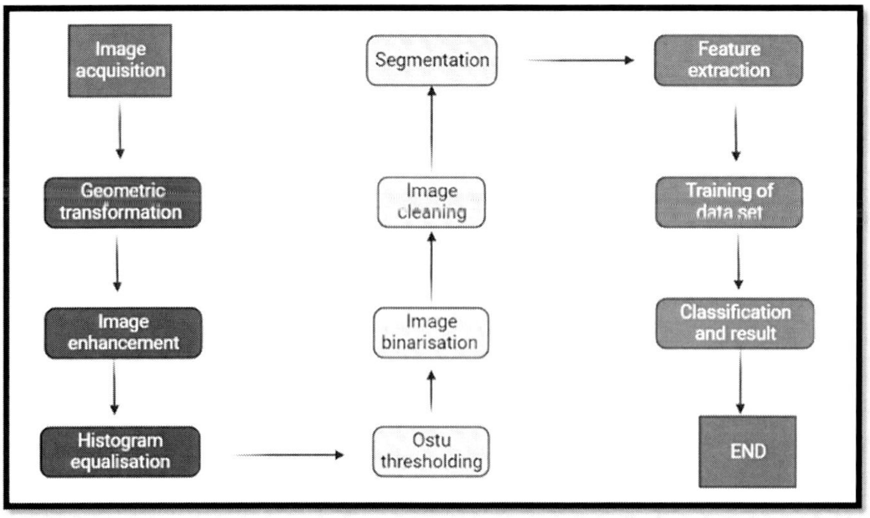


**Figure 2.** Flowchart of the process of detection of PCOS. The first step demonstrates image acquisition and follows histogram equalization with segmentation and feature extraction. Finally, data training comes to the end of the process and reports classification and result of PCOS.

### 3.7. Rotterdam Criteria for PCOS Diagnosis

A new recommendation from the International PCOS Network supported the Rotterdam criteria for adults and the requirement for both oligo-anovulation and hyperandrogenism for the diagnosis of PCOS in teenagers. Hyperandrogenism is an important clinical characteristic of the syndrome due to its worse prognosis and higher risk of heart and metabolic disease. However, recent genetic discoveries imply that it could not be the main cause of PCOS symptoms. About 60 to 80% of cases are hyperandrogenic, as determined by the Rotterdam criteria (Jeevitha & Priya, 2022). Because there are still no established diagnostic cut-offs for biochemical hyperandrogenism and several free testosterone measurement techniques are inaccurate, diagnosing the condition remains difficult.

### 3.8. Weight Management to Control Issues of PCOS

There is no doubt that having a healthy weight is important for anyone, but it is especially important for people with PCOS. PCOS is a hormonal condition that is caused by an imbalance of the hormones that control ovulation. This can lead to irregular periods, infertility, and obesity. PCOS affects more than five million women globally who are of reproductive age. It is an endocrine condition defined by alterations in the levels of female hormones and aberrant male hormone synthesis. Ovarian dysfunction brought on by this illness increases the risk of infertility and miscarriage. Obesity, an irregular menstrual cycle, excess production of acne, the male hormone, and hirsutism are all signs of PCOS. The good news is that there are many things that patients can do to help improve their health if they have PCOS and are overweight or obese (Joham et al., 2022).

According to the National Women's Health Information Centre (2010), Physical activity has been linked with a decreased risk of developing polycystic ovary syndrome (PCOS) (Ma et al., 2021). Regular physical activity is protective against the development of PCOS in both women with the condition and those without it. Physical activity has been linked with a decreased risk of developing polycystic ovary syndrome (PCOS). Regular physical activity is protective against the development of PCOS in both women with the condition and those without it.

## 4. Mitigation to Solve the PCOS Issues

Menstrual cycle irregularities and skin conditions are the two disorders most frequently linked to PCOS. The symptoms of PCOS are exacerbated by high blood pressure and excessive cholesterol. Serum Anti-Müllerian Hormone (AMH) levels and follicle count are associated with PCOS-affected women. According to certain studies, there is a strong link between serum AMH levels and the outcomes of PCOM ultrasonography. Our findings suggest that serum AMH may act as a stand-in for ovarian follicle count and a substitution marker of PCOS for ultrasonography, depending on the availability of both variables. Recent research is demonstrated a strong association between high AMH concentrations (>35 pmol/L) and the ultrasound-based diagnosis of PCOS. Additionally, high blood sugar is seen as the disease progresses (Moran et al., 2011). A crucial issue is the early diagnosis of this serious illness.

### 4.1. Consequential Discussion of Machine Learning for Earlier Detection of PCOS

Early detection can benefit from the use of machine learning. Not every woman can afford the medical costs. Some people experience anxiety about discussing such a subject with doctors. In such a circumstance, a functional forecasting system can be quite beneficial. With the aid of machine learning, numerous prognostication techniques have been developed for the early detection of PCOS, also known as polycystic ovary syndrome. The detection of PCOS is categorized in two ways. Using just a Supervised Dimensionality Reduction method can provide us with a new advantage to address this issue because Dimensionality Reduction methods have a stronger impact on the performance of Machine Learning. Ultrasound is another way to detect PCOS using technology. During Days 2–7 of the menstrual cycle, it should be preferred to use ultrasound for the scan. As a result, no growing follicle can conceal or alter the volume of an ovary. Scanning can be done at random or 2–5 days after progesterone-induced bleeding in cases of oligo or amenorrhoeic women (Hosain et al., 2022). A doctor can examine the womb and ovaries much more closely with an internal transvaginal ultrasound, which is also the most popular way to identify PCOS. A reduction diet is a great way to manage PCOS if a patient feels like a diet is not helping to regulate their cycles (Nasim et al., 2022).

### 4.2. Consequence of Reduction Diet in PCOS

A reduction diet is a stricter version of a healthy diet that helps to control weight and blood sugar levels. One of the first things PCOS women will want to do when starting a reduction diet is to calculate their daily calorie intake. They will need to reduce their overall caloric intake by about 25%. This might mean cutting out some high-calorie foods or increasing the consumption of lower-calorie alternatives. They will also want to make sure to include plenty of fruits, vegetables, and whole grains in their diet.

The primary goal of the optimal segmentation technique is to find every follicle that might be present in the dark area of the ultrasound pictures. This method also eliminates the automated system's ability to detect errors due to the subpar ultrasound pictures used to diagnose follicle counts. In PCOS, the AI employs ultrasound waves to determine the stage of PCOS and the health of the uterus and Fallopian tube (Parker et al., 2020). Additionally, it measures the quantity and size of ovarian cysts. Even though the specific cause of PCOS is yet unknown, studies claim that the condition is often inherited. It is difficult to forecast polycystic ovaries using automatic follicle detection (PCO). Because of the ultrasound pictures' increased noise and low contrast, frequently leads to erroneous detection.

### 4.3. Significance of Insulin-Sensitizing Medications in PCOS

Insulin-sensitizing drugs should be used by the majority of PCOS patients as they lower insulin resistance, hirsutism, obesity, irregular menstrual periods, and ovulation. Compared to other drugs used to treat PCOS symptoms, metformin (Glucophage) has the strongest evidence to support its efficacy. A balanced hormonal system and nutritious food both support regular menstrual cycles. Iron is the main and best-explained relationship between nutrition and menstruation. Iron is a crucial mineral that supports the body in performing several tasks. Meals can have a direct impact on the gut, trigger reflexes in the neurological system, alter the concentration of different metabolites in the blood, or alter the amounts of circulating gut hormones indirectly. Avoiding this ailment requires eating the correct meals and leading a healthy lifestyle. Women with PCOS can get the same hirsutism treatments as women without the condition, such as those who suffer from idiopathic hirsutism (Purohit & Venugopalan, 2009). Numerous non-pharmacological treatment alternatives exist, such as electrolysis, waxing, bleaching, plucking, depilatory lotions, thermolysis, and laser therapy.

### 4.4. Importance of Glucagon-Like Peptide Receptor 1 for PCOS Treatment

Liraglutide is a glucagon-like peptide receptor 1 agonist approved for the management of type 2 diabetes and obesity. Liraglutide was effective in helping obese PCOS patients lose a significant amount of weight and shrink their waistlines (Rachana et al., 2021). Following an oral glucose load, the incretin hormones glucagon-like peptide-1 and glucose-dependent insulinotropic polypeptide (GIP), which are both inactivated by dipeptidyl peptidase-4 (DPP-4), promote insulin production. This process may be slowed or perhaps cease to exist in people with PCOS and type 2 diabetes, however, using pharmaceutical doses of GLP-1 can restore insulin excretion. A lipase inhibitor with the indication of treating obesity is called orlistat. Orlistat is effective at causing weight loss in overweight or obese women with PCOS and at enhancing clinical and biological indicators of hyperandrogenism and IR. PCOS typically appears in women while they are of reproductive age when concerns like finding a partner, starting a relationship, and starting a family are frequently highly important. Unbalances in the psychosexual sphere might result from factors that have a detrimental impact on physical beauty, femininity, or fertility. The effects of PCOS on the mind could potentially outweigh.

## 4.5. Use of Metformin for PCOS

Patients with PCOS who use metformin see lower serum testosterone levels and more frequent spontaneous ovulation and regular menstrual cycles compared to those who take a placebo (Radosh, 2009). However, metformin is no longer advised to promote ovulation because it achieves poorer live birth rates when compared to CC. Furthermore, there is inconclusive information about whether live birth rates are different when metformin is added to CC compared to CC alone. This makes sense because, compared to CC alone, the addition of metformin to CC raises the rates of clinical pregnancy, ovulation, and miscarriage. Limited research is suggested that providing metformin may raise the pregnancy rate in women who are resistant to CC.

Women with PCOS may be treated for hirsutism with insulin-sensitizing medications such as metformin, acarbose (Precose), and rosiglitazone (Avandia). Based on Ferriman-Gallwey hirsutism ratings, spironolactone, and rosiglitazone are more efficient than metformin. For the treatment of hirsutism in women with PCOS, a Cochrane study found that metformin is equally effective as oral contraceptives; however, a more recent systematic review found that metformin is ineffective. FDA-approved for the treatment of unsightly facial hair, topical eflornithine cream has no published data on its usage specifically in PCOS-affected women. Sibutramine (Meridia), a medication authorized for the treatment of obesity, can help lessen hirsutism. The best medication to take is probably metformin since it reduces insulin resistance, which is indicated by high fasting blood glucose or fast glucose/insulin ratios in PCOS patients (Rocha et al., 2019). The most popular medication for these patients' metabolic control is metformin. In women with PCOS, the effectiveness of metformin as an insulin-sensitizing and hypoglycaemic medication has been well established. Metformin may be more effective for PCOS patients who are not fat than for those who are. FDA maternity category B applies to metformin.

According to anecdotal evidence, oral contraceptives are the most popular medications used to treat irregular menstruation in women with PCOS. Few researchers have, however, looked at how they affect PCOS women's menstrual periods. Although cyproterone acetate plus progestin has undergone significant research, it is not offered in the US. According to studies, spironolactone, acarbose, rosiglitazone, and metformin may help with menstrual irregularities (such as oligomenorrhea). The best option is likely metformin, which may reduce insulin resistance and menstrual abnormalities. Even though PCOS recurs, the symptoms can be managed by controlling the hormones. A balanced hormonal system and nutritious food both support regular menstrual cycles. Avoiding this ailment requires eating the correct meals and leading a healthy lifestyle.

## 5. Challenges to Mitigate This Concern in Lifestyle

The ability to be resilient is acquired via problem-solving. Knowing that one can overcome obstacles, learn from obstacles, and profit from mistakes is a good foundation for success in later life. Lifestyle planning, psychological support, and metabolic screening with fertility counselling are multiple disciplinary teams for PCOS care as illustrated in Figure 3. In general, machine learning is a technique that enables computer systems to learn from data. This can be used to improve the accuracy of predictions made by the system or to improve the speed with which the system can make predictions (Shrivastava et al., 2019). One issue with using machine learning in PCOS is that the system is not well-suited to the type of data that is typically found in this condition. PCOS is characterized by high levels of circulating testosterone, which can make it difficult for the system to learn from data.

There is growing evidence that suggests high sugar and processed foods in a regular diet are harmful to people with PCOS. A diet that is high in sugar and processed foods is associated with an increased risk of developing PCOS (Wagh et al., 2021). A study published in the journal Metabolism found that women with PCOS who ate a high-sugar diet had a threefold increased risk of developing the condition compared to women who ate a low-sugar diet. A high-sugar diet is also associated with an increased risk of developing other health problems, such as insulin resistance, obesity, and type 2 diabetes (Xenou & Gourounti, 2021). Body mass index, insulin and glucose levels, and triglycerides were all connected with the development of T2D in a favourable way while having more children was associated with it in a negative one. It is vital to know that PCOS can cause gestational diabetes, which happens when pregnant women experience glucose problems. Birth complications include premature birth, breathing problems, jaundice, and more may result from this.

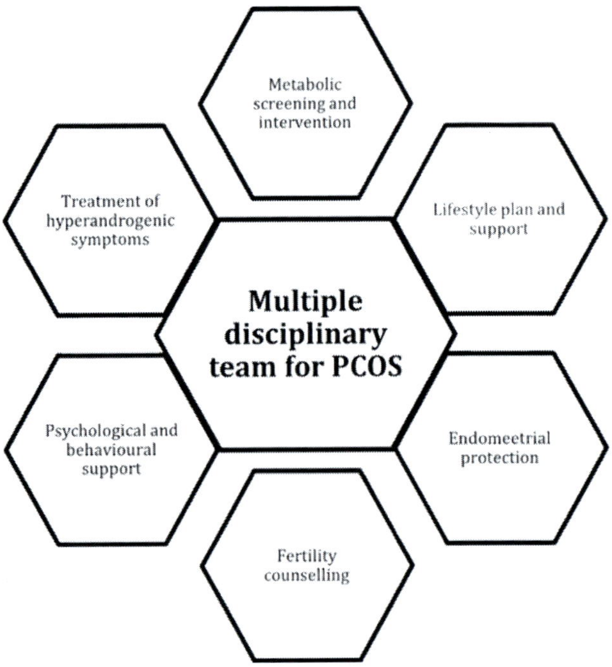


**Figure 3**. List of challenges to mitigate PCOS concerns from lifestyle.

### 5.1. Connection of Comorbidity and PCOS

Many lifestyle factors, including the consumption of alcohol and cigarettes, eating habits, and physical activity, are directly linked to several chronic health conditions, including obesity, cancer, diabetes, and cardiovascular disease. Once more, the positive challenge is not about attempting to be more optimistic than they are. It involves examining their negativity so that they can make conscious decisions to view some situations more positively (Xue et al., 2019). Patients with PCOS have higher rates of non-traditional cardiovascular risk factors, such as mood disorders like sorrow and anxiety, in addition to classic cardiovascular risk factors including hypertension, dyslipidaemia, and type 2 diabetes mellitus. A sizable component of the problem is due to insulin resistance, which affects 1 in 4 persons and is the modern world's most prevalent ailment. Insulin resistance is caused by a diet high in sucrose (concentrated fructose), as well as by smoking, being overweight, stress, trans fats, and environmental toxins. Changes to long-standing patterns, usually including food or exercise, are referred to as lifestyle modifications, and the new behaviour must be maintained for weeks, months, or even years. One of the many ailments that can be cured with a lifestyle change is obesity.

### 5.2. Physical Challenges of PCOS

Infertility, melancholy, anxiety, mood swings, weight gain, irregular menstruation cycles, acne, and PCOS are all indications of endocrine conditions. Estimates place the prevalence of PCOS at 15 to 20% of women who are of childbearing age. They found that women with PCOS had a 77%, 53%, and 17% higher risk of eating disorders, anxiety, and depression, respectively, than did those without PCOS and twice as much. Mood swings are common in polycystic ovary syndrome (PCOS). They can be a sign that our hormones are out of balance and the patient has an underlying problem, such as an endometrial problem or an issue with the thyroid.

PCOS is a condition that affects the ovaries and can cause an imbalance of hormones. Health education is important for people with PCOS because it can help them learn about the condition and how to manage it. One way to help manage PCOS is to learn about the foods that are good for the patient's health and the diet that is best for PCOS. One of the best diets for PCOS is the Mediterranean diet. This diet is high in fruits, vegetables, and fish. It is also low in saturated fats and cholesterol (Xue et al., 2019). The diagnosis of PCOS can be a very heart-wrenching experience. For many women, it means that they have an illness that is associated with a high risk of developing high blood pressure, diabetes, and other health problems. One of the most common symptoms of PCOS is an elevated level of the hormone estrogenic. Oestrogen can contribute to an increased propensity for melancholy, as well as other mood problems. This is because oestrogen can increase levels of the hormone cortisol, which can lead to feelings of depression and anxiety.

### 5.2. Effect of Exercise to Improve PCOS Conditions

Another way to manage PCOS is to exercise which can help to improve patients' moods and reduce the risk of diabetes. High cholesterol and triglyceride levels are more prevalent in

PCOS-affected women. This can also exacerbate other issues like metabolic syndrome, which is more common in PCOS-affected women. Combining exercise with a healthy, low-fat diet can help lower cholesterol (Woodward et al., 2020). The leading cause of death for women is heart disease, and women with PCOS are considerably more likely to experience atherosclerosis, high blood pressure, and high cholesterol. Frequent cardio workouts dramatically reduce the chance of these issues by strengthening the heart muscle. Cardio or aerobic exercise strengthens the heart muscle, considerably reducing the risk of cardiovascular disease and illnesses like atherosclerosis or hypertension. This is crucial for PCOS-affected individuals because they have a higher risk of cardiovascular disease. There is still much that is unknown about PCOS, but there is mounting evidence that suggests that the condition is associated with abnormalities in the way that the brain functions. Studies have shown that women with PCOS have a higher rate of experiencing problems with cognitive functions such as poor memory, and decision-making skills (Barrea et al., 2023). Medical practitioners are an important part of the PCOS education process. They can provide education about the condition and provide access to treatments and therapies. They can also provide support and guidance during treatment.

Type 2 diabetes, hypertension, and impaired glucose tolerance are all more common in PCOS-afflicted women. Women with PCOS are thought to have a higher prevalence of cardiovascular illness, and it has been predicted that they also have a much higher risk of myocardial infarction (Mirabelli et al., 2020). The main treatments for PCOS are regular exercise, wholesome eating, and weight management. If patients have trouble getting pregnant, the doctor may recommend fertility medications in addition to birth control pills to ease their symptoms and control their periods. Treatment might lessen symptoms and aid in avoiding future health issues. Women with PCOS continue to experience psychological issues like fear and depression even after they have reached fertile age.

## Conclusion

The inclusion of exercise, diet charts, and lifestyle modifications can improve the health condition of PCOS patients. Exercise has been shown to improve insulin sensitivity and reduce the symptoms of PCOS, such as obesity, high blood pressure, and diabetes. One study found that obese patients who exercised lost more weight and had better blood sugar control than obese patients who did not exercise. Exercise can also help to improve mood and energy levels in people with PCOS. One study found that women with PCOS who exercised reported feeling more in control of their lives and had improved mental health. As per the discussion, PCOS might not work similarly for all patients, it may vary as per the health conditions. One of the Principles of Therapeutics is the fact that treatment should be tailored to the individual. This means that the same approach to diet and health care that works for one person may not work for another. In the case of PCOS, this means that different people may require different types of diet and exercise to manage their symptoms. There is a growing body of evidence demonstrating the benefits of eating green foods for women with polycystic ovary syndrome (PCOS). An overweight woman with PCOS who ate more green vegetables and fruits had a decrease in insulin resistance, a better lipid profile, and a decrease in body weight and waist circumference. Eating a healthy diet is key to managing PCOS. Plenty of whole grains, fruits and vegetables, and low-fat foods are part of a balanced diet that can aid digestion and lessen the impact of fat deposition in the body.

Some research has shown that lifestyle choices can have a big impact on the development of polycystic ovary syndrome (PCOS). Smoking is one of the biggest risk factors for developing PCOS. Smoking can increase the risk of developing PCOS by up to 40%. Quitting smoking can help improve fertility and overall health. In addition to that, the hormone insulin aids in the body's control of blood sugar levels. In people with PCOS, insulin resistance can mean that the body does not respond as well to insulin, which can lead to elevated blood sugar levels. This can lead to obesity and other health problems. Treatment with insulin can help to improve blood sugar levels and reduce the risk of PCOS-related health problems. Hence, to improve the health condition of PCOS patients they need to change their food habits and lifestyle which contain low-fat foods and improve blood circulation throughout the body. Proper medication and treatment are important to control the effects of PCOS. AI-based detection reduces the time for detection and provides an accurate result that helps the medical system to provide better treatment in earlier diagnosis conditions. Thus, physical challenges with comorbidity enhance the chance of PCOS and machine learning-based detection initiates fast medical interventions to improve the quality of life for PCOS women.

## References

Alshammari, S. A., AlDhayan, A. Z., Al-Essa, O. M. S., Alosaimi, M. M., Al-Badr, B. M., Ali, A. B., & Ajlan, Q. A. (2020). Challenges to lifestyle modification of chronic disease patients attending primary health care centers in Riyadh. *Journal of Family Medicine and Primary Care*, *9*(12), 6186.

Barrea, L., Camajani, E., Cernea, S., Frias-Toral, E., Lamabadusuriya, D., Ceriani, F., Savastano, S., Colao, A., Muscogiuri, G., & Verde, L. (2023). Ketogenic Diet as Medical Prescription in Women with Polycystic Ovary Syndrome (PCOS). *Current Nutrition Reports*, 1-9.

Brutocao, C., Zaiem, F., Alsawas, M., Morrow, A. S., Murad, M. H., & Javed, A. (2018). Psychiatric disorders in women with polycystic ovary syndrome: a systematic review and meta-analysis. *Endocrine*, *62*, 318-325.

Chang, R. J., & Coffler, M. S. (2007). Polycystic ovary syndrome: early detection in the adolescent. *Clinical obstetrics and gynecology*, *50*(1), 178-187.

Couillaud, B. M., Espeau, P., Mignet, N., & Corvis, Y. (2019). State of the art of pharmaceutical solid forms: from crystal property issues to nanocrystals formulation. *ChemMedChem*, *14*(1), 8-23.

Denny, A., Raj, A., Ashok, A., Ram, C. M., & George, R. (2019). i-hope: Detection and prediction system for polycystic ovary syndrome (pcos) using machine learning techniques. TENCON 2019-2019 IEEE Region 10 Conference (TENCON),

Guan, Y., Wang, D., Bu, H., Zhao, T., & Wang, H. (2020). The effect of metformin on polycystic ovary syndrome in overweight women: a systematic review and meta-analysis of randomized controlled trials. *International journal of endocrinology*, *2020*.

Guerain, M. (2020). A review on high pressure experiments for study of crystallographic behavior and polymorphism of pharmaceutical materials. *Journal of Pharmaceutical Sciences*, *109*(9), 2640-2653.

Gupta, A., Soni, H., Joshi, R., & Laban, R. M. (2022). Discriminant analysis in contrasting dimensions for polycystic ovary syndrome prognostication. *arXiv preprint arXiv:2201.03029*.

Hosain, A. S., Mehedi, M. H. K., & Kabir, I. E. (2022). PCONet: A convolutional neural network architecture to detect polycystic ovary syndrome (PCOS) from ovarian ultrasound images. 2022 International Conference on Engineering and Emerging Technologies (ICEET),

Jeevitha, S., & Priya, N. (2022). Optimized Segmentation Technique for Detecting PCOS in Ultrasound Images. Congress on Intelligent Systems: Proceedings of CIS 2021, Volume 1,

Joham, A. E., Norman, R. J., Stener-Victorin, E., Legro, R. S., Franks, S., Moran, L. J., Boyle, J., & Teede, H. J. (2022). Polycystic ovary syndrome. *The Lancet Diabetes & Endocrinology*.

Ma, R., Ding, X., Wang, Y., Deng, Y., & Sun, A. (2021). The therapeutic effects of glucagon-like peptide-1 receptor agonists and metformin on polycystic ovary syndrome: A protocol for systematic review and meta-analysis. *Medicine*, *100*(23).

Mirabelli, M., Chiefari, E., Arcidiacono, B., Corigliano, D. M., Brunetti, F. S., Maggisano, V., Russo, D., Foti, D. P., & Brunetti, A. (2020). Mediterranean diet nutrients to turn the tide against insulin resistance and related diseases. *Nutrients*, *12*(4), 1066.

Moran, L. J., Hutchison, S. K., Norman, R. J., & Teede, H. J. (2011). Lifestyle changes in women with polycystic ovary syndrome. *Cochrane Database of Systematic Reviews (7)*.

Nasim, S., Almutairi, M. S., Munir, K., Raza, A., & Younas, F. (2022). A Novel Approach for Polycystic Ovary Syndrome Prediction Using Machine Learning in Bioinformatics. *IEEE Access*, *10*, 97610-97624.

Parker, M., Warren, A., Nair, S., & Barnard, M. (2020). Adherence to treatment for polycystic ovarian syndrome: A systematic review. *PloS one*, *15*(2), e0228586.

Purohit, R., & Venugopalan, P. (2009). Polymorphism: an overview. *Resonance*, *14*, 882-893.

Rachana, B., Priyanka, T., Sahana, K., Supritha, T., Parameshachari, B., & Sunitha, R. (2021). Detection of polycystic ovarian syndrome using follicle recognition technique. *Global Transitions Proceedings*, *2*(2), 304-308.

Radosh, L. (2009). Drug treatments for polycystic ovary syndrome. *American family physician*, *79*(8), 671-676.

Rocha, A. L., Oliveira, F. R., Azevedo, R. C., Silva, V. A., Peres, T. M., Candido, A. L., Gomes, K. B., & Reis, F. M. (2019). Recent advances in the understanding and management of polycystic ovary syndrome. *F1000Research*, *8*.

Shrivastava, V., Batham, L., Mishra, S., & Mishra, A. (2019). Management of symptoms associated with obsessive-compulsive disorder (ocd) and polycystic ovarian disease (pcod) through an integrated approach including yagya therapy. *Interdisciplinary Journal of Yagya Research*, *2*(1), 39-51.

Wagh, P., Panjwani, M., & Amrutha, S. (2021). Early detection of PCOD using machine learning techniques. In *Artificial Intelligence and Speech Technology* (pp. 9-20). CRC Press.

Woodward, A., Klonizakis, M., & Broom, D. (2020). Exercise and polycystic ovary syndrome. *Physical Exercise for Human Health*, 123-136.

Xenou, M., & Gourounti, K. (2021). Dietary patterns and polycystic ovary syndrome: a systematic review. *Maedica*, *16*(3), 516.

Xue, J., Li, X., Liu, P., Li, K., Sha, L., Yang, X., Zhu, L., Wang, Z., Dong, Y., & Zhang, L. (2019). Inulin and metformin ameliorate polycystic ovary syndrome via anti-inflammation and modulating gut microbiota in mice. *Endocrine journal*, *66*(10), 859-870.

# About the Editors

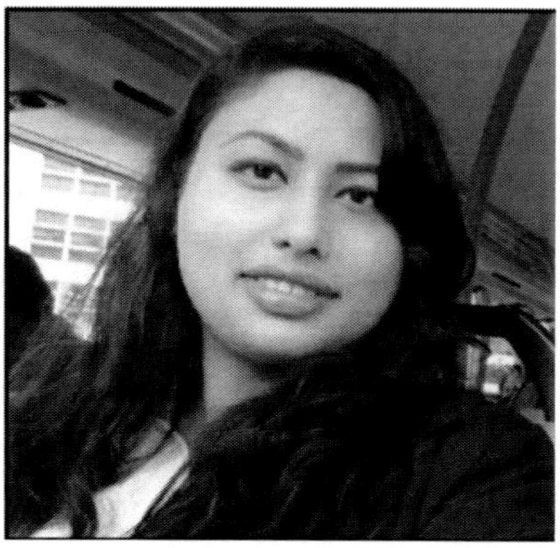

**Dr. Arpita Roy** is currently working as an Assistant Professor in Department of Biotechnology, Sharda University, Greater Noida, India. She has specialization in "Plant Biotechnology, Nanobiotechnology, Environmental Biotechnology and Microbiology". She has been teaching graduates/post graduates Biotechnology. She has taught topics related to Plant Biotechnology, Microbiology, Bioprocess Engineering and Solid Waste Management. She has authored more than 90 scientific articles and 25 book chapters from international publishers. She has presented and participated in numerous State, National and International conferences, seminars, workshops and symposium. She has received the Commendable Research Award for excellence in research during the year 2019, 2020 and 2021- Delhi Technological University. She has served as editorial board member and reviewer of reputed international journals. Recently she has been enlisted in Enlisted in **Top 2% scientists in the world** (Stanford University report published by Elsevier). She has published three edited books and worked as guest editor in various reputed journals.

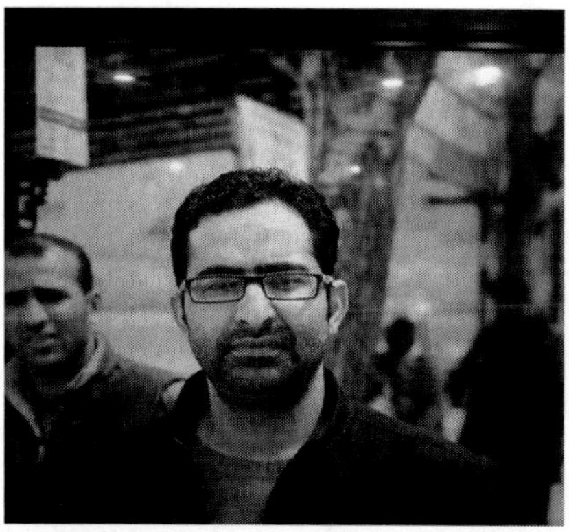

**Dr. Gowhar Rashid** is working as an Assistant Professor in the Amity Medical School at Amity University Haryana. Born and raised in the beautiful region of Srinagar, Kashmir, Dr. Gowhar has developed a passion for advancing the field of medical science. His educational journey led him to complete his BSc, MSc, and Ph.D. in Biochemistry from the prestigious Sher I Kashmir Institute of Medical Sciences in Kashmir, India.

With a specialization in diagnostics and cancer research, Dr. Gowhar Rashid has become a recognized expert in his field. His in-depth knowledge and dedication to his work have earned him recognition and respect from both his peers and students. His research endeavors focus on finding innovative solutions and breakthroughs in cancer diagnostics, aiming to improve patient outcomes and contribute to the field's advancements.

Dr. Gowhar's expertise is widely acknowledged, and his contributions to the scientific community are well-documented. He has authored numerous papers published in reputed, high-impact journals, further establishing his reputation as a distinguished researcher. Additionally, he holds the esteemed position of Editorial Fellow in Innovation in Digital Health, Diagnostics, and Biomarkers (IDDB), showcasing his commitment to staying at the forefront of cutting-edge developments in these crucial areas.

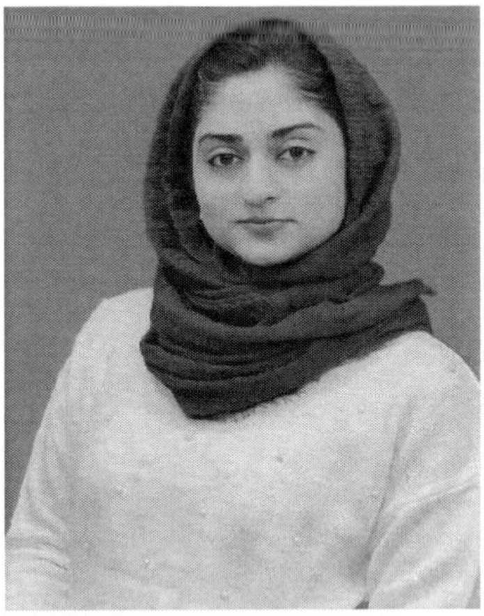

**Miss Nihad Ashraf Khan** is an alumni of Jamia Millia Islamia, New Delhi, India from where she completed her Master's in Biosciences. She has completed her Bachelor's from India's most reputed University, Delhi University, Ramjas College in 2020. She has been part of several projects during her Bachelor's and Master's and has gained expertise in Bio-informatics, a booming platform for scientific researches. Her research interests include **Microbiology, Cell and Molecular Biology** and **Bioinformatics** . She has worked on a research project during her master's on "***Mechanistic insight into anti-candidal effects of Methyl eugenol"*** and even done a computational study on ***Alzheimer's Disease, an approach towards phytochemicals for drug designing***. She is interested to contribute in scientific researches through her novel ideas.

# Index

## D



## E



## F



## G

## L



## M

## S



## T



## U



## V



## W



## Y